Oxford Textbook of

Communication in Oncology and Palliative Care

Oxford Textbook of
Communication in Oncology and Palliative Care

SECOND EDITION

Edited by

David W. Kissane

Barry D. Bultz

Phyllis N. Butow

Carma L. Bylund

Simon Noble

Susie Wilkinson

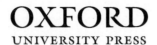

OXFORD

UNIVERSITY PRESS

Great Clarendon Street, Oxford, OX2 6DP,
United Kingdom

Oxford University Press is a department of the University of Oxford.
It furthers the University's objective of excellence in research, scholarship,
and education by publishing worldwide. Oxford is a registered trade mark of
Oxford University Press in the UK and in certain other countries

Published in the United States of America by Oxford University Press
198 Madison Avenue, New York, NY 10016, United States of America

British Library Cataloguing in Publication Data
Data available

Library of Congress Cataloging in Publication Data
Data available

ISBN 978-0-19-873613-4 (Hbk.)
ISBN 978-0-19-883201-0 (Pbk.)

Printed and bound by
CPI Group (UK) Ltd, Croydon, CR0 4YY

Oxford University Press makes no representation, express or implied, that the
drug dosages in this book are correct. Readers must therefore always check
the product information and clinical procedures with the most up-to-date
published product information and data sheets provided by the manufacturers
and the most recent codes of conduct and safety regulations. The authors and
the publishers do not accept responsibility or legal liability for any errors in the
text or for the misuse or misapplication of material in this work. Except where
otherwise stated, drug dosages and recommendations are for the non-pregnant
adult who is not breast-feeding

Links to third party websites are provided by Oxford in good faith and
for information only. Oxford disclaims any responsibility for the materials
contained in any third party website referenced in this work.

Foreword

Communication is at the very essence of our being. Every human being is interconnected with others and, as such, communicates. Looking at babies, they establish communication rapidly with their mothers, others in speaking to them use 'baby talk' and higher pitch but quieter voice, long before the baby can distinguish meaning from the sounds other than 'calm or fright'.

Although language is often considered as the main means of communication, in fact the majority of communication is non-verbal. Even when words are used, much of the message comes through the tone of voice; when written down, such tone is more difficult to discern, but syntax and punctuation often reveal tenderness of tone, anger, or even aggression.

In clinical practice in recent years, there has been a tendency to focus on communication in terms of conveying information to patients—and, with their permission, to those important to them. But all too often such communication has gone wrong because the fundamental step of listening has had less importance in curricula than verbal construct. Without careful listening to all the non-verbal cues as well as the words that our patients utter, we will almost inevitably miscommunicate and will fail to give the information the person needs, or may give it in a way they cannot understand and interpret, retain, and use for decision-making.

In modern media, we have so much information transmitted, but so little check on how it has been received or 'heard'. Social media has overtaken the simple model of radio transmitter and receiver, and brought with it ever greater dangers, as the messages portrayed are often value-laden, opinionated, and devoid of scrutiny for accuracy or applicability.

In the clinical setting, listening, with all one's senses, becomes the quintessential part of communicating. The wise clinician will listen with eyes—noticing the changing expressions on a person's face, the transient diverted gaze of embarrassment or fear, their gait, a slight tremor, small beads of sweat, or pallor—as well as listening to sounds and words uttered. But there are deeper layers to listening too. As the Chinese symbol for listening portrays, one listens with undivided attention and with one's heart, with one's whole being. A slight odour, a dishevelled look, a hesitant speech that takes time to fill the void of silence with whatever is critically important to the person—all these give enormous clues to the clinician, who can better tailor diagnostic acumen to ensure the message given to the patient is appropriate and one that can be understood in the least traumatic way, while of course being truthful and not misleading the patient.

Even without language, enormous amounts of communication can occur. When an interpreter is used, no one should forget the importance of monitoring the non-verbal cues from the patient as he or she listens to the translated word. So much can be conveyed by those expressive gestures and sounds that transcend nationality, race, and culture.

This book is all about communication in one of the most feared areas of medicine: oncology. Fear of the diagnosis represents a lingering hopelessness from years gone by, with a reality of the seriousness and harshness of many treatments, the assault they pose to personhood, body image, and self-esteem. Of course, it is not only a patient who is affected by a diagnosis of cancer. Their family, adults and children alike, are deeply affected too in a myriad of ways as they see their world fall apart and their future uncertain.

Of course, communication of messages needs sensitive decisions about who needs to know what and when—too often failures in care are attributed to poor communication between services. When it comes to communication with patients, many complaints and law suits have resulted from poor and insensitive talking, telling, and ways of giving messages. But clinicians are not sued for listening sensitively and carefully—listening is the 'failsafe mechanism' of communication.

So read on, dip in and out of this textbook, use it, and above all, enjoy it. However brilliant we might believe we are at communication, we never see ourselves as others do and we always need to learn, both from the experience and evidence from what went before and from what the next generation have learnt from us, improved upon, and developed. Our duty is to the wholeness of the person in front of us. When they feel their world has been shattered by cancer, our sensitive and careful communication can help them understand what is and needs to happen, to make sense of it, and then to communicate with their own family, friends, employers—whomever they wish—to plan for the worst and hope for the best. Big conversations have big benefits.

Ilora Finlay
Professor Baroness Finlay of Llandaff FRCP,
FRCGP, FMedSci, FHEA, LSW

Preface

Cancer remains one of the most dreaded diagnoses because of the enormous threat it brings to the well-being and survival of the patients it afflicts. Challenged to adapt with courage and cope with complex treatments, patients and their families need the support of the whole multidisciplinary team to deal optimally with their predicament. Communication is at the heart of the effective delivery of this care.

With the development of genetic profiling of every tumour, personalized medicine aims to exquisitely tailor therapies to the uniqueness of the patient's disease. The same level of individualized care is essential in responding humanely to each person. What has become known as patient-centred care is that which is not only empathically and compassionately delivered, but also fashioned to suit the values and preferences of the person. The resultant message framing delivers information in a customized manner to suit the cultural, ethnic, educational, social, spiritual, and philosophical needs of each person. The challenge to communicate effectively is huge.

Whether information is being delivered electronically, via print media, or in the face-to-face consultation, use of the science of communication becomes mandatory to ameliorate suffering, facilitate adjustment, and promote healing. A considerable evidence-base has emerged from research that can guide strategies to optimize information delivery and support patient adaptation. Included here are the models and curricula of communication skills training, the use of decision aides, relationally-focused ethics, and shared decision-making. In this book, we have aimed to bring together the science and practice of communication for the disciplines engaged in oncology and palliative care.

In 2010, we published the successful *Handbook of Communication in Oncology and Palliative Care*. In this second edition, which Oxford University Press have brought into its textbook series, we have added to the core curriculum for communication skills training a new section that focuses on communication challenges for nurses. Spanning the training of student and specialist nurses, this curriculum covers acute settings, chronic illness, and end-of-life care. New perspectives have also been incorporated into this edition

about discussing risk, responding to third parties present in clinical consultations, facilitating family meetings, talking about survivorship, and discussing death and dying. To enrich care delivery, our specialty curriculum considers the multidisciplinary team, treatment adherence, unproven therapies, genetics, infertility and sexuality, while presenting optimal ways to work with an interpreter. The needs of the varied disciplines include a focus on surgeons, radiologists, social workers, and chaplains, as well as attention to the specific needs of the very young and the elderly. We conclude with research methodology and approaches being undertaken by leading research groups across Europe and North America.

The syllabus that we offer through this book is unashamedly applied to the specialties of cancer and palliative care, recognizing that while generic communication skills will be taught at the undergraduate level, specialists benefit from an applied approach that targets their specific clinical challenges. Our audience is multidisciplinary and inclusive of all of the disciplines engaged in cancer care. The resultant scope is international in perspective, drawing upon the leading scholars engaged in communication research.

We thank our authors for their scholarship and generous contribution to this text, their collegiality, friendship, and goodwill. We also thank the staff supporting the editors, the commissioning and production teams at Oxford University Press, and all who, in however small a manner, have assisted in bringing this book to publication. A special thanks to Caroline Smith at OUP for her patience and collaborative style in supporting us all.

We trust that this textbook will advance the quality of the care delivered by aiding clinicians to sensitively and effectively personalize their communication in response to the needs of their patients and families.

David W. Kissane, AC
Barry D. Bultz, PhD
Phyllis N. Butow, PhD
Carma L. Bylund, PhD
Simon Noble, MD
Susie Wilkinson, PhD

Contents

SECTION F
Education and international initiatives in communication training

SECTION G
Research in cancer communication

Abbreviations

AA	African American	EOL	end of life
AACH	American Academy on Communication in Healthcare	EPAAC	European Partnership for Action Against Cancer
AAMC	Association of American Medical Colleges	ESAS	Edmonton Symptom Assessment System
ACGME	Accreditation Council for Graduate Medical Education	FDA	Food and Drug Administration
		FP	fertility preservation
ACR	American College of Radiology	FTC	facilitator training course
ACST	advanced communication skills training	GPA	goals, plans, and action
ADL	activities of daily living	GPVTS	General Practitioner Vocational Training Scheme
ALOBA	agenda-led outcome-based analysis	GSR	galvanic skin response
AMA	American Medical Association	GTA	gynaecological teaching associates
AND	Allow Natural Death	GUIDE	Get ready, Understand, Inform, Deepen, and Equip
APN	advanced practice nurses	HBOC	hereditary breast and ovarian cancer
APS	American Pain Society	HCP	healthcare professional
ART	assisted reproduction techniques	HIPAA	Health Insurance Portability and Accountability Act
ASCO	American Society of Clinical Oncology	HMC	Hamad Medical Corporation
ASPE	Association of Standardized Patient Educators	IAS	interaction analysis systems
AYAC	adolescents and young adults with cancer	ICE	Ideas, Concerns, and Expectations
BMI	body mass index	ICSI	intracytoplasmic sperm injection
CA	conversation analysis	ICU	intensive care unit
CAM	complementary and alternative medicine	IOM	Institute of Medicine
CE	continuing education	IPDAS	International Patient Decision Aid Collaboration
CEA	carcinoembryonic antigen	IPE	interprofessional education
CHF	chronic heart failure	IPOS	International Psycho-Oncology Society
CMSDM	communication model of shared decision-making	IVF	*in vitro* fertilization
CNS	central nervous system	JCAHO	Joint Commission on Accreditation of Healthcare Organizations
COPD	chronic obstructive pulmonary disease		
CPG	clinical practice guidelines	LOC	locus of control
CRCWEM	Cancer Research Campaign Workshop Evaluation Manual	LOS	length of stay
		MAOI	monoamine oxidase inhibitors
CRP	communication-and-resolution programmes	MCC	Medical Council of Canada
CRRT	continuous renal replacement therapy	MCI	mild cognitive impairment
CST	communication skills training	MDT	multidisciplinary team
CT	computed tomography	MENA	Middle East and North Africa
CTIMP	clinical trials in therapeutic medicinal products	MIPS	Medical Interaction Process System
DA	decision aids	MPCC	Measure of Patient-Centred Communication
DNACPR	Do Not Attempt Cardiopulmonary Resuscitation	MPM	mortality predicted model
		MRI	magnetic resonance imaging
DNR	Do-Not-Resuscitate	MSKCC	Memorial Sloan Kettering Cancer Cente
DoH	Department of Health	MUE	medication use evaluation
DRP	drug-related problems	NBME	National Board of Medical Examiners
DUE	drug use evaluation	NCCIH	National Center for Complementary and Integrative Health
ECG	electrocardiogram		
eGFR	estimated glomerular filtration rate	NCCN	National Comprehensive Cancer Network

NCCS	National Coalition for Cancer Survivorship		RT	radiation therapy
NCI	National Cancer Institute		SACT	systemic anti-cancer therapy
NHMRC	National Health and Medical Research Council		SBAR	Situation, Background, Assessment, and Recommendations
NI	Northern Ireland		SCCAP	Siminoff Communication Content and Affect Program
NICE	National Institute for Health and Care Excellence		SCL	Swiss Cancer League
NIH	National Institutes of Health		SCP	survivor care plan
NMC	Nursing and Midwifery Council		SCT	stem cell transplant
NQF	National Quality Forum		SDM	shared decision-making
NSCLC	non-small cell lung cancer		SEGUE	Set the stage; Elicit information; Give information; Understand the patient's perspective; End the encounter
NVS	newest vital sign			
OCS	Office of Cancer Survivorship			
ODF	overall defensive functioning			
OPTION	Observing Patient Involvement Scale		SHCP	senior healthcare professionals
OSCE	objective structured clinical examination		SHO	senior house officer
PACS	picture archiving and communication systems		SMART	Specific, Measurable, Achievable, Realistic and Timely
PACT	Partner, Assess, Care, and Transition		SNF	Swiss National Science Foundation
PARIHS	Promoting Action on Research Implementation in Health Services		SOP	standard operating procedures
			SP	standardized patient
PCP	primary care provider		SPA	standardized patient assessment
PECT	patient emotion cue test		SPIKES	Setting, Preparation, Information, Knowledge, Empathy, Strategy
PEGASUS	Patients' Expectations and Goals: Assisting Shared Understanding of Surgery			
PET	positron emission tomography		SSMO	Swiss Society of Medical Oncology
PFCC	Partnering with Families in Cancer Care		SSRI	selective serotonin reuptake inhibitors
PRISM	Physical Pleasure—Relational Intimacy Model of Sexual Motivation		TAPPA	Test of Accurate Perception of Patients' Affect
PROTAN	PROTocol ANalyser		UICC	Union for International Cancer Control
PSOC	psychosocial oncology care		UK	United Kingdom
PYLL	potential years of life lost		US	United States (of America)
QOL	quality of life		USMLE	United States Medical Licensing Examination
QPL	question prompt lists		VCCCP	Victorian Cancer Clinicians Communications Program
RCGP	Royal College of General Practitioners			
RCN	Royal College of Nursing		VCM	values clarification method
RCT	randomized controlled trial		VLE	virtual learning environment
RIAS	Roter Interactional Analysis System		WTHD	wish to hasten death

Contributors

Ronald D. Adelman, Professor of Geriatric Medicine, Division of Geriatrics and Palliative Medicine, Weill-Cornell College of Medicine, New York, NY, USA

Terrance Albrecht, Professor and Division Chief for Population Sciences in the Wayne State University School of Medicine, Department of Oncology; Professor and Associate Center Director for Population Sciences, and Leader of the Population Studies and Disparities Research Program at the Karmanos Cancer Institute, Detroit, MI, USA

Khalid Alyafei, Senior Consultant, Paediatric Emergency, Hamad Medical Corporation; Assistant Professor of Clinical Paediatrics at Weill Cornell Medicine—Qatar, Doha, Qatar

Robert M. Arnold, Professor and Medical Director, Palliative and Supportive Institute, University of Pittsburgh Medical Center, University of Pittsburgh, Pittsburgh, PA, USA

Kimlin Tam Ashing, Professor and Director, Center of Community Alliance for Research and Education, Department of Population Sciences, City of Hope Medical Center, California, CA, USA

Sylvie Aubin, Associate Professor, Department of Oncology, McGill University; and Psychologist and Research Associate, Louise Granofsky Psychosocial Oncology Program, Segal Cancer Centre, Jewish General Hospital, QC, Canada

Anthony L. Back, Co-Director, University of Washington's Cambia Palliative Care Center of Excellence, Seattle, WA, USA

Walter F. Baile, Professor of Behavioral Science and Psychiatry, Director of the Interpersonal Communication and Relationship Enhancement (I*CARE) program, MD Anderson Cancer Center, The University of Texas, Houston, TX, USA

Kinta Beaver, Professor of Cancer Care, School of Health Sciences, University of Central Lancashire, Preston, UK

Jürg Bernhard, Associate Professor, Psychooncology Service, Department of Medical Oncology, Inselspital, Bern University Hospital, Bern, Switzerland

Gabriella Bianchi, Clinical Psychologist and Psychotherapist, Psycho-Oncology Consultant, Breast Centre of the Italian Switzerland (CSSI), Lugano, Switzerland

Céline Bourquin, Senior Research Fellow, Psychiatric Liaison Service, Department of Psychiatry, Lausanne University Hospital, Lausanne, Switzerland

Frances Boyle, Professor of Medical Oncology and Director of Patricia Ritchie Centre for Cancer Care and Research, Mater Hospital, North Sydney, NSW, Australia

Marie O'Boyle-Duggan, Associate Professor, Birmingham City University, School of Nursing, Midwifery and Social Work, Birmingham, England, UK

Richard F. Brown, Associate Professor, Department of Health Behavior and Policy, Virginia Commonwealth University School of Medicine, Richmond, VA, USA

Barry D. Bultz, Professor and Head, Division of Psychosocial Oncology; Daniel Family Leadership Chair in Psychosocial Oncology, Department of Oncology, Cumming School of Medicine, University of Calgary; and, Department of Psychosocial Oncology, Tom Baker Cancer Centre, Calgary, AB, Canada; and Conjoint Professor, School of Medicine and Public Health, Faculty of Medicine and Health, University of Newcastle, Australia

Melanie Burton, Head of Technology Enhanced Learning Development, Education for Health, Warwick, UK

Phyllis N. Butow, Professor and Founding Director, Centre for Medical Psychology and Evidence-based Decision Making (CeMPED), School of Psychology, University of Sydney, Sydney, NSW, Australia

Carma L. Bylund, Associate Professor, College of Journalism and Communications, and College of Medicine, UF Health Cancer Center, University of Florida, Gainesville, FL, USA

Linda E. Carlson, Enbridge Research Chair in Psychosocial Oncology, Alberta Innovates-Health Solutions Health Scholar, Professor, Division of Psychosocial Oncology, Department of Oncology, Cumming School of Medicine, University of Calgary, Calgary, AB, Canada

Valérie Carrard, Department of Organizational Behavior, Faculty of Business and Economics, HEC Lausanne, University of Lausanne, Lausanne, Switzerland

Peter Chan, Urological Surgeon, Royal Victoria Hospital; Director of Male Reproductive Medicine, and Associate Professor, Department of Urology, McGill Faculty of Medicine, Montreal, QC, Canada

Cathy Charles†, Late Professor Emeritus, Centre for Health Economics and Policy Analysis, Department of Clinical Epidemiology and Biostatistics, McMaster University, Hamilton, ON, Canada

Noé Rubén Chávez, Community Psychologist and Research Fellow, Division of Outcomes Research, Department of Population Sciences, City of Hope Medical Center, California, CA, USA

Betty Chewning, Apple Professor, Director, Sonderegger Research Center; School of Pharmacy, University of Wisconsin-Madison, Madison, WI, USA

Grace H. Christ, Professor Emeritus of Social Work, Columbia School of Social Work, Columbia University, New York, NY, USA

Alex Clarke, Consultant Clinical Psychologist, Visiting Professor, Centre for Appearance Research, Department of Health and Social Sciences, University of the West of England, Bristol, UK

Josephine M. Clayton, Palliative Care Physician and Associate Professor of Palliative Care, Hammond Care Palliative and Supportive Care Service, Greenwich Hospital, Greenwich; and Sydney Medical School, University of Sydney, NSW, Australia

Kathy Cole-Kelly, Professor of Family Medicine, Director of Communication in Medicine Program, Director of Foundations of Clinical Medicine Seminars, Case Western Reserve University School of Medicine, Cleveland, OH, USA

Michael Connolly, Consultant Nurse, Supportive and Palliative Care, University Hospital of South Manchester NHS Foundation Trust, Manchester, UK

Lara J. Cooke, Senior Income Manager, American Cancer Society, Philadelphia, PA, USA

Lauren M. Czaplicki, Johns Hopkins Bloomberg School of Public Health, Baltimore, MD, USA

Thomas A. D'Agostino, Post-Doctoral Fellow, Department of Psychiatry and Behavioral Sciences, Memorial Sloan Kettering Cancer Center, New York, NY, USA

Donna D'Alessio, Associate Attending Radiologist, Department of Radiology, Memorial Sloan Kettering Cancer Center, New York, NY, USA

Anthony De La Cruz, Research Nurse Practitioner, Memorial Sloan Kettering Cancer Center, Department of Nursing, New York, NY, USA

M. Robin DiMatteo, Distinguished Professor Emerita, Department of Psychology, University of California, Riverside, USA

Barbara Lubrano di Ciccone, Associate Professor, Moffitt Cancer Center, Tampa, FL, USA

Lilo Dietrich, Outpatient Psycho-oncological Counseling, Kantonsspital St. Gallen, Switzerland

Stewart Dunn, Professor of Psychological Medicine, Pam McLean Centre, Sydney Medical School Northern and Royal North Shore Hospital, Sydney, NSW, Australia

John Encandela, Yale Department of Psychiatry, Yale School of Medicine, Teaching and Learning Center, New Haven, CT, USA

Kimberly Feigin, Department of Radiology, Memorial Sloan Kettering Cancer Center, New York, NY, USA

Anne Finn, National Co-Lead, Advanced Communication Skills Training Programme (ACST), Nurse Education Consultant, Clinical Education Centre, Altnagelvin Hospital, Derry, Northern Ireland, UK

Kelly A. Edwards, Professor, Department of Bioethics and Humanities, University of Washington School of Medicine, Seattle, WA, USA

Clara Gaff, Executive Director, Melbourne Genomics Health Alliance, the Walter and Eliza Hall Institute, Melbourne, VIC, Australia; and Honorary Principal Fellow, University of Melbourne, VIC, Australia

Amiram Gafni, Professor, Centre for Health Economics and Policy Analysis, Department of Clinical Epidemiology and Biostatistics, McMaster University, Hamilton, ON, Canada

Thomas H. Gallagher, Professor and Associate Chair, Department of Medicine; and Professor, Department of Bioethics and Humanities, University of Washington, Seattle, WA, USA

Marshalee George, Oncology Nurse Practitioner, Johns Hopkins University School of Medicine, Baltimore, MD, USA

Janine Giese-Davis, Associate Professor, Division of Psychosocial Oncology, Department of Oncology, Cumming School of Medicine, University of Calgary, Calgary, AB, Canada

Lauren Goldstein, Doctoral Candidate in Social Psychology, UCLA Department of Psychology, Teachers College, Columbia University, New York, NY, USA

Luigi Grassi, Professor and Chair of Psychiatry, Dean of the Department of Biomedical and Specialty Surgical Sciences, University of Ferrara; and Head of the University Unit of Hospital Psychiatry, Integrated Department of Mental Health and Addictive Disorders, S. Anna University Hospital and Health Authorities, Ferrara, Italy

Michele G. Greene, Professor, Department of Health and Nutrition Sciences, Brooklyn College, CUNY School of Public Health, Brooklyn, NY, USA

Thomas F. Hack, Professor, College of Nursing, Faculty of Health Sciences, University of Manitoba; Canadian Breast Cancer Foundation (Prairies/NWT), Chair in Psychosocial and Supportive Care Oncology Research; Director, Psychosocial Oncology and Cancer Nursing Research, I.H. Asper Clinical

---

† It is with regret that we report the death of Cathy Charles during the preparation of this edition of the textbook

Research Institute; Research Associate, Manitoba Palliative Care Research Unit, Canada; and Visiting Professor, University of Central Lancashire, Preston, UK

Judith A. Hall, Professor of Social Psychology, Department of Psychology, Northeastern University, Boston, MA, USA

Diana Harcourt, Professor of Appearance and Health Psychology, Centre for Appearance Research, Department of Health and Social Sciences, University of the West of England, Bristol, UK

Kelly B. Haskard-Zolnierek, Associate Professor, Department of Psychology, Texas State University, San Marcos, TX, USA

Joshua Hauser, Associate Professor, Department of Medicine, Palliative Care, Feinberg School of Medicine, Northwestern University, Chicago, IL, USA

Paul Heinrich, Consultant, Medical Communication, Founding Creative Director, Pam McLean Centre, University of Sydney, Sydney, NSW, Australia

Courtney Hempton, Department of Psychiatry, School of Clinical Sciences at Monash Health, Monash University, Clayton, VIC, Australia

Christopher Herbert, The Bishop of St Albans (1995–2009) and Former Chair of the Hospital Chaplaincies Council, St Albans, Herts, UK

Shira Hichenberg, Research Manager, Memorial Sloan Kettering Cancer Center, Department of Psychiatry and Behavioral Sciences, New York, NY, USA

Christoph Hürny, Professor, Geriatric Clinic, St. Gallen, Switzerland

Sarina R. Isenberg, Department of Health, Behavior and Society, Johns Hopkins Bloomberg School of Public Health, Baltimore, MD, USA

Paul B. Jacobsen, Professor and Chair, Department of Health Outcomes, Moffitt Cancer Center and Research Institute, Tampa, FL, USA

Michael Jefford, Deputy Head, Department of Medical Oncology, Peter MacCallum Cancer Centre, Melbourne; Director of the Australian Cancer Survivorship Centre; and Principal Fellow, The University of Melbourne, Parkville, VIC, Australia

Louise Keogh, Associate Professor, Melbourne School of Population and Global Health, University of Melbourne, Parkville, VIC, Australia

Emma King, Macmillian Palliative Care Facilitator, Western Health and Social Care Trust, Omagh, County Tyrone, Northern Ireland, UK

Alexander Kiss, Professor and Head, Division of Psychosomatic Medicine, Basel University Hospital, Basel, Switzerland

David W. Kissane, AC, Professor and Chair, Department of Psychiatry, School of Clinical Sciences at Monash Health, Monash University, Clayton, VIC, Australia; Professor of Psychiatry, Weill Medical College of Cornell University; and Memorial Sloan Kettering Cancer Center, New York, NY, USA

Lyuba Konopasek, Designated Institutional Official, New York Presbyterian Hospital; Associate Professor of Pediatrics, Weill Cornell Medical College, New York, NY, USA

Suzanne M. Kurtz, Clinical Professor, Director of Clinical Communication, College of Veterinary Medicine, Washington State University, Pullman, WA, USA

Lauren Latella, Research Assistant, Department of Psychiatry and Behavioral Sciences, Memorial Sloan Kettering Cancer Center, New York, NY, USA

Carrie Lethborg, Senior Social Worker, Department of Social Work, St Vincent's Hospital, Melbourne; Research Fellow, Department of Psychiatry, Monash University, Clayton, VIC, Australia

Tomer T. Levin, Associate Professor of Psychiatry, Director of Collaborative and Integrative Care and the Psychiatry Collaborative Care Center, Weill Cornell Medicine, New York, NY, USA

Deborah Lewis, Senior Lecturer, School of Nursing and Midwifery, Faculty of Health, Education and Life Sciences, Birmingham City University, Birmingham, UK

Yves Libert, Psychologist, Psycho-Oncology Clinic, Institut Jules Bordet, Université Libre de Bruxelles; and Professor, Faculty of Psychology and Educational Sciences, Université Libre de Bruxelles, Belgium

Aurore Liénard, Psychologist, Psycho-Oncology Clinic, Institut Jules Bordet, Brussels, Belgium

Renee Lim, Director of Program Development, Pam McLean Centre; Lecturer, Sydney Medical School Northern and Royal North Shore Hospital, Sydney, NSW, Australia

Mack Lipkin Jr, Professor of Medicine, New York University School of Medicine, Bellevue Hospital Center, New York, NY, USA

Elizabeth Lobb, Professor of Palliative Care, Adjunct Professor, School of Medicine, the University of Notre Dame, Sydney; and Calvary Health Care Kogarah; and Cunningham Centre for Palliative Care, St Vincent's Hospital, Sydney, NSW, Australia

Matthew Loscalzo, Professor and Executive Director Department of Supportive Care Medicine, Professor Population Sciences, City of Hope National Medical Center, Duarte, CA, USA

Joshua J. Lounsberry, Department of Psychosocial Oncology, Tom Baker Cancer Centre, Calgary, AB, Canada

Melanie Lovell, Palliative Care Staff Specialist, Greenwich Hospital, Hammond Care; and Clinical Associate Professor, Northern Clinical School, University of Sydney, Sydney, NSW, Australia

E. Jane Maher, Joint Chief Medical Officer, Macmillan Cancer Support and NHS Clinical Leader, Consultant Clinical Oncologist, Mount Vernon Cancer Centre and Hillingdon Hospital, Northwood, UK

Gregory Makoul, PatientWisdom, New Haven, CT, USA; University of Connecticut School of Medicine, Farmington, CT, USA

Rebecca L. Malhi, Psychologist and Research Associate, Department of Oncology, Division of Psychosocial Oncology, Cumming School of Medicine, University of Calgary, Calgary, AB, Canada

Ruth Manna, Manager, Comskil Program, Communication Skills Training and Research Laboratory, Department of Psychiatry and Behavioral Sciences, Memorial Sloan Kettering Cancer Center, New York, NY, USA

Marianne Schmid Mast, Psychologist and Professor, Department of Organizational Behavior, Faculty of Business and Economics, HEC Lausanne, University of Lausanne, Lausanne, Switzerland

Isabelle Merckaert, Professor, Psychosomatic and Psycho-Oncology Research Unit, Faculty of Psychology and Educational Sciences, Université Libre de Bruxelles, and Psychologist, Psycho-Oncology Clinic, Institute Jules Bordet, Brussels, Belgium

Tricia A. Miller, Psychologist, Department of Psychology, University of California, Riverside, CA, USA

Cynthia W. Moore, Associate Psychologist, Division of Child and Adolescent Psychiatry, Massachusetts General Hospital, Harvard Medical School, Boston, MA, USA

Julia Neal, Director of Education, Education for Health, The Athenaeum, Warwick, UK

Simon Noble, Marie Curie Professor in Supportive and Palliative Medicine, Division of Population Medicine, Cardiff University, Cardiff, Wales, UK

Patricia A. Parker, Associate Member and Associate Attending Psychologist; Director, Communication Skills Training and Research Laboratory, Memorial Sloan Kettering Cancer Center, New York, NY, USA

Steve Passik, Vice President, Clinical Research and Advocacy, Millennium Health, San Diego, CA, USA

Nicola Pease, Consultant Palliative Medicine Physician, Palliative Medicine Department, Velindre NHS Trust, Cardiff, UK

Emily B. Peterson, Doctoral Candidate, Department of Communication, George Mason University, Fairfax, VA, USA

Jennifer Philip, Associate Professor and Co-Deputy Director, Centre for Palliative Care, St Vincent's Hospital, University of Melbourne, Melbourne, VIC, Australia

Susan Poultney, Senior Lecturer, Birmingham City University, School of Nursing, Midwifery and Social Work, Birmingham, UK

Paula K. Rauch, Attending Psychiatrist, Department of Psychiatry, Massachusetts General Hospital, Harvard Medical School, Boston, MA, USA

Darius Razavi, Professor and Head, Psychosomatic and Psycho-Oncology Research Unit, Faculty of Psychology and Educational Sciences, Université Libre de Bruxelles; Psychiatrist and Head, Psycho-Oncology Clinic, Institute Jules Bordet, Brussels, Belgium

Anita Roberts, Senior Lecturer, Marie Curie Palliative Care Institute Liverpool, University of Liverpool, Liverpool, UK

Felicia Roberts, Professor, Brian Lamb School of Communication, Purdue University, West Lafayette, IN, USA

John W. Robinson, Clinical Psychologist, Department of Psychosocial Oncology, Tom Baker Cancer Centre; and Associate Professor, Department of Oncology, Cumming School of Medicine and Department of Psychology, University of Calgary, Calgary, AB, Canada

Zeev Rosberger, Associate Professor, Department of Oncology, McGill Faculty of Medicine; and Director, Psychosocial Oncology Program, Institute of Community and Family Psychiatry, Jewish General Hospital, Montreal, QC, Canada

Marcy Rosenbaum, Professor of Family Medicine, Office of Consultation and Research in Medical Education, University of Iowa College of Medicine, Iowa City, IA, USA

Debra L. Roter, University Distinguished Service Professor, Department of Health, Behavior and Society, Johns Hopkins University, Bloomberg School of Public Health, Baltimore, MD, USA

Lidia Schapira, Associate Professor, Stanford School of Medicine, Director, Cancer Survivorship Program, Stanford Comprehensive Cancer Institute, Stanford, CA, USA

Henry Schneiderman, Palliative Care Physician Champion, Saint Francis Hospital and Medical Center; Professor of Medicine, University of Connecticut Health Center; and Clinical Professor, Nursing, Yale University, Hartford, CT, USA

Penelope Schofield, Professor, Department of Psychology, School of Health Sciences, Swinburne University of Technology, Hawthorn; Department of Cancer Experiences Research, Peter MacCallum Cancer Centre, Melbourne; and Sir Peter MacCallum Department of Oncology and Faculty of Health Sciences, Dentistry, and Medicine, The University of Melbourne, Parkville, VIC, Australia

Stephen Scott, Associate Professor, Associate Dean for Student Affairs, Weill Cornell Medicine-Qatar, Doha, Qatar

Linda Sheahan, Palliative Medicine Consultant, St George Hospital Cancer Care Centre, University of Sydney, Sydney, NSW, Australia

Megan J. Shen, Assistant Professor of Psychology in Medicine, Weill Cornell Medicine, New York, NY, USA

Milagros D. Silva, Weill Cornell Medicine and New York Presbyterian, Department of Medicine, Division of Geriatrics and Palliative Medicine, New York, NY, USA

Laura A. Siminoff, Dean of the College of Public Health, Laura H. Carnell Professor of Public Health, Temple University, Philadelphia, PA, USA

Peter Speck, Former Health Care Chaplain; and Honorary Senior Lecturer, King's College London, Department of Palliative Care, Policy and Rehabilitation, Guy's, King's and St Thomas' Medical School, London, UK

Friedrich Stiefel, Professor and Head, Psychiatric Liaison Service, Department of Psychiatry, Lausanne University Hospital, Lausanne, Switzerland

Martin Stockler, Professor of Oncology and Clinical Epidemiology, Central Clinical School and NHMRC Clinical Trials Centre, University of Sydney, Concord Repatriation General and Royal Prince Alfred Hospitals, Sydney, NSW, Australia

Andy S.L. Tan, Assistant Professor of Social and Behavioral Sciences, Department of Social and Behavioral Sciences, Harvard T. H. Chan School of Public Health; and Center for Community-Based Research, Division of Population Sciences, Dana-Farber Cancer Institute, Boston, MA, USA

Martin H.N. Tattersall, Professor of Cancer Medicine, Department of Medicine, Central Clinical School, University of Sydney, Sydney, NSW, Australia

Bejoy C. Thomas, Adjunct Associate Professor, Department of Oncology, Cumming School of Medicine; and Coordinator, Department of Psychosocial and Rehabilitation Oncology, Tom Baker Cancer Centre, Alberta Health Services, Calgary, AB, Canada

Maria D. Thomson, Assistant Professor, Health Behavior and Policy, Virginia Commonwealth University, School of Medicine, Richmond, VA, USA

Bethan Tranter, Head, Medicines Management, Velindre Hospital, Cardiff, Wales, UK

Luzia Travado, Head of Psycho-oncology Service, Clinical Center of the Champalimaud Center for the Unknown, Champalimaud Foundation, Lisbon, Portugal

Amanda Tristram, Clinical Senior Lecturer, Gynaecological Cancer Surgery, Cardiff University, Cardiff, Wales, UK

James A. Tulsky, Chair, Department of Psychosocial Oncology and Palliative Care, Dana-Farber Cancer Institute; Chief, Division of Palliative Medicine, Brigham and Women's Hospital; and Professor of Medicine, Harvard Medical School, Boston, MA, USA

Jane Turner, Professor, Discipline of Psychiatry, School of Medicine, Faculty of Medicine and Biomedical Sciences, The University of Queensland, Brisbane, QLD, Australia

A. Katalin Urban, Staff Specialist, Department of Palliative Medicine, Concord Repatriation General Hospital, Sydney, NSW, Australia

Lauren M. Walker, Research Assistant, Professor and Clinical Psychologist, Department of Oncology, Division of Psychosocial Oncology, Cumming School of Medicine, University of Calgary, Calgary, AB, Canada

Hannah Waterhouse, Education for Health, The Athenaeum, Warwick; and Heart Failure Specialist Nurse, Derbyshire Community Health Services NHS Foundation Trust, UK

Jennifer Gueguen Weber, Staff Psychologist, CHE Senior Psychological Services, Brooklyn, NY, USA

Alison Wiesenthal, Assistant Attending Palliative Medicine Physician, Department of Medicine, Memorial Sloan Kettering Cancer Center, New York, NY, USA

Susie Wilkinson, International Liaison Lead, Honorary Senior Lecturer Marie Curie Palliative Care Institute Liverpool (MCPCIL), Cancer Research Centre, University of Liverpool, Liverpool, UK

Brigitta Wössmer, Senior Psychologist, Division of Psychosomatic Medicine, Basel University Hospital, Basel, Switzerland

Alexander Wuensch, Psychologist, Department of Psychosomatic Medicine and Psychotherapy, Comprehensive Cancer Center Freiburg, Psychosocial Support for Cancer Patients, Medical Center, Faculty of Medicine, University of Freiburg, Germany

Patsy Yates, Professor, Head of School of Nursing, Faculty of Health, Queensland University of Technology (QUT), Brisbane, QLD, Australia

Lai Cheng Yew, Specialist Registrar in Clinical Oncology, University College London NHS Foundation Trust, London, UK

Talia Zaider, Assistant Attending Psychologist, Director, Family Therapy Clinic, Department of Psychiatry and Behavioral Sciences, Memorial Sloan Kettering Cancer Center, New York, NY, USA

SECTION A

Introduction to communication studies in cancer and palliative medicine

Section editor: Carma L. Bylund

CHAPTER 1

The history of communication skills knowledge and training

Mack Lipkin, Jr.

Introduction to the history of communication skills

This chapter attempts to provide the reader with a concise and personal journey that recalls how we got to where we are in the field of communication in medicine, which inheres an implicit 'where we are' (Lipkin 2008). For mutual sanity, it does not attempt to be encyclopaedic, comprehensive, or complete. Any accuracy it has derives from the author's experience of 40 years' participation in the field. It attempts to steer between the Scylla of what Dunn describes as 'evidence-based navel gazing' and those Charybdis of self-indulgent, evidence-free, charismatic pronouncement. A talented reader might extract an historical sense of why we are where we are, and so have a skeletal perspective from which to hang what follows in the highly focused subsequent chapters.

Most of the history of communication skills knowledge and teaching derives from work and studies done in general medicine, or further afield, rather than in cancer care. This chapter includes such material because much of our knowledge and skill about communication is generic, crosses specific applications and content areas like cancer care and because the most useful conceptual frameworks and approaches began elsewhere and have only partially been rendered cancer specific. Nevertheless, cancer care has been advanced in attempting, as this book reflects, to codify the processes required to accomplish some key goals: to help patients to accept their diagnosis and prognosis; to accept or reject tests and difficult treatments according to their core preferences; to participate in studies; to enable them to participate meaningfully when curative care is futile; and to facilitate dying with dignity. This is why much of the remainder of the book speaks specifically of cancer-derived work which has been relatively underrepresented to date.

The importance of communication in medicine generally was understood by prehistoric human healers. Fabrega emphasized that even in the smallest social units, such as isolated tribal groups of as few as five, sick people need to show their sickness in order to seek and get help (Fabrega 1999). Healers need also to understand their diseases and illnesses and to plan and execute their healing rituals and treatments (Kleinman *et al.* 1978).

Communication plays an important role in classical accounts of medicine

Hippocrates' first aphorism speaks of compliance, thus:

> Life is short and the art long; the occasion fleeting; experience fallacious, and judgment difficult. The physician must not only

be prepared to do what is right himself, but also to make the patient, the attendants, and externals cooperate (Hippocrates and Adams 1849).

Hippocrates speaks about prognosis like someone who lived daily with the dying beyond help:

> … by foreseeing and foretelling, in the presence of the sick, the present, past, and the future, … he will be the more readily believed to be acquainted with the circumstances of the sick; so that men will have more confidence to entrust themselves to such a physician (Hippocrates and Adams 1849).

Galen in his account of caring for Marcus Aurelius uses observation and communication to win the Emperor's loyalty. He says the Emperor said of him:

> … there is one physician who is not hide-bound by rules … He is the first of Physicians … and of Philosophers. For Marcus (says Galen) had already had experience with many, not only desirous of money, but contentious, vain-glorious, envious and malignant (Clendening 1942).

And so it goes, through most of the greatest, Maimonides (Nuland 2005), Paracelsus, Peabody, *ad scholarum infinitum*. In the pre-scientific era, communication had an honoured place in the physician's work.

The stepchild status of communication in medicine: Or is it the runt of the litter?

In the course of the gradual empiricism of medicine, the counting of dead bodies leading to vital statistics, the cutting of corpses leading to pathology, which in turn led to understandings of organs and disease specificities, communication remained a stepchild. On the one hand, it was and is the medium of care, and so as little noticed as water by fish. On the other, ambitious and righteous pioneers, striving to render their approach the orthodox one, tended to overstate the importance of whatever was their focus and to diminish, or even dismiss, the thing not counted (by them) as soft, subjective, trivial, or unnecessary, a still prevalent attitude of reductionist thinkers, who magically (tragically) believe all levels of science can be reduced to the lowest.

Nor did the shaky nature of the business (up to 1910 or so, according to Henderson, the average patient meeting the average physician lacked an average chance of benefit), the presence in the field of the epidemiologically expected but nonetheless highly visible presence of scoundrels, fakes, and opportunists, and the ubiquity of physicians, including the weakest, fail to earn its comeuppance (Henderson 1987). Take Chaucer's Doctour of Phisik:

> In al this world ne was ther noon hym lyk
> To speke of phisik and of surgerye,
> For he was grounded in astronomye;
> He kepte his pacient a ful greet deel
> In hours, by his magik naturel …
> Therefore he loved gold in special (Gray 2003).

Reproduced from Gray D, *The Oxford Companion to Chaucer*, p. 26, Oxford University Press, Oxford, UK, Copyright © 2003, with permission from Oxford University Press.

Or consider Moliere's *Médecin Malgré Lui*, a mock doctor full of himself and absurd in spite of himself. Literature up to this moment is rife with fictional takes on medicine's and doctors' frailties. So is history, with the *Oxford Illustrated Companion to Medicine* featuring a section on doctor-murderers (Locke *et al.* 2001).

The nature of the work leads also to doctors playing important literary roles, from Chekov's dyspeptic, yet quiet, hero victims of life's small inevitabilities, to the bystander in the *Death of Ivan Illych*, and to Drs Jekyll, Manette, and Zhivago. Our modern doctor heroes tend to be self-identified, such as William Carlos Willliams, Oliver Sachs, Vergese, and their literary sibs. The straw-doctor has been the pawn of many from myriad fields, his communication especially vulnerable as the outward manifestation of his being, up to and including current authors on such topics as narrative medicine, medical ethics, or healthcare reform.

Education about communication reflects the greater world

Medical education on the subject of doctor's talk and behaviour reflects this greater world context consistently, from Flexner forward to the present. There is tedious consistency to the critiques of their peers by sensitive physician-authors writing about what is wrong with how doctors work and communicate, and about how they should and might improve. On the one hand, these pathedocs are illiterate. They don't listen, care, take time, admit error, or behave decently … On the other, they are too technical and scientific: they lack art!

So teaching about communication was ignored, left to advocates, seconded to psychiatry, and given short shrift in curricula and in study. At Harvard Medical School in 1966, the introduction to 'taking a history' was bimodal. First, students were given 'a little red book' (not Mao's), with a 'several hours long' laundry list of specialist-asserted 'essential' questions, to be asked in order, on penalty of incompleteness. Then, small groups of clueless students in new white coats were told things like, 'Taking a history is like playing music … now, go do it'.

The history of communication teaching and standard dogma (i.e. prevailing views) has evolved through a series of phases: the prehistoric, classical and ancient, rhetorical, exhortative/charismatic, descriptive empirical, experimental empirical, and the consensus dulled by the dismal meta-analytic.

The rhetorical phase was marked by authors such as Osler and exemplified by Peabody in his 'The care of the patient' (1927) with its dictum, '… for the secret of the care of patients is in caring for the patient' (Peabody 1927). I dub this phase 'rhetorical' because its promulgators tended to great seniority, and they did not directly involve themselves in the creation or oversight of curriculum to

ensure the promulgation of the values and behaviours they advocated from their experiential bases.

Next came great clinician-educators such as William Morgan and George Engel, who codified in 1969 an approach described as *The Clinical Approach to the Patient* (Morgan and Engel 1969), which embodies the content of 'the little red book', the wisdom of wise, psychoanalytic teachers such as Sullivan, Frank, and Engel himself, and the implicit charismatic notion, 'do as I do and you will be as good as I am'. Such teachers were like those of prior eras in exhorting students to do well and right. They differed, however, from prior eras in including an overarching approach to care, claiming to set a standard, and carving time into the curriculum to teach the mandated skills. What was lacking from a current perspective were objective data that what they exhorted was of demonstrated value, concerning such outcomes as knowledge gained, skills acquired, skills enduring, and skills applied in practice. In addition, communication was embedded in a broader approach and so relegated once again to hind tit, getting the few remaining drops of curricular milk after 'auscultating the heart' and 'examining the retina' had gorged on hours of teaching time about their highly specific skills (and as recent studies have shown, also not positively and durably changing behaviour: the dysfunction of curricular obesity). Down the road, several charismatic authors evolved highly specific, but not empirically derived methods, for talking with cancer patients. Over time, some of these have been partially, although usually not independently, evaluated.

While Morgan and Engel's approach (1969) was being published and a powerful, charismatic series of papers were added by Engel (Engel 1980), a small revolution began, unnoticed by the senior exhorters. This was in the systematic examination of actual interviews, foreshadowed by John Stoeckle and pioneered by Korsch and colleagues in 1968 (Korsch *et al.* 1968). Korsch captured sequential interviews in a paediatric emergency department and showed what was really happening through application of a rudimentary but empirically derived classification scheme. The bottom line was that the doctors and the parents were speaking different languages, with arbitrary and unpredictable points of intersection. This work permanently changed the communication analysis business.

Prior to that, there was an enormous literary (narratives with embellishments) literature, with the tone set by psychosomaticians like Groddeck and psychoanalysts like Freud, Jung, and their acolytes. For 70 years or so, schools of thought and care were fashioned, based upon interviews, with sequences of them remembered in scholarly tranquillity by towering figures of unassailable authority, whose actual speech and interaction were unavailable for validation, correction, or bias filtration. Of course, there were sporadic recordings made on audio and video recorders, often analysed endlessly and tendentiously. But it was the advent of practical, real, medical world recording that marked the modern era of communication investigation.

Modern communication analysis

The innovation which ensured that a valid and reproducible empirical base of information would evolve into semi-quantitative analysis eventually justifying models and theory was invented by Bales who crafted an *Interactional Analysis* method (Bales 1950) for sociological research. In this method, an encounter was captured on tape and then every thought or phrase, technically an *utterance*, was arranged into categories that were mutually exclusive (every utterance went into just one bin) and exhaustive (a bin could be found for every utterance). In the early 1970s, Deborah Roter adapted the Bales method to medical interviews; first for her doctoral thesis, and subsequently in print (Roter 1977).

The Roter Interactional Analysis System (RIAS) became the gold standard method of evaluating what is actually happening verbally in interviews (see Chapter 62). Highly reliable, reproducible (at higher reproducibility and coding reliability rates than most research or clinical tests), and relevant, the RIAS categorizes every utterance into one of 34 categories that most subsequent authors have found adequate for their thinking and analysis. Since then, Roter and her colleagues have added items and subscales to especially reflect content needs of particular areas, such as the emergency room or palliative care. In 2000, Fallowfield and Ford added the ability to analyse utterances in sequence and for meaning, thus creating an analytic tool (the MIPS, or Medical Interaction Process System) specifically evolved for evaluation of cancer care communication quality and education (Ford et al. 2000). But the RIAS also is used in cancer care studies.

Currently, there is a vast array of such instruments that has been created by investigators striving to pin something particular down or simply to do it their way (see Chapter 61). Pendleton characterized these systems as being of five types: sociolinguistic, non-verbal, clinical process, verbal content, or evaluative (Pendleton 1973). The differing nuances, while permitting researchers finesse and subtlety, sometimes render fraught comparison across studies. Nevertheless, using such schema, researchers have demonstrated that when communication is done better, health outcomes (such as blood pressure and glycaemic control) and systems outcomes (such as patient and practitioner satisfaction, return visit rate, medical error rates, and malpractice lawsuits) can result in considerable improvement.

Inui and colleagues strikingly critiqued this approach as stripping the meaning away from rich interactions, reproaching RIAS and related interactional schema as being like a critic who would describe Hamlet as a '… play with 21 principal characters, a ghost, a group of players …' and numerous what-ho's (Wasserman and Inui 1983; Inui and Carter 1985). This is rather like attacking physics as stripping a rainbow of its colour by describing it as the refraction of light by the atmosphere. Readers of Roter and her followers (Stewart and Roter 1989) and users of RIAS and MIPS will have noted that the attempt to create an empirical, reproducible, and valid method need not preclude awareness or valuing of meaning. What Inui was onto is that studying meaning lags behind other aspects of understanding how doctors and patients ought to talk together to optimize outcomes of their mutual work. In reviewing such systems, Wasserman and Inui asserted that schema such as Roter's ought to '… take into account the salient dimensions of interpersonal communications … characterize information exchange that occurs through several channels: through tone of voice, sighing, pauses … (and) gesture, facial expression … the context … and the sequencing of communication behaviors … and attempt to change behavior in light of such lessons …' (Wasserman and Inui 1983), a tall order not yet fulfilled by a single system. The reader is urged to recall Peabody in considering the application of scientific methods to the processes of medicine and of medical education. He wrote, in 'The care of the patient':

> There is no more contradiction between the science of medicine and the art of medicine than between the science of aeronautics and the art of flying. Good practice presupposes an understanding of the sciences which contribute to the structure of modern medicine, but it is obvious that sound professional training should include a much broader equipment (Peabody 1927).

The Lipkin model and the American Academy on Communication in Healthcare

It was in pursuit of 'much broader equipment' that in 1979, Lipkin and Putnam initiated the first interest group in the Society of General Internal Medicine (then SREPCIM), which came to be called the 'Task Force on the Doctor and Patient', growing in 1993 into the current American Academy on Communication in Healthcare (AACH). Lipkin, a mentee and then colleague of George Engel, and Putnam, a collaborator with William Stiles in creating an interactional process analytical method, recognized that the then evolving new science required an innovative basis for teaching and practice. They and their colleagues believed that precisely as in cardiology or chemotherapy, what is said and done by doctors and by teachers of doctors should, where feasible, have an empirical basis, a theoretical structure, a common language, sound values, and be taught using demonstrably effective methods.

The 'Task Force on the Doctor and Patient' began to do bootstrap self-education. In 1984, Lipkin et al. published a comprehensive curriculum for the medical interview which provided a roadmap for the field (Lipkin 1984). The curriculum had four general objectives: patient-centred interviewing and treatment; an integrated approach to clinical reasoning and patient care; personal development of humanistic values; and psychosocial and psychiatric medicine. Each objective had extensive, empirical (where possible) knowledge, skills, and attitudes specified. It discussed teaching strategies, options, and evaluation. In the same time frame, two Task Force participants, Cohen-Cole and Bird, described three functions of the interview: (a) gathering information; (b) developing a relationship; and (c) communicating information, noting that specific teachable behaviours could be allocated to each function (Cohen-Cole and Bird 1991). Regular meetings of this developing, invisible college of interested persons led to the unexpected recognition that even the best teachers and biggest experts needed significant work on their own skills.

In response to this need, Lipkin in 1982 (Lipkin et al. 1995) invented a course model that synthesized educational ideas from Engel (1980), Freire (1986), Rogers (1970; 1983) and Knowles (1980). It used small groups to both learn about personal skills and how to improve them, and how to integrate such learning into the real world and daily practice. It used Rogerian group methods to help the learner overcome any personal barriers to progress, which appeared rooted in his or her own development and psychological structures. It used a task focus to synthesize and foster integration of these learnings. Over several iterations a method evolved that used specifically appropriate teaching methods to accomplish explicit, higher order learning challenges, and proceeded to help the learner synthesize and integrate these.

In 1983, Novack and Clark initially directed what became a still ongoing annual course on teaching interviewing (Novack et al. 1993), which spawned similar courses in the United Kingdom, under the auspices of the Medical Interview Teachers Association and now has offshoots in Scandinavia, Switzerland, and Italy.

The Lipkin model used in these courses has been documented to change knowledge, skills, and attitudes (Lipkin *et al.* 1995); to demonstrate a dose response (Fallowfield *et al.* 1998); to change real world behaviour in the short term and durably; to elicit personal growth and transformational experiences in learners (Kern *et al.* 2001); and to be applicable across higher order learning situations, such as in cancer care, substance abuse, disaster response (Zabar *et al.* 2004), pain management, and education itself (Pololi *et al.* 2001). It grew and evolved as the major model of the AACH and many of its trainees. Thorough the heightened standing of the work, the proliferation of trained teachers, and the consequent cultural evolution, the place of communication teaching in medical school curricula shifted from being present in roughly 35% of US schools in 1978 to about 75% in 1992 (Novack *et al.* 1993).

Cancer research campaign studies in the United Kingdom

In the United Kingdom during the 1980s, Peter Maguire showed that teaching students about communication processes early in medical school changed behaviour, that the changes endured, and that they generalized over time (Maguire *et al.* 1986). The gap between the experimental, well-taught groups of students and those taught in the usual (charismatic) manner was not only meaningful and significant, but over five years it continued to widen. Maguire's curriculum, however, was rather general, his main technique being focused on feedback, with the rest undocumented. When tested in varied health practitioners (doctors, nurses, social workers) with cancer care experience, greater patient disclosure of information resulted from the use of empathic statements, open directive questions, focus on the psychological, and summarizing (Maguire 1996). For this purpose, he developed a new Cancer Research Campaign rating system (Maguire 1991).

Fallowfield translated the Lipkin model into the cancer care setting in the United Kingdom, and over the next decade, evolved it in her team's ongoing studies of its effectiveness (Fallowfield *et al.* 1998; 2002). She set out to use real patient outcomes with practicing cancer specialists. She first showed that her adaptation of the Lipkin model had a dose response and worked better in three days than in 1.5 day courses (Fallowfield *et al.* 1998). She went on to show experimentally in follow-up at one year that cancer doctors made good use of focused questions (34%), open questions (27%), fewer inappropriate interruptions and more empathic statements (69%), fewer leading questions (24%), and more recognition of non-verbal and affective cues (Fallowfield *et al.* 2003). This remains the most powerful rigorously documented result of communication training in medicine.

European and other studies

In Belgium, Razavi's group showed subsequently that some communication skills training outcomes are enhanced by follow-up consolidation workshops (Merckaert *et al.* 2008). In Chapter 55, the Swiss model makes particular use of post-training supervision to consolidate gains in skills. Other approaches have been developed which overlap with those described. For example, in Chapter 54, the 'Oncotalk' model describes improvement in giving bad news and discussing transitions to palliative care. While showing skills improvement, the use of a non-experimental design and only

immediately post-training, standardized patient evaluations limits the validity of claims of superiority of this system.

Rao *et al.* (2007) performed a systematic review of 36 randomized controlled trials in which educational interventions were evaluated using objective measures of verbal communication behaviours on physician (Wasserman and Inui 1983), patient (Roter 1977), or both (Kleinman *et al.* 1978). This meta-analytic review reduces these rather complex studies to their least common denominator, concluding that higher ratings by physicians occurred when skills practice with feedback occurred and that outcomes included commonly taught behaviours, such as those reported above (see Fig. 1.1).

One synthesis of communication skills training was expressed in a highly condensed form in two Kalamazoo consensus statements (Makoul 2001; Duffy *et al.* 2004). These were significantly influenced by the more extensive Macy Project in Health Communication (Kalet *et al.* 2004). In this project, a process of faculty survey, literature review, and expert opinion was used to evolve a set of 63 'competencies' or behaviours, expressed so as to be measurable, and believed to be essential for graduating physicians (Kalet *et al.* 2004). These were organized in a logical schema depicting the flow of the medical interview, as shown in Figure 1.1. Each of the major headings contains sub-items which are behaviourally expressed, measurable using simple techniques, and empirically derived. A cohort, controlled study demonstrated that this complex set of skills (the evaluation measured some 30, which had been blinded to the curricular designers) could be taught and significantly changed behaviour over a year (Yedida *et al.* 2003).

Areas of growth and need for communication knowledge and education

The most striking deficiency in communication knowledge and training is a gap that continues to widen. The information technology revolution has changed practice markedly and obviously, at least in those parts of the world with full access to both computers and the internet.

Computers have intruded into examination rooms and preliminary studies lament their intrusion as taking the practitioner's attention away from the patient; costing time, an average of two minutes—which in a world of six-minute encounters is major; interfering with eye and other contact; and fostering impersonality. In fact, patients like computers, talk with them more easily than with doctors, and see them as a sign of being up to date.

Similarly, the advance of the smartphone has permitted major positive change. Patients can text and get through asynchronously. This means they can get onto their doctor's screen in short order. Much routine business can be done through email. Video makes possible Skype or other video chats, while apps exist that allow HIPAA (i.e. meeting federal US privacy standards) compliant video discussion. New apps are permitting a variety of examinations from the electrocardiogram (ECG) to visual acuity testing, to translation between common languages. In the next few years, much more care will be done at home, including what is now done in hospital. The impact on the verbal and non-verbal aspects of communication will be extraordinary and is only now being begun to be imagined.

Finally, the internet permits patients to access both valuable information and overwhelming misinformation, some commercially

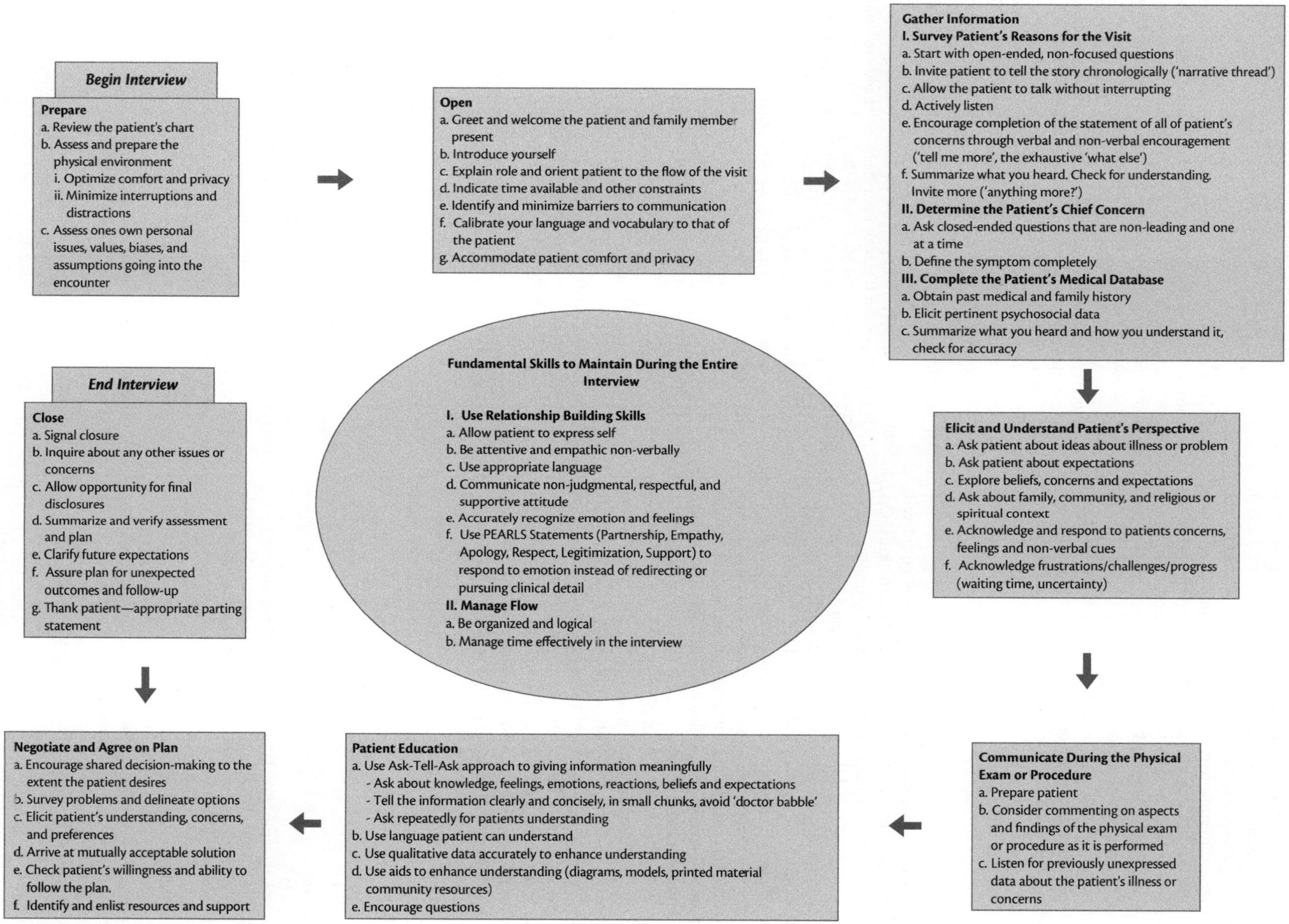

Gather Information

I. Survey Patient's Reasons for the Visit
a. Start with open-ended, non-focused questions
b. Invite patient to tell the story chronologically ('narrative thread')
c. Allow the patient to talk without interrupting
d. Actively listen
e. Encourage completion of the statement of all of patient's concerns through verbal and non-verbal encouragement ('tell me more', the exhaustive 'what else')
f. Summarize what you heard. Check for understanding. Invite more ('anything more?')

II. Determine the Patient's Chief Concern
a. Ask closed-ended questions that are non-leading and one at a time
b. Define the symptom completely

III. Complete the Patient's Medical Database
a. Obtain past medical and family history
b. Elicit pertinent psychosocial data
c. Summarize what you heard and how you understand it, check for accuracy

Elicit and Understand Patient's Perspective
a. Ask patient about ideas about illness or problem
b. Ask patient about expectations
c. Explore beliefs, concerns and expectations
d. Ask about family, community, and religious or spiritual context
e. Acknowledge and respond to patients concerns, feelings and non-verbal cues
f. Acknowledge frustrations/challenges/progress (waiting time, uncertainty)

Communicate During the Physical Exam or Procedure
a. Prepare patient
b. Consider commenting on aspects and findings of the physical exam or procedure as it is performed
c. Listen for previously unexpressed data about the patient's illness or concerns

Open
a. Greet and welcome the patient and family member present
b. Introduce yourself
c. Explain role and orient patient to the flow of the visit
d. Indicate time available and other constraints
e. Identify and minimize barriers to communication
   i. Optimize comfort and privacy
   ii. Minimize interruptions and distractions
f. Calibrate your language and vocabulary to that of the patient
g. Accommodate patient comfort and privacy

Fundamental Skills to Maintain During the Entire Interview

I. Use Relationship Building Skills
a. Allow patient to express self
b. Be attentive and empathic non-verbally
c. Use appropriate language
d. Communicate non-judgmental, respectful, and supportive attitude
e. Accurately recognize emotion and feelings
f. Use PEARLS Statements (Partnership, Empathy, Apology, Respect, Legitimization, Support) to respond to emotion instead of redirecting or pursuing clinical detail

II. Manage Flow
a. Be organized and logical
b. Manage time effectively in the interview

Patient Education
a. Use Ask-Tell-Ask approach to giving information meaningfully
   - Ask about knowledge, feelings, emotions, reactions, beliefs and expectations
   - Tell the information clearly and concisely, in small chunks, avoid 'doctor babble'
   - Ask repeatedly for patients understanding
b. Use language patient can understand
c. Use qualitative data accurately to enhance understanding
d. Use aids to enhance understanding (diagrams, models, printed material community resources)
e. Encourage questions

Begin Interview

Prepare
a. Review the patient's chart
b. Assess and prepare the physical environment
   i. Optimize comfort and privacy
   ii. Minimize interruptions and distractions
c. Assess ones own personal issues, values, biases, and assumptions going into the encounter

End Interview

Close
a. Signal closure
b. Inquire about any other issues or concerns
c. Allow opportunity for final disclosures
d. Summarize and verify assessment and plan
e. Clarify future expectations
f. Assure plan for unexpected outcomes and follow-up
g. Thank patient—appropriate parting statement

Negotiate and Agree on Plan
a. Encourage shared decision-making to the extent the patient desires
b. Survey problems and delineate options
c. Elicit patient's understanding, concerns, and preferences
d. Arrive at mutually acceptable solution
e. Check patient's willingness and ability to follow the plan.
f. Identify and enlist resources and support

Fig. 1.1 Structure and sequence of effective doctor–patient communication.

This model is reproduced with permission from the Macy Initiative in Health Communication.

driven, other parts ideology or idiocy driven. Perhaps the most salutary information now becoming available is the patient's own medical history and record. The OpenNotes project is pioneering and assessing the impact of making notes available to patients in real time. So far, satisfaction is high, mistakes are identified and eliminated, and counterintuitively, time is not expanded (Walker *et al.* 2015). A second salutary and now long-standing use of the internet is as a way to unburden the suffering families of cancer and other patients undergoing medical tragedy via a bulletin board mode of permitting broad-scale communication to the friends and colleagues of those concerned. A well-established example of this is CaringBridge, which allows anyone to create a website that enables those with permission to join to read updates and to provide notes and comments (https://www.caringbridge.org). The relief this provides is extraordinary, yet not well understood, or appreciated.

Conclusion

By 1993, a consensus emerged concerning what was empirically validated as the core of teach-worthy communication skills. One example was the Toronto consensus statement (Simpson *et al.* 1991). In 1995, the AACH published its authoritative reference text, which covered clinical care, education, and research as an exposition of communication knowledge, skills, and training for internal and family medicine (Lipkin *et al.* 1995). Since then, although there have been serial syntheses and consensus efforts (always a moving target), the core principles of communication skills training have remained quite stable, once one translates the babble of new language into common core concepts.

Thus, at this point in the evolution of work between doctors and patients, we can fairly say we know what ought to be done, we can teach it to medical students, residents, and practitioners, and doing so improves important outcomes of care, as well as patient and practitioner satisfaction in their mutual and important work. The future holds predictable transformations related to how new science and technology will move medicine back into the home and away from hospitals and offices. What is unknown is how revolutions in the detection of emotion, in our understanding of cognitive processing, and real-time text processing will move us towards deeper ability for doctors and patients to understand and empathize, and therefore connect.

References

Bales RF (1950). *Interaction Process Analysis*. Addison Wesley, Cambridge, MA.

CaringBridge website. Available at: https://www.caringbridge.org

Clendening L (1942). Galen Prognostics XI. In: Clendening L (ed.). *Source Book of Medical History, compiled with notes by Logan Clendening*. pp. 51–2. Dover, New York, NY.

Cohen-Cole SA, Bird J (1991). *The Medical Interview: The Three-Function Approach*. Mosby, St. Louis, MS.

Duffy FD, Gordon GH, Whelan G, Cole-Kelly K, Frankel R and all the participants in the American Academy on Physician and Patients Conference on Education and Evaluation of Competence in Communication and Interpersonal Skills (2004). Assessing competence and interpersonal skills. The Kalamazoo II report. *Acad Med* **79**.

Gray D (2003). *The Oxford Companion to Chaucer*. p. 26. Oxford University Press, Oxford, UK.

Engel GL (1980). The clinical application of the biopsychosocial model. *Am J Psychiatry* **137**, 107–11.

Fabrega Jr HF (1999). *Evolution of Sickness and Healing*. University of California Press, Berkeley, CA.

Fallowfield L, Jenkins V, Farewell V, et al. (2003). Enduring impact of communication skills training: results of a 12-month follow-up. *Br J Cancer* **89**, 1445–9.

Fallowfield L, Jenkins V, Farewell V, Saul J, Duffy A, Eves R (2002). Efficacy of a cancer research UK communication skills training model for oncologists: A randomized controlled trial. *Lancet* **359**, 650–7.

Fallowfield L, Lipkin M, Hall A (1998). Teaching senior oncologists communication skills: Results from phase I of a comprehensive longitudinal program in the United Kingdom. *J Clin Onc* **16**, 1961–8.

Ford S, Hall A, Ratcliff D, Fallowfield L (2000). The Medical Interaction Process System (MIPS): An instrument for analyzing interviews of oncologists and patients with cancer. *Soc Sci Med* **50**, 553–66.

Freire P (1986). *Pedagogy of the Oppressed*. Continuum, New York, NY.

Henderson LJ (1987). Quoted in Stoeckle JD (ed.). Encounters between patients and doctors. pp. 1–2. MIT Press, Cambridge, MA.

Hippocrates, Adams F (1849). *The Genuine Works of Hippocrates*. Translated by Francis Adams, Sydenham Society. Kessinger, New York, NY.

Inui TS, Carter WB (1985). Problems and prospects for health services research on provider-patient communication. *Med Care*, **23**, 521–38.

Kalet A, Pugnaire MP, Cole-Kelly K, et al. (2004). Teaching communication in clinical clerkships: Models from the Macy initiative in health communications. *Acad Med* **79**, 511–20.

Kern DE, Wright SM, Carrese JA, et al. (2001). Personal growth in medical faculty: a qualitative study. *West J Med* **175(2)**, 92–8.

Kleinman A, Eisenberg M, Good B (1978). Culture, illness, and care: clinical lessons from anthropologic and cross-cultural research. *Ann Int Med* **88**, 251–8.

Knowles MS (1980). *The Modern Practice of Adult Education: from Pedagogy to Androgogy*. Adult Education Company, New York, NY.

Korsch BM, Gozzi E, Francis F (1968). Gaps in doctor patient communication. *Pediatrics* **42**, 855–71.

Lipkin M (2008). The medical interview. In: Feldman M, Christiansen J (eds). *Behavioral Medicine*, 3rd edition, pp. 1–9. McGraw Hill Medical, New York, NY.

Lipkin M, Kaplan C, Clark W Novack DH (1995). Teaching medical interviewing: the Lipkin Model. In: Lipkin MJr., Putnam S, Lazare A (eds). *The Medical Interview: Clinical Care, Education and Research*. Springer-Verlag, New York, NY.

Lipkin Jr M, Putnam S, Lazare A (eds). (1995). *The Medical Interview: Clinical Care, Education and Research*. Springer-Verlag, New York, NY.

Lipkin M, Quill T, Napadano RJ (1984). The medical interview: A core curriculum for residencies in internal medicine. *Ann Int Med* **100**, 277–83.

Locke S, Last JM, Dunea G (2001). *Oxford Illustrated Companion to Medicine*. pp. 310–11. Oxford University Press, Oxford, UK.

Maguire P, Fairbairn S, Fletcher C (1986). Consultation skills of young doctors—benefits of feedback training in interviewing as students persists. *Br Med J* **292**, 1573–8.

Maguire P, Faulkner A, Booth K, Elliott C, Hillier V (1996). Helping cancer patients disclose their concerns. *Euro J Cancer* **32A**, 78–81.

Maguire P, Booth K (1991). Development of a rating system to assess interaction between cancer patients and health professionals. Report to the Cancer Research Campaign. CRC, London, UK.

Makoul G (2001). Participants in the Bayer-Fetzer Conference on Physician Patient Communication in Medical Communication. Essential elements of communication in medical encounters: the Kalamazoo consensus statement. *Acad Med* **76**, 390–3.

Merckaert I, Libert Y, Delvaux N, et al. (2008). Factors influencing physicians' detection of cancer patients' and relatives' distress: can a communication skills training program improve physicians' detection? *Psycho-Oncology* **17**, 260–9.

Morgan WL, Engel GL (1969). *The Clinical Approach to the Patient*. Saunders, New York, NY.

Novack DH, Volk G, Drossman DA, Lipkin MJr (1993). Medical interviewing and interpersonal skills teaching in US medical schools: progress, problems, and promise. *JAMA* **269**, 2101–5.

Nuland SB (2005). *Maimonides (Jewish Encounters)*. Schocken, New York, NY.

Peabody FW (1927). The care of the patient. *JAMA* **88**, 877–82.

Pendleton D (1983). Doctor-patient communication. A review. In: Pendleto7n D, Hasler J (eds). *Doctor-patient Communication*. Academic Press, London, UK.

Pololi L, Clay MC, Lipkin Jr M, Hewson M, Kaplan C, Frankel R (2001). Reflections on integrating theories of adult education into a medical school faculty development course. *Med Teach* **23**, 276–83.

Rao JK, Anderson LA, Inui TS, Frankel RM (2007). Communication interventions make a difference in conversations between physicians and patients. *Med Care* **45**, 340–9.

Rogers CR (1970). *On Encounter Groups*. Harper and Row, New York, NY.

Rogers CR (1983). *Freedom to Learn for the 80s*. Merrill, Columbus, OH.

Roter DL (1977). Patient participation in the patient-provider interaction: the effects of patient question asking on the quality of interaction, satisfaction and compliance. *Health Educ Monogr* **5**, 281–315.

Simpson M, Buckman R, Stewart M, *et al.* (1991). Doctor-patient communication: the Toronto consensus statement. *BMJ* **303**, 1385–7.

Stewart M, Roter D (1989). *Communicating with Medical Patients*. Sage, London, UK.

Walker J, Meltsner M, Delbanco T (2015). US experience with doctors and patients sharing clinical notes. *BMJ* **10**, 350:g7785.

Wasserman RC, Inui TS (1983). Systematic analysis of clinician-patient interactions: a critique of recent approaches with suggestions for future research. *Med Care* **21**, 279–312.

Yedidia MJ, Gillespie CC, Kachur E, *et al.* (2003). Effect of communications training on medical student performance. *JAMA* **290**, 1157–65.

Zabar S, Kalet AL, Kachur EK, *et al.* (2004). Practicing bioterrorism-related psychosocial skills with standardized patients. *J Gen Intern Med* **19**(s1), 109–241.

CHAPTER 2

Journeys to the centre of empathy: The authentic core of communication skills

Renee Lim and Stewart Dunn

Introduction to communication skills

As a species we are programmed to respond to the situations and emotions of others. Mirror neurons, a specialized class of neurons in the premotor cortex and the inferior parietal cortex, provide a neurobiological basis for translating actions we observe in others into internal representations in the observer's brain (Riess 2010). Sadly, simulation-based communication training compared with usual education does not appear to improve the quality of communication about end-of-life care, nor the quality of end-of-life care (Curtis *et al*. 2013). Moreover, a Cochrane Systematic Review found no evidence to support a beneficial effect of communication skills training on professional burnout, patients' mental or physical health, and patient satisfaction (Moore *et al*. 2013).

How then do we use this innate capacity to engage with people as they struggle to bypass the road from cancer diagnosis to palliative care? The authors propose that authenticity is the key to how we develop, sustain, and teach empathic communication.

'Houston, we've had a problem here'

On April 11, 1970, a well-prepared team of three men sat within the Apollo 13, and were launched into space with the intention of landing on the Moon. This would be NASA's third manned mission, with many unmanned trips previously successful as well. Unfortunately, two days into the mission, an oxygen tank exploded and crippled the service module, which was the mainstay of much of the mission's resources.

The team of three were forced to move into the lunar module (a transport module intended for one to two people for a maximum of 36 hours). And then NASA ground control had the job of getting them home ... alive.

When three men (and a major scientific organization) who had done everything by the book found themselves sitting in what was essentially a scooter in space, the world could not believe it. But it was how it was dealt with that made the story amazing.

Three major issues stand out:

◆ The lunar module contained lithium hydroxide to remove exhaled carbon dioxide from the chamber. However, this was not sufficient for three men for many days. The oxygen tanks in the command module had a cube-shaped connection, and the receiving sockets in the lunar module were round. So a team of engineers on the ground had to first determine what was available on the Apollo 13, and then create something that would 'fit a square peg into a round hole'.

◆ After completely shutting down the command module to preserve power, a restart was needed to get the crew home. The powering up process was never intended to be accomplished mid-flight. The limited power available also meant that the normal processes could not be followed. Condensation which had developed on the solid surfaces of the module threatened to short-circuit the electrical systems even if the power-up was successful. So designers on the ground worked against the clock, with no certainty of success, to design a new way to restart the command module, a way that had never been done before. And then cross their fingers.

◆ The final part of the trip was particularly stressful. The difficulty of any re-entry was compounded, in this case, by the need for the team to use the lunar module, and disconnect from the remainder of the Apollo 13. This involved very specific timing, to prevent the pressure of the separation of the modules damaging the hatches and potentially burning the astronauts. A calculation was made—purely theoretical—and the team implemented it. But due to a well-known phenomenon called the communications blackout, there was a period where nobody, except the team in the lunar module, could actually know what was going on. It was not until many minutes after the success or the failure of the calculated procedure that those at ground control actually knew the outcome.

Fortunately for all involved, it was a success. And a success in many ways beyond the landing of the module with the astronauts alive on board. It was a celebration in ingenuity and adaptability, in dealing with pressure, and using respectful and effective communication in a high stake, time-pressured, life or death situation. Sound familiar?

The world has changed

Medicine has developed over the years—from basic faith and witchcraft, through to scientifically supported theories enacted on people's bodies, through to modern evidence-based medicine where proof is essential before implementation. The understanding and teaching of communication, once it was finally added to the list of skills necessary to be a good doctor, has followed suit. Initially considered a gift, then slowly rationalized into a series of tick boxes, and recently, assumed to be teachable as a complex process because we have learned how to break it down, test it, and prove over time that, as a general rule, the individual components work.

As long as medicine remained an expert field, this was almost enough. In the role of expert information and service provider, with control of the interview, use of the behavioural checklists developed for 'communication' often successfully created and maintained the right environment—safety, acknowledgement, and structure. An environment where the patient could see the attempt to care and safely assume that the effort to behave in all those 'empathic ways' reflected the effort to be the best doctor, and therefore, also choose the best treatment for the patient. In fact, if this was not a natural skill, it was almost all the more reflective of the doctor's desire to care. And for many years, medicine has existed comfortably within this structure, with varying degrees of personal care but a huge professional responsibility undertaken by the clinical individual. Life carried on shoulders therefore often understandably too weary to pull upright, or even shrug, in response to exposure to emotion.

Modern-day medicine has changed. In the progression to a patient-centred care model, the way medicine has functioned for centuries is no longer possible. As patients become more educated, as doctors become both more plentiful and more disparate in their opinions, as health becomes a service determined not just by need but by desire and financial capacity, and the multidisciplinary team is the norm, rather than a novelty, the individual clinician is no longer essential, or as easily forgivable. The ability to perform empathic behaviours within a structured interview is no longer an option, because we no longer have control of the interview. This is how the world is in general—a consumer society with international accessibility and immediate internet information, accompanied by hyperstimuli and interaction. The world has changed and we in the health profession are taking too long to catch up. We've been put on the Apollo 13, and we need to learn to adapt.

So what is the single most useful communication tool to the modern-day clinician? The obvious answer is probably empathy. And empathy is not unimportant. However, we recommend a trait that has not played too prominently in any previous iteration of the attributes of the good doctor: authenticity.

There's something about empathy

Empathy is a key component of a meaningful relationship. It increases understanding, equality, and respect. And in medicine, where significant relationships must develop between clinician and patient, we have struggled with it for many years. From whether it is necessary, through to whether it is teachable. And if taught, is it effective and safe?

Of course, there are those who naturally are empathic—especially at the start (Chen et al. 2012).

However, we all find ourselves overwhelmed by other factors: time pressure; litigation risk; ongoing training requirements; administrative roles and job instability. Health professionals don't stop being empathic; they just stop having the resources to engage with that empathy to develop the relationships they would like to with their patients and colleagues.

And then there are those who sit somewhere on the spectrum between professional through to inappropriate. There are many within education who want to weed these people out of the system. And we hope this never happens. Just because your heart is not on your sleeve getting sprayed with blood, phlegm, vomit, and melena, does not mean that you are not a good doctor. In fact, some patients don't want to see their doctors get dirty. The 'House's of the world can be quite popular in saving people's lives.

So why is empathy failing our students in learning about effective medical communication (Neumann et al. 2011)?

One of the key problems with empathy as a word is its multiple definitions. We do not disagree with what is being taught, but we worry it is being labelled inappropriately.

Psychologists discriminate between *affective empathy*, our sensations and feelings in response to others' emotions, and *cognitive empathy*, our ability to identify and understand other peoples' emotions (Reniers et al. 2011).

Others have gone much further, adding the ability to understand the patient's situation, perspective and feelings (and their attached meanings), to communicate that understanding and check its accuracy, and to act verbally and non-verbally on that understanding (Mercer and Reynolds 2002).

The second issue is the way we ascribe empathy a series of actions, as mentioned in the more academic definitions. By trying to create identifiable teachable 'empathic behaviours', we encourage students to believe, like a pulmonary embolism protocol, that if you follow these behaviours you will be communicating with empathy.

But there is no correlation between saying 'You seem upset' and giving a box of tissues (because you know it is the right thing to do) and the complex understanding and integration of another's experience that (some of) the definitions of empathy imply. The problem is not that the behaviours are not useful, or that empathy at a higher order does not improve relationships. It is that by identifying the behaviours as empathy, we leave our clinicians feeling one of two things: either that these behaviours are a poor substitute for empathy and therefore they don't take the teaching seriously; or that these behaviours will convince the world, and even themselves, that they are empathic, and therefore assume the teaching is all they need to learn. Ever.

Either way, we have failed to provide clinicians with useful tools that are clear, accessible to everyone, and safe. We have launched them into space with no true understanding of the processes that might save them when protocols break down.

Because we know that empathy is not a series of behaviours and acknowledgement, but a true understanding, not just of the existence of, but also the reasons behind, a response to a situation. And that only time, experience, choice, and sometimes personality will make one truly empathic, in the way that most of the world understands that word.

To ask our doctors, especially at the early stages of their lives and careers to 'just do it' is unfair. Especially when we are well aware in the literature of the patient's ability to see through the false niceties and often respond negatively to these, even if the medical situation itself is fine. And then there is that fine distinction between caring and paternalism. If we convince our clinicians these behaviours are empathy, we set them up to fail. They do their best, tick all the boxes, the patient does not believe them, or feels condescended to—and therefore, the clinician is left in an untrusting relationship, and a sense of failure despite doing everything right. The oxygen tank blew up anyway.

What is authenticity?

Authenticity is

- 'The quality of being authentic; genuineness' (Dictionary.com, Merriam-Webster).
- 'A mode of existence arising from self-awareness, critical reflection on one's goals and values, and responsibility for one's own actions; the condition of being true to oneself' (Oxford English Dictionaries).

The communication skills and frameworks we teach are incredibly useful and important. And they improve the patient experience and clinical outcomes, as many studies have shown. We should try as hard as we can to acknowledge and understand what our patients (and colleagues) are going through.

However, perhaps we are coming at this from the wrong direction. Asking someone to 'have empathy' expects them to recognize, acknowledge, appreciate, and understand the reasons behind people's emotions, and then provide solutions that sit within the other person's framework and capacity. Can we ask that of our clinicians? Probably not at the universal level we talk about. But can we ask them to be empathic about the things they understand themselves. That they have experienced. That is a fair request. And we should probably also make it okay for them to not always understand why another person responds the way they do.

Because that would be human

Our proposition is to teach clinicians to communicate with authenticity. To be honest with themselves, their patients, and their colleagues. To use their authenticity and the communication skills they have learned to house a sharing of feelings and information. This does not override the professional relationship of a doctor with their patient. But it gives the clinician the freedom to acknowledge their own limitations and needs, re-establishes both the patient's own empathy for the situation and their expectations, and creates a more equal opportunity for discussion. We do not believe this will decrease the empathy shown by most doctors—if anything, the ability to say that they don't know or understand what is going on could provide, from the patient's response to this admission, an increase in the clinician's understanding of the patient's situation. In fact, encouraging authenticity should increase a clinician's engagement and potential sharing of their own emotions and experiences, which can be a way of showing empathy.

When you try to teach communication, you have a choice. You either make it 'medical communication', give it a strict set of parameters so it is a 'new skill', and then ensure that what you teach will almost always be right. *Or*, knowing it is an already established skill within the clinician as a person equipped with previous experiences and emotional outcomes, we use *our* empathy to recognize their situation and skills, acknowledge their present state, appreciate and understand why it is like that and what the process of communication means to them, and then come up with a solution that is based on their knowledge, needs, experience, and goals.

Student-centred communication teaching. And it must begin with authenticity. Because the foundations are *you*. They are 'Knowing yourself'. Authenticity requires the student to know how their lives have shaped them, why they react the way they do, and what their strengths and weaknesses are. It requires mindfulness, honesty, and sharing. It requires strength to commit to following a path that is appropriate for you, and sometimes realizing you are not like those around you. And it requires acceptance from those others, similar to yourself or not.

This is a culture change. To teach it, you as the teacher, must also travel down this path. Colleagues must share their own stories, and this could lead to more complementary team structures and collaboration. And patients, too, must acknowledge their roles within the new patient-centred model, communicate differently with the clinician, and engage in the uncertainty of modern medicine as an equal traveller on the journey.

So what can we learn from a spaceship?

So let's go back to Apollo 13 because it's always nice to know something you want to try has worked before.

Work with what you've got

Like the engineers reconnecting the oxygen tanks, we have to realize that authenticity comes from knowing who you are. Most aspects of good communication are about the outcome of that communication, rather than a single behaviour that is considered right or wrong. Successful people come in all shapes and sizes. And it is possible to develop behaviours in most people that achieve a particular outcome, but connected to their authenticity. Suited to their style. Accommodated to their limitations. And embracing of their strengths.

Authenticity is sustainable. Even the best actors will tell you that maintaining a character far removed from your natural preferences is difficult. Stanislavski, who developed a well-regarded and oft-used acting technique, believed that authenticity in acting stemmed from 'listen[ing] internally to your body and externally to your fellow actors' (Merlin 2007). Rather than asking clinicians to 'fake it till they make it', we can develop strong foundations of core skills that can be expanded, because they are based on the clinician's natural skillset.

First time, every time, and the road is fraught with danger

It is hard in medicine to admit uncertainty, to have accounted for all the variables, and still put lives at risk. But, like the command module, there are always going to be things outside our control. And in the case of a patient-centred care relationship, the variable is the patient.

In the past, medical decision-making was essentially based on disease. And, with some exceptions, most disease is moderately predictable and has a specific number of parameters with normal and abnormal ranges. Thus, using either personal or evidence-based experience, there was a high probability that a set of actions would produce a known result.

But our patient-centred care model changes that. Not only is it often the first time for the patient, which makes their reaction unpredictable, it is also always now going to be the first time for the doctor. Because we are not treating just the disease. We are treating a person … and their disease … and their emotional needs … and their history … and their psychosocial situation … and their future plans. Our job is to help them integrate all these into a set of decisions. So the reality is, we will never have 'seen this before'.

For the clinician the challenge is becoming authentic because it is a continuous process, not an event. It involves not just knowing oneself, but also recognizing others and the mutual influence between individuals.

It is possible that authenticity might protect against professional burnout. Being authentic is about being who you are in the moment in an evolving relationship with the real world. And psychological research has shown that being authentic and mindful of the present allows us to interact with others in a way that incorporates self-relevant information in a relatively non-defensive manner (Lakey *et al.* 2008). Sometime around 1624 the poet John Donne wrote 'Any man's death diminishes me, because I am involved in mankind'. There is a corollary: 'Any authentic human contact enriches me because I am involved in mankind'.

By being authentic, we achieve two things: we accept that we don't know what is in front of us. And we create realistic expectations. Everyone at NASA knew that there was a chance the reboot might not be possible. And then even when it was, that there was a high risk that the condensation would fry the system, so all the work would be for nothing. But the commitment was to the effort, the attempt. And if ground control had pretended everything was definitely going to work, then the time delays, and the obvious problems the astronauts saw in front of them, would have made them stop trusting the things that were said down on Earth. They would have felt placated, ignored, and unsafe. Instead, by being honest—both about the effort and the potential outcomes—the decision was made by both parties equally. Is this not what patient-centred care is about?

The communications blackout

We all want to help. And especially for those of us who naturally empathize, we feel like we are on that journey with the other. All doctors experience physiological arousal in their interactions with patients (Brown *et al.* 2009; Shaw *et al.* 2013). The spectrum of ways in which doctors deal with this is considerable. Emotional arousal can be denied, sublimated, or repressed, ignored, tolerated—and it can overwhelm. Professional burnout is a very high risk for oncology professionals (Shanafelt *et al.* 2012) and possibly higher for palliative care professionals (Kamal *et al.* 2014). Along this spectrum, however, it can also be used judiciously to enhance empathy and rapport.

All of these responses are appropriate at different times. What then does it mean for a doctor to be 'authentic'? The reality is that, for most of us, we will never really understand what the patient is going through. The ability to say 'I know how you feel' is limited by a fortunate reality that for most working-age individuals, death is not imminent, and severe pain, nausea, or dyspnoea are not day-to-day occurrences.

This is why authenticity is perhaps a more useful tool than empathy. Because while we can share much of the journey, and provide information and options, it is those astronauts that must then choose and actually follow those instructions, without assurance of an outcome. And we cannot be there during those blackouts. We cannot know, we can only perceive and interpret. But we can feel, and authenticity allows us to share our understanding and feelings. It is a small, but distinct, difference, and one that takes the pressure off both the clinician and the patient to somehow believe that we are capable of complete understanding. Or that anything less should be considered equivalent.

In practice

In communication teaching, role play is a common technique. In fact, it is well known to be a more effective teaching technique than didactic information provision. A combination of modelling and experiential learning creates the foundations of most communications teaching around the world.

In this context, there are four key components—the content, the 'patient', the teacher, and the student. And each can be used to ensure a development of authenticity in our clinicians.

The content

Adult and higher education models reflect often on motivation in ensuring effective engaging teaching (Pintrich 2003). Within medicine, little content is reliant on specific student interests and motivations, as it is all essential to be a competent doctor. Similarly, the importance of learning tasks that utilize self-determination and efficacy are relatively new to medical teaching, and often connected to non-core content, despite clear evidence that engaging these aspects of students increases both their approach to and outcomes of learning (Urdan and Schoenfelder 2006).

In teaching communication, it is essential to 'empathize' with your student—to recognize, acknowledge, and validate the different reasons why a student would consider this an essential part of being a competent doctor. Throwaway lines like 'Of course you all care about your patients', or 'Good communication is essential to being a good person' will not engage that group of students you are most hoping to reach.

The content of communication teaching needs to acknowledge the individual experiences and styles, and also the plethora of reasons why good communication counts, including:

- improved clinical outcomes;
- improved patient satisfaction;
- better clinician well-being;
- decreased litigation;
- time-saving.

And if litigation is the key driver for a student, then that is okay. Acknowledging the legitimacy of that reason will make them more authentic in both their learning, and, in the future, their communication style than any judgement of that reason, and a concerted effort and 'hope that they will develop a heart'. Because you have found what matters to them, you can adjust the context of the teaching to make sure that what you are teaching is important to their future.

Similarly, a cookie-cutter approach towards communication methods disempowers individuals who do not already communicate in a particular way. By focusing on the individual's skills, and encouraging them to both explore their own choices, and perhaps try other options in a safe space, you encourage both self-determination and efficacy, and the onus of the outcomes of the communication rest more squarely on the student's shoulders.

The 'patient'

If authenticity is the aim, then the learning task must itself be authentic. Research into simulation and authentic tasks has had varied results, though most would agree that psychological fidelity is more important than engineering fidelity (McGaghie *et al.* 2010) and also that while authentic tasks do not necessarily show improved practice, increased exposure to patients does (Durning 2012). One of the ways this can be done is by increasing the authenticity of the simulated patient. The more complex and real the 'patient' is, the less option the student has to use the 'checklist' and succeed. It also means that the 'patient interaction' will have more authentic outcomes. This is more likely with the initiation of (any or all of) the following:

- well-developed character briefs and scenarios specifically aimed at not responding to false attempts at care, or where it is difficult to engage the patient with superficial behaviours;

- the use of trained actors or real patients;

- rehearsal or development time prior to the task.

The student, who often comes in with bravado and 'It's not real' barriers aplenty, has no choice but to be authentic in response to such a real and complex individual.

The benefit of this style of role play is twofold:

It encourages students to drop the checklist, and instead initiate a problem-solving model to understand the individual patient and develop an effective communication method.

The specificity of the character limits the student's ability to now generalize the learning from that role play to be 'relevant to all patients'. Thus the learning is about the process of understanding the patient, and themselves, and not on the individual actions that were effective.

The teacher

See one, do one, teach one. The well-known medical teaching mantra. While said with laughter, the truth is that it is often the case. But at its core, there is a bigger truth—teaching by example.

To teach authenticity is hard. Because as the teacher, you must relinquish two things: the role of the expert … and the answers. And most medical educators feel uncomfortable engaging in a non-expert role, as their training is usually as the content expert, rather than as a teacher. Ibarra cites Stanford psychologist Deborah Gruenfeld who describes this as managing the tension between authority and approachability:

> To be authoritative, you privilege your knowledge, experience, and expertise over others, maintaining a measure of distance. To be approachable, you emphasize your relationships with people, their input, and their perspective, and you lead with empathy and warmth (Ibarra 2015).

True exploration of authenticity must be facilitated, rather than taught, as the building blocks come from within the student—a constructivist approach which increases authentic integration and application of learning outcomes (Grabinger and Dunlap 1995). To do this, the teacher must themselves be authentic about their own knowledge, limitations, and needs in the context of communication, both with the students, and also with the 'patients' who will walk into the room. The desire to 'tell them how to do it' must be withheld with the aim that they will develop their own version, with your guidance, of communication with that patient. One that is based on their own skills, and therefore is not only reproducible and sustainable, but also often fulfilling (Krasner *et al.* 2009), rather than fabricated from a memory bank.

With that in mind, facilitation skills are recommended for anyone teaching communication to students who does not want to rely on checklists and memorizing frameworks. The following phrases often help to reset when the expert-teacher in all of us rears its ugly head.

- 'I'm standing next to you.'

- 'I don't know.'

- 'It's up to you.'

- 'There's no right or wrong, just choices.'

- 'How do you feel?'

The student/trainee

Here, like the patient, we have to accept that some things are out of our control. We cannot force them to be authentic, but by offering both an example of, and a safe space to engage with, authenticity, we create a new framework of honest reflection, sharing, and collaboration. In many ways we are preparing them for the new world of medicine—that of the patient-centred care model, where the doctor doesn't *tell* the patient what to do, and they cannot control the relationship. Instead, they must simply exist within it. But they deserve to do so as themselves, obviously within professional boundaries, but as equal human beings bringing much to the table, and with their own humanity.

We all want them to come home safe. But, honestly, we don't know if they will. And perhaps that's okay, if we can share the load.

References

Brown RF, Dunn SM, Byrnes K, Morris R, Heinrich P, Shaw JM (2009). Doctors' stress responses and poor communication performance in simulated bad-news consultations. *Acad Med* **84** (11), 1595–602.

Chen DC, Kirshenbaum DS, Yan J, Kirshenbaum E, Aseltine RH (2012). Characterizing changes in student empathy throughout medical school. *Med Teach* **34** (4), 305–11.

Curtis JR, Back AL, Ford DW, *et al.* (2013). Effect of communication skills training for residents and nurse practitioners on quality of communication with patients with serious illness: A randomized trial. *JAMA* **310** (21), 2271–81.

Dictionary.com, Merriam-Webster. Authenticity. Available at: http://dictionary.reference.com/browse/authenticity?s=t

Durning SJ, LaRochelle J, Pangaro L, *et al.* (2012). Does the authenticity of preclinical teaching format affect subsequent clinical clerkship outcomes? A prospective randomized crossover trial. *Teach Learn Med* **24**, 177–82.

Grabinger RS, Dunlap JC (1995). Rich environments for active learning: A definition.. *Res Learn Tech* **3**, 5–34.

Ibarra H (2015). The authenticity paradox: Why feeling like a fake can be a sign of growth. *Harvard Business Review* Jan-Feb, 1–9.

Kamal A, Bull J, Wolf S, Samsa G, Ast K, Swetz KM, Shanafelt TD, Abernethy AP (2014). Prevalence and predictors of burnout among specialty palliative care clinicians in the United States: Results of a national survey. *J Clin Oncol* **32**, suppl 31; abstr 87.

Krasner MS, Epstein RM, Beckman H, *et al.* (2009). Association of an educational program in mindful communication with burnout, empathy, and attitudes among primary care physicians. *JAMA* **302**(12), 1284–93.

Lakey CE, Kernis MH, Heppner WJ, Lance CE (2008). Individual differences in authenticity and mindfulness as predictors of verbal defensiveness. *J Res Personality* **42**, 230–8.

McGaghie WC, Issenberg SB, Petrusa, ER, Scalese, RJ (2010). A critical review of simulation-based medical education research: 2003–2009. *Med Educ* **44**, 50–63.

Mercer SW, Reynolds WJ (2002). Empathy and quality of care. *Br J Gen Pract* **52** Suppl, S9–12.

Merlin B (2007). *The Complete Stanislavski Toolkit*. Nick Hern Books Ltd, London, UK.

Moore PM, Rivera Mercado S, Grez Artigues M, Lawrie TA (2013). Communication skills training for healthcare professionals working with people who have cancer (Review). *Cochrane Database Syst Rev* **28**, 3, CD003751.

Neumann M, Edelhäuser F, Tauschel D, *et al.* (2011). Empathy decline and its reasons: a systematic review of studies with medical students and residents. *Acad Med* **86** (8), 996–1009.

Oxford English Dictionaries. Authenticity. Available at: http://www.oed.com/view/Entry/13325?redirectedFrom=Authenticity#eid

Pintrich, PR (2003). A motivational science perspective on the role of student motivation in learning and teaching contexts. *J Ed Psychol* **95**, 667–86.

Reniers RLEP, Corcoran R, Drake R, Shryane NM, Völlm BA (2011). *J Pers Assess* **93** (1), 84–95.

Riess H (2010). Empathy in medicine: a neurobiological perspective. *JAMA* **304** (14), 1604–5.

Shanafelt TD, Gradishar WJ, Kosty M, *et al.* (2012). Burnout and career satisfaction among US Oncologists. *J Clin Oncol* **30**, 1235–41.

Shaw JM, Brown RF, Heinrich P, Dunn SM (2013). Doctors' experience of stress during simulated bad news consultations. *Patient Ed Couns* **93**, 203–8.

Urdan T, Schoenfelder, E (2006). Classroom effects on student motivation: Goal structures, social relationships, and competence beliefs. *J School Psychol* **44**, 331–49.

CHAPTER 3

Models of communication skills training and their practical implications

Richard F. Brown, Alexander Wuensch, and Carma L. Bylund

Introduction to models of communication: Skills training and their practical implications

Several models of physician–patient communication that have served as conceptual frameworks for communication skills training have been described over recent years. Studies have explored the efficacy of such training in altering physician behaviours. We begin this chapter with an overview of the current research in communication skills training. Afterwards, we discuss different models in their strengths and weaknesses. We then focus on a model of communication skills training, which was developed at Memorial Sloan Kettering Cancer Center in New York, NY, in an effort to address critiques of these earlier models.

Overview of current research in communication skills training

Communication skills training for healthcare professionals (CST) is an effective means to ensure high-quality communication. These effects are well studied in standardized settings (Brown and Bylund 2008; Fallowfield *et al.* 2003; Goelz *et al.* 2011; Razavi *et al.* 2003). Early positive results of such research studies triggered several programmes for improving communication over the past 20 years. Different reviews, including a Cochrane review (Fellowes *et al.* 2004), emphasize that physicians' communication skills can be altered through training with small to medium effect sizes.

Physician–patient consultation communication is a dynamic, individual process. The personality, attitudes, values, and beliefs of individuals influence the communication process. This interaction can be further complicated by the presence of family members and caregivers in the consultation. Furthermore, culture plays an important role in determining how communication proceeds. There is an increasing interest focused on understanding differences in the culture of consultation communication between Western and non-Western cultures, for example the Far East or the Middle East (Salem and Salem 2013; Wuensch *et al.* 2013). In Western cultures, consultation communication focuses on ensuring that the autonomy of an individual patient is preserved and ensuring that patients are well informed and are thus well equipped to make treatment decisions.

Conversely, in Eastern countries the focus of communication is to ensure that patients, within the context of their family, understand the goal of beneficence and preventing patients from harm. In this context, historical and cultural norms often lead to family members being informed about a cancer diagnosis before, or instead of, the patient. Often the family members make decisions about disclosure of the diagnosis to the patient and make treatment decisions on the patient's behalf. Our experience teaching communication skills in such cultures leads us to believe that these cultural norms are slowly changing. New physicians, often trained in Western models, are uncomfortable with the disregard for patient autonomy.

Taking cultural diversity into account, it is important to have an understanding of the various models that exist for teaching communication skills.

Review of existing models

Our review of the literature indicated seven established models of physician–patient communication. These models have helped to guide communication skills training programmes and provide information about assessment: the Bayer Institute for Healthcare Communication E4 Model; the Three-Function Model/Brown Interview Checklist; the Calgary–Cambridge Observation Guide; Patient-Centred Clinical Method; SEGUE Framework for Teaching and Assessing Communication Skills; The Four Habits Model; and SPIKES. For each of these, we briefly summarize first the conceptualization of the model, and then the way in which its application is assessed.

The Bayer Institute for Healthcare Communication E4 Model

This model describes four important elements of communication as: Engage, Empathize, Educate, and Enlist.

◆ Engage includes eliciting the patient's story and setting an agenda.

◆ Empathize ensures awareness and acceptance of the patient's feelings and values.

◆ Educate seeks to assess the patient's understanding, answer questions, and ensure realistic appreciation.

◆ Enlist establishes decision-making and encouragement of adherence, keeping the patient's understanding and involvement central (Keller and Carroll 1994).

The Three-Function Model/Brown Interview Checklist

Here there is emphasis on three functions of effective medical interviewing: building the relationship; assessing the patient's problem; and managing the patient's problem. The relationship is established with basic skills like empathy, support, and respect. The physician collects information by non-verbal listening, asking open-ended questions, facilitating, and clarifying. The patient's ideas about aetiology are elicited before the clinician provides the diagnosis, checks understanding, describes treatment goals and plans, and checks willingness to proceed (Cole and Bird 2000).

The Calgary–Cambridge Observation Guide

This model divides the consultation into five tasks: initiating the session; gathering information; building the relationship; giving information; explanation and planning; and closing the session. Establishing rapport and identifying reasons for attendance initiates the session, then problems are explored to understand the patient's perspective. As the patient is involved, the relationship is built. The process of giving information includes aiding accurate recall, achieving a shared understanding, and planning treatment. The session is closed by summarizing and contracting (Kurtz and Silverman 1996).

The Patient-Centred Clinical Method

The Patient-Centred Clinical Method is based on six interactive components: exploring both the disease and the illness experience; understanding the whole person; finding common ground regarding management; incorporating prevention and health promotion; enhancing the patient–doctor relationship; and being realistic. These six components are integrated with a skilled clinician using patient cues to move flexibly between each element (Stewart et al. 1995).

SEGUE Framework for Teaching and Assessing Communication Skills

The acronym for this approach is derived from the first letter for each step: Set the stage; Elicit information; Give information; Understand the patient's perspective; End the encounter. Within each domain are identified communication tasks. For instance, set the stage includes creating an agenda and making a personal connection. Elicit information seeks the patient's view of the problem, including both physical and psychosocial factors. Giving information includes providing explanations, while understand the patient's perspective acknowledges their accomplishments respectfully. The next steps are reviewed during closure (Makoul 2001b).

The Four Habits model

Four sequential, interrelated patterns of behaviour form a family of attitudes and skills. The four habits are: invest in the beginning; elicit the patient's perspective; demonstrate empathy; and invest in the end. Habits are interrelated. If the clinician does not elicit all of the patient's concerns and assess their importance at the beginning, empathy may be misplaced, diagnoses based on erroneous hypotheses, or patient concerns left unresolved. Investing upfront in the patient's issues while planning the visit ensures due attention to the patient's needs and the impact of the illness on their lifestyle. Such a person-centred approach depends on empathic exchanges. The closure is also crucial in establishing the diagnosis and buy-in to the management plan (Frankel and Stein 1999; Krupat et al. 2006).

The SPIKES Model

The SPIKES protocol was initially developed to train oncologists in a sequential communication skills method to aid in breaking bad news discussions (Baile et al. 2000). The model has subsequently been extended to cover other communication challenges in the oncology setting, such as providing complex information during discussions about joining a clinical trial (Wuensch et al. 2011) and in emotionally challenging task such as talking about the shift from curative to palliative care (Goelz et al. 2011). The SPIKES acronym refers to six steps: Setting up the interview; assessing the patient's Perception; obtaining the patient's Invitation; giving Knowledge and information to the patient ; Addressing the patient's emotions with Empathic Response; and Strategy and Summary. Each step emphasizes skills that target different aspects of the communication challenge: step one promotes a safe and private consultation setting with a minimum of disturbances; step two assesses the patient's perception; and step three assesses the patient's information needs before disclosing information. Step four emphasizes skills to structure information that meets the needs assessed in step three; step five focuses on empathic responses to emotional cues of the patient, step six provides skills to summarize the content of the consultation either by the physician or the patient. The SPIKES protocol can be seen as a tool box. Skills should be applied flexibly and oriented to the patient. It also can be enriched by other models (Baile et al. 2000; Back et al. 2005; van Vliet and Epstein 2014).

Strengths and limitations

These models have been extremely valuable in implementing and assessing communication skills training programmes. Each provides a set of components, further defined by more specific communication skills or behaviours. Each also has an accompanying assessment tool. These models are well suited to primary care consultations, wherein a patient's problem needs to be diagnosed, understood, and then managed. They are ideal for teaching in medical schools.

However, for healthcare professionals working in oncology settings, these models have limitations. They often represent a generic approach to the first consultation, but not continuing care. For instance, a typical cancer patient at a comprehensive cancer centre may come to a first visit already knowing their diagnosis. The focus is not on eliciting information and trying to make a diagnosis. Instead, these visits often have complicated discussions about treatment options and can include difficult conversations about prognosis and end-of-life care. The models presented above may not be appropriate for these types of applied cancer consultations. Mindful of this, we undertook a further review of the communication skills training literature in search of an approach better suited to the highly specialized fields of cancer and palliative care.

In a seminal systematic review of 26 communication intervention studies, Cegala and Broz (2002) concluded there is good evidence that communication training is effective in improving skills. However, they also raised several concerns. First, they pointed out that very little information is usually provided about which skills were actually taught. Without such detail, it is impossible to judge if correct outcome assessments were used. Second, where the skills being taught were named, there were several occasions of misalignment between the intervention's objectives (e.g. promoting patient-centred interviewing) and the assessment tool. Third, they asserted that 'little effort has been made to provide an over-arching framework for organizing communication skills' (Cegala and Lenzmeier Broz 2002; p. 1005).

To these limitations, we add that the term 'communication skill' is used inconsistently across studies and is often ambiguous within studies. Terms such as: 'task' (Makoul 2001*b*), 'element' (Makoul 2001*a*), 'approach and technique' (Roter and Hall 1992), 'strategy' (Razavi *et al.* 2003), 'step', and 'component' (Baile *et al.* 2000) are found commonly. In some cases, these words are used interchangeably without explanation (Makoul 2001*a*; Razavi *et al.* 2003). We found only one textbook definition of communication skills: 'the numerous acts that health workers express in caring for their patients' (Fielding 1995). Others, while offering no explicit definition, list skills of varying abstractness such as 'effective care', 'question style', and 'making eye contact' (Fielding 1995). Additionally, differing degrees of complexity are present in clinical encounters, ranging from 'greet and obtain patient name' to 'set consultation agenda', to 'determine and acknowledge patient's ideas' (Girgis 1997; Girgis and Smith 1998; Kurtz *et al.* 1998).

In order to address some of the limitations found in the previous literature, we developed the Comskil model, initially to be used in cancer communication skills training (Brown and Bylund 2008).

Theoretical foundations of the Comskil model

Physician–patient communication is interpersonal communication in a particular context. Thus, as interpersonal communication scholars have developed a body of theory to aid in the understanding of this process, we have drawn on this work to inform our conceptual model. Two theories help explain how people formulate their communication:

◆ goals, plans, and action (GPA) theories; and

◆ sociolinguistic theory.

Communication theorists provide a clear ordering of the components of interpersonal communication in GPA theories (Miller 2002). These theories distinguish between communication elements that vary in abstractness. Originating in fields of communication and psychology (Austin and Vancouver 1996; Clark and Delia 1979), the premise is that people rely on goals and plans (Kellermann 1992), to guide their communication. Goals have been defined as the 'future states of affairs that individuals desire to attain or maintain' (Wilson and Morgan 2006; p. 68). Plans are more concrete than goals-they are mental representations of actions needed to achieve a goal (Berger 1997). Plans vary in complexity and specificity. Actions are even more concrete, as they are the enacting of the behaviour that is planned.

As a second theoretical foundation, sociolinguistic theory clarifies communication styles. Two basic orientations are the position-centred and person-centred approaches. The position-centred communicator relies on a restricted code of communication, following the rules and norms of the predicament. The person-centred communicator adapts his or her communication in response to the perspectives, feelings, and intentions of others (Miller 2002) and is one characteristic of being a 'mindful practitioner' (Epstein 1999). In the Comskil model, we recognize, as do GPA theories, that there is more than one way to meet a particular communication goal. The Comskil model offers potential strategies and skills that individuals can use, while adapting them to a variety of challenging situations (e.g. breaking bad news, discussing prognosis, or treatment options) and allowing them to be congruent with each clinician's own interpersonal communication style. In using this theory, we concur with Kurtz and colleagues, who note that 'communication training should increase rather than reduce flexibility by providing an expanded repertoire of skills that physicians can adeptly and intentionally choose to use as they require' (Kurtz *et al.* 1998; p. 45).

In order to address the difficulties inherent in earlier programmes of communication skills training, we have adapted the GPA and sociolinguistic theoretical frameworks as the basis of an innovative approach within which each component is defined, explicit, and unambiguous. This approach also enables more accurate and specific assessment to be made about how well trainees learn these skills, thus addressing an important limitation in the current literature.

Defining the core components of the Comskil model

In order to make the teaching of communication skills more explicit and to aid in the evaluation of the outcome of training, we present four communication components in the typical consultation:

◆ goals;

◆ strategies;

◆ skills;

◆ process tasks.

In this section, we define these terms and describe how the components are integrated (Brown and Bylund 2008).

Communication goals

A communication goal is defined as the desired outcome of the consultation or portion of the consultation. For example, the communication goal of a breaking bad news module (Bylund and Brown 2006) is: 'To convey threatening information in a way which promotes understanding, recall, and a sense of ongoing support'. As GPA theories explain, this definition of a goal focuses on the desired state that the individual is attempting to attain. The communication goal is achieved through the use of communication strategies, skills, process tasks, and cognitive appraisals.

Communication strategies

Communication strategies are defined as plans that direct communication behaviour toward the successful realization of a communication goal. The cumulative use of several strategies facilitates goal achievement. For example, 'Respond empathically to emotion' and 'Provide information in a way that it will be understood' are both strategies that may help to achieve the communication goal for breaking bad news. As with the plans in GPA theories, strategies are more concrete than goals. Furthermore, a strategy can be accomplished in more than one way.

Communication skills

A communication skill is defined as a discrete unit of speech by which a physician can further the clinical dialogue, and thus achieve fulfilment of a strategy. This definition describes the communication skill as verbal, concrete, teachable, and observable. Skills are similar to the notion of actions in GPA theories; they are the most concrete elements of the hierarchy. In addition, a variety of communication skills may be utilized in the attainment of any particular strategy. For example, the strategy of 'Respond empathically to emotion' could be accomplished through choice of skills like acknowledgement, validation, normalization, or praising patient's efforts. The strategy of 'Provide information in a way that it will be understood' could be accomplished through previewing information, summarizing information, and/or checking patient understanding. Communication skills exist and are expressed in certain contexts. As we have explored both the literature and various teaching modules (Back *et al.* 2003; Brown *et al.* 2004; Girgis and Sanson-Fisher 1995; Girgis and Smith 1998), we have compiled a list of 26 discrete communication skills (see Table 3.1). We have organized these skills into six higher-order categories to assist both teaching and assessment and to aid learners' understanding and recall. These are:

1. Establishing the consultation framework skills.
2. Information organization skills.
3. Checking skills.
4. Questioning skills.
5. Empathic communication skills.
6. Shared decision-making skills.

The five core categories of basic skills vs. advanced skills

A modification we made to the model was to separate the skills that could be used in any type of communication context with those that were specific to a particular type of discussion. Referring back to Table 3.1, we now consider the 'shared decision-making' skills and a new group of skills focused on conducting family meetings to be in a separate group of advanced skills.

Process tasks

Process tasks are defined as sets of dialogues or non-verbal behaviours that create an environment for effective communication. These are similar to skills as they are concrete, while goals and strategies are abstract. Together with skills, process tasks help an individual enact a strategy as a means to meet a goal. Process tasks require thoughtful consideration and can range on a continuum from basic to more complex. Examples of basic process tasks include:

- introducing self to patient;
- providing a private space in which to break bad news; and
- ensuring that the doctor is at eye level.

Examples of more complex process tasks include:

- avoiding premature reassurance;
- paying attention to information framing (words or numbers); and
- using a randomization story to help explain a randomized clinical trial (Brown *et al.* 2004; Butow *et al.* 2002).

Integrating the core communication components

Clearly, our definitions of communication goals, strategies, skills, process tasks, and cognitive appraisals are related to one another.

The communication strategy is a higher-order category and is accomplished through the use of communication skills and/or process tasks. Communication skills differ from strategies and process tasks, as they provide a building block for complex communication tasks. As noted by Kurtz, Silverman, and Draper, core skills are fundamental: 'Once core skills are mastered, specific communication issues are much more readily tackled' (Kurtz *et al.* 1998) (p. 38). The components influence each other in a dynamic process to achieve the communication goal. In order to make the relationships between these components clear, we have developed comprehensive modular blueprints that provide the essential communication components for each of our applied modules, taught using the model described here. We have included as an example the modular blueprint for a breaking bad news module (see Table 3.2).

Evaluation

In order to collect objective skill uptake data, we recommend video-recording two actual patient consultations before and after each learner has participated in training. Self-reported data can be collected by asking the learners to provide evaluations of the value of the training modules.

Coding of strategies, skills, and process tasks

We have operationalized the Comskil coding scheme to measure the use of the strategies, skills, and process tasks described in this model (Bylund *et al.* 2009). These are described in a coding manual that provides coding rules and multiple examples of each of the component parts. Coders are trained to use the manual to identify the presence of strategies, skills, or process tasks while viewing consultation video recordings. The particular strength of this method is that we are able to ensure that the skills taught are directly matched to those measured as part of the evaluation process. This coding system is applied to these recordings to assess participants' baseline skills and post-training uptake. Inter-rater reliability for this coding has been established (kappa = 0.76).

Table 3.1 Communication skills in six categories with descriptions

Skill	Description
Check patient understanding	Ask the patient about his or her understanding of previously conveyed information or the current situation. Optimally, understanding will be checked on more than one occasion and patients will be asked to reframe in their own words the information conveyed.
Check patient medical knowledge	Ask the patient about his or her understanding of the medical words used.
Check patient preference for information	Ask the patient about the amount and type of information desired. This needs to be done on more than one occasion. It is an iterative process—patients' information needs may vary throughout the consultation and across the course of the illness.
Introduce joint decision-making	Offer joint decision-making and say why it is important.
Check patient preference decision-making	Ask the patient about his or her preferred role in decision-making. This needs to be done on more than one occasion. It is an iterative process— patients' preferred roles may change throughout the consultation and across the course of the illness.
Reinforce joint decision-making	If joint decision-making has been introduced, review the concept at a later point in the illness or consultation (unless the patient has opted out of joint decision-making).
Make partnership statements	Convey alliance with the patient.
Offer decision delay	Reinforce time to make treatment decision if applicable. If used, reassure patient that this delay will not affect treatment efficacy.
Declare agenda items	State what you would like to accomplish in the consultation.
Invite patient agenda items	Ask patient what items he or she would like to discuss today.
Negotiate agenda	Ask patient to help you prioritize agenda items.
Invite patient questions	Make it clear to the patient that you are willing to answer questions and address concerns.
Endorse question asking	Express to the patient the importance of asking questions; provide a rationale for asking questions (i.e. that patients can gain salient information).
Clarify	Ask a question to try to better understand what a patient is saying.
Restate	State in your own words what you think the patient is saying.
Make a 'take stock' statement	Pause in the dialogue to review the prior discussion. Seek the patient's permission to move on.
Acknowledge	Make a statement that indicates recognition of the patient's emotion or experience.
Normalize	Make a comparative statement that expresses that a particular emotional response is not out of the ordinary.
Validate	Make a statement expressing that a patient's emotional response to an event or an experience is appropriate and reasonable.
Encourage expression of feelings	Express to the patient that you would like to know how he or she is feeling.
Praise patient efforts	Make a statement that validates a patient's attempts to cope with treatment or side effects, to make lifestyle changes, or to be adherent to treatment regime.
Express a willingness to help	Make a specific offer of help or a general statement about being available for future help.
Preview information	Give an overview of the main points that you are about to cover.
Summarize	Recap the main details conveyed. As with checking behaviours, this should occur at various points during the consultation where appropriate.
Review next steps	Go over with the patient the next things that the patient will do (e.g. make a follow-up appointment).

Source: data from Brown RF *et al.*, 'Developing ethical strategies to assist oncologists in seeking informed consent to cancer clinical trials', *Social Science and Medicine*, Volume 58, Issue 2, pp. 379–90, Copyright © 2004 Elsevier Science Ltd. All rights reserved.

Conclusion

The Comskil model of communication skills training is a flexible, conceptual framework that can be adapted to meet the education requirements in a variety of healthcare contexts. Although initially developed for cancer communication between physicians and patients, it is now used internationality a variety of specialties (e.g. medicine, psychiatry, emergency medicine, paediatrics) as well as with nurses. The model provides discrete and unambiguous definitions and hierarchy of communication strategies, skills, and process tasks enabling a systematic assessment process that is carefully matched to the Comskil curriculum.

Table 3.2 Modular blueprint—breaking bad news

(*Goal:* To convey threatening information in a way that promotes understanding, recall, and support for the patient's emotional response and a sense of ongoing support.)

Strategies	Skills	Process tasks
Establish the consultation framework	Declare your agenda items Invite patient agenda items Negotiate agenda Check shared agreement about illness	Greet patient appropriately Make introductions Ensure patient is clothed Sit at eye level
Tailor the consultation to the patient's needs	Check patient understanding Check patient preference-information	Avoid interruptions Invite appropriate third party
Provide information in a way that it will be understood	Preview information Invite patient questions Check patient understanding	Avoid jargon Address all questions Draw diagrams Categorize
Provide information in a way that it will be recalled	Summarize	Write information down Repeat
Respond empathically to emotion	Encourage expression of feelings Acknowledge Normalize Validate Ask open questions	Maintain eye contact Allow time to integrate Offer tissues Provide hope and reassurance
Check readiness to discuss management options	Check patient preference—decision-making Preview information	Provide literature
Close the consultation	Check patient understanding Invite patient questions Endorse question asking Reinforce joint decision-making Summarize Review next steps	Offer to talk to relatives Offer follow-up phone calls or consultation

Reproduced from Brown RF and Bylund CL, 'Communication skills training: describing a new conceptual model', *Academic Medicine*, Volume 83, Number 1, pp. 37–44, Copyright © 2008 Association of American Medical Colleges, with permission from Wolters Kluwer Health, Inc.

References

Austin JT, Vancouver JB (1996). Goal constucts in psychology: structure, process and content. *Psychol Bull* **120**, 338–75.

Back AL, Arnold RM, Baile WF, Tulsky JA, Fryer-Edwards K (2005). Approaching difficult communication tasks in oncology. *CA Cancer J Clin* **55**, 164–77.

Back AL, Arnold RM, Tulsky JA, Baile WF, Fryer-Edwards KA (2003). Teaching communication skills to medical oncology fellows. *J Clin Oncol* **21**, 2433–6.

Baile WF, Buckman R, Lenzi R, Glober G, Beale EA, Kudelka AP (2000). SPIKES-A six-step protocol for delivering bad news—application to the patient with cancer. *Oncologist* **5**, 302–11.

Berger CR (1997). *Planning Strategic Interaction: Attaining Goals Through Communicative Action.* Lawrence Erlbaum, Mahwah, NJ.

Brown RF, Butow PN, Butt DG, Moore AR, Tattersall MHN (2004). Developing ethical strategies to assist oncologists in seeking informed consent to cancer clinical trials. *Soc Sci Med* **58**, 379–90.

Brown RF, Bylund CL (2008). Communication skills training: Describing a new conceptual model. *Acad Med* **83**, 37–44.

Butow PN, Brown RF, Cogar S, Tattersall MHN, Dunn SM (2002). Oncologists' reactions to cancer patients' verbal cues. *Psychooncology* **11**, 47–58.

Bylund CL, Brown RF (2006). *Breaking Bad News.* Memorial Sloan Kettering Cancer Center, New York, NY.

Bylund CL, Brown RF, Gueguen J, Diamond C, Bianculli J, Kissane DW (2009). The implementation and assessment of a comprehensive communication skills training curriculum for oncologists. *Psychooncology* **19**, 583–93.

Cegala DJ, Lenzmeier Broz S (2002). Physician communication skills training: a review of theoretical backgrounds, objectives and skills. *Med Educ* **36**, 1004–16.

Clark RA, Delia JG (1979). 'Topoi' and rhetorical competence. *Q J Speech* **65**, 187–206.

Cole SA, Bird J (2000). *The Medical Interview: the Three Function Approach.* Mosby Inc, St. Louis, MO.

Epstein RM (1999). Mindful practice. *JAMA* **282**, 833–9.

Fallowfield LJ, Jenkins VA, Farewell V, Solis-Trapala I (2003). Enduring impact of communication skills training—results of a 12-month follow-up. *Br J Cancer* **89**, 1445–9.

Fellowes D, Wilkinson S, Moore P (2004). Communication skills training for health care professionals working with cancer patients, their families and/or carers. *Cochrane Database Syst Rev* **2**, CD003751.

Fielding R (1995). *Clinical Communication Skills.* Hong Kong University Press, Hong Kong, China.

Frankel RM, Stein T (1999). Getting the most out of the clinical encounter: the four habits model. *Permanente J* **3**, 79–88.

Girgis A (1997). Overview of consensus guidelines on breaking bad news. Available at: http://www.nbcc.org.au/bestpractice/commskills/modules.html

Girgis A, Sanson-Fisher RW (1995). Breaking bad news: consensus guidelines for medical practitioners. *J Clin Oncol* **13**, 2449–56.

Girgis A, Smith J (1998). *Communication Skills Training Program.* Newcastle, NSW, University of Newcastle.

Goelz T, Wuensch A, Stubenrauch S, *et al.* (2011). Specific training program improves oncologists' palliative care communication skills in a randomized controlled trial. *J Clin Oncol* **29**, 3402–7.

Keller VF, Carroll JG (1994). A new model for physician-patient communication. *Patient Educ Couns* **35**, 121–40.

Kellermann K (1992). Communication: inherently strategic and primarily automatic. *Commun Monogr* **61**, 210–35.

Krupat E, Frankel R, Stein T, Irish J (2006). The Four Habits Coding Scheme: validation of an instrument to assess clinicians' communication behavior. *Patient Educ Couns* **62**, 38–45.

Kurtz SM, Silverman JD (1996). The Calgary-Cambridge Referenced Observation Guides: an aid to defining the curriculum and organizing the teaching in communication training programmes. *Med Educ* **30**, 83–9.

Kurtz SM, Silverman JD, Draper J (1998). *Teaching and Learning Communication Skills in Medicine.* Radcliff Medical Press Ltd., Oxford, UK.

Makoul G (2001*a*). Essential elements of communication in medical encounters: the Kalamazoo consensus statement. *Acad Med* **76**, 390–3.

Makoul G (2001*b*). The SEGUE Framework for teaching and assessing communication skills. *Patient Educ Couns* **45**, 23–34.

Miller K (2002). *Communication Theories: Perspectives, Processes, and Contexts.* McGraw-Hill, Boston, MA.

Razavi D, Merckaert I, Marchal S, *et al.* (2003). How to optimize physicians' communication skills in cancer care—results of a randomized study assessing the usefulness of posttraining consolidation workshops. *J Clin Oncol* **21**, 3141–9.

Roter DL, Hall JA (1992). *Doctors Talking with Patients, Patients Talking with Doctors: Improving Communication in Medical Visits.* Greenwood, Westport, CT.

Salem A, Salem AF (2013). Breaking bad news: current prospective and practical guideline for Muslim countries. *J Cancer Educ* **28**, 790–4.

Stewart M, Belle Brown J, Weston WW, McWhinney IR, McWilliam CL, Freeman TR (1995). *Patient-Centered Medicine: Transforming the Clinical Method.* Sage Publications, Thousand Oaks, CA.

van Vliet LM, Epstein AS (2014). Current state of the art and science of patient-clinician communication in progressive disease: patients' need to know and need to feel known. *J Clin Oncol* **32**, 3474–8.

Wilson SR, Morgan WM (2006). *Goals-Plans-Action Theories: Theories Of Goals, Plans and Planning Processes in Families.* Sage Publications, Thousand Oaks, CA.

Wuensch A, Goelz T, Bertz H, Wirsching M, Fritzsche K (2011). Disclosing information about randomised controlled trials in oncology: training concept and evaluation of an individualised communication skills training for physicians COM-ON-rct. *Euro J Cancer Care* **20**, 570–6.

Wuensch A, Tang L, Goelz T, *et al.* (2013). Breaking bad news in China—the dilemma of patients' autonomy and traditional norms. A first communication skills training for Chinese oncologists and caretakers. *Psychooncology* **22**, 1192–5.

CHAPTER 4

Shared decision-making, decision aids, and the role of values in treatment decision-making

Amiram Gafni and Cathy Charles[†]

Introduction to shared decision-making

Over the past two decades, shared decision-making (SDM), a specific approach to making decisions in the medical encounter, has received considerable conceptual and practical attention among physicians, social scientists, and ethicists. In addition, governments and professional associations in different countries are developing patient charters/bills of rights to promote responsiveness to, and involvement of, patients in treatment decision-making (Charles and Gafni 2010). In this chapter we describe (i) the key characteristics of a SDM approach; (ii) the clinical contexts for SDM; (iii) the definition and use of decision aids (DA), as well as their relationship to SDM; and (iv) the vexing problem of defining the meaning and role of values/preferences in treatment decision-making.

SDM: What is it?

Despite the widespread interest in promoting SDM, there does not seem to be as yet a universally accepted consensus on the meaning of this concept. Many authors have attempted to define shared treatment decision-making. There has been some overlap in the dimensions identified as key characteristics of this approach. Two articles, one by Makoul and Clayman (2006) and another by Moumjid and colleagues (2007), reviewed the most commonly cited definitions in the literature. Both found that the definition by Charles and colleagues (1997, 1999) was the most commonly cited and we will use this definition here. The particular clinical context that this definition pertains to is one of potentially life-threatening illness, such as cancer, where there are important decisions to be made at key points in the disease process, and several treatment options exist, with different possible outcomes and substantial uncertainty.

Charles and colleagues (1997) initially defined shared treatment decision-making as having four key characteristics:

◆ that at least two participants—physician and patient—be involved;

◆ that both parties share information;

◆ that both parties take steps to build a consensus about the preferred decision; and

◆ that an agreement is reached on the decision to implement.

[†] It is with regret that we report the death of Cathy Charles during the preparation of this edition of the textbook.

In a subsequent follow-up paper (Charles *et al.* 1999), Charles and colleagues expanded on this initial formulation by explicitly identifying different analytic steps in the treatment decision-making process and identifying and comparing how, in implementation, these steps differ depending on whether the approach adopted to decision-making is paternalistic, shared, informed, or lies somewhere in-between. The authors also pointed out the dynamic nature of the treatment decision-making process by recognizing that the approach adopted at the outset of a medical encounter may change as the interaction evolves.

In Table 4.1 (from Charles *et al.* 1999) the different analytic steps that define the treatment decision-making process are presented: information exchange, deliberation or discussion of treatment options and preferences, and deciding on the treatment to implement. The three most prominent approaches to treatment decision-making are also presented in this table and compared in terms of how the different analytic steps are implemented in each model. The table also makes clear that the prominent approaches, as depicted in Table 4.1, are 'ideal' or 'pure' types and that, in reality, actual decision-making approaches may well lie somewhere in-between. The framework does not assume that there is a right or wrong approach to arriving at a decision. Rather, it attempts to highlight the distinctive characteristics of each of the prominent approaches, which are described in more detail below.

Paternalistic approach of treatment decision-making

In the purest form of the paternalistic approach, information flow is one-way—from physician to patient—and is limited to medical information about the disease and its treatment, about which physicians are legally required to inform the patient.. The physician alone, or in consultation with colleagues, decides on the treatment to implement and the patient passively acquiesces to professional authority by agreeing to the physician's decision. An assumption underlying this approach, which has increasingly been challenged in recent years, is that physicians will make the best treatment decision for their patients and can do so without eliciting from the latter information about their cultural beliefs, personal preferences for different treatment outcomes, and values that might influence the meaning that patients attribute to their illness and preferred ways of coping with it.

Table 4.1 Comparison of treatment decision-making approaches

Analytical stages	Models	Paternalistic	(in between approaches)	Shared	(in between approaches)	Informed
Information exchange	Flow	One way (largely)		Two way		One way (largely)
	Direction	Physician → patient		Physician ⇌ patient		Physician → patient
	Type	Medical		Medical and personal		Medical
	Amount[a]	Minimum Legal required		All relevant for decision-making		All relevant for decision-making
Deliberation		Physician alone or with other physicians		Physician and patient (plus potential others)		Patient (plus potential others)
Deciding on treatment to implement		Physicians		Physician and patient		Patient

[a] Minimum required.

Reprinted from *Social Science and Medicine*, Volume 49, Issue 5, Charles C, Gafni A, and Whelan T, 'Decision-making in the physician–patient encounter: revisiting the shared treatment decision-making model,' pp. 651–661, Copyright © 1999 Elsevier Science Ltd., with permission from Elsevier, http://www.sciencedirect.com/science/journal/02779536. Source: data from Charles C, Whelan T, Gafni A, *et al.*, 'Doing nothing is no choice: lay constructions of treatment decision-making among women with early-stage breast cancer', *Sociology of Health and Illness*, Volume 20, Number 1, pp. 71–95, Copyright © Blackwell's Publishers Ltd/Editorial Board 1998.

Informed model of treatment decision-making

At the other end of the spectrum lies the informed model of treatment decision-making. Here the patient is the sole decision-maker and the physician's role is to communicate to the patient all relevant treatment options and their potential risks and benefits. The amount and type of information communicated includes, at a minimum, all relevant information on the above issues to enable the patient to make an informed choice. Communication of such information is one-way—from physician to patient. In its pure type, this decision-making process involves a division of labour, whereby the physician communicates information to the patient and the latter adds her preferences in order to make the decision that is right for her. This model is thought to enhance patient control and autonomy over the decision-making process.

Some believe that the 'physician as a perfect agent' to her patient is an example of a paternalistic approach, where the choice of treatment that the physician makes for the patient will be the same as the choice that the patient would have made herself (an informed model). Note that in such a case, the treatment chosen by the patient in the informed decision-making process and by the physician, if she is a perfect agent, will be the same. While this is true in theory, Gafni and colleagues (1998) have argued that this is not likely to happen in practice. They describe the 'physician as perfect agent' approach as one where the patient delegates authority to her physician to make medical decisions—and the challenge is to encourage the physician to find out the patient's preferences. In the informed approach, the patient retains the authority to make medical decisions and the challenge is to encourage the physician to transfer knowledge about treatment options to the patient in a clear and non-biased way. Gafni and colleagues argue that for several reasons it is simpler for physicians to transfer technical knowledge to the patient than it is for patients to transfer their preferences to physicians. Because of this difference in the feasibility of implementation, while each of these approaches in the abstract would be expected to yield a similar result (i.e. the same decision), this is unlikely to be true in reality.

Shared approach to treatment decision-making

The pure-type shared decision-making approach lies between the other two (i.e. paternalistic and informed) described above. The

essential characteristic of this approach is its interactional nature, in that the physician and patient share all stages of the decision-making process simultaneously. There is a two-way exchange of information. The physician communicates to the patient evidence-based information about the various relevant treatment options (including no treatment) and their potential risks and benefits, elicits information from the patient about her values, lifestyle and preferences, and, in the typical case, provides a treatment recommendation, taking into account both of the above sets of factors, plus the physician's own values about what is the best treatment for this particular patient. The patient communicates what she knows about her disease, and the risks and benefits of various treatment options she has heard about, as well as her values, life circumstances, and preferences that may influence which treatment she thinks would be best for her. Both parties agree on the decision to implement. This approach assumes that the physician and patient each have a legitimate investment in the treatment decision. Hence, both declare treatment preferences and their rationale for these, while trying to build consensus on the most appropriate treatment to implement. If a consensus cannot be reached, SDM will not occur.

Clinical contexts for SDM

The above discussion has focused on what SDM is; that is, the defining characteristics of this approach to decision-making in the context of other prominent approaches and in the context of acute care, such as cancer care. Even within a single disease, for example cancer, the decision-making context can vary substantially in terms of the nature, manifestations, and progress of the disease, as well as available treatment options, depending on the particular disease site and disease stage. Some form of SDM may be appropriate in all these situations. Increasingly, SDM is also seen as appropriate for clinical contexts other than acute care, such as primary care (Murray *et al.* 2006) and chronic care (Montori *et al.* 2006), in a modified form and tailored to fit the specific clinical characteristics of that context.

Whether SDM will actually occur in any given encounter depends on patient and physician preferences for different treatment decision-making approaches, and the extent to which barriers and facilitators exist in a given care setting to facilitate or inhibit use of this approach (Charles *et al.* 2004; Ford *et al.* 2002; Holmes-Rovner *et al.* 2000). A number of studies undertaken in different countries have found that patient preferences for involvement in treatment decision-making vary (Gattellari *et al.* 2001; Charles *et al.* 1998; Salked *et al.* 2004; Davey *et al.* 2004; Belcher *et al.* 2006; Nguyen *et al.* 2014). There is no one approach that fits everyone. For this reason, it is important to assess not simply the extent to which SDM occurs, but also the match between what approach the patient wants to use with her physician and what she receives.

The relationship between physician and patient is not symmetrical. The physician typically has more power by virtue of her greater knowledge, expertise, and professional authority, and the fact that she is not sick; yet it is the patient who bears the consequences of implementing the treatment decision. For these reasons, we feel that the onus is on the physician to ascertain the patient's preferences for the role she wants to play in decision-making, and to facilitate patient involvement in decision-making as much as she wants.

It is increasingly argued that shared or informed treatment decision-making models are better than more paternalistic approaches, and should be universally promoted. Such statements are normative in nature, involving value judgements. If the underlying goal of this type of promotion is to allow patients to make decisions in a way that is consistent with their preferences, then we think that patients should be allowed to choose their preferred approach of decision-making, including the option of choosing a paternalistic approach, if that is what they want.

It is not always clear from the literature whether SDM is being promoted because it is seen as a positive end in itself, or rather as a means to achieve other ends. SDM has been proposed, for example, as a means to increase patient autonomy and control in decision-making, to improve patient satisfaction, to enhance patient compliance with decisions made, to increase the extent to which decisions made are consistent with patient values, and to reduce healthcare costs (Charles *et al.* 2005). Many hoped-for patient outcomes are thus 'loaded on' to the concept of patient involvement in treatment decision-making, a concept that, when implemented in the clinical context, is expected to achieve multiple goals (Charles *et al.* 2005). As we will see in the next section, this expectation is also true of various forms of treatment decision aids designed to help promote SDM in the medical encounter.

Definition and use of treatment DA and their relationship to SDM

In this chapter we use O'Connor and colleagues' (2007) definition of DA:

> Patient decision aids are interventions designed to help people make specific, deliberative choices among options (including the status quo) by providing information on the options and outcomes (e.g. benefits, harms) in sufficient detail that an individual could judge their value implicitly (O'Connor *et al.* 2007; p. 554).

Two key components are inherent in this definition: first that decision aids are designed to transfer technical information on available treatments and their potential benefits and risks to the patient; and, second, that such information is a necessary prerequisite for creating an informed patient, who is thereby enabled to participate in making a treatment decision that fits with her values. These two components are commonly cited in definitions of decisions aids. In addition, such aids are thought to be of benefit in establishing

rapport between physicians and patients, and in providing a structure that would encourage input from both parties in the treatment decision-making process (Charles *et al.* 2005).

In the cancer field, in particular, the number of decision aids developed over the last 20 years has proliferated for several reasons (O'Brien *et al.* 2009). First, studies have shown that the transfer of technical information on treatment options from physicians to cancer patients is often problematic; second, the introduction of new cancer treatments has increased the number of options available; third, many treatments offer varying mixes of potential benefits and side effects, whose subjective value varies from patient to patient. For this reason, cancer patients are now encouraged to make these preferences known in the encounter, so that the decision made will reflect not only evidence on effective treatment, but also patient preferences for different outcomes.

There are many forms of decision aids, most of which present information visually to patients on treatment options and the potential risks and benefits associated with each (Charles *et al.* 2005). Decision aids may also include some form of values clarification exercise intended to help the patient clarify her preferences for various treatment outcomes and the kinds of trade-offs she is willing to make between the risks and benefits associated with each, to arrive at her preferred decision (O'Connor *et al.* 1999). We will expand on the role of these exercises later in the separate section on the vexing problem of defining the meaning, role, and measurement of values/preferences in treatment decision-making.

Decision aids incorporate a number of assumptions that may or may not be made clear to the patient at the time of their use. For example, the developers of decision aids determine which treatment options to include for the patient to consider, as well as which risks and benefits (outcomes), the specific method (e.g. trade-off) that patients are to use to process the information presented, and the theoretical foundations of the method specified for making the treatment decision, (e.g. expected utility theory; Charles *et al.* 2005). As long as both the physician and patient are aware of these assumptions, explicitly buy into them, and agree that the method presented is the best way to make treatment decisions, there is no problem. However, the extent to which physicians are aware of these assumptions and communicate them to patients, and the extent to which patients understand and accept these, are unknown and thus cast doubt on the validity of such exercises (Charles *et al.* 2005).

Underlying decision aids are cultural beliefs that frame their development and use. For example, decision aids are firmly embedded in a biological model of illness, an evidence-based medicine paradigm, medical concepts of risk, ethical precepts of informed choice, and a defined approach to decision-making (Charles *et al.* 2006). These common features of decision aids are not surprising given the Western medicine-oriented clinical and research contexts in which they have been developed. However, an interesting question for future research is the extent to which such aids are perceived as useful by patients from different cultural groups, whose beliefs about health and illness and the factors influencing these, as well as legitimate pathways to, and types of, healthcare may differ from those that underlie the development of current decision aids (Charles *et al.* 2006).

The terms 'SDM' and 'DA' are often used interchangeably in the academic literature. This might be due to the fact that like the concept of SDM, treatment decision aids have been defined in different ways with different emphases, depending on the author. But the relationship between SDM and DA can actually take diverse forms. For example, in any given clinical encounter, a SDM process could be used with a DA or without a DA. Similarly, a DA could be used in any given clinical encounter whether the decision-making approach taken is a SDM process or not. We view SDM and DA as two distinct concepts and assume that a SDM approach does not require the use of a DA. Where a DA is used in a SDM process it is typically introduced because it is seen to be helpful in implementing a SDM approach.

The role of values in SDM/DA

According to the International Patient Decision Aid Collaboration (IPDAS 2012), composed of leaders in the field of SDM, the ultimate goal of a DA is to improve the quality of a decision. A quality decision is defined as 'the extent to which patients choose and/or receive healthcare interventions that are congruent with their informed and considered values' (IPDAS). However, the term 'values' is not defined. It should be noted that the terms 'values' and 'preferences' are commonly used in documents and papers but with no clear description of the difference, if any, between the two. Hence in this chapter we use both interchangeably. The lack of good definition represents in our mind the somewhat fuzzy thinking characterizing discussions of the meaning, role, and measurement of value/preference in SDM/DA, and in treatment decision-making in general. A simple example is the fact that in the definition of a good decision (see above) there is no mention of physician values/preferences. Whether physician values/preferences for treatment outcomes should be considered a legitimate part of a *shared* process (e.g. Charles *et al*. 1999) is left undiscussed and hence remains ambiguous.

IPDAS, along with many SDM advocates, see decision-making as a division of labour. The option set of treatments to be included in a DA is based on available clinical evidence about the most effective treatments and their potential risks and benefits. The physician's role is to communicate this information to patients, with or without a DA. The patient contributes his/her values/preferences about the desirability of potential outcomes of the various options presented. A 'values clarification method' (or exercise) (VCM) has been incorporated into some DA with the goal of helping the patient reveal her true values/preferences so that a treatment decision can be made which is congruent with these values (a requirement for a quality decision). The use of VCMs is based on the assumption that patients do not know their own values and need help in both ascertaining and communicating these to others, because IPDAS actually uses the term VCM.

There are important problematic issues about the use of VCMs that we think have not been addressed in the academic literature. In order to determine whether a VCM is required and would help a given patient, the clinician needs to know that the patient is not clear on what his/her values are. This raises the issue of how the clinician is to know whether the patient is clear or not—a question that, to our knowledge, has not been addressed. If the physician is somehow able to ascertain that the patient is not clear on what her values are and needs help in clarifying these, then the physician could try and find an exercise that would allow the patient to reveal her true preferences/values. The process of matching a given decision process theory with the patient's preference structure requires that the physician knows the latter. But if the clinician knows this, then he/she could tell the patient rather than asking the patient to engage in a VCM. In this case the physician also needs to explain to the patient how he/she knows the patient's preference structure when the patient does not. Finally, if the clinician does not know what the patient's preference structure is, then he/she can offer the patient some type of VCM based on a theory they think is useful. However, in this case the clinician would need to explain to the patient that the decision process theory underlying this VCM may be different from the way the patient usually makes decisions, and hence may not reveal his/her true preferences. In this scenario, the patient would also need to be asked, given the above, whether s/he would agree to proceed with the exercise or not.

If there is a mismatch between the decision process theory underlying a particular values clarification method given to a patient and the patient's usual way of making decisions, then the exercise is more likely to impose a particular decision-making process onto the patient, rather than support the patient's usual approach—that is the exercise will impede the patient from making a decision that is consistent with his/her true preferences. In addition, any given patient may not know which theory, if any, he/she subscribes to and in this case may not realize that a given VCM is based on a particular theory, or recognize that he/she is being steered to think about decision-making in a particular way (Charles *et al*. 2005).

Conclusion

Shared decision-making between physicians and patients is often advocated as the 'best' approach to treatment in the clinical encounter. In reality, what is defined as 'best' can vary depending on whose perspective is being solicited and the criteria by which 'best' is judged. One rationale that is often cited for the promotion of shared decision-making is the achievement of greater patient autonomy and control in decision-making. But if this is the primary goal, then an informed model, where the patient has full control over decision-making, would seem to be better able to meet this objective. We think that the merit of a shared approach, or variant thereof, is that it incorporates physician transfer of key information on treatment options and their benefits and risks to the patient, and enables the latter to share in decision-making as much as she wants, rather than defining an ideal standard of participation that is thought to be best for everyone. The 'best' model is not some abstract and decontextualized blueprint—but rather a much more fluid, contextualized approach that fits with the patient's preferences and experiential comfort level, with different approaches to decision-making.

We have seen from the above discussion of decision aids that they were originally designed as a means of implementing shared decision-making, by facilitating information transfer from physician to patient, thereby enabling more informed patient choice. Increasingly, decision aids are expected to positively affect a wide variety of additional outcomes (e.g. the health of the patient, the cost of providing the intervention), even though the rationale for these expectations and the mechanisms by which decision aids are to achieve these outcomes are rarely presented. Given the evidence of variability in the success of decisions aids to yield positive results in the areas cited here, and the overwhelmingly consistent evidence of positive effects of decision aids on patient knowledge acquisition, we wonder whether expectations of what such aids should and can achieve have been overly optimistic. Perhaps we need to focus research attention more on developing decision aids for different clinical and cultural contexts, with the more limited goal of increasing patient knowledge of treatment options and their outcomes (which we know such aids are good at already), rather than attempting to search for an ever-expanding number of outcome measures that decision aids might possibly affect, but which were never included as up-front goals in the design of these instruments.

Early decision aids were developed to be used in the context of the physician–patient relationship (Levine *et al.* 1992). Such aids were often thought to be of benefit in establishing rapport between physicians and patients, and in providing a structure that would encourage input from both parties in the process of treatment decision-making. One of the more interesting trends in the use of these tools has been an increase in the number of non-physicians who are now administering decision aids to patients, and the use of various take-home versions of such aids. To the extent that this trend continues, decision aids will, increasingly, be taken out of the context of the physician–patient encounter. An interesting question is whether this trend reflects an underlying assumption that anyone can administer such tools, with or without prior training, and that patient engagement in this process with the physician is not that important. In this case, decision aids may well become more of a stand alone and standardized intervention, more appropriate to an informed approach to treatment decision-making, rather than a tool to encourage discussion and consensus building on the treatment to implement (i.e. shared decision-making) between physician and patient in the clinical encounter.

Confusion still exists in the academic literature on the meaning of SDM. Part of the problem stems from the fact that the same label—SDM—is used to describe different approaches to treatment decision-making. Thus identifying empirically what is and what is not a SDM approach is difficult to pin down in practice. Also because there is no consensus on the meaning of the concept, it is not clear whose values count. In some SDM models, physician values and preferences are seen as a legitimate input into the decision-making process, while in others they are not. However, we argue that physicians should not be excluded from expressing their treatment preferences during the deliberation process because to do so fails to recognize the vulnerability of many patients who want either implicit or explicit guidance about what their physicians think is the best treatment for them in a given situation.

We have illustrated in this chapter that there are important problematic issues about the meaning and role of VCMs in DA. There is a need for additional conceptual thinking to try to resolve these issues. There is also a need for more empirical research to assess the extent to which VCMs help or hinder patients in clarifying and expressing their true preferences about different treatment options and their risks and benefits.

References

Belcher VN, Fried TR, Agostini JV, *et al.* (2006). Views of older adults on patient participation in medication-related decision-making. *J Gen Intern Med* **21**, 298–303.

Charles C, Gafni A (2010). Shared treatment decision-making and the use of decision-aids. In: Kissane DW, Bultz BD, Butow PN, Finlay IG (eds). *Handbook of Communication in Oncology and Palliative Care.* Oxford University Press: London, UK.

Charles C, Gafni A, Whelan T (1997). Shared decision-making in the medical encounter: what does it mean? (Or it takes at least two to tango). *Soc Sci Med* **44**, 681–92.

Charles C, Gafni A, Whelan T (1999). Decision-making in the physician-patient encounter: revisiting the shared treatment decision-making model. *Soc Sci Med* **49**, 651–61.

Charles C, Gafni A, Whelan T (2004). Self-reported use of shared decision-making among breast cancer specialists and perceived barriers and facilitators to implementing this approach. *Health Expect* **7**, 338–48.

Charles C, Gafni A, Whelan T, *et al.* (2005). Treatment decision-aids: conceptual issues and future directions. *Health Expect* **8**, 114–25.

Charles C, Gafni A, Whelan T, *et al.* (2006). Cultural influences on the physician-patient encounter: the case of shared treatment decision-making. *Patient Educ Couns* **63**, 262–7.

Charles C, Whelan T, Gafni A, *et al.* (1998). Doing nothing is no choice: lay constructions of treatment decision-making among women with early-stage breast cancer. *Sociol Health Illn* **20**, 71–95.

Davey HM, Lim J, Butow P, *et al.* (2004). Women's preferences for and views on decision-making for diagnostic tests. *Soc Sci Med* **58**, 1699–707.

Ford A, Schofield T, Hope T (2002). Barriers to the evidence-based patient choice (EBPC) consultation. *Patient Educ Couns* **47**, 179–85.

Gafni A, Charles C, Whelan T (1998). The physician–patient encounter: the physician as a perfect agent for the patient *versus* the informed treatment decision-making model. *Soc Sci Med* **47**, 347–54.

Gattellari M, Butow P, Tattersall M (2001). Sharing decisions in cancer care. *Soc Sci Med* **52**, 1865–78.

Holmes-Rovner M, Valade D, Orlowski C, *et al.* (2000). Implementing shared decision-making in routine practice: barriers and opportunities. *Health Expect* **3**, 182–91.

International Patient Decision Aids Standards (IPDAS) Collaboration (2012). What are patient decision aids? Available at: http://ipdas.ohri.ca/what.html

Levine MN, Gafni A, Markham B, *et al.* (1992). A bedside decision instrument to elicit a patient's preference concerning adjuvant chemotherapy for breast cancer. *Ann Intern Med* **117**, 53–8.

Makoul G, Clayman ML (2006). An integrative model of shared decision-making in medical encounters. *Patient Educ Couns* **60**, 301–12.

Montori V, Gafni A, Charles C (2006). A shared treatment decision-making approach between patients with chronic conditions and their clinicians: the case of diabetes. *Health Expect* **9**, 25–36.

Moumjid N, Gafni A, Brémond A, *et al.* (2007). Shared decision-making in the medical encounter: are we all talking about the same thing? *Med Decis Making* **27**, 539–46.

Murray E, Charles C, Gafni A (2006). Shared decision-making in primary care: tailoring the Charles *et al.* model to fit the context of general practice. *Patient Educ Couns* **62**, 205–11.

Nguyen F, Moumjid N, Charles C, *et al.* (2014). Treatment decision-making in the medical encounter: Comparing the attitudes of French surgeons and their patients in breast cancer care. *Patient Educ Couns* **14**, 123–9.

O'Brien MA. Whelan TJ, Villasis-Keever M, *et al.* (2009). Are cancer-related decision aids effective? A systematic review and meta-analysis. *J Clin Oncol* **27**, 974–85.

O'Connor A, Wells G, Tugwell P, *et al.* (1999). The effect of an explicit values clarification exercise in a woman's decision aid regarding postmenopausal hormone therapy. *Health Expect* **2**, 21–32.

O'Connor AM, Stacey D, Barry MJ, *et al.* (2007). Do patient decision aids meet effectiveness criteria of the international patient decision aid standards collaboration? A systematic review and meta-analysis. *Med Decis Making* **27**, 554–74.

Salkeld G, Solomon M, Butow P (2004). A matter of trust—patient's views on decision-making in colorectal cancer. *Health Expect* **7**, 104–14.

CHAPTER 5

The ethics of communication in cancer and palliative care

Laura A. Siminoff and Maria D. Thomson

Introduction to cancer communication and ethics

There are two approaches to cancer communication and ethics. First, ethics in cancer communication can refer to the *ethical implications* of cancer communication. Second, it can refer to the *ethics of* cancer communication research, which entails the obligations of researchers working in this field of research. Cancer communication research is especially salient, as cancer patients and practitioners have been one of the major laboratories for research in, and application of, bioethical theory. The majority of this chapter will focus on the importance and role of cancer communication research on our knowledge and understanding of bioethics.

Overview of ethical theories

Principlism

Bioethics as a field is based in moral reasoning. The major theoretical framework is 'Principlism', in which four basic principles of bioethics—beneficence, non-malfeasance, justice, and autonomy—are applied to the decisions made about healthcare, whether therapeutic or preventive. This approach is generally referred to as 'normative' ethics, in that it considers which rules or principles have merit. It is beyond the scope of this chapter to argue whether this is the best approach to moral reasoning; rather, it is the one most commonly applied within the field of bioethics.

Autonomy is a form of personal liberty where the individual is the agent determining his or her own course of action (Beauchamp and Childress 2004). Analogous to this is the concept of respect for autonomy, in which others acknowledge that persons are ends in themselves and should not be treated as a means. The assumption is that the individual has the capacity to act intentionally, with understanding, and without controlling influences that would hamper the individual acting as a free and voluntary agent (Beauchamp and Childress 2004).

The principle of non-malfeasance is best drawn from the maxim, 'above all, do no harm'. This principle affirms the need for medical competence as the minimum standard for providing patient care. This principle is frequently combined with that of beneficence, referring to a duty to act in the interest of another. Healthcare providers must not only refrain from harming patients, but are also obligated to aid them (Beauchamp and Childress 2004).

The principle of justice has probably received the least attention from bioethicists and policy makers. Justice in healthcare is usually defined as a form of fairness, and implies the fair distribution of goods and services in society.

Casuistry

'Casuistry' is an alternative approach to moral reasoning. Casuistry is a case-based method of moral reasoning that does not rely on basic principles to guide decisions. Casuistry asserts that moral knowledge develops incrementally through analysis of specific cases through moral triangulation. An analogy is the development of English Common Law (Arras 1991). A distinct advantage of casuistry is its rejection of the trend toward reductionism and the individualism of principlist-based ethics. It also lends itself to greater inclusivity of varying cultural perspectives and values, but can be criticized on the grounds that it is too 'relativist' and situationally dependent.

Virtue ethics

Another framework guiding the thinking of bioethicists is 'virtue' theory in which the character of the person, with their 'internal goods' or values, is seen to guide the behaviour and integrity of the clinician (Beauchamp and Childress 2004). Virtue ethics is a valuable addition to approaching moral conflicts, especially when principles are in conflict. In addition, virtue ethics can be seen as taking a more holistic, flexible, and relational approach to healthcare ethics (Benner 1997). Compassion, practical wisdom, sincerity, trustworthiness, honesty, conscientiousness, and competence are some of the key virtues guiding medical practice. Medical education increasingly promotes recognition of these values that guide the principle of beneficence, yet recognize the relational nature of the encounter and form a motivating force for effective communication (Benner 1997; Randall and Downie 1996).

Doctrine of informed consent

The concept of informed consent derives from the basic principles of beneficence, non-malfeasance, autonomy, and justice. The most important principle is respect for autonomy, which provides the basis for the practice of 'informed consent' in the healthcare provider–patient interactions regarding healthcare decisions. Ideally, informed consent is the process through which patients are fully informed about their health (diagnosis) and healthcare options (treatment choices), such that it enables them to participate in making decisions about their healthcare. There are five essential elements of informed consent:

1. discussion about the rationale for the procedure;

2. communicating the potential benefits of the procedure;

3. understanding the risks involved;

4. explanation of any treatment alternatives available; and

5. assuring the decision of the subject is voluntary (Siminoff 2003).

Informed consent by definition implies communication in both oral and written forms. Informed consent has at least two goals: to promote individual autonomy and to promote rational decision-making (Lidz *et al.* 1984). The main mechanism of informed consent is communication, and the quality of the communication will determine the quality or 'trueness' of the consent.

Perhaps one of the most difficult issues, and most germane to health communication, is coercion. Coercion is defined as the imposition of another's will by means of a serious threat or even an irresistible offer or as influence by means of rational argument (Faden and Beauchamp 1986). The ability to differentiate persuasion from coercion, or even manipulation, can be difficult. Persuasion is the use of techniques or reasonable incentives to change an individual's way of thinking (Beauchamp and Childress 2004). It can appear controlling, as it may be used to elicit a desired decision; for example, if a patient chooses to participate in a clinical trial, but it is not defined as coercion if the decision is the result of appeal to reason (Benner 1997; Siminoff 2003). However, excessive threat or manipulation may not be necessary for patients to feel coerced into making certain decisions. Thus, Allmark and Mason (2006) acknowledged that recruiting desperate participants to trials was not ethical because their decisions were essentially coerced. If participants believe that the trial is their only hope, and they cannot receive treatment without participating, it makes the decision less than voluntary and interferes with patient autonomy. In this example, patients may believe that they will suffer negative consequences if they do not consent, and that the incentives of survival or better quality of life fall outside of the realm of the 'reasonable' incentives used in persuasion. Thus, medical research, especially interventional research, must carefully consider whether the techniques used to obtain informed consent are persuasive or coercive.

Finally, research on informed consent has examined how much information is needed for adequate consent. To date, most approaches to informed consent take a legalistic, rather than an empirical, approach to this question. Standard texts (Beauchamp and Childress 2004; Lidz *et al.* 1984) all identify three standards.

♦ There is a 'reasonable physician standard' that asks, 'What would a typical physician say about this intervention?'. This standard allows the physician to determine what information is appropriate to disclose. Most research has shown that the typical physician tells the patient very little, making this a standard of dubious value.

♦ The 'reasonable patient standard' asks, 'What would the average patient need to know in order to make an informed decision?'. This standard focuses on considering what a patient would need to know in order to understand the choices he or she is presented.

♦ Finally, there is a 'subjective standard' that asks, 'What would a specific patient need to know and understand in order to make an informed decision?'. This standard requires tailoring information to each patient.

None of these standards truly answer the question of how much information patients need to make informed decisions, and they evade altogether the question of how information should be delivered. Communication research can help answer these questions.

Communication and consent

Communication is the seminal activity to attain informed decision-making. Proper communication about the patient's illness and treatment options, including clinical trials, is necessary in order to respect patient autonomy and to ensure that participation is voluntary. Communication research has been a vital tool for providing observational data that have informed ethicists and policy makers about consent practices. The advisory committee formed by President Clinton in 1994 uncovered serious ethical violations in a series of radiation studies performed by the government approximately 50 years ago (Kass and Sugarman 1996). This commission found that many consent forms did not properly address risks and may have overemphasized benefits (Kass and Sugarman 1996). Some patients believed it was a treatment option that was better than standard therapy, while others thought they had no choice. Consent forms were too complicated for many to read and understand—using technical language, small fonts, lengthy and technical descriptions, and requiring a high reading level. People involved in the radiation studies were hurt physically but also emotionally because they were deceived (Faden 1996). Today, people are still confused about the difference between research and medical care.

The ways physicians must present patients with information during the informed consent process is twofold: first, they need to provide all information to the patient as mandated by legal requirements; and, second, they must introduce and explain the information in an unbiased fashion, to ensure that patients can make an informed, voluntary choice (Siminoff 1992). Studies continue to show that many physicians and researchers do not communicate all the domains of legal informed consent to patients. For example, a study by Sankar (2004), examining the informed consent process for phase 1 clinical trials, found that compensation for injury was never discussed orally, and that confidentiality and the right to withdraw were discussed in only 6% of consent sessions. While most consent information is also covered in the consent form, the forms often have high reading levels, use technical or medical jargon, and may minimize risks and exaggerate potential benefits.

Sankar (2004) also found that communication problems existed in the way investigators framed the information in their discussions with patients (leaving out or emphasizing certain information), discussed benefits that were unlikely, did not clearly discriminate between research and treatment, and mixed the unproven with the known (e.g. by making something seem effective, while also saying that the research is still needed). Other studies have found that this ambiguous presentation of information is not uncommon during the informed consent process, which underscores the importance of information being communicated clearly and effectively to patients in order for them to make their own informed, autonomous decisions (Applebaum 2002; Applebaum *et al.* 1982). It also underscores that clinicians struggle with understanding and incorporating the concept of equipoise (belief that it is unknown whether or not one arm of a trial is better than the other) into their belief system. While some physicians have a good understanding of this concept and find it useful in conceptualizing clinical trials both for themselves and their patients (Garcia *et al.* 2004), other physicians do not appear to understand the concept and report describing the experimental arm of a trial as if it is new, distinctive, or revolutionary to the patient, rather than explaining that it is not yet known if one arm of the study is better than the other (Ziebland *et al.* 2007).

Conversely, comprehensible, unambiguous communication between physicians and patients can aid the informed consent process. Research has shown that there are ways of communicating information that patients perceive as more understandable and personally tailored than others, which can reduce confusion in informed consent and decision-making. One study (Studts *et al.* 2005) reported that participants were better able to understand, and found it easier to make a decision, when chemotherapy-risk information was presented in a more personal manner and with a concise, positive framing, than when the same information was presented in a manner that was negative, impersonal, persuasive, ambiguous, or wordy. Thus, communication must be clear and unbiased in order to aid in the decision-making process.

Intersection of cancer communication, decision-making, and consent

Cancer patients face several challenges when making decisions. Despite the advances in prevention, early detection, and treatment, the public still ranks cancer as the illness of which they are most afraid. Paradoxically, with advances in cancer treatment has come the challenge of choice between multiple treatment options, making the decision-making process of weighing the risks and benefits of each treatment more difficult for patients (Siminoff and Step 2005). As greater responsibility is placed on patients for their own care, patients are, therefore, making decisions that they may not be prepared or qualified to make (Siminoff and Step 2005). For example, as interest in the creation of biospecimen repositories to aid cancer research grows (Vaught *et al.* 2011), patients undergoing surgery are increasingly being asked to donate biological specimens to these repositories (otherwise known as biobanks). Donating to biobanking registries have important ethical implications for patients, including safeguarding health information privacy and understanding how their samples will be stored and used in the future (Koskan *et al.* 2012). One proposed remedy to this situation is the use of decision aids. Introduced in the 1980s, these tools are designed to provide objective information to patients about various treatment options. Decision aids can assist in decision-making by helping patients make treatment choices that are consistent with their own values, increasing patient knowledge about risks and benefits, and allowing patients to participate in the decision-making process (Weinstein *et al.* 2007).

The use of decision aids also raises ethical questions. For example, Nelson and colleagues suggest that the structure of decision aids may actually interfere with patients' own decision-making strategies (Nelson *et al.* 2007). When people scrutinize their decisions too closely or too much, they may actually be less likely to focus on information relevant to the situation at hand. If patients do not have strong and stable values, decision aids cannot help

them reach the decision that is most consistent with their values; rather, patients may construct temporary values while using the decision aid, and thus are susceptible to forming values based on the way the information is portrayed (Nelson *et al.* 2007). When one option is enrolling in a clinical trial, researchers must be especially careful. In order to be ethical, decision aids and interventions in communication research in general must focus on helping patients make informed decisions, not just helping patients see how particular decisions, such as the decision to enrol in a trial or participate in a biobank, may fit with their value system. Finally, more basic research is needed to know what types of information are most valuable and influential to medical decision-making. These data could help to guide the design of better decision aids.

The decision to participate in a research study is a unique kind of decision in healthcare. Most decisions faced by patients are regarding what types of treatments will be the most likely to aid their medical problems or help maintain a high quality of life while ill. Informed participation in a clinical trial generally means that subjects must understand the diagnosis, the relationship between the illness and their future health and functioning, and the benefits of standard therapy options. They need to also obtain some understanding of how treatment received within the context of a clinical trial differs from standard care. Other exigencies are time constraints and dealing with medical uncertainty. For example, even when there is no medical reason to make the decision quickly, patients often feel pressured to do so by their fears for their health or by their physicians. Simply handing a patient a written consent form does not constitute adequate consent. The information needs to be communicated in a meaningful way, so that the patient is prepared to participate in the decision-making process. Clinical trials aim to test new medications or medical regimens that may be helpful to society and other patients in the future, rather than directly helping the patients actually participating in the study. Many patients still agree to participate in clinical trials with the belief that they may be getting 'better' treatment than they would receive from standard treatment, or that the purpose of the trial is to provide them with better treatment. This misunderstanding has been termed the 'therapeutic misconception' (Applebaum *et al.* 1982). In order for communication between clinicians and patients to be effective, the essential elements of informed consent must be addressed, yet these five basic topics are not always discussed (Finucane *et al.* 1993). Although physicians are now providing patients with much more information than they did just 30 years ago (Applebaum *et al.* 1982; Garcia *et al.* 2004; Ziebland *et al.* 2007), many physicians are still hesitant to disclose all relevant information to their patients fearing full disclosure as potentially burdensome or provoking unnecessary anxiety (Studts *et al.* 2005; Siminoff and Step 2005). Thus, physicians struggle with deciding what information to convey to patients, as opposed to (what they perceive to be) harmful or overwhelming, for patients.

Physicians may also be unclear about what they should or should not communicate to patients. Until 10 years ago, there were gag clauses that could prevent physicians from discussing treatment options that insurance companies would not cover. Similarly, health maintenance organizations would prohibit referral to medical specialists if they were not included in the insurance company's group of providers (Faden 1997). Although these restrictive clauses have since been prohibited, some still believe that in order to maximize efficiency, physicians should not discuss options in which the benefit to the patient does not outweigh the cost of the therapy. Withholding information and options in this manner threatens the concept of informed consent.

While most patients desire information about their diagnosis and possible treatment options, there is great variability regarding the extent to which they would like to participate in the decision-making process. Moreover, it must be recognized that while the majority of patients prefer a reasonable amount of detailed information, others do not. Matching studies, which examine the extent to which a patient's level of desire for information is met and the effect on patient outcomes, have somewhat mixed findings; however, the likelihood of positive outcomes (such as more satisfaction or less depression) is increased if treatment interventions are tailored to provide patients with the amount or method of providing information that they desire (Kiesler and Auerbach 2006; Hotta et al. 2010). These studies demonstrate the importance of tailoring information preferences to each individual, as meeting patients' desire for information and decision-making can have a beneficial effect on patient outcomes. Health communication research can help develop mechanisms for intelligently tailoring information for individual patients.

Ethically challenging communication in palliative care

Many physicians are uncomfortable discussing poor prognoses with their patients, particularly when it comes to a terminal prognosis. While physicians will answer patient questions truthfully when asked, they are often less likely to volunteer information about poor prognoses. A common rationale for this practice is to preserve hope for patients with late-stage disease. In addition, there is a fear that these patients are already psychologically fragile and explicit discussions of prognosis will damage an already delicate psyche. Moreover, many physicians are concerned as to how accurate their prognosis really is, whether or not patients understand probabilities, and if these discussions hurt the doctor–patient relationship (Christakis 1999; Glare et al. 2003; Gordon and Daugherty 2003). However, if patients are not provided with sufficient information, or misinterpret the vague or optimistically-framed information provided by the physician, patients and their families frequently continue to hope for, or expect, a miracle. Some seek out futile care and endure advanced treatments for what may be small, if any, benefits, and some patients could undergo chemotherapy for a survival benefit of just one week (Matsuyama et al. 2006).

Communication between patients and their family members at the end of life also raises certain ethical dilemmas. When patients are incapacitated, surrogates are often called upon to make medical decisions for patients. There is a presumption that these surrogates will carry out the patients' wishes. However, it is not uncommon for a patient's preferences for end-of-life care to be unknown to family members. This may be due to the patient's failure or inability to convey their preferences to family members before loss of capacity, or the absence of written advance directives. Often surrogates project their own preferences onto patients; that is, surrogates are more likely to predict that patients would want the same end-of-life treatments that the surrogates themselves would want, rather than what the patients would actually prefer (Fagerlin et al. 2001). Even if surrogates do know patient preferences based on previous conversations, surrogates may not base their decisions for patient

care on these preferences, but instead base the decision on their own beliefs about quality of life, possibility of change or recovery, or family burden (Arnold and Kellum 2003; Rothchild 1994; Vig et al. 2006). Therefore, clinicians need to be aware that the use of surrogates as decision-makers for patients is an imperfect ethical instrument.

Models of decision-making in communication research

Patients vary in the extent to which they want to participate in the decision-making process about their care. There is a range of desire for information but, in general, studies show that about 92% want information about their illness and treatment options. Patients vary more in their wish to participate in treatment decisions (Benbassat et al. 1998). Before the 1980s, a paternalistic approach dominated, and patients accepted the physician's recommendation. In this model, the flow of information passed unidirectionally from physician to patient, rather than both contributing to the discussion (Charles et al. 1999). The focus was medical in orientation, with the physician providing sufficient information to meet legal requirements for informed consent, but rarely full disclosure. While some individuals, particularly those who are older, less educated, and having a more severe illness still prefer the paternalistic style of decision-making (Auerbach 2001), the development of a wider range of treatment options has led most patients to now prefer to participate in the decision-making process, to at least some degree.

At the other end of the spectrum is the fully informed model. This is more consumer-oriented, as patients learn about their illness and treatment options so that they can make their autonomous choice. The content of the consultation focuses more on medical and other relevant information that informs patients about all treatment options, with their risks and benefits. This model assumes that patients will make the best decision for themselves, so that the deliberation is undertaken by the patient.

Falling in between these two extremes is the model of shared decision-making. Shared decision-making is characterized by bidirectional information exchange and joint participation in decision-making (Siminoff and Step 2005). The physician and patient (and possibly the patient's family) discuss options and come to a treatment decision together. One specific paradigm of shared decision-making, the communication model of shared decision-making (CMSDM), puts emphasis on the transactional process that occurs between the physician and patient when communicating to come to a decision about cancer treatment (Siminoff and Step 2005). This model is based on four assumptions:

1. the physician and patient (as well as any others participating in decision-making, such as family members) work as a system and communicate with one another;

2. both verbal and non-verbal messages are exchanged;

3. physicians introduce patients to the consultation process and set the communication climate; and

4. patients must convey their preferences regarding the extent to which they will participate in the decision-making process.

This model highlights three influential factors involved in the interactional process between the physician and the patient. The first factor is patient–physician communication antecedents. Each individual has background characteristics that affect communication; namely, sociodemographic characteristics, personality traits (i.e. argumentative or docile), and communication competence (i.e. knowing what to communicate and how to do so). The second factor is the communication climate, which influences what happens during the consultation and takes the emotional, cognitive, and decisional preferences of each individual into account. The communication climate is affected by the patient's and physician's information and decision-making preferences, the severity of disease (i.e. patients tend to be more passive when illness is more severe), each participant's emotional state, and the role expectations of each person. The third factor is the treatment decision in which the physician and patient, having hopefully established a relationship characterized by trust, jointly contribute to making a treatment decision. These models provide a framework to guide the development of clear and objective cancer communication materials and interventions.

Future directions

Communication research is the major vehicle for understanding the ethics of cancer communication, especially informed consent to treatment and to participation in clinical trials. Health communication researchers are deeply involved in attempting to develop 'better' ways for clinical communication to unfold and to help with treatment decision-making. The ethical obligations of communication researchers need to be sensitive concerning whose values are being upheld or promoted, and how we use effective models of communication persuasively but not coercively.

References

Allmark P, Mason S (2006). Should desperate volunteers be included in randomised controlled trials? *J Med Ethics* **32**, 548–53.

Applebaum PS (2002). Clarifying the ethics of clinical research: a path toward avoiding the therapeutic misconception. *Am J Bioethics* **2**, 22–3.

Applebaum PS, Roth LH, Lidz CW (1982). The therapeutic misconception: informed consent in psychiatric research. *Int J Law Psychiatry* **5**, 319–29.

Arnold RM, Kellum J (2003). Moral justifications for surrogate decision making in the intensive care unit: implications and limitations. *Crit Care Med* **31** (5 Suppl), S347–53.

Arras JD (1991). Getting down to cases: the revival of casuistry in bioethics. *J Med Philosophy* **16**, 29–51.

Auerbach SM (2001). Should patients have control over their own healthcare?: empirical evidence and research issues. *Ann Behav Med* **22**, 246–59.

Beauchamp T, Childress J (2004). *Principles of Medical Ethics*, 6th edition. Oxford University Press, New York, NY.

Benbassat CE, Pipel D, Tidhar M (1998). Patients' preferences for participation in clinical decision making: a review of published surveys. *Behav Med* **24**, 81–8.

Benner P (1997). A dialogue between virtue ethics and care ethics. *Theor Med* **18**, 47–61.

Charles C, Gafni A, Whelan T (1999). Decision-making in the physician-patient encounter: revisiting the shared treatment decision-making model. *Soc Sci Med* **49**, 651–61.

Christakis NA (1999). Prognostication and bioethics. *Daedalus* **128**, 197–214.

Faden RR (1996). Chair's perspective on the work of the advisory committee on human radiation experiment. *Kennedy Inst Ethics J* **6**, 215–21.

Faden RR (1997). Managed care and informed consent. *Kennedy Inst Ethics J* **7**, 377–9.

Faden RR, Beauchamp TL (1986). *A History and Theory of Informed Consent*. Oxford University Press, New York, NY.

Fagerlin A, Ditto PH, Danks JH, Houts RM, Smucker WD (2001). projection in surrogate decisions about life-sustaining medical treatments. *Health Psychol* **20**, 166–75.

Finucane TE, Beamer BA, Roca RP, Kawas CH (1993). Establishing advance medical directives with demented patients: a pilot study. *J Clin Ethics* **4**, 51–4.

Garcia J, Elbourne D, Snowdon C (2004). Equipoise: A case study of the views of clinicians involved in two neonatal trials. *Clin Trials* **1**, 170–8.

Glare P, Virik K, Jones M, et al. (2003). A systematic review of physicians' survival predictions in terminally ill cancer patients. *BMJ* **327**, 195–8.

Gordon EJ, Daugherty CK (2003). Hitting You Over the Head: Oncologists' Disclosure of Prognosis to Advanced Cancer Patients. *Bioethics* **17**, 142–68.

Hotta K, Kiura K, Takigawa N, et al. (2010). Desire for information and involvement in treatment decisions: lung cancer patients' preferences and their physicians' perceptions: results from okayama lung cancer study group trial 0705. *J Thoracic Oncology* **5**, 1668–72.

Kass NE, Sugarman J (1996). Are research subjects adequately protected? A review and discussion of studies conducted by the advisory committee on human radiation experiments. *Kennedy Inst Ethics J* **16**, 271–82.

Kiesler DJ, Auerbach SM (2006). Optimal matches of patient preferences for information, decision-making and interpersonal behaviour: evidence, models and interventions. *Patient Educ Couns* **61**, 319–41.

Koskan A, Arevalo M, Gwede CK, et al. (2012). Ethics of clear health communication: Applying the CLEAN look approach to communicate biobanking information for cancer research. *J Health Care Poor Underserved* **23**, 58–66.

Lidz CW, Meisel A, Zerubavel E, et al. (1984). *Informed Consent: A Study of Decision Making in Psychiatry*. Oxford University Press, New York, NY.

Matsuyama R, Reddy S, Smith TJ (2006). Why do patients choose chemotherapy near the end of life? a review of the perspective of those facing death from cancer. *J Clin Oncol* **24**, 3490–6.

Nelson WL, Han PKJ, Fagerlin A, et al. (2007). Rethinking the objectives of decision aids: a call for conceptual clarity. *Med Decis Making* **27**, 609–18.

Randall F, Downie R (1996). *Palliative Care Ethics*. Oxford University Press, Oxford, UK.

Rothchild E (1994). Family dynamics in end-of-life treatment decisions. *Gen Hos Psych* **16**, 251–8.

Sankar P (2004). Communication and miscommunication in informed consent to research. *Med Anthropol Q* **18**, 429–46.

Siminoff LA (1992). Improving communication with cancer patients. *Oncology* **6**, 83–7.

Siminoff LA (2003). Toward improving the informed consent process in research with humans. *IRB: Ethics & Human Research* **25**, S1–3.

Siminoff LA, Step MM (2005). A communication model of shared decision making: accounting for cancer treatment decisions. *Health Psychol* **24**, S99–105.

Studts JL, Abell TD, Roetzer LM, et al. (2005). Preferences for different methods of communicating information regarding adjuvant chemotherapy for breast cancer. *Psychooncology* **14**, 647–60.

Vaught J, Rogers J, Myers K, et al. (2011). An NCI perspective on creating sustainable biospecimen resources. *J Natl Cancer Instit Monogr* **2011**, 1–7.

Vig EK, Taylor JS, Starks H, Hopley EK, Fryer-Edwards K (2006). Beyond substituted judgment: how surrogates navigate end-of-life decision-making. *J Am Geriatr Soc* **54**, 1688–93.

Weinstein JN, Clay K, Morgan TS (2007). Informed patient choice: patient-centered valuing of surgical risks and benefits. *Health Aff (Millwood)* **26**, 726–30.

Ziebland S, Featherstone K, Snowdon C, et al. (2007). Does it matter if clinicians recruiting for a trial don't understand what the trial is really about? qualitative study of surgeons' experiences of participation in a pragmatic multi-centre RCT. *Trials* **8** (4).

CHAPTER 6

Gender, power, and non-verbal communication

Marianne Schmid Mast, Valérie Carrard, and Judith A. Hall

Introduction to communication in cancer care

The importance of communication in cancer care has been well documented. Communication is a challenging process which unfolds between two persons in a particular situation. As such, it has a great variety of determinants. In the present chapter, we propose a summary of the literature on three communication-related factors that have been studied scarcely in the palliative or oncology setting: non-verbal communication, power, and gender. To approach these issues, we will first discuss findings from the field of general practice on the importance of non-verbal communication in the provider–patient interaction. We will then explore how dominance and power affect the communication process between providers and their patients and how gender affects all of these aspects. Finally, we will relate these findings to the particular setting of oncology and palliative care.

Importance of non-verbal communication in the medical setting

With the growing interest of researchers for the communication process in medical interactions, researchers have paid relatively more attention to the verbal than the non-verbal content of communication (Schmid Mast 2007). However, depending on the situation, non-verbal behaviour can matter more than verbal messages as a source of information. For example, in the case of an ambiguous verbal message or one of doubtful honesty, non-verbal cues provide key understanding. They become especially salient when they contradict the words being spoken, or when the context is highly emotional. Non-verbal cues serve not just to express emotions but also to signal attention or physical symptoms like pain, to convey attitudes about friendliness or dominance, and to reveal personality characteristics such as shyness or extraversion (Knapp et al. 2013).

The general definition of non-verbal behaviour is a 'communication effected by means other than words' (Knapp et al. 2013, p. 8). However, the distinction between verbal and non-verbal communication is not always clear-cut. Sign language, for instance, is non-verbal behaviour through its use of gestures, but it is also verbal in that each gesture has a distinct linguistic meaning. Voice modulation, pitch, and rate, or speech duration are interconnected with the verbal content of the communication, but are considered non-verbal communication because they add information beyond the words alone. Besides such speech-related non-verbal cues, non-verbal behaviours include facial expressions conveying emotions, or eye gaze, gestures, posture, touch, and interpersonal distance (Knapp et al. 2013). One challenging issue in the study of communication is that the same non-verbal behaviour can mean different things depending on context. A smile, for example, can mean joy as well as empathy or uneasiness.

Several tools are used to test non-verbal decoding skills. The Patient Emotion Cue Test (PECT; Blanch-Hartigan 2011) and the Test of Accurate Perception of Patients' Affect (TAPPA; Hall et al. 2014) for instance are both designed for assessing this skill in healthcare providers. In a typical test of this kind, short videos are shown and the test taker is asked to infer the emotions or intentions of the person in the videotape. In the PECT, test takers have to evaluate the emotions displayed by a videotaped actress portraying a patient, and in the TAPPA one guesses the thoughts and feelings of real medical patients during their visits. Research reveals that people can be rather accurate when assessing what others feel or think based on non-verbal cues but that there are huge individual differences in this ability. Skill at accurately 'reading' others has been shown to be linked to self and other-rated social-emotional competence, communality, prosocial behaviour, and positive personality traits (Hall et al. 2009a). Medical students scoring higher in interpersonal accuracy tests seem also to be advantaged in their relationships with patients and analogue patients (participants asked to put themselves in the shoes of a patient) rating them as having better interpersonal skills (Hall et al. 2014), being more compassionate and likeable, as well as showing more dominant, more engaged, and less distressed behaviours (Hall et al. 2009b).

Importance of patient non-verbal behaviour

How patients behave non-verbally during the medical encounter has scarcely been studied. It is however an important source of information for the provider. In order to diagnose a patient's illness, healthcare providers use different approaches: objective measurement (e.g. blood cells analysis); a physical examination; and also the verbal and non-verbal signals of the patient. For example, pain recognition is essential for providers and can be achieved through the observation of patients' facial expressions (Patrick *et al.* 1986). Also, some coronary illnesses have been shown to be linked to expressing more anger by patients (Rosenberg *et al.* 2001). So clinicians who are astute in decoding the patient's non-verbal behaviour might be at an advantage for reaching an accurate diagnosis. The correct interpretation of a patient's non-verbal cues by the provider is also linked to other positive medical interaction outcomes. Hall's literature review (2011) concludes that the better healthcare providers are at accurately decoding non-verbal cues, the more positive the outcomes in terms of satisfaction, appointment keeping, and evaluation of the physician's clinical skills, and the provider's warmth and engagement.

Importance of provider non-verbal behaviour

The scarcity of studies on the effects of provider non-verbal communication in the medical encounter is astonishing, given that existing empirical evidence shows that the clinician's non-verbal behaviour impacts patients' outcomes. A systematic review indeed showed that better patient outcomes (e.g. satisfaction, trust, compliance, adherence, and long-term health effects) are linked to the physician showing more affiliative non-verbal behaviours like nodding, forward leaning, direct body orientation, uncrossed legs and arms, arm symmetry, and less mutual gaze (Beck *et al.* 2002). In the same vein, the distancing behaviour of physical therapists, such as absence of smiling and looking away from the patient, was related to decreases in patients' physical and cognitive functioning (Ambady *et al.* 2002*a*). Also, surgeons with a more dominant tone of voice were more likely to have been sued for medical malpractice than surgeons with a less dominant tone (Ambady *et al.* 2002*b*).

The non-verbal behaviours of a provider that convey caring and low dominance are linked to better patient outcomes. This supports findings showing that the provider communication style with the best patient outcomes is patient-centred communication, characterized by high caring (perspective taking and expressing emotions) as well as low dominance. In the next section, we consider the control, power, and dominance distribution in the medical encounter and its impact on patient outcomes.

Power and dominance in the medical encounter

In many ways, the provider can be defined as having more power and control over the patient than vice versa. The provider typically has higher status, in terms of social standing and earning capacity. In general, providers have more medical knowledge, thus more clinical competence than patients. Furthermore, help-seeking is fundamentally a position of powerlessness. Discomfort, pain, or anxiety about the prognosis or treatment might contribute to the patient's loss of power and control over the situation.

The distribution of power between patients and providers can vary. Roter and Hall (2006) conceptualize alternative relationship styles between doctor and patient as falling into four prototypes. In one, called *paternalistic*, the doctor is in control while the patient plays a traditional, passive role. Being in control covers establishing legitimate topics for discussion, making key decisions, and conveying only as much information as the doctor chooses. The opposite, which Roter and Hall (2006) call *consumerist*, reverses these

roles. The patient is now in control and the doctor plays the weaker role. A third style they call *default*, in which both participants take a fairly laissez-faire and uninvolved stance, without a clear definition of roles, obligations, and prerogatives. Finally, they can be in a relationship called *mutuality*, where both of them participate in an active and balanced way; they negotiate goals and agenda, they are both involved in decision-making, and respect for the patient's values and perspective is high. This style is called patient-centred (Roter and Hall 2006).

Roter and Hall's classification (2006) is a useful framework for studying communication between a clinician and patient. It indicates also that either medical partner can show a more or less dominant stance. Moreover, even within one type of power relationship between provider and patient, the way the provider behaves towards the patient can still vary in dominance.

Non-verbal indicators of dominance

Hall *et al.* (2005) investigated with a meta-analysis which non-verbal behaviours are related to the perception of dominance in the general population. Their meta-analysis showed that people are perceived as dominant when they display less self-touch as well as more other-touch, when they gesture more and show more body openness, adopt a more erect or tense posture, shift more their body or their legs, use smaller interpersonal distance, lower their eyebrows more, nod more, have a more expressive face, and gaze more. Concerning cues related to voice, the authors showed that louder voice, more voice variation and relaxation, more interruptions, less pausing, faster speech rate, and lower voice pitch are perceived as dominant.

In the medical encounter, Schmid Mast and colleagues (2011) showed that people often use the same non-verbal indicators to judge dominance in clinicians as they do for the general population in different social settings. Providers' non-verbal behaviours perceived as being dominant included: more indirect body orientation; more gesturing; more forward leaning; less self-touch; less gazing at the patient; more gazing at the notes or computer; more frowning; less smiling; less nodding; longer speaking time; louder voice; more voice modulation; and more talking while doing something else. All in all, expansive gestures and less caring behaviours of the provider are perceived as dominance cues in the medical setting.

Impact of dominance behaviours on the provider–patient encounter

As one may guess, more provider dominance is usually related to poorer medical encounter outcomes (Ambady *et al.* 2002*a*; Ambady *et al.* 2002*b*) and it affects how the medical encounter unfolds. Schmid Mast *et al.* (2008*b*) found that patients spoke less, provided less medical information, and agreed more when interacting with 'high dominance' compared to 'low dominance' providers. The clinician who adopts a dominant style might, therefore, be at a disadvantage because the diagnosis is largely based on medical information provided by the patient.

Interestingly, certain dominance behaviours have been shown to be differently linked to satisfaction when they are displayed by female as compared to male providers. For instance, more interruptions correlate with less patient satisfaction in a male–male dyad, but with more satisfaction in a female–female dyad (Hall *et al.* 1994). Gender differences seem thus to be an important factor for the understanding of provider–patient communication and its effect on medical outcomes. In the following, we present a review of gender influences on medical encounters.

Impact of gender in the medical encounter

In this section, we will see that the provider's gender affects the way they communicate with their patients, as well as the way their patients communicate with them. Moreover, we will present how female and male patients are addressed and behave according to their gender.

Provider gender

Female and male providers show some communality in their ways of communicating with patients. They share the same amount and quality of medical information, as well as social conversation (medically irrelevant information) with their patients (Roter *et al.* 2002). However, female providers talk more about the psychosocial impact of a diagnosis or treatment and use more partnership building (e.g. soliciting expectations from and including the patient in the decision-making processes). Moreover, female clinicians use more positive communication (e.g. encouragement), emotionally focused talk (e.g. emotional probes, empathy), and supportive behaviours such as smiling and nodding. Last but not least, consultations with female providers are on average two minutes longer than with male providers (Roter *et al.* 2002). All in all, women clinicians seem to display more of the patient-centred typical behaviours. Indeed, compared to men, they show both more partnership building and more warmness through verbal as well as non-verbal communication (Roter *et al.* 2002).

The gender of the provider also affects patient behaviour. In a meta-analysis, Hall and Roter (2002) showed that patients of female providers talked more and conveyed more biomedical and psychosocial information than did patients seeing a male provider. Patients communicate more positively (e.g. statement of agreement) with a female clinician, use more partnership building statements, and behave more assertively. In sum, female clinicians appear to enhance patient participation and empowerment in the medical interaction.

Patient gender

On average, women seek medical advice more often than men. Female patients ask more questions and show more interest during the conversation with the provider than their male counterparts (Hall and Roter 1995). The provider's behaviour also changes according to the patient's gender. Compared to male patients, female patients receive more emotionally concerned statements and more information from their providers (Hall and Roter 1998). This is most likely the result of the providers' tendency to ask female patients more questions about their feelings and thoughts (Hall and Roter 1998). Importantly, clinicians use a calmer and less dominant voice when speaking to a woman (Hall *et al.* 1994). In sum, providers communicate with female patients in a more emotional and partnership-oriented way.

Gender composition of the dyad

Because both patient and provider gender affect medical communication, studies that consider both aspects simultaneously prove helpful in extricating the role of gender. Female–female interactions seem to follow the patient-centred model, with female providers showing more concern about the female patient, her situation, and treating her as a partner in decision-making (Roter and Hall 2004). In female–female dyads, providers and patients talk for fairly equivalent periods of time, whereas in male dyads, the provider typically speaks more than the patient (Hall *et al.* 1994). The male–male dyads are more hierarchical also, in that patients are less included in decision-making (Kaplan *et al.* 1995).

The female clinician and male patient dyads seem to be the most challenging. When female providers interact with men, they adopt a potentially ambiguous style: although they smile more and use less jargon, they convey more dominance and less friendliness through their voices (Hall *et al.* 1994). The male patients also respond ambiguously to female clinicians, in that they make more partnership statements while at the same time they use a more dominant and bored tone of voice (Hall *et al.* 1994). The ambiguity of the interaction partners' behaviours in this dyad may reflect an uneasiness with a situation in which a woman endorses a high power position and a man a low power position, a constellation that goes against common gender stereotypes. We will come back to the gender stereotypes issue below and try to shed more light on the observed ambiguities.

Gender and patient satisfaction

We just showed how gender can influence providers and patients' behaviours and one may wonder whether those differences can also affect consultation outcomes. Most of the studies on communication in healthcare use self-reported patient satisfaction as a consultation outcome. Patient satisfaction is widely recognized as a valid measure of positive medical interaction outcomes because it is linked to patients' medical improvements (Wickizer *et al.* 2004).

A meta-analysis by Hall, Blanch-Hartigan, and Roter (2011) showed that female providers have more satisfied patients than male providers, but the effect size was so small (r < 0.04) that the difference between male and female providers cannot be interpreted. The lack of a female provider's advantage in patient satisfaction is surprising because, as we have seen, female providers display a more patient-centred interaction style than male providers and the female providers' patients seem to respond to it with a more empowered interaction style. Because patient-centredness has been shown to be beneficial for the patients, we would expect female providers to have more satisfied patients as compared as their male counterparts. It seems that somehow female providers are not rewarded for their adoption of a good medical interaction style. One explanation for this astonishing finding could be the gender stereotypes and role expectations that patients bring into the medical encounter. In order to understand this phenomenon, we will now present how gender, power, and stereotypes can influence performance evaluation in the general population before focusing more specifically on the provider–patient situation.

Gender and power interplay

Research shows that women are less likely to be found in leadership positions or to emerge as group leaders compared to men (Eagly 2007). Women behave less dominantly, are less competitive, and are more interpersonally oriented; they are more communal (Eagly 2007). Those styles of behaviour are not only descriptive, but they are also prescriptive, in that they shape what we expect from women and men in terms of behaviour. Female leaders typically find themselves in a double bind situation. If they behave according to what is expected from women (more communal, caring, or gentle), their behaviour does not correspond to the one expected from a leader and thus these women are devalued (Eagly 2007; Heilman 2001). However, if women behave in a role-consistent way (dominant, challenging, or entrepreneurial), the expectations linked to their gender are in contradiction to their behaviour. In both cases, female leaders will be poorly evaluated, because of the lack of fit between gender stereotypes and role expectations (Heilman 2001).

Gender and power in the medical encounter

Similar to what happens for female leaders, female physicians are in a double bind situation. They are perceived in a negative light if they adopt gender-incongruent behaviours. Burgoon *et al.* (1991) showed that variations in aggressive communication (non-aggressive, moderately aggressive, and aggressive) affected patients differently depending on the physician's gender. Patient satisfaction decreased with greater aggressiveness in female physicians, whereas patient satisfaction was less affected by male physicians' aggression. Meanwhile, Schmid Mast *et al.* (2007) showed that in male–male dyads, the communication style of the physicians did not influence analogue patients' evaluation of the consultation, whereas in female–female dyads less caring physicians received less positive evaluation. In same-sex dyads, female physicians are thus badly evaluated if they adopt an interaction style incongruent with gender stereotypes.

Also, there is evidence that the greater the dissonance between gender stereotypes and job expectations, the less positively female physicians are evaluated. Indeed, the younger the physician, and the older the patient, the less satisfied the patient is with a female physician (Hall *et al.* 1994).

Interestingly, patients expect physicians to show caring and empathic behaviours which are stereotypically female behaviours (Eagly 2007). And indeed, female physicians are rewarded for endorsing the typically feminine caring style of communication. Schmid Mast and colleagues (2008*a*) found that patient satisfaction correlated with stereotypically female behaviours (e.g. more gazing, less interpersonal distance, softer voice) when displayed by women physicians. For male physicians, satisfaction was high when they adhered to stereotypically male behaviours (e.g. more interpersonal distance, greater expansiveness, louder voice) but this link was less pronounced than the one between stereotypically female behaviours and satisfaction with female physicians.

This strong link to behavioural expectations in female physicians might explain why they do not get the credit they deserve, given the fact that they use a more patient-centred interaction style. Hall and colleagues (2015), compared the evaluation of high and low patient-centred female and male physicians. Analogue patients were asked to evaluate videotapes of male and female actors each displaying either high or low patient-centredness while interacting with a patient. The results show that low patient-centred female physicians were not evaluated differently from low patient-centred male physicians. However, when the analogue patients watched a male physician displaying high patient-centredness, they evaluated him much more positively than the female physician displaying exactly the same behaviours. The authors concluded that the female physicians do not get credit for their use of patient-centred care, because it is a pattern of behaviours expected from every woman

and so female physicians do not get extra credit for it. In contrast, patient-centred male physicians are seen as exceptionally good, because they show behaviours that are not expected from them according to gender stereotypes, and the behaviour corresponds to the state of art in physician–patient communication.

Significance in the cancer and palliative care setting

So far we have presented a literature review on non-verbal communication, power, and gender in general medical settings. In oncology or palliative settings, care delivery is different from standard medical settings with respect to the length of the provider–patient relationship, nature of the treatment decisions, and the complexity of medical issues. In this context, the emotional dimension is omnipresent, and especially fear and depression are prevalent given that end-of-life decisions are at stake. Research shows that symptoms of distress are often not detected and go untreated (Ryan *et al.* 2005). Given that affect is mostly expressed non-verbally, the correct assessment of a patient's demeanour and non-verbal cues is crucial to the provision of responsive care. It has indeed been shown that more interpersonally accurate providers detect more anxiety and depression in their patients with rare false–positive evaluations (Robbins *et al.* 1994).

In oncology and palliative care, the severity of the illnesses and the related impairments and weaknesses place the patient in an even more submissive and passive role compared to the provider, who has the power to potentially alleviate the patients' health concerns and pain, and even possibly save their lives. The hierarchical difference between patient and provider are thus most likely intensified by the particularities of oncology and palliative care. It is also important to note that severely ill patients on average prefer more paternalistic and dominant providers (Kiesler and Auerbach 2006). So we would expect oncology and palliative patients to be more tolerant towards a dominant interaction style from their physicians, and maybe even prefer this kind of interaction, instead of a more patient-centred one.

The role that gender plays in communication in oncology has been insufficiently explored. But as the power difference between patient and provider is intensified, we would expect that the dissonance between role expectations and gender stereotypes is exacerbated in oncology and palliative care. Female providers in those settings would therefore be even more negatively evaluated if they showed a dominant interaction style, or would receive even less credit when showing a patient-centred interaction style.

Depending on the type of cancer, there might be preferences for one gender or the other, which could influence the patient's evaluation of the provider. We know that patients prefer a female obstetrician (Plunkett *et al.* 2002) and that they are on average more satisfied with female obstetricians than with their male counterparts (Roter *et al.* 1999). It is thus likely that women with cervical cancer, for instance, might prefer a female provider and would also be more satisfied with a female provider.

These reflections are driven by the existing literature, but unless we have empirical evidence, the question of how power and gender affect the particular setting of oncology and palliative care still remains open. Given the importance of non-verbal communication in the patient–provider relationship, providers and especially oncologists might want to consider non-verbal decoding training

(Blanch-Hartigan and Ruben 2013). Oncologists could benefit from a better understanding of their patients' non-verbal cues for the accuracy of the diagnosis, the adequacy of the treatment decisions, and the optimization of the relationship with their patients. Another important factor to consider in oncology training is the different characteristics of providers and patients such as age, gender, and ethnicity because, as the preceding section outlined, individual provider characteristics can affect the quality of the medical interaction and the relationship between healthcare providers and their patients.

References

Ambady N, Koo J, Rosenthal R, Winograd CH (2002a). Physical therapists' nonverbal communication predicts geriatric patients' health outcomes. *Psychol Aging* **17**, 443–52.

Ambady N, Laplante D, Nguyen T, Rosenthal R, Chaumeton N, Levinson W (2002b). Surgeons' tone of voice: A clue to malpractice history. *Surgery* **132**, 5–9.

Beck RS, Daughtridge R, Sloane PD (2002). Physician-patient communication in the primary care office: A systematic review. *J Am Board Fam Pract* **15**, 25–38.

Blanch-Hartigan D (2011). Measuring providers' verbal and nonverbal emotion recognition ability: reliability and validity of the Patient Emotion Cue Test (PECT). *Patient Educ Couns* **82**, 370–6.

Blanch-Hartigan D, Ruben MA (2013). Training clinicians to accurately perceive their patients: Current state and future directions. *Patient Educ Couns* **92**, 328–36.

Burgoon M, Birk TS, Hall JR (1991). Compliance and satisfaction with physician-patient communication an expectancy theory interpretation of gender differences. *Human Comm Res* **18**, 177–208.

Eagly AH (2007). Female leadership advantage and disadvantage: resolving the contradictions. *Psychology of Women Quarterly* **31**, 1–12.

Hall JA (2011). Clinicians' accuracy in perceiving patients: Its relevance for clinical practice and a narrative review of methods and correlates. *Patient Educ Couns* **84**, 319–24.

Hall JA, Andrzejewski SA, Yopchick JE (2009a). Psychosocial correlates of interpersonal sensitivity: a meta-analysis. *J Nonverbal Behav* **33**, 149–80.

Hall JA, Blanch-Hartigan D, Roter DL (2011). Patients' satisfaction with male versus female physicians: A meta-analysis. *Med Care* **49**, 611–617.

Hall JA, Coats EJ, Smith Lebeau L (2005). Nonverbal behavior and the vertical dimension of social relations: A meta-analysis. *Psychol Bull* **131**, 898–924.

Hall JA, Irish JT, Roter DL, Ehrlich CM, Miller LH (1994). Gender in medical encounters: An analysis of physician and patient communication in a primary care setting. *Health Psychology* **13**, 384–92.

Hall JA, Roter DL (1995). Patient gender and communication with physicians: Results of a community-based study. *Women's Health* **1**, 77–95.

Hall JA, Roter DL (1998). Medical communication and gender: A summary of research. *J Gend Specif Med* **1**, 39–42.

Hall JA, Roter DL (2002). Do patients talk differently to male and female physicians? A meta-analytic review. *Patient Educ Couns* **48**, 217–224.

Hall JA, Roter DL, Blanch DC, Frankel RM (2009b). Nonverbal sensitivity in medical students: Implications for clinical interactions. *J Gen Internal Med* **24**, 1217–22.

Hall JA, Roter DL, Blanch-Hartigan DC, Schmid Mast M, Pitegoff CA (2015). How patient-centered do female physicians need to be? Analogue

patients' satisfaction with male and female physicians' identical behaviors. *Health Commun* **30**, 894–900.

Hall JA, Ship AN, Ruben MA, et al. (2014). The Test of Accurate Perception of Patients' Affect (TAPPA): an ecologically valid tool for assessing interpersonal perception accuracy in clinicians. *Patient Educ Couns* **94**, 218–23.

Heilman ME (2001). Description and prescription: How gender stereotypes prevent women's ascent up the organizational ladder. *J Social Issues* **57**, 657–74.

Kaplan SH, Gandek B, Greenfield S, Rogers W, Ware JE (1995). Patient and visit characteristics related to physicians' participatory decision-making style: Results from the Medical Outcomes Study. *Med Care* **33**, 1176–87.

Kiesler DJ, Auerbach SM (2006). Optimal matches of patient preferences for information, decision-making and interpersonal behavior: Evidence, models and interventions. *Patient Educ Couns* **61**, 319–41.

Knapp M L, Hall JA, Horgan TG (2013). *Nonverbal Communication in Human Interaction*, 8th edition. Cengage Learning, Boston, MA.

Patrick CJ, Craig KD, Prkachin KM (1986). Observer judgments of acute pain: facial action determinants. *J Pers Soc Psychol* **50**, 1291–8.

Plunkett BA, Kohli P, Milad MP (2002). The importance of physician gender in the selection of an obstetrician or a gynecologist. *Am J Obstet Gynecol* **186**, 926–8.

Robbins JM, Kirmayer LJ, Cathébras P, Yaffe MJ, Dworkind M (1994). Physician characteristics and the recognition of depression and anxiety in primary care. *Med Care* **32**, 795–812.

Rosenberg EL, Ekman P, Jiang W, et al. (2001). Linkages between facial expressions of anger and transient myocardial ischemia in men with coronary artery disease. *Emotion* **1**, 107–15.

Roter DL, Geller G, Bernhardt BA, Larson SM, Doksum T (1999). Effects of obstetrician gender on communication and patient satisfaction. *Obstet Gynecol* **93**, 635–41.

Roter DL, Hall JA (2004). Physician gender and patient-centered communication: A critical review of empirical research. *Ann Rev Public Health* **25**, 497–519.

Roter DL, Hall JA (2006). *Doctors Talking with Patients/Patients Talking with Doctors: Improving Communication in Medical Visits*, 2nd edition. Praeger, Westport, CT.

Roter DL, Hall JA, Aoki Y (2002). Physician gender effects in medical communication: A meta-analytic review. *J Am Med Assoc* **288**, 756–64.

Ryan H, Schofield P, Cockburn J, et al. (2005). How to recognize and manage psychological distress in cancer patients. *Euro J Cancer Care* **14**, 7–15.

Schmid Mast M (2007). On the importance of nonverbal communication in the physician–patient interaction. *Patient Educ Couns* **67**, 315–18.

Schmid Mast M, Hall JA, Cronauer CK, Cousin G (2011). Perceived dominance in physicians: Are female physicians under scrutiny?. *Patient Educ Couns* **83**, 174–9.

Schmid Mast M, Hall JA, Köckner C, Choi E (2008a). Physician gender affects how physician nonverbal behavior is related to patient satisfaction. *Med Care* **46**, 1212–18.

Schmid Mast M, Hall JA, Roter DL (2007). Disentangling physician sex and physician communication style: Their effects on patient satisfaction in a virtual medical visit. *Patient Educ Couns* **68**, 16–22.

Schmid Mast M, Hall JA, Roter DL (2008b). Caring and dominance affect participants' perceptions and behaviors during a virtual medical visit. *J Gen Int Med* **23**, 523–7.

Wickizer TM, Franklin G, Fulton-Kehoe D, Turner JA, Mootz R, Smith-Weller T (2004). Patient satisfaction, treatment experience, and disability outcomes in a population-based cohort of injured workers in Washington state: Implications for quality improvement. *Health Serv Res* **39**, 727–48.

CHAPTER 7

Medical student training in communication skills

Gregory Makoul, Joshua Hauser,
and Henry Schneiderman

Introduction to medical student training in communication skills

Communication is now recognized as a fundamental and indispensable clinical skill. Effective communication is critical to appropriate diagnosis and management in every specialty, and absolutely essential for connecting with patients on a cognitive and emotional level. Indeed, effective communication is associated with improved satisfaction, adherence, and outcomes as well as fewer malpractice claims (Stewart *et al.* 1999; Cegala *et al.* 2000; Stewart 2005). Moreover, poor physician communication skills discerned in a medical licensing exam have been shown to predict subsequent patient complaints to regulatory authorities (Tamblyn *et al.* 2007).

Accordingly, communication skills are a basic competency advocated by the General Medical Council in the UK (General Medical Council 2013), by accrediting bodies in the US (Liaison Committee on Medical Education 2013; Batalden *et al.* 2002; Horowitz 2000; The Joint Commission 2010), and by similar organizations in other countries. In this chapter, we review approaches to teaching communication skills at the medical school level, explicating special considerations for effective communication in the context of oncology and primary care.

Approaches to teaching and assessment

Like any skill, communication is best learned through a combination of practice, feedback, and reflection. For medical students, communication skills training generally begins early and extends into clinical training, where increasing levels of sophistication and more robust patient experiences often compete with a hidden curriculum marked by cynicism and a focus on expediency that slights interactional skills (Hafferty 1998). Explicit reinforcement of communication skills throughout medical school—with dedicated opportunities for students to reflect, obtain constructive feedback, and voice concerns about the challenges they encounter—is a powerful counter to the hidden curriculum (Makoul *et al.* 2010).

The primary approaches to communication teaching and assessment in medical school couple small group teaching with either *role play* or *interviews with simulated patients*. While both methods have value, neither mirrors the uncertainty, fear, and pain of encounters with real patients, especially patients with co-morbidities and deep miseries. Thus, the goal of these modalities is to help students develop the skills and strategies they will refine when working with patients and families in clinical situations.

Role play

Role play is a simple and inexpensive form of simulation. It provides an opportunity to learn, practice, and receive feedback on communication skills in a familiar environment, without the complexity of interacting with real or simulated patients. In role play, a specific case is developed and key roles—such as patient, oncologist, family member—are assigned to students. Role plays should be based on a scenario but not scripted, have a clearly delineated objective (i.e. 'discuss a new biopsy that shows breast cancer' rather than 'talk to this patient'), and include debriefing immediately following the session. When constructing role plays, it is important to remember that the goal is to help students experience a role and work towards accomplishing particular communication tasks, rather than to understand minute details of a clinical case.

A major challenge in any type of role play is that it can feel artificial to students (Nestel and Tierney 2007). They might not take the exercise seriously or might speak in ways that actual patients would not (e.g. 'the pain is radiating from my supraspinatus'). Role plays are meant to parallel actual events; being clear that the goal is to try to feel what it is like to be in a particular role—patient, family member, or physician—can help to redirect and focus attention. In our palliative care teaching, we use role plays to discuss challenging topics such as revealing a new diagnosis of cancer, conveying the challenge of treatment options, discussing poor prognosis, and introducing discussion of hospice with patient and family. As these are difficult topics, many students benefit from practice and thoughtful, constructive feedback before seeing actual patients.

Simulated patients

A variety of techniques involving simulated patients have been used for teaching and assessing communication skills, ranging from the basic up to more advanced topics such as breaking bad news, genetic counselling, pain management, and shared decision-making (Mavis *et al.* 2002; Wakefield *et al.* 2003; Windish *et al.* 2005; McGovern *et al.* 2006). The same people who are trained to portray patients can also be trained to portray family members, a role that is especially important in palliative medicine and critical care, where over 60% of advance directive discussions occur with a proxy (Lorin *et al.* 2006).

When simulated patients are incorporated into teaching, they serve as 'patient instructors' who modulate their demeanour, change personal details of the role they portray (e.g. relationships, coping styles, emotions, lifestyles, work situations, family dynamics), and provide feedback. In contrast, when involved in assessments, simulated patients function as 'standardized patients'. The term 'standardized' means just that: Standardized patients invoke a consistent demeanour and the same set of information—during each student encounter. They are, in essence, the test. Accordingly, they employ consistent criteria for evaluating each student.

While potential disadvantages of simulated patients include cost as well as the need for training and support staff, there are considerable advantages ranging from validity (Colliver *et al.* 1999) to opportunities for direct feedback, multiple observation points, and focused practice of basic and advanced skills in a safe environment. Moreover, they afford a level of authenticity that is rarely achieved in traditional role play. Consider this excerpt from *Cutting the Cord: Five Stories about the First Year of Medical School* (Makoul and Malinowski 1998), a documentary that features the experiences of medical students:

> The coolest part about medical school so far was the first time we went in for our patient instructor session. The first session we had, I'd just be coming in and introducing myself—meeting the patient. Before I knocked on the door I thought to myself: This is it. This is like the real thing. This is, you know—not even that it was just practice or play or just an exercise, but this is really what it's all about. This is me going in, meeting a patient for the first time, starting to make a relationship, learning everything about that patient, and starting to analyze what is going on with that patient—what we can do to make that patient's life better. And it was like this whole revelation that happened before I knocked on the door, before I walked in the room.

> Text extracts reproduced with permission from video produced by Makoul, G. and Malinowski, D., *Cutting the Cord: Five Stories about the First Year of Medical School*, Northwestern University, Feinberg School of Medicine, Chicago, Illinois, USA, Copyright © 1998 Gregory Makoul.

This example illuminates a key issue: Students know that interactions with simulated patients are an 'exercise', but they take them very seriously when their patient instructors and standardized patients are well prepared.

The SEGUE Framework

A key need for students is a conceptual framework that is flexible enough for diverse situations yet sufficiently specific to afford practical guidance. One example is the SEGUE Framework for Teaching and Assessing Communication Skills (Makoul 2001), a well-validated and widely used approach that parallels the flow of a clinical encounter in most specialties. The SEGUE Framework has been adopted for undergraduate medical education in many countries over the past 20 years, and is in widespread use across the continuum of training today.

As illustrated in Figure 7.1, the SEGUE Framework outlines specific communication tasks that comprise effective encounters, organized within the acronymic rubric (Set the stage, Elicit information, Give information, Understand the patient's perspective,

and End the encounter). There is also a section delineating tasks that relate directly to discussing a new or modified treatment plan. Makoul and Schofield have noted that:

> Focusing on tasks provides a sense of purpose for learning communication skills. The task approach also preserves the individuality of students by encouraging them to develop a repertoire of strategies and skills, and respond to patients in a flexible way (Makoul and Schofield 1999).

For instance, if one task is defined as 'make a personal connection with the patient', students and physicians can proceed in a variety of equally effective ways, choosing one that fits their own personal style, the particular patient, and the situation. This built-in flexibility with respect to the skills and strategies required for each task reflects the individuality of human communication. The task approach directs attention towards communication content and process, rather than bedside manner per se. While it focuses on observable behaviour, this approach can facilitate discussion and exploration of attitudes relevant to each task as well.

Using the SEGUE Framework in oncology and palliative care

Both oncology and palliative care emphasize understanding the patient, the family, and the dynamics around illness. The recognition that suffering is multidimensional—embodying physical, emotional, spiritual, and existential pain—is a fundamental observation of Dame Cicely Saunders, the nurse and social worker who became a physician and founder of the hospice movement (Saunders and Baines 1983). This theme has been extended to emphasize how much healthcare, in any context, can alleviate or exacerbate suffering (Lee and Hut 2014).

By focusing attention on communication tasks associated with setting the stage, eliciting and giving information, understanding the patient perspective, and properly ending encounters, the SEGUE Framework is an important tool in oncology and palliative care, where the importance of addressing multiple frames of reference (e.g. patient, family, medical team) is heightened. Moreover, the tasks associated with discussing a new or modified treatment plan are often more complex in this context, as there are trade-offs between length of life and quality of life. For instance, for some patients in the oncology setting, relevant options include surgery, chemotherapy, radiation, off-label therapies, and emerging genomic therapies, as well as purely palliative care.

What is unique about oncology and palliative care as a context for communication?

Several noteworthy differences make communication fundamentally challenging and particularly important for medical students and experienced physicians alike:

1. *Role of the physician.* Oncology and palliative care physicians are almost always consultants to patients and their families, and consequently do not have a long-term relationship that facilitates shared expectations. Palliative care physicians are also consultants to other providers and, these days, patients tend to have numerous providers. Serving as a 'new set of eyes' can help the palliative team work towards reconciling divergent perspectives. This makes eliciting information to assess the extent of shared

understanding all the more crucial, magnifying the importance of each encounter and adding pressure to build human connections quickly and effectively.

2. *Severity of illness*. Although patients are referred to palliative and hospice care for a number of different reasons, the predominant trigger is life-threatening or life-limiting illness, often with multiple co-morbidities requiring coordinated, compassionate management. This clearly distinguishes palliative care from most other specialties. Accordingly, communication must focus on the primary reason for palliative care as well as on other conditions, needs, and limitations.

3. *Interdisciplinary teams*. Oncology and palliative care emphasize interdisciplinary teamwork. This calls for enhanced incorporation of the strengths of different team members: integrative practitioners, nurses, nurse practitioners, pharmacists, physician assistants, physicians, social workers, and spiritual care providers. While such cooperation requires much more than just assembling a group of providers and clarifying roles, limited data address how teamwork 'works' in palliative care (Goebel *et al.* 2015). At a fundamental level, expectations for communication, coordination, and functional leadership need to be transparent for teams at every stage of development.

The SEGUE Framework   Patient: _____   Physician or Student: _____

Set the stage

		Yes	No
1.	Greet patient appropriately		
2.	Establish reason for visit _____		
3.	Outline agenda for visit (e.g. 'anything else?', issues, sequence)		
4.	Make a personal connection during visit (e.g. go beyond medical issues at hand)		
→5.	Maintain patient's privacy (e.g. close door)		

Elicit information

		n/a	Yes	No
6.	Elicit patient's view of health problem and/or progress			
7.	Explore physical/physiological factors			
8.	Explore psychosocial/emotional factors (e.g. living situation, family relations, stress)			
9.	Discuss antecedent treatments (e.g. self-care, last visit, other medical care)			
10.	Discuss how health problem affects patient's life (e.g. quality-of-life)			
11.	Discuss life-style issues/prevention strategies (e.g. health risks)			
→12.	Avoid directive/leading questions			
→13.	Give patient opportunity/time to talk (e.g. don't interrupt)			
→14.	Listen. Give patient undivided attention (e.g. face patient, verbal acknowledgement, non-verbal feedback)			
→15.	Check/clarify information (e.g. recap, ask 'how much')			

Give information

		n/a	Yes	No
16.	Explain rationale for diagnostic procedures (e.g. exam, tests)			
17.	Teach patient about his/her own body and situation (e.g. provide feedback from exam/tests, explain rationale)			
18.	Encourage patient to ask questions/check understanding			
→19.	Adapt to patient's level of understanding (e.g. avoid/explain jargon)			

Fig. 7.1 The SEGUE Framework.

Note: Items without an arrow focus on *content*; mark 'Yes' if done *at least one time* during the encounter.

Items with an arrow (→) focus on *process* and should be maintained throughout the encounter; mark 'No' if at least one relevant instance when *not* done.

Understand the patient's perspective

		n/a	Yes	No
20.	Acknowledge patient's accomplishments/progress/challenges			
21.	Acknowledge waiting time			
→22.	Express caring, concern, empathy			
→23.	Maintain a respectful tone			

End the encounter

		Yes	No
24.	Ask if there is anything else patient would like to discuss		
25.	Review next steps with patient		

If suggested a new or modified treatment/prevention plan:

		n/a	Yes	No
26.	Discuss patient's expectation/goal for treatment/prevention			
27.	Involve patient in deciding upon a plan (e.g. options, rationale, values, preferences, concerns)			
28.	Explain likely benefits of the option(s) discussed			
29.	Explain likely side-effects and risks of the option(s) discussed			
30.	Provide complete instructions for plan			
31.	Discuss patient's ability to follow plan			
32.	Discuss importance of patient's role in treatment/prevention			

Fig. 7.1 Continued

4. *Dying and death.* Many patients or families conflate palliative care with hospice, and perceive that hospice is where you go to die. Feelings and fears of 'throwing in the towel' or 'giving up' are common. The crucial strategy here is to avoid the trap and distraction of defending hospice, instead exploring sources of feelings and helping people cope with the sense of sadness, loss, and grief that are often present.

5. *Involvement of families.* Palliative care explicitly views the family as vital to the care of patients. Practical reasons apply: many patients cannot communicate; many patients rely on family members to give medications and other forms of care. Compelling humanistic and philosophical reasons also apply (Gawande 2014). Yet it is important to recognize that family members of seriously ill patients carry increased risk for morbidity of their own, as well as mortality and financial hardship (Christakis and Allison 2006). Students must expand their view beyond the traditional doctor–patient paradigm to one that fully engages third parties, as discussed in Chapter 17.

Advanced communication skills for medical students

Oncology and palliative care present many predicaments that require advanced communication skills to augment the approach to accomplishing basic communication tasks outlined in the SEGUE Framework. While training for these skills begins in medical school, they must grow apace throughout residency and beyond if they are to be deployed efficiently and effectively. Although we focus on cancer in this book, these advanced skills serve all clinicians with patients facing difficult situations. In the remainder of this chapter,

we explore several domains of advanced communication skills and consider implications for medical student training.

Each of the areas addressed can be taught to medical students in small groups with role play and/or with simulated patients. Medical students on clinical rotation can observe and participate in these interactions, and reflect upon them with peers and preceptors. Advanced medical students with adequate support and preparation can even 'take the lead' on some of these conversations if accompanied by an experienced mentor, whether physician, physician assistant, nurse practitioner, or clinical social worker.

Bad news

Although a new diagnosis of cancer is often held up as the paradigm for breaking bad news, more common situations include referral to hospice, referral to a long-term care facility, and even mere palliative care consultation. Medical students and residents clearly recognize the myriad forms of bad news, ranging from mundane to highly charged (Makoul 1998). They recognize the need for training about how to approach the topic, how to be sensitive, how to be direct, how to be clear/informative, how to read/predict patient reactions, how to handle patient reactions, how to handle their own reactions, how to minimize harm/pain, how to help/support the patient, what to tell, when to tell, where to tell, who to tell, how much to tell, appropriate emotion to convey, appropriate non-verbal communication, and appropriate verbal communication (Makoul 1998).

As detailed in Chapter 12, a widely disseminated approach is called SPIKES (Baile *et al.* 2000). SPIKES has much in common with the SEGUE Framework, but is tailored specifically to disclosure of bad news. More specifically, SPIKES reinforces basic communication principles such as providing privacy, minimizing interruptions, checking patient understanding about his illness, asking how much detail is desired, providing information clearly and simply, and encouraging questions. SPIKES offers a guideline for any segment of a clinical interview in which new and difficult information needs to be revealed. As with any guideline, it serves as a resource for learning, not a rigid prescription. Medical students become increasingly effective as they move from regarding models (e.g. SEGUE Framework or SPIKES) as scripts, to using them as scaffolds to build meaningful conversations and relationships.

Prognosis/uncertainty

While communicating prognosis is a challenging topic for physicians-in-training and physicians-in-practice, patients and families seem to have an increasingly insistent desire to receive this information (Butow *et al.* 2002; Bernacki and Block 2014). The relative neglect of prognosis in medical textbooks is only partially offset by improvements in prognostic rules and scales (Lamont and Christakis 2003, Glare *et al.* 2004), which can be used to teach medical students to estimate prognosis. By definition, these apply to populations, not to individual patients. Accordingly, two extremes are best avoided: first, giving a specific number ('You have 6 months'), and second, saying only 'I don't know'. While it is literally true that one can never know exactly what the future will bring, saying nothing beyond 'I don't know' discredits physician knowledge and expertise, and makes it more difficult for patients and families to plan (see Chapter 13 for detailed material on discussing prognosis).

When teaching medical students about prognosis, we favour a process akin to that used in breaking bad news: ask what patients already know and what level of detail they would like to have, then present a prognostic estimate using time ranges such as 'days to weeks' or 'weeks to months'. While acknowledging uncertainty, students can learn to give patients and families a general idea about the future without undue vagueness or misplaced pseudo-specificity. The work of the Serious Illness Care Program reinforces this concept vividly (Ariadne Labs 2015; Bernacki and Block 2014).

Goals of care/introducing palliative care

As hospice and palliative services continue to expand worldwide, the communication task of transitioning patients and families to palliative care takes on added importance and urgency. There are data associating hospice with attitudes of 'giving up' or 'not being appropriately treated' (Daugherty and Steensma 2002; Friedman *et al.* 2002). Maintaining hope in the face of life-threatening illness is a core skill and an ongoing challenge for every practitioner (Casarett and Quill 2007; Boyd and Murray 2014). To introduce the topic, medical students can ask questions that revolve around goals of care, which is particularly important because patients, families, and care teams often talk about the plan of care before ascertaining whether they have different goals in mind. Indeed, a recent review notes that 'Communication about the goals of care is a low-risk, high-value intervention for patients with serious and life-threatening illness' (Bernacki and Block 2014). Questions along the lines of 'What are you hoping for?' or 'What are you expecting to happen?' afford an open-ended way of doing this. In response, some patients may begin sharing their views about not dying in hospital, or the value of good symptom control.

When such an open-ended approach proves unfruitful, it can be helpful to frame the situation more narrowly: 'We are concerned that things have worsened and that, at this point, chemotherapy may do more harm than good. I imagine that you might have thought about this too'. A follow-up question might be: 'Given the current picture, what is most important for you?'. For some patients, endorsement of the palliative approach could be a natural next step: 'In these situations, we often find that a focus on comfort, quality of life, and support for you and your family is the most helpful'. The specific words are less important than the beginning with an open-ended elicitation of patient perspective and, if necessary, moving to a more focused inquiry that broaches death and the need for palliative care.

Conflict management

Conflict is a challenge in oncology situations, especially around decisions regarding medical futility, once again highlighting frames of reference as a critical factor in human communication. Indeed, many conflicts arise from differences in understanding, values, and goals between patient, family members, and healthcare professionals (Goold *et al.* 2000). Moreover, pre-existing family conflict is often exacerbated when a loved one has a life-threatening illness (Kramer *et al.* 2010).

Given this state of affairs, focusing on conflict management—with attention to specific tasks and skills such as facilitation, negotiation, and understanding multiple perspectives—makes excellent sense. Curricular materials addressing conflict management for medical students have improved student confidence in navigating conflict (Ang 2002). Of course, in addition to conflict within families, there may be conflicts between families and healthcare professionals, and between the healthcare professionals themselves.

Family meetings

Conducting family meetings is a core competency, and the associated skill set is increasingly recognized as critical throughout medical practice (see Chapter 18). A fundamental tenet of palliative care is the strong belief that patients and family members—together—form the unit of care. Although definitions of families vary, we and others find it most useful to consider anyone who is important to a patient, whether related by blood or marriage or neither, as a family member. This definition deliberately accommodates both friends and significant others. While it is beyond the scope of this chapter to explore the variety of family types and dynamics, two basic points are critical:

1. *Family members have different frames of reference.* Given varied educational and professional backgrounds—and relational histories—family members have differing perspectives on the patient and on relevant medical decisions, goals, and preferences.

2. *Families may have pre-existing conflicts.* In addition to different opinions about dealing with illness, families often carry long-term disagreements or conflicts, which worsen under the stress of illness. Over time, families develop their own styles of negotiating, coping, and reaching consensus, some of which are more functional and adaptive than others. Family members need time and space to work through decisions; and they may be looking for help—and even a referee of sorts.

Accordingly, normalizing disparate perspectives ('We often see families having different points of view about things') and acknowledging conflict ('Some families have different perspectives that lead to strong disagreements') enhance efficacy.

Although there are various forms of contact between families and healthcare professionals, one common setting is a family meeting. Here, a team gathers with the family to discuss the patient's condition and treatment, as well as goals and next steps. As in any meeting, a clear agenda, strong leadership, and defined roles improve the likelihood of positive process and outcome. There are three stages of a family meeting: (i) preparation to clarify who will attend and their roles, including who will lead the meeting; (ii) the meeting itself, during which all are introduced, the agenda is followed, and recommendations are summarized; (iii) the post-meeting phase, during which the plan is carried out. Well-structured and effectively facilitated family meetings allow expression of and making headway on emotions, conflict, and difficult decisions (Cook and Rocker 2014; Weissman 2010a–f).

Communication and teamwork

It is not unusual for patients in palliative care to have many professional caregivers. On the medical side, these include medical students, residents, nurse practitioners and physician assistants, fellows/registrars, attending physicians, and a seemingly endless stream of hospitalists and consultants. On the nursing side, hospitalized patients receive care from multiple staff nurses and nursing assistants. Within a week on a typical hospital-based palliative care programme, patients may be seen by 8 physicians, 2–4 staff nurses, 2 nursing assistants, and 1–2 social workers. Accordingly, effective communication between professional caregivers is indispensable and rate-limiting for any degree of coordinated, cohesive care. In addition to systemic interventions that support such communication (e.g. daily huddles and interdisciplinary team meetings), it is vital that all clinicians involved with care strive to enhance interpersonal communication skills with each other, as well as with patients and families. The realization that patients and families need help with coordination of care (i.e. they can't and shouldn't have to do it themselves), is an essential touchstone for medical students and all members of the team.

In terms of improving communication among providers, use of a daily goals checklist in the intensive care unit (ICU) has been shown to be an effective intervention (Pronovost et al. 2003). In addition, efforts to train ICU staff in interdisciplinary communication around end-of-life care and family meetings have also been successful (Shaw et al. 2014). At least one study has revealed significant difficulties in communication between medical students and nurses (Nadolski et al. 2006). A first step to better communication—and better care—is basic awareness of the roles and strengths that different professionals bring to the team (Schneiderman 2015). More active strategies for efficient and focused communication include explicitly involving nurses, social workers, and other team members in critical decisions about care, eliciting perspectives of multiple team members, and actively listening during multidisciplinary team meetings (see Chapter 33).

Conclusion

This overview of communication education for medical students introduces subsequent chapters that offer further curriculum guidance. The overarching goal is a continuum of training to grow the skills of young clinicians as they perform increasingly sophisticated clinical tasks and learn to cope with increasingly complex patients. At root, attention to their own humanity and frame-of-reference—as well as the humanity and unique perspectives of patients, families, and colleagues—will enhance learning and care throughout this continuum. In every country that trains medical students, efforts to build excellence in both basic and advanced communication skills must be explicitly recognized and commensurately resourced as the very core of establishing a truly healing profession.

References

Ang M (2002). Advanced communication skills: conflict management and persuasion. *Acad Med* **77**, 1166.

Ariadne Labs. 2015. *Serious Illness Care* [Online]. Boston: Ariadne Labs. Available at: http://www.ariadnelabs.org/programs/serious-illness-care/ [Accessed February 21, 2015].

Baile W F, Buckman R, Lenzi R, Glober G, Beale EA, Kudelka AP (2000). SPIKES-A six-step protocol for delivering bad news: application to the patient with cancer. *Oncologist* **5**, 302–11.

Batalden P, Leach D, Swing S, Dreyfus H, Dreyfus S (2002). General competencies and accreditation in graduate medical education. *Health Aff (Millwood)* **21**, 103–11.

Bernacki RE, Block SD (2014). Communication about serious illness care goals: a review and synthesis of best practices. *JAMA Intern Med* **174**, 1994–2003.

Boyd K, Murray SA (2014). Why is talking about dying such a challenge? *BMJ* **348**, g3699.

Butow PN, Dowsett S, Hagerty R, Tattersall MH (2002). Communicating prognosis to patients with metastatic disease: what do they really want to know? *Support Care Cancer* **10**, 161–8.

Casarett DJ, Quill TE (2007). "I'm not ready for hospice": strategies for timely and effective hospice discussions. *Ann Intern Med* **146**, 443–9.

Cegala DJ, Marinelli T, Post D (2000). The effects of patient communication skills training on compliance. *Arch Fam Med* **9**, 57–64.

Christakis NA, Allison PD (2006). Mortality after the hospitalization of a spouse. *N Engl J Med* **354**, 719–30.

Colliver JA, Swartz MH, Robbs RS, Cohen DS (1999). Relationship between clinical competence and interpersonal and communication skills in standardized-patient assessment. *Acad Med* **74**, 271–4.

Cook D, Rocker G (2014). Dying with dignity in the intensive care unit. *N Engl J Med* **370**, 2506–14.

Daugherty CK, Steensma DP (2002). Overcoming obstacles to hospice care: an ethical examination of inertia and inaction. *J Clin Oncol* **20**, 2752–5.

Friedman BT, Harwood MK, Shields M (2002). Barriers and enablers to hospice referrals: an expert overview. *J Palliat Med* **5**, 73–84.

Gawande A (2014). *Being Mortal: Medicine and What Matters Most in the End*. Metropolitan Books, New York, NY.

General Medical Council (2013). *Domain 3: Communication, partnership and teamwork* [Online]. General Medical Council. Available at: http://www.gmc-uk.org/guidance/good_medical_practice/communication_partnership_teamwork.asp [Accessed January 14, 2015].

Glare PA, Eychmueller S, Mcmahon P (2004). Diagnostic accuracy of the palliative prognostic score in hospitalized patients with advanced cancer. *J Clin Oncol* **22**, 4823–8.

Goebel J, Guo W, Chong K (2015). A team of experts or an expert team: interdisciplinary teamwork and perceptions of palliative care quality. *J Pain Symptom Manage* **49**, 429.

Goold SD, Williams B, Arnold RM (2000). Conflicts regarding decisions to limit treatment: a differential diagnosis. *JAMA* **283**, 909–14.

Hafferty FW (1998). Beyond curriculum reform: confronting medicine's hidden curriculum. *Acad Med* **73**, 403–7.

Horowitz SD (2000). Evaluation of clinical competencies: basic certification, subspecialty certification, and recertification. *Am J Phys Med Rehabil* **79**, 478–80.

Kramer BJ, Kavanaugh M, Trentham-Dietz A, Walsh M, Yonker JA (2010). Predictors of family conflict at the end of life: the experience of spouses and adult children of persons with lung cancer. *Gerontologist* **50**, 215–25.

Lamont EB, Christakis NA (2003). Complexities in prognostication in advanced cancer: "to help them live their lives the way they want to." *JAMA* **290**, 98–104.

Lee T, Hut N (2014). Thomas Lee: the value of alleviating patient suffering. *Healthc Financ Manage* **68**, 50–3.

Liaison Committee on Medical Education (2013). *Functions and Structure of a Medical School: Standards for Accreditation of Medical Education Programs Leading to the M.D. Degree*. Liaison Committee on Medical Education, Washington DC, WA.

Lorin S, Rho L, Wisnivesky JP, Nierman DM (2006). Improving medical student intensive care unit communication skills: a novel educational initiative using standardized family members. *Crit Care Med* **34**, 2386–91.

Makoul G (1998). Medical student and resident perspectives on delivering bad news. *Acad Med* **73**, S35–7.

Makoul G (2001). The SEGUE Framework for teaching and assessing communication skills. *Patient Educ Couns* **45**, 23–34.

Makoul G, Malinowski D (1998). *Cutting the Cord: Five Stories about the First Year of Medical School*. Northwestern University Feinberg School of Medicine, Chicago, IL.

Makoul G, Schofield T (1999). Communication teaching and assessment in medical education: an international consensus statement. Netherlands Institute of Primary Health Care. *Patient Educ Couns* **37**, 191–5.

Makoul G, Zick AB, Aakhus M, Neely KJ, Roemer PE (2010). Using an online forum to encourage reflection about difficult conversations in medicine. *Patient Educ Couns* **79**, 83–6.

Mavis BE, Ogle KS, Lovell KL, Madden LM (2002). Medical students as standardized patients to assess interviewing skills for pain evaluation. *Med Educ* **36**, 135–40.

Mcgovern MM, Johnston M, Brown K, Zinberg R, Cohen D (2006). Use of standardized patients in undergraduate medical genetics education. *Teach Learn Med* **18**, 203–7.

Nadolski GJ, Bell MA, Brewer BB, Frankel RM, Cushing HE, Brokaw JJ (2006). Evaluating the quality of interaction between medical students and nurses in a large teaching hospital. *BMC Med Educ* **6**, 23.

Nestel D, Tierney T (2007). Role-play for medical students learning about communication: guidelines for maximising benefits. *BMC Med Educ* **7**, 3.

Pronovost P, Berenholtz S, Dorman T, Lipsett PA, Simmonds T, Haraden C (2003). Improving communication in the ICU using daily goals. *J Crit Care* **18**, 71–5.

Saunders C, Baines M (1983). *Living with Dying: The Management of Terminal Disease*. Oxford University Press, Oxford, UK.

Schneiderman H (2015). A piece of my mind: Efficacy at the bedside. *JAMA* **313**, 569–70.

Shaw DJ, Davidson JE, Smilde RI, Sondoozi T, Agan D (2014). Multidisciplinary team training to enhance family communication in the ICU. *Crit Care Med* **42**, 265–71.

Stewart M (2005). Reflections on the doctor-patient relationship: from evidence and experience. *Br J Gen Pract* **55**, 793–801.

Stewart M, Brown JB, Boon H, Galajda J, Meredith L, Sangster M (1999). Evidence on patient-doctor communication. *Cancer Prev Control* **3**, 25–30.

Tamblyn R, Abrahamowicz M, Dauphinee D, *et al.* (2007). Physician scores on a national clinical skills examination as predictors of complaints to medical regulatory authorities. *JAMA* **298**, 993–1001.

The Joint Commission (2010). *The Joint Commission: Advancing Effective Communication, Cultural Competence, and Patient- and Family-Centered Care: A Roadmap for Hospitals*. The Joint Commission, Oakbrook Terrace, IL.

Wakefield A, Cooke S, Boggis C (2003). Learning together: use of simulated patients with nursing and medical students for breaking bad news. *Int J Palliat Nurs* **9**, 32–8.

Weissman DE, Quill TE, Arnold RM (2010*a*). The family meeting: causes of conflict #225. *J Palliat Med* **13**, 328–9.

Weissman DE, Quill TE, Arnold RM (2010*b*). The family meeting: end-of-life goal setting and future planning #227. *J Palliat Med* **13**, 462–3.

Weissman DE, Quill TE, Arnold RM (2010*c*). The family meeting: starting the conversation #223. *J Palliat Med* **13**, 204–5.

Weissman DE, Quill TE, Arnold RM (2010*d*). Helping surrogates make decisions #226. *J Palliat Med* **13**, 461–2.

Weissman DE, Quill TE, Arnold RM (2010*e*). Preparing for the family meeting #222. *J Palliat Med* **13**, 203–4.

Weissman DE, Quill TE, Arnold RM (2010*f*). Responding to emotion in family meetings #224. *J Palliat Med* **13**, 327–8.

Windish DM, Price EG, Clever SL, Magaziner JL, Thomas PA (2005). Teaching medical students the important connection between communication and clinical reasoning. *J Gen Intern Med* **20**, 1108–13.

CHAPTER 8

Training patients to reach their communication goals: A concordance perspective

Thomas A. D'Agostino, Carma L. Bylund, and Betty Chewning

Introduction to training patients to reach their communication goals

As the volume of literature in this book suggests, improving clinicians' communication is currently the subject of much scholarship throughout the world. Improving clinicians' communication is necessary, but on its own is not sufficient to achieve the best possible communication in a clinical encounter. This chapter focuses on an area that has received less attention—training patients to be good communicators. The physician–patient interaction is a dynamic, socially-constructed, and reciprocal process (Parker *et al.* 2005; Street 2003) that relies on at least two participants. Effective communication requires both parties to be actively involved and competent communicators. Moreover, patients' communication may influence physicians' responses (Roter *et al.* 1997). Thus, to fully understand and improve physician–patient communication requires a focus on both sides of the interaction.

Such a focus is particularly important given that patients face many challenges in their clinical consultations, including physicians' ethnic or cultural biases (Street 2003), interruptions (Marvel *et al.* 1999), lack of empathic communication (Bylund and Makoul 2005), minimal tolerance for patients' desires to talk about internet information (Street 2003), and a lack of physician–patient concordance (Chewning and Wiederholt 2003; Parker *et al.* 2005). Despite the research and teaching efforts that have gone into physician training, patient communication training must also be addressed in order to achieve optimal physician–patient communication. Considerable research has indicated that there is room for improvement in patients' communication skills, including asking questions (Brown *et al.* 2001), explicitly stating concerns (Butow *et al.* 2002), and verifying information (Cegala *et al.* 2000*b*). The ineffective use of these skills may contribute to patients' misunderstanding of information given to them (Cegala *et al.* 2000*b*) and/or lack of treatment adherence (Golin *et al.* 1996).

This chapter begins with a review of studies of patient communication training. We then move to an explanation of the concept of concordance in the physician–patient relationship and how concordance provides a fruitful conceptual grounding for patient communication training.

Review of patient communication training studies

Published studies on patient communication training in the cancer setting are sparse. Consequently, we have chosen to review literature on patient communication training more broadly. Patient communication training studies differ in both method and content of training, as well as reported outcomes.

Method of training

We have expanded upon the definition of Parker and colleagues (Parker *et al.* 2005) in describing the methods of patient communication training. The three methods of training present in the literature are materials only, materials plus coaching, and group-based interventions.

Materials only

Materials-only communication interventions include those in which patients are given written materials to use on their own. Such methods usually include the use of question prompt lists, which have been shown to increase the number of questions patients ask their oncologist, particularly around the topics of tests, treatment, and prognosis (Brown *et al.* 1999; Brown *et al.* 2001). Since question prompt lists are comprehensively reviewed elsewhere, they will not be covered in detail here. The most widely used patient communication skills curriculum was developed by Cegala and colleagues (Cegala *et al.* 2000*a*; Cegala *et al.* 2000*b*). Initially designed as an educational booklet, the PACE System expanded the focus of materials-only interventions beyond just asking questions and has been used in several empirical studies (Cegala *et al.* 2000*a*; Cegala *et al.* 2000*b*; Cegala *et al.* 2001; Post *et al.* 2001). Katz *et al.* (2012) evaluated an educational video intervention to facilitate colorectal cancer screening discussions and adherence in low-income minority patients. Entitled *Ask your doctor about colon cancer* *screening*, the 12-minute video was supplemented by two brochures and included the PACE curriculum. More recently, Meropol *et al.* (2013) incorporated the PACE curriculum into an interactive web-based communication aid for cancer patients. Details regarding content of the PACE System will be discussed below.

Materials plus coaching

The second type of intervention category is materials plus coaching. This method involves the use of a one-on-one intervention in which a researcher interacts directly with a patient to discuss specific communication strategies or skills that can be used during consultations. Such methods may utilize some elements described in materials-only interventions (e.g. question prompt sheets), but differ in that they also include a component of rehearsal or coaching (Parker *et al.* 2005).

Cegala and colleagues have tested an intervention comparing patients receiving the PACE System booklet with patients who received the booklet and also had individual coaching (Cegala *et al.* 2001; Cegala *et al.* 2000a; Cegala *et al.* 2000b; Post *et al.* 2001). The coaching process involved asking patients if they experienced any problems using the training booklet, going over the booklet page by page, and helping patients organize how they would approach the consultation (Cegala *et al.* 2001).

Street *et al.* (2010) conducted a randomized controlled trial evaluating a tailored education-coaching intervention designed to assist cancer patients in discussing pain-related questions, concerns, and preferences with physicians. Each intervention patient met with a trained health educator for 20 to 40 minutes prior to their scheduled oncology visit and received a set of individualized messages and skill-building exercises. Patients randomized to the enhanced usual care arm met with a health educator to review educational materials on pain control.

Bylund *et al.* (2011) piloted a workshop aimed at improving healthcare communication skills in a minority cancer patient population. The communication skills training workshops were delivered to patients by the lead author, a communication specialist, on-site at a community-based oncology clinic. Each face-to-face workshop consisted of a 20 to 30 minute didactic presentation and open discussion with video clips demonstrating communication skills. Control group participants completed surveys only.

Group-based interventions

The third patient communication intervention method found in the literature is group-based interventions. To follow, we summarize four articles that have described the development and evaluation of such group-based interventions.

Within an oncology setting, Fisch and colleagues (2003) conducted a one-day workshop called *My Life, My Choice*, held to educate cancer patients and family members about improving communication with their cancer care providers. The eight-hour workshop made use of a combination of lectures, as well as both large and small group discussions facilitated by healthcare professionals.

Other group-based interventions have been open to individuals beyond cancer. Tran and colleagues (2004) described a community education forum aimed at improving active patient communication. Entitled *How to Talk to Your Physician*, the two-hour programme was presented by a physician and non-physician, in an effort to establish the collaborative nature of the physician–patient interaction. Towle and colleagues (2003) designed and implemented interactive workshops for seniors at a community centre with the goal of promoting active participation in consultations. The workshops were about two hours in duration and involved participants receiving a booklet of communication skills, which were then modelled by simulated physicians and patients.

Peek and colleagues (2012) tested a ten-session, culturally-tailored patient empowerment intervention for low-income African American patients with diabetes. Lasting approximately 90 minutes each, weekly sessions included a variety of interactive educational components, including group discussions, role play, individual testimonies, and more.

Content of training

Many patient communication interventions focus almost exclusively on patient question asking. Although asking questions is critically important to effective physician–patient communication, other interventions have included a more comprehensive range of skills.

The PACE System, developed by Cegala (Cegala *et al.* 2000a; Cegala *et al.* 2000b), proposes that effective patient communication involves four components: *Presenting Detailed Information; Asking Questions; Checking Understanding; and Expressing Concerns. Presenting Detailed Information* involves being prepared before the consultation to give a focused and extensive breadth of information about symptoms, history, reasons for visit, needs, etc. *Asking Questions* pertains to having a preset list of questions prepared that will deepen understanding of any information, treatments, tests, or diagnoses that may be presented in the consultation. *Checking Understanding* is a form of information verification, and can involve skills such as asking the physician to clarify information that is unclear, repeating aloud the information that is provided to improve retention, and summarizing the information back to the physician in order to check understanding. Finally, *Expressing Concerns* aims to bring to light any conflicts or concerns (e.g. religious, cultural) that may hinder treatment or the physician–patient interaction. Through open expression of these concerns, a mutual effort of resolution can be reached.

The PACE System has been included in a number of patient communication interventions. For example, Towle and colleagues (2003) used Cegala's PACE curriculum in their group-based workshops for seniors. The PACE System was also incorporated into a colorectal cancer screening video intervention (Katz *et al.* 2012). The educational video included physicians describing facts about colorectal cancer and the importance of screening. The informational section was followed by a narrative portion that focused on communication skills and offered patient testimonials to reinforce the importance of completing screening tests. In addition to viewing the 12-minute video, intervention participants received a brochure that focused on asking their provider for a colorectal cancer screening test.

Other research studies have adapted the PACE System. Cegala *et al.* (2013) altered the PACE curriculum, keying content to suit an intervention for parents of paediatric surgery patients. Meropol *et al.* (2013) adapted the PACE System in designing a theory-guided, interactive web-based communication aid for cancer patients. Referred to as CONNECT, this communication aid includes an assessment of patient values, goals, and communication preferences, a communication skills training component, and a pre-consultation summary report for physicians.

Bylund *et al.* (2011) built upon the PACE System, incorporating a fifth communication strategy focusing on *Stating Preferences* concerning communication, treatment, and role responsibilities in decision-making. This communication skill allows each patient to take an active role in shaping the dynamic of the physician–patient relationship and flow of information.

A different patient communication training curriculum was designed and utilized by Fisch and colleagues (2003). The community-based workshop for cancer patients and their families was divided into three sessions. Session one was entitled *Getting Through the Diagnosis/Prognosis Phase* and involved presentation of skills relevant to reviewing healthcare insurance, choosing the right physician, and slowing down to verify diagnosis, seek second opinions, and clarify information. Session two, *Exploring Treatment Options*, consisted of informing patients of barriers to understanding and then skills training to overcome them. Often problems such as being flooded with information, losing a sense of control within a consultation, and unfamiliar jargon can hinder understanding. This session helped inform patients of such issues that they may not be aware of, as well as teaching skills like asking questions and bringing support to visits. Furthermore, this session also aimed to expand patients' knowledge regarding the importance of exploring treatment options. Finally, session three, *Asking the Difficult Questions*, focused on dealing with terminal illness and death. Patients were provided with information regarding emotional responses they may encounter, coping strategies, informing loved ones, preparing for death, and self-assessment of faith, life, and final goals.

Another patient communication training curriculum has been developed and used in community educational forums (Tran *et al.* 2004). Each forum involved attendees receiving a 20-page orientation guidebook and engaging in an interactive discussion facilitated by co-educators, including trigger videos, provocative questions about physician–patient interactions, and suggestions for improving communication. Most relevant to effective patient communication training are the tips for improving patient/physician communication. These are similar to Cegala's concept of PACE, and use an 'ABC' mnemonic to improve recall: *Asking questions to receive information, Being prepared for each visit,* and *expressing one's Concerns.*

The tailored education-coaching intervention offered by Street *et al.* (2010) included several components designed to increase self-efficacy, enhance physician–patient communication, and improve care of cancer-related pain. Patients met with a health educator who provided each patient with a copy of the National Cancer Institute's booklet *Pain Control: A Guide for Patients with Cancer and their Families*; examined current knowledge, attitudes, and preferences regarding pain management; corrected misconceptions about cancer pain control; taught relevant pain control concepts and communication skills (e.g. asking questions, expressing concerns, stating opinions and preferences); guided planning (e.g. identifying goals, matching effective strategies); and facilitated the development of a list of questions and concerns about pain. Patients were also offered the opportunity to role play.

Finally, the culturally-tailored patient empowerment intervention developed by Peek *et al.* (2012) included three content areas addressed across ten sessions. The first six class sessions consisted of general diabetes education and self-management skills, including disease-related information and dietary/nutrition choices. Patients participated in several experiential exercises. For example, a mock grocery store was created, allowing patients an opportunity to practice food choice and lifestyle skills. The next three sessions focused on shared decision-making and physician–patient communication. These sessions addressed perceived barriers, behavioural beliefs, and subjective norms around decision-making, as well as covering communication and negotiation skills (e.g. asking more questions, providing more details). The final session provided an opportunity to review materials and practice self-care, shared decision-making, and communication skills.

Outcomes of patient communication training

With few comprehensive patient communication training programmes published to date, our report on outcomes is limited. The outcomes reported in these studies can be divided into several categories, including patient self-efficacy, behavioural intention, patient satisfaction, observations of patient skill usage, and adherence.

One simple outcome that can be assessed is how the communication training affected patients' self-efficacy. Results of the community education forum described by Tran *et al.* (2004) indicated that participants' confidence in their ability to communicate effectively with their physician increased. Bylund *et al.* (2011) observed that workshop participants demonstrated significant improvements on a measure of healthcare communication behaviour. Specifically, patients who completed the intervention showed increases in their self-rated healthcare communication skills as measured by behavioural intention. Furthermore, the majority expressed a belief that these skills would improve their healthcare. However, in both of the aforementioned studies, post-test evaluations were given immediately following the intervention, so it is unclear if the change in patient confidence levels was sustained over time, or whether actual communication behaviour matched intention.

The impact of communication training on patients' ratings of satisfaction and communication have also been reported. Meropol *et al.* (2013) found that patients who participated in the CONNECT intervention found treatment decisions easier to reach and were more likely to be satisfied with their decisions. In addition, intervention patients reported higher levels of satisfaction with physician communication and discussions of support services and quality of life concerns.

An important outcome of patient communication intervention studies is the extent to which training changes patient behaviour. Cegala and colleagues found that compared to patients receiving materials-only or standard care, patients who received materials plus coaching were significantly engaged in more effective and efficient information seeking, provided physicians with more detailed information, and used more summarizing utterances to verify information (Cegala *et al.* 2000b). Similar results were repeated in a study involving older patients (Cegala *et al.* 2001). Patients receiving materials plus coaching engaged in significantly more information seeking and provision, and obtained more information. In their trial evaluating a tailored education and coaching intervention, Street *et al.* (2010) found that intervention patients discussed their pain concerns at a higher rate.

If indeed a communication training programme can improve communication skills, it follows that this should have some effect on more distal outcomes—such as treatment adherence. Cegala and colleagues found that patients who received materials plus coaching were significantly more compliant overall (Cegala *et al.*

2000*a*). Patients who viewed an educational video addressing colorectal cancer screening information and communication skills reported discussing screening with their provider, had screening tests orders, and completed screening tests at significantly higher rates (Katz *et al.* 2012). Similarly, diabetes patients who completed a ten-session, culturally-tailored empowerment intervention demonstrated significant improvements in diabetes self-efficacy (i.e. confidence and ability to manage one's diabetes), self-care behaviours (e.g. following a healthy eating plan), and clinical outcomes (e.g. haemoglobin A1c levels) (Peek *et al.* 2012).

Other research has shown the importance of considering patient characteristics such as race and culture when formulating patient communication training programmes. The culturally-tailored curriculum discussed above (Peek *et al.* 2012) provides one example. In another study, subjects received either a 14-page communication workbook two to three days pre-visit, or a two-page patient communication handout in the waiting room. Significant differences in the effect of the interventions on Caucasian patients and African American patients were noted. The workbook had a significant effect on Caucasian patients compared to minimal or no effect on African American patients. Workbook-trained Caucasians asked more questions, obtained more information, had greater delayed recall, and greater adherence than their Caucasian counterparts in either of the other two groups. No such significant differences were found for African American patients (Post *et al.* 2001).

In summary, the limited literature on comprehensive patient communication training interventions indicates promising findings of the effect of these interventions on patient outcomes. Additional studies are necessary to continue to build an evidence base for effective patient communication training programmes.

One particular limitation of the current research in this area is a lack of a unifying theoretical or conceptual model. Grounding communication training programmes in such a framework is useful in providing coherence to the curriculum, a rationale for the skills being taught and the assessment of those skills. To move patient communication training work forward, we advocate adopting concordance as a conceptual framework.

Concordance as a conceptual framework for patient communication interventions

Our approach to patient communication training is founded upon the same perspective that good provider communication is founded upon—concordance, or a shared agreement between the clinician and patient. With concordance as the goal, training for both clinicians and patients should be directed at attaining that goal. Current communication training focused on patient-centredness and shared decision-making (Brown *et al.* 2007) attend to the clinician's role in achieving concordance. We believe that patient communication training programmes that are grounded in the notion of concordance will be the most effective in producing a good physician–patient relationship.

The concept of concordance with respect to regimen decision-making was introduced in 1997 by the Royal British Pharmaceutical Society. Joining calls for greater patient-centred care and shared decision-making, concordance was introduced as a cooperative communication style to decrease the continuing 30–50% medication non-adherence rates. Concordance is defined as an agreement reached after negotiation between a patient and a healthcare professional that respects the beliefs and wishes of the patient in determining whether, when, and how medicines are to be taken (RPSGB 1997). The concordance framework depends on a two-way process, where shared meaning is negotiated between participants (Shah and Chewning 2006). In this model, more attention is paid to mutual responsibility of actors for the effect and effectiveness of the transaction. An underlying assumption is that the context and history of the physician and patient, as well as the other person's behaviour will influence each person's behaviour (Shah and Chewning 2006). The final product of the healthcare encounter is an agreed upon regimen to address the patient's health quality of life priorities. We propose that concordance should be the goal of any physician–patient consultation, even when there is no need for a specific decision to be made, or a regimen to be decided upon. If we think of physician–patient communication as something that happens over a course of many individual consultations, it becomes clear that concordance transcends a discrete visit.

As Pollock (2005) discusses, 'People seek to contain the disruption of illness, to reduce its significance and engage in lives that are fulfilling and, as far as possible, normal' (p. 146). However, to do this implies a partnership with clinicians during the healthcare encounter that respects the patient's priorities and quality of life preferences. It is helpful to view the encounter as a communication pathway in which: a clinician may offer options and ask for patient preferences; patients may or may not state preferences in response to provider requests; both parties offer rationale; and agreement may be reached (Chewning *et al.* 2006). The concordance perspective recognizes that a patient may quite appropriately choose to delegate the decision role to the clinician. However, in one recent observational study, decisional deferral occurred in only 7% of visits (Chewning *et al.* 2007). Furthermore, a systematic review of 115 studies published since 2000 found that the majority of patients (in 71% of studies examined) wished to have shared decision roles (Chewning *et al.* 2012).

At its best, regimen agreement is sought during the encounter by a clinician who communicates much needed expertise and information and by a patient who communicates priorities, concerns, symptoms, and preferences. From this perspective, the patient's responsibility for observation, self-reflection, and communication is central to the communication framework. Patient as well as provider training is needed for the potential partnership process to result in concordance. While providers need training to offer options and ask for patient preferences, patients in turn may even need help recognizing that the clinician gave an option or the opportunity to state a preference. In a recent observational study, patients underreported the number of times a physician was observed presenting them with an option or asking their preference (Chewning *et al.* 2006).

Returning to the PACE curriculum (Cegala *et al.* 2000*a*; Cegala *et al.* 2000*b*), we see how each of these four skills is important to reaching concordance. First, patients need to be able to present information in a clear way in order for physicians to offer the right choices. Second, patients may need more information before offering a preference and therefore need to be able to ask questions. Third, patients may have concerns or criteria relevant to the decision that inform a preference or inform what the physician recommends. Learning how to effectively express concerns may be important. Fourth, in order to ensure that decisions are being made based on a shared understanding of information, patients should check their understanding of the information. These correspond with the four PACE skills. An emphasis that we believe should be added to this curriculum is training patients to articulate a clear preference when one is held (Bylund *et al.* 2011).

The concordance concept of an encounter in which a decision is to be made involves negotiation. Each party exchanges their rationale and expertise to reach a mutually agreeable recommendation for care. The clinician who makes the decision without input from the patient does so in the dark. Expectations can be established to have the patient monitor regimens and report at the next visit. For example, a side effect monitoring tool of chemotherapy symptom cycles can assist shared decision-making and calibration of regimens (Hermansen-Kobulnicky *et al.* 2004; Hermansen-Kobulnicky 2002). Monitoring is not simply about adverse effects or symptom relief, but also how well the intervention serves the patient's quality of life priorities. It can inform the ongoing regimen decisions and the administration of care, such as scheduling chemotherapy to minimize disruption in order to maintain a quality life (Wiederholt 1997). Self-stylized symptom monitoring by cancer patients is already common (Hermansen-Kobulnicky 2009). While clinician behaviours are critical to encourage this involvement, patient training can help patients to have reasonable self-efficacy to share their results with providers as part of the decision process.

Conclusion

Physician–patient communication is a dynamic, socially-constructed process that must have competent communication on both sides of the equation. Although work in training physicians remains critical, we need to expand our thinking to include how to best prepare patients to participate in consultations in ways that will lead to concordance. There is a paucity of published reports of comprehensive patient communication training interventions that move beyond question asking to include other important skills. Growing this area of training and research will contribute in vital ways to scholarship on physician–patient communication, and to patients' experiences (Street 2003).

References

Brown RF, Butow PN, Boyer M J, Tattersall MHN (1999). Promoting patient participation in the cancer consultation; evaluation of a prompt sheet and coaching in question asking. *Br J Cancer* **80**, 242–8.

Brown RF, Butow PN, Boyle F, Tattersall MH (2007). Seeking informed consent to cancer clinical trials; evaluating the efficacy of doctor communication skills training. *Psychooncology* **16**, 507–16.

Brown RF, Butow PN, Dunn SM, Tattersall MHN (2001). Promoting patient participation and shortening cancer consultations; a randomised trial. *Br J Cancer* **85**, 1273–9.

Butow PN, Brown RF, Cogar S, Tattersall MHN, Dunn SM (2002). Oncologists' reactions to cancer patients verbal cues. *Psychooncology* **11**, 47–58.

Bylund CL, Goytia EJ, D'Agostino TA, *et al.* (2011). Evaluation of a pilot communication skills training intervention for minority cancer patients. *J Psychosoc Oncol* **29**, 347–58.

Bylund CL, Makoul G (2005). Examining empathy in medical encounters: an observational study using the empathic communication coding system. *Health Commun* **18**, 123–40.

Cegala DJ, Marinelli T, Post D (2000*a*). The effects of patient communication skills training on compliance. *Arch Fam Med* **9**, 57–64.

Cegala DJ, Mcclure L, Marinelli TM, Post DM (2000*b*). The effects of communication skills training on patients' participation during medical interviews. *Patient Educ Couns* **41**, 209–22.

Cegala DJ, Post DM, Mcclure L (2001). The effects of patient communication skills training on the discourse of older patients during a primary care interview. *J Am Geriatr Soc*, 49, 1505–11.

Chewning B, Bylund CL, Shah B, Arora NK, Gueguen JA, Makoul G (2012). Patient preferences for shared decisions: a systematic review. *Patient Educ Couns* **86**, 9–18.

Chewning B, Sleath B, Shah BK, *et al.* (2007). Comparing patient interviews to a concordance observational coding tool of the medication decision process. *Oral presentation at the International Conference on Communication in Healthcare.* Charleston, SC.

Chewning B, Sleath B, Shah BK, Devellis B, Yon AS (2006). Concordance in medication decisions for reheumatoid arthritis: patient-provider discussion pathways. *Oral presentation at the European Association for Healthcare Communication.* Basel, Switzerland.

Chewning BA, Wiederholt JB (2003). Concordance in cancer medication management. *Patient Educ Couns* **50**, 75–8.

Fisch M, Cohen MZ, Rutledge C, Cripe LD (2003). Teaching patients how to improve communication with their health care providers: A unique workshop experience. *J Cancer Educ* **18**, 18–193.

Golin CE, Dimatteo MR, Gelberg L (1996). The role of patient participation in the doctor visit: Implications for adherence to diabetes care. *Diabetes Care* **19**, 1153–64.

Hermansen-Kobulnicky CJ (2009). Symptom-monitoring behaviors of rural cancer patients and survivors. *Support Care Cancer* **17**, 617–26.

Hermansen-Kobulnicky CJ, Chewning B (2002). Teaching cancer patients to monitor side effects: an exploratory test to increase shared decision making. *European Conference on Communication in Healthcare.* Warwick, UK.

Hermansen-Kobulnicky CJ, Wiederholt JB, Chewning B (2004). Adverse effect monitoring: opportunity for patient care and pharmacy practice. *J Am Pharm Assoc (2003)* **44**, 75–86; quiz 87–8.

Katz ML, Fisher JL, Fleming K, Paskett ED (2012). Patient activation increases colorectal cancer screening rates: a randomized trial among low-income minority patients. *Cancer Epidemiol Biomarkers Prev* **21**, 45–52.

Marvel MK, Epstein RM, Flowers K, Beckman HB (1999). Soliciting the patient's agenda: Have we improved? *J Am Med Assoc* **281**, 283–7.

Meropol NJ, Egleston BL, Buzaglo JS, *et al.* (2013). A web-based communication aid for patients with cancer: the CONNECT Study. *Cancer* **119**, 1437–45.

Parker PA, Davison BJ, Tishelman C, Brundage MD, Team TSC (2005). What do we know about facilitating patient communication in the cancer care setting?. *Psychooncology* **14**, 848–58.

Peek ME, Harmon SA, Scott SJ (2012). Culturally tailoring patient education and communication skills training to empower African-Americans with diabetes. *Transl Behav Med* **2**, 296–308.

Pollock K (2005). *Concordance in Medical Consultations: a critical review.* Radcliffe Publishing Ltd., Abingdon, UK.

Post DM, Cegala DJ, Marinelli TM (2001). Teaching patients to communicate with physicians: The impact of race. *J Nat Med Assoc* **93**, 6–12.

Roter DL, Stewart M, Putnam SM, Lipkin MJ, Stiles W, Inui TS (1997). Communication patterns of primary care physicians. *JAMA* **277**, 350–6.

RPSGB (1997). *From Compliance to Concordance: achieving shared goals in medicine taking* [Online]. Available: http://www.concordance.org [Accessed October 15, 2008].

Shah B, Chewning B (2006). Conceptualizing and measuring pharmacist-patient communication: a review of published studies. *Res Social Adm Pharm* **2**, 153–85.

Street R (2003). Communication in medical encounters: an ecological perspective. In: Thompson TL, Dorsey AM, Miller KI, Parrott R (eds). *Handbook of Health Communication* (pp. 63–89). Lawrence Erlbaum Associates, Mahway, NJ.

Street RL, Slee C, Kalauokalani DK, Dean DE, Tancredi DJ, Kravitz RL (2010). Improving physician-patient communication about cancer pain with a tailored education-coaching intervention. *Patient Educ Couns* **80**, 42–7.

Towle A, Godolphin W, Manklow J, Wiesinger H (2003). Patient perceptions that limit a community-based intervention to promote participation. *Patient Educ Couns* **50**, 231–3.

Tran AN, Haidet P, Street RL Jr, O'Malley KJ, Martin F, Ashton CM (2004). Empowering communication: a community-based intervention for patients. *Patient Educ Couns* **52**, 113–21.

Wiederholt J W, Wiederholt PA (1997). The patient: Our teacher and friend. *Am J Pharmaceut Educ* **61**, 415–23.

CHAPTER 9

Cancer patients' use of the internet for cancer information and support

Emily B. Peterson, Megan J. Shen, Jennifer Gueguen Weber, and Carma L. Bylund

Introduction to seeking information

The internet has significantly transformed the way in which patients meet their health-related information needs, with consumers increasingly going online for help with diagnosing, understanding, and even treating medical concerns. A recent Pew Research report found that 72% of internet users said they looked for health information online within the past year, with 35% of users saying that they have gone online specifically to try to figure out what medical condition they or a loved one might have (Pew Forum 2013).

Nearly two-thirds (63%) of cancer patients report going online to seek information about their diagnosis (Castleton et al. 2011). For cancer patients and their caregivers, the rate of active information seeking both on and off the web is influenced by both tumour type and disease stage (Eheman et al. 2009; Nagler et al. 2010; van de Poll-Franse and van Eenbergen 2008). For example, one study found that breast and prostate cancer patients reported more information seeking than colorectal cancer patients, and these differences were most pronounced in early stages of cancer (Nagler et al. 2010). Such differences may be explained by variances in the amount of information available for different cancer types and stages of interest, and the degree of medical uncertainty or controversy surrounding various treatment options.

Individual differences in information seeking are also highly significant; patients who search for cancer-related internet information differ considerably from those who do not. Age is often one of the strongest predictors of internet usage, with younger patients, sometimes labelled 'digital natives', consistently reporting higher levels of internet information seeking than their older counterparts (Kontos et al. 2014). Studies of mixed groups of cancer patients have found that patients who search for information tend to be female, married, own a computer, have internet access at home, and have a higher income and education level than cancer patients who do not search for cancer-related internet information (Eheman et al. 2009; Kontos et al. 2014; Wallace et al. 2014). Additionally, disparities in health information seeking persist among ethnic minority patients with cancer. A number of studies report that the internet is used less frequently as a source of information by racial/ethnic minority patients (Helft et al. 2005; Wallace et al. 2014) and minority cancer survivors (Chou et al. 2011).

Online health-seeking rates tend to be particularly high at cancer diagnosis and during follow-up cancer care (Hesse et al. 2008; Shea-Budgell et al. 2014). Despite a preference to get information from their healthcare providers first, cancer survivors report using the internet as a first, and sometimes primary, source of information about their cancer (Hesse et al. 2008). Cancer-related internet information is also often accessed by those caring for loved ones with the disease. Two-thirds of people searching the internet for health information report doing so for someone else (Cutrona et al. 2014). These caregivers play a key role in obtaining cancer-related health information (Cutrona et al. 2014). Some studies have found that more caregivers than patients access the internet directly for information about cancer (James et al. 2007) and that caregivers tend to use internet resources differently than patients searching for information about themselves. Namely, caregivers are more likely to report activities requiring user-generated content, such as participation in social networking sites (Cutrona et al. 2014). Patients are then exposed to this information as their caregivers provide it to them.

Seeking support

Online social support serves as an essential coping resource for many patients with cancer, often promoting both physical and psychological well-being (Shim et al. 2011). Online support groups provide a way for patients with cancer to talk to and learn from others with similar health experiences, despite geographical restrictions. Because participants in cancer support groups are likely going through similar health experiences, they are well-positioned to offer unparalleled empathy and advice (Rains et al. 2015). Indeed, the literature about cancer support groups has suggested that participation in such groups can positively affect patients' adaptation to illness, including decreasing feelings of alienation, anxiety, isolation and misinformation (Klemm et al. 1999). Cancer patients vary in their use of online support groups, with men primarily seeking information and women primarily seeking encouragement and support (Im *et al.* 2007). Studies also suggest that online support-seeking may be a particularly important coping strategy for stigmatized diseases, such as lung cancer, where patients may become disconnected with their existing social network (Rains *et al.* in press).

Benefits and drawbacks

There are several reported benefits associated with cancer patients or their caregivers searching for cancer-related internet information. As noted above, many patients find support through online cancer support groups. In a study of mixed-type cancer patients, 62% of patients reported that cancer-related internet information made them feel more hopeful (Helft *et al.* 2005). Further, health-related internet searches can empower patients who are seeking information about their cancer to become active participants in their care. An additional potential benefit of the internet in helping cancer patients and their caregivers lies in its ability to provide a wealth of information from various sources about frequently misunderstood topics. For example, while cancer clinical trials are critical to cancer patient care and outcomes, participation is low, and patient understanding of the topic is limited. Thus, websites devoted to information on clinical trials can have a positive impact (Dolinsky *et al.* 2006).

It has also been suggested that there are potentially detrimental effects associated with patients searching for cancer-related information on the internet. Patients, even those comfortable using the internet, may have a difficult time distinguishing between reliable and unreliable sites (Balka *et al.* 2010). One study of colorectal cancer patients found that the majority of patients began information seeking by using search engines and had a difficult time discerning the best sites from the many options returned from the searches (Sajid *et al.* 2011). Some patients may become overwhelmed, aware of conflicting medical information, and more nervous, anxious, and confused (Helft *et al.* 2005).

The impact of the internet on the physician–patient relationship

Increased access to health-related internet information has provided patients access to information that was previously either unavailable or difficult to access, causing a significant shift in physician–patient communication and relationships. One of these shifts has come in the form of a levelling effect of the power imbalance in the physician–patient relationship, specifically in terms of expert power (Bylund *et al.* 2007*b*). Namely, the increased presence of web-acquired cancer-related information has also shifted the long-standing notion of physicians as the traditional medical authority (Wald *et al.* 2007). This shift in power can provide a positive impact on the physician–patient relationship, such as helping patients make more informed healthcare choices, engage in better shared decision-making, and have increased access to their own health information (Wald *et al.* 2007). It is important to note, however, that while some cancer patients report feeling empowered by internet information (Fleisher *et al.* 2002), internet information is only empowering to the extent that the oncologist is receptive to the patient being involved in the decision-making process (Broom 2005*b*).

Alternatively, access to health-related internet information can have negative or harmful effects on the physician–patient

relationship. This occurs when patients directly challenge physicians' opinions (Broom 2005*a*), or when their views about health-related internet information are contrary to physicians' views (Sommerhalder *et al.* 2009). However, relatively few healthcare providers (16%) report concern that internet information will cause their patients to question their authority (Emond *et al.* 2013). Another potentially negative effect of health-related internet information is that internet discussions may result in longer consultations (Helft *et al.* 2003), which can be frustrating for physicians who have limited time with each patient. Despite these potential negative effects on the physician–patient relationship, one study found that 93% of physicians acknowledge that their patients use the internet to seek out health-related information and 80% of physicians expressed a positive opinion about their patients bringing up internet information during the consultation (Emond *et al.* 2013).

With the increased use of the internet, the disparities between what patients and physicians believe to be considered 'good' or 'reliable' forms of internet information have decreased. For instance, studies conducted in 2005 suggested that oncologists had concerns about the accuracy of cancer-related internet information, with one study indicating that 91% of oncologists reported that the internet had the potential to cause harm to patients (Broom 2005; Newnham *et al.* 2005). However, more recent studies have indicated that few health professionals (8%) indicate concern that health-related internet information could have a harmful effect on the physician–patient relationship (Emond *et al.* 2013).

Communication about internet information

Because cancer patients and their caregivers are increasingly using the internet to find health information (Bylund *et al.* 2010), some oncological healthcare providers advocate that providers should consider providing guidance in helping patients find reliable information on the internet and engaging them in conversations about what they have found. This guidance and support may increase patient satisfaction and enhance physician–patient communication (Penson *et al.* 2002).

Examining physician–patient interactions from an interpersonal communication framework can help illuminate the communication occurring in clinical consultations. Facework theories (Brown and Levinson 1987) are a useful guide within this interpersonal communication framework. *Face* is defined by Cupach and Metts (1994) as 'the conception of self that each person displays in particular interactions with others' (p. 3). These theories explain that in interpersonal communication, an individual's communication may threaten his or her face, which is called a face-threatening act (Brown and Levinson 1987). The conversational partner may respond in a manner that further threatens the other person's face, or works to support the other person's face.

In prior work, the patient's act of introducing internet information into a physician–patient consultation has been conceptualized as a 'face-threatening' act (Bylund *et al.* 2007*a*; Shen *et al.* 2015). The physician may feel his or her face is threatened by the patient looking for information elsewhere. Alternatively, the patient may feel his or her face is threatened by acknowledging that s/he has looked elsewhere. How a physician responds to the patient introducing the internet information, and the course of the discussion that follows, can prove to either support the patient's face (by validating the patient's efforts or taking the information seriously), or further threaten the patient's face (by warning the patient about the dangers of the internet or being dismissive of the information without any validation of efforts).

Consistent with the facework theories framework, our work in this area has focused specifically on describing these discussions and understanding how patients introduce information, how physicians respond, and how this affects the physician–patient relationship (Bylund and Gueguen 2006; Shen *et al.* 2015; D'Agostino *et al.* 2012; Bylund *et al.* 2007a). One of our studies (Bylund and Gueguen 2006) demonstrated that cancer patients and their caregivers introduced internet information in a variety of ways. A little more than half reported asking a question to the oncologist, 28% reported making a statement of fact, and 13% made an assertive statement. The majority of oncologists used face-saving responses, such as taking the information the patients presented seriously (61%) or showing active interest (13%), while 28% disagreed with the information or the patient's request, which may be face-threatening to the patient.

To better understand how patients introduce cancer-related internet information and how physicians respond, we conducted a qualitative study examining clinical consultations between patients and oncologists in which cancer-related internet information was discussed (Shen *et al.* 2015). In line with our prior work, results from this study were consistent with facework theories. Namely, patients often engaged in face-saving techniques, such as implicitly introducing information or noting that the information they looked up came from reputable sources. Oncologists, in turn, engaged in response techniques designed to reduce face threat, such as encouraging patients' utilization of the internet, validating their use of the internet, and providing them with detailed information to aid in patients' decision-making.

Another study from our team (Bylund *et al.* 2010) indicated that, again consistent with facework theories, physicians' responses to patients' introduction of internet information influenced patients' satisfaction. Namely, when physicians showed an interest and involvement in patients' introduction of internet information and took the information seriously, patients were less likely to report a desire to change the physician's response and reported higher levels of satisfaction with communication. When patients experience difficulties interpreting the meaning of health-related internet information, which it has been suggested that they often do, physicians discussing patients' concerns and answering their questions are critical to successful clinical consultations with internet-informed patients (Sommerhalder *et al.* 2009). In order to maximize patient-centred communication, physicians should take a shared approach by utilizing internet information as a means of improving the physician–patient relationship. To this end, they should be encouraged to take their patients and the information they present seriously, show their patients that they are interested and involved, and address patients' questions and concerns.

Although patients frequently report looking up health-related internet information (Bylund *et al.* 2010), they do not always introduce it within the clinical consultation. In fact, one study found that only 50% of patients who had read cancer-related internet information actually reported discussing it with their physicians (Shen *et al.* 2015). When they do choose to discuss the internet information, the three most frequent reasons for doing so include: being proactive in their own health, appealing to the physician as an expert, and becoming more educated (Bylund *et al.* 2009). Additionally, patients frequently ask their physicians for feedback on the

information they look up on the internet (Shen *et al.* 2015), suggesting that patients seek their physicians' involvement in understanding the information they find online.

One study examined why patients decide not to talk with their providers about the health-related internet information that they have read (Imes *et al.* 2008). The following reasons were listed: attribution about the information (29%), healthcare systems or personal circumstances (20%), patient perceptions of their clinician as not being open to discussing internet information (14%), fear of intruding on the providers' domain (13%), and saving face (8%). The authors concluded that the majority of reasons that patients do not speak with their physicians about internet information are resolvable barriers, with many of the reasons related to concerns about with the physician–patient relationship.

Of concern is that few physicians (20%) refer patients to reputable internet sources without a request for such information, whereas the majority (64%) of physicians do when asked (Emond *et al.* 2013). Given the high rates of patients reporting looking up health-related internet information but inconsistently introducing it within the clinical consultation, it may be helpful for physicians to refer their patients pre-emptively to trusted sources to ensure the quality of health-related internet information consumed by patients.

Improving provider–patient communication about internet health information

Suggested guidelines

Based on the research reviewed in this chapter, this section will introduce suggested guidelines to help structure and support provider–patient discussions about internet health information. The suggestions that follow could be applied to a workshop focused particularly on discussing internet information, or adapted for discussions that are raised in other workshops (Box 9.1).

Explore the patient's experiences with internet information

Because oncology patients have reported sharing online health information more than patients seeing other specialists (Rider *et al.* 2014), this first strategy can be used after a patient introduces internet information. Alternatively, this could be done routinely as a way to introduce such a discussion with new patients, many of whom have likely looked for information online prior to their appointment. Communication skills that might be useful in achieving this strategy include asking open questions, clarifying, and restating.

Box 9.1 Guidelines for provider–patient communication
1. Explore the patient's experience with internet information.
2. Validating patient efforts.
3. Respond empathically to patient's experience.
4. Correct misunderstandings.
5. Provide guidance.
6. Reinforce the provider–patient relationship.

Exemplary statements

'You mentioned that you had found some information online. It's helpful for me to understand your experiences with looking up information about your cancer on the internet. Tell me about that.'

'I'd just like to take a minute to talk about internet health information, as I do with all my patients. Tell me about your experience with looking up information about your cancer online.'

Validating the patient's efforts

Research on this topic has indicated that validating a patient's efforts in searching for internet health information is important (Bylund et al. 2007a; Wald et al. 2007). It is expected that this validation can create a buffer of sorts if the information found was incorrect by allowing the patient to save face. It also sets the tone for an empathic response to the patient's experience and then the correction of any misunderstanding, and the provision of additional information as appropriate.

Exemplary statements

'It's great that you are actively searching for information about your treatment options.'

'I'm glad to see you've done some homework on your father's condition.'

Respond empathically to the patient's experience

If a patient discloses emotions surrounding the experience of reading internet information, the provider should respond empathically (Wald et al. 2007). Empathic communication skills include: acknowledging, validating or normalizing the patient's emotion or experience, and encouraging the patient to express feelings.

Exemplary statements

'I'm happy to hear that you've found some websites that have been helpful for you.'

'Yes, finding conflicting information on different websites can be really frustrating.'

Correct misunderstandings or incorrect information

It may be necessary to correct a patient's misunderstandings or incorrect information that the patient has found. We recommend that this be done after validating efforts and responding empathically to the patient's experience (Box 9.1) to reduce the amount of face threat that patients may experience. Communication skills that may be helpful in achieving this include: previewing information, inviting patient questions, and checking patient understanding. At times, the provider can benefit from negotiating the agenda in order to defer the patient's questions about internet information until the end of the consultation.

Exemplary statements

'There are a couple aspects of this information you found on the internet that I think we should talk about. First … '

'What do you see as the difference between what you read and what you and I have talked about?'

Provide guidance

Although providers may experience discomfort in providing guidance to patients about internet information, it is critical to do so because patients and their families demonstrate the desire for this guidance (Domínguez and Sapiña 2014). Those who are familiar with the internet have found useful websites, or developed effective strategies for searching for internet health information may feel comfortable providing guidance. Encouraging the use of credible internet sources for medical information and providing recommendations of such sites can be very helpful for patients (Wald et al. 2007). Not only do a substantial proportion of patients demonstrate a desire for such vetted informational resources, but the provision of trustworthy websites may benefit not only the patients but the providers as well (Katz et al. 2014). Doing so acknowledges patients' preferences for searching for health-related information online while providing some parameters for doing so.

Exemplary statements

'One of the websites that some of my patients have found useful is … '

'Our institution's website gives some internet resources for patients with breast cancer. Have you looked at those?'

Reinforce the provider–patient partnership

It has been suggested that the discussion of information that patients have found online leads to increased satisfaction for both parties (Hay et al. 2008). At the end of the discussion about the internet information, it may be helpful to reinforce the provider–patient partnership. This strategy can set a foundation for the future of this relationship by advocating for mutual open sharing of information. To do this, a provider may use communication skills such as making a partnership statement, endorsing question asking, and asking open-ended questions.

Exemplary statement

'I think it's very important that we talk about the information that you are reading on the internet about your cancer to ensure that we are on the same page. In our future visits, please let me know if you have questions about what you have been reading. What do you think?'

Suggestions for teaching

Teaching students or other learners about how to talk with patients about internet information can be integrated easily into an ongoing communication skills training programme. For instance, a module on shared decision-making could add a small component about how to respond to patient-initiated internet conversations. Alternatively, a separate short module on the topic of internet discussions could be added to a larger curriculum.

Preparing standardized patients (SPs) to participate in these types of trainings is important. We have found it useful in working with actors to have them take in printed results from online health searches that fit the role play scenario. This takes some background work in finding materials and working with the actors to integrate them into the role plays. However, we have found in our own work that this improves the believability of the scenario. SPs can also be guided to either ask a direct question about the internet information (e.g. 'I have a question about something I read online') or to give a more indirect cue (e.g. 'I got really upset after I looked on the internet about the prognosis.').

References

Balka E, Krueger G, Holmes BJ, Stephen JE (2010). Situating internet use: information-seeking among young women with breast cancer. *J Comput Mediat Commun* 15, 389–411.

Broom A (2005a). Medical specialists' accounts of the impact of the Internet on the doctor/patient relationship. *Health* 9, 319–38.

Broom A (2005b). Virtually He@lthy: The impact of internet use on disease experience and the doctor-patient relationship. *Qual Health Res* 15, 325–45.

Brown P, Levinson S (1987). *Politeness: Some Universals in Language Use.* Cambridge University Press, Cambridge, UK.

Bylund C, Gueguen J (2006). Physician-patient conversations about internet cancer information. *Psychooncology* 15, S189.

Bylund C L, Gueguen JA, D'agostino TA, Imes RS, Sonet E (2009). Cancer patients' decisions about discussing Internet information with their doctors. *Psychooncology* 18, 1139–46.

Bylund CL, Gueguen JA, D'agostino TA, Li Y, Sonet E (2010). Doctor-patient communication about cancer-related Internet information. *J Psychosoc Oncol* 28, 127–42.

Bylund CL, Gueguen JA, Sabee CM, Imes RS, Li Y, Sanford AA (2007a). Provider–patient dialogue about Internet health information: an exploration of strategies to improve the provider–patient relationship. *Patient Educ Couns* 66, 346–52.

Bylund CL, Sabee CM, Imes RS, Sanford AA (2007b). Exploration of the construct of reliance among patients who talk with their providers about internet information. *J Health Commun* 12, 17–28.

Castleton K, Fong T, Wang-Gillam A, et al. (2011). A survey of Internet utilization among patients with cancer. *Supportive Care in Cancer* 19, 1183–90.

Chou WY, Liu B, Post S, Hesse B (2011). Health-related Internet use among cancer survivors: Data from the Health Information National Trends Survey, 2003–2008. *J Cancer Surviv* 5, 263–70.

Cupach W, Metts S (1994). *Facework.* Thousand Oaks, London, UK.

Cutrona S, Mazor K, Vieux S, Luger T, Volkman J, Finney Rutten L (2014). Health information-seeking on behalf of others: characteristics of "surrogate seekers." *J Cancer Educ* 30, 1–8.

D'Agostino TA, Ostroff JS, Heerdt A, Dickler M, Li Y, Bylund CL (2012). Toward a greater understanding of breast cancer patients' decisions to discuss cancer-related internet information with their doctors: An exploratory study. *Patient Educ Couns* 89, 109–115.

Dolinsky CM, Wei SJ, Hampshire MK, Metz JM (2006). Breast cancer patients' attitudes toward clinical trials in the radiation oncology clinic versus those searching for trial information on the Internet. *Breast Jl* 12, 324–30.

Domínguez M, Sapiña L (2014). Pediatric cancer and the internet: exploring the gap in doctor-parents communication. *J Cancer Educ* 30, 145–51.

Eheman CR, Berkowitz Z, Lee J (2009). Information-seeking styles among cancer patients before and after treatment by demographics and use of information sources. *J Health Commun* 14, 487–502.

Emond Y, Groot J, Wetzels W, Osch L (2013). Internet guidance in oncology practice: determinants of health professionals' Internet referral behavior. *Psychooncology* 22, 74–82.

Fleisher L, Bass S, Ruzek S (2002). Relationships among internet health information use, patient behaviour and self-efficacy in newly diagnosed cancer patients who contact the National Cancer institute's (NCI) Atlantic Region Cancer Information Service (CIS). *AMIA Annual Fall Symposium.*

Hay MC, Cadigan RJ, Khanna D, et al. (2008). Prepared patients: Internet information seeking by new rheumatology patients. *Arthritis Rheum* 59, 575–82.

Helft PR, Eckles RE, Johnson-Calley CS, Daugherty CK (2005). Use of the Internet to obtain cancer information among cancer patients at an urban county hospital. *J Clin Oncol* 23, 4954–62.

Helft PR, Hlubocky F, Daugherty CK (2003). American oncologists' views of internet use by cancer patients: a mail survey of American Society of Clinical Oncology members. *J Clin Oncol* 21, 942–7.

Hesse BW, Arora NK, Burke Beckjord E, Finney Rutten LJ (2008). Information support for cancer survivors. *Cancer* 112, 2529–40.

Im EO, Chee W, Liu Y, et al. (2007). Characteristics of cancer patients in internet cancer support groups. *Comput Inform Nurs* 25, 334–43.

Imes RS, Bylund CL, Sabee CM, Routsong TR, Sanford AA (2008). Patients' reasons for refraining from discussing internet health information with their healthcare providers. *Health Communication* 23, 538–47.

James N, Daniels H, Rahman R, McConkey C, Derry J, Young A (2007). A study of information seeking by cancer patients and their carers. *Clin Oncol (R Coll Radiol)* 19, 356–62.

Katz JE, Roberge D, Coulombe G (2014). The cancer patient's use and appreciation of the internet and other modern means of communication. *Technol Cancer Res Treat* 13, 477–84.

Klemm P, Reppert K, Visich L (1999). A nontraditional cancer support group: the internet. *Comput Nurs* 16, 31–6.

Kontos E, Blake KD, Chou WY, Prestin A (2014). Predictors of eHealth usage: insights on the digital divide from the health information national trends survey 2012. *J Med Internet Res* 16, e172.

Nagler RH, Gray SW, Romantan A, et al. (2010). Differences in information seeking among breast, prostate, and colorectal cancer patients: Results from a population-based survey. *Patient Educ Couns* 81, S54–S62.

Newnham GM, Burns WI, Snyder RD (2005). Attitudes of oncology health professionals to information from the Internet and other media. *Med J Aus* 183, 197–200.

Penson RT, Benson RC, Parles K, Chabner BA, Lynch TJ (2002). Virtual connections: internet health care. *Oncologist* 7, 555–68.

Pew Forum. 2013. *Pew Internet and American Life Project* [Online]. Available at: http://www.pewinternet.org/fact-sheets/health-fact-sheet/

Rains S, Peterson EB, Wright K (2015). Communicating social support in computer-mediated contexts among individuals coping with illness: a meta-analytic review of content analyses examining support messages shared online. *Commun Mono* 28, 403–30.

Rider T, Malik M, Chevassut T (2014). Haematology patients and the internet—The use of on-line health information and the impact on the patient–doctor relationship. *Patient Educ Couns* 97, 223–38.

Sajid MS, Shakir AJ, Baig MK (2011). Information on the Internet about colorectal cancer: patient attitude and potential toward Web browsing. A prospective observational study. *Can J Surg* 54, 339–43.

Shea-Budgell MA, Kostaras X, Myhill KP, Hagen NA (2014). Information needs and sources of information for patients during cancer follow-up. *Curr Oncol* 21, 165–73.

Shen MJ, Dyson RC, D'Agostino TA, et al. (2015). Cancer-related internet information communication between oncologists and breast cancer patients: A qualitative study. *Psychooncology* 24, 1439–47.

Shim M, Cappella JN, Han JY (2011). How does insightful and emotional disclosure bring potential health benefits? Study based on online support groups for women with breast cancer. *J Commun* 61, 432–54.

Sommerhalder K, Abraham A, Zufferey MC, Barth J, Abel T (2009). Internet information and medical consultations: experiences from patients' and physicians' perspectives. *Patient Educ Counsel* 77, 266–71.

Van De Poll-Franse LV, Van Eenbergen M (2008). Internet use by cancer survivors: current use and future wishes. *Support Care Cancer* 16, 1189–95.

Wald HS, Dube CE, Anthony DC (2007). Untangling the Web—the impact of Internet use on health care and the physician–patient relationship. *Patient Educ Couns* 68, 218–24.

Wallace L, Lilley L, Lodrigues W (2014). Analysis of internet usage among cancer patients in a county hospital setting: a quality improvement initiative. *JMIR Res Protoc* 3, e26.

CHAPTER 10

Audio-recording cancer consultations for patients and their families—putting evidence into practice

Thomas F. Hack, Kinta Beaver, and Penelope Schofield

Introduction to audio-recording cancer consultations

The experience of cancer is one of the most challenging and potentially devastating events that can befall a person. Physical and psychosocial threats abound throughout the disease continuum; from when the presence of cancer is suspected, through the diagnostic period and treatment phase(s), and either into survivorship, or to palliation and the final breaths of life. The process of adjustment to cancer involves a myriad of coping responses, many of which involve processing information to inform treatment decisions or the management of symptoms or treatment side effects. Effective communication between the patient, family, and healthcare professional is pivotal to adequately informing the patient about disease and treatment options, promoting patient participation in medical decision-making, and fostering psychosocial adjustment in the patient. It is through patient–professional discourse that patients come to better understand the specific nature of their disease, as well as their unique treatment needs. These professional consultations are the vehicle by which patients can participate knowledgeably in the treatment decision-making process; yet patients commonly enter the consultation room in a state of elevated anxiety and leave with a weak recollection of information provided. For this reason, health professionals frequently encourage patients to ask a family member to accompany them to important consultations. Family members can be a source of emotional support and provide assistance with decision-making but they, like patients, have poor memories of consultation content. If the information that is imparted during any given consultation is essential for making informed decisions, then interventions are needed to enhance information comprehension and retention, thereby fostering patient and family participation in medical care decisions. One such intervention that holds empirical promise is furnishing patients and their families with audio recordings of important consultations.

The purpose of this chapter is threefold:

1. to briefly review the empirical literature on the value of consultation audio recordings for patients and families;

2. to conduct a theory-driven examination of the factors that limit practice uptake of this intervention; and

3. to provide practical suggestions for how these factors might best be addressed to enhance clinical uptake of consultation audio-recording.

Review of empirical evidence

Patients must understand their disease and treatment options sufficiently to be effective treatment consumers. While not all patients may express a wish to have greater control over the medical decisions that affect their well-being, research evidence suggests it is in their best interest to do so: patients who adopt a passive role in decision-making have overall poorer adjustment to their cancer than patients who are actively involved (Hack *et al.* 2006). Many factors are likely to contribute to this passive role; lack of disease knowledge, lack of general education, lack of ability to respond assertively, and fears of death, which all serve to silence patients during consultations. If the values we espouse for communication during oncology consultations include patient–professional collaboration, fully informed patient consumers, and greater decision-making control by patients, then efforts are needed to enhance the processes involved in conveying information to patients.

One intervention that holds empirical promise in addressing the unmet needs and concerns of newly diagnosed and follow-up cancer patients is consultation audio-recording (Pitkethly *et al.* 2008). The evidence supports the conclusion that audio recordings of oncology consultations provide valuable benefits to patients. These recordings allow for memories to be refreshed; for the learning of information not recalled from the consultation; for a clearer understanding of one's cancer treatment; for greater confidence that critical aspects of the disease and treatment have been discussed; and for greater information recall. Consultation recordings provide patients with a means by which to initiate disease and treatment discussions with family members and helps patients assume a significantly more active role in subsequent consultations. Consultation recordings are well received by the majority of cancer patients. In a recent qualitative analysis of patient interviews, patients reported four primary benefits: anxiety reduction; enhanced retention of information; better informed decision-making; and improved communication with family members (Hack *et al.* 2013).

From the research conducted in this area, we can conclude that consultation recordings improve information recall, reduce anxiety, enhance patient satisfaction with communication, and increase patients' perceptions that essential aspects of their disease and treatment have been addressed during the consultation. The Cochrane Collaborative Group, in its revised systematic review of the consultation recording research literature, concluded that 'the provision of recordings or summaries of key consultations may benefit most adults with cancer. Although more research is needed to improve our understanding of these interventions, most patients find them very useful. Practitioners should consider offering people tape recordings or written summaries of their consultations' (Pitkethly *et al.* 2008, p. 1).

Theoretical considerations

Despite the empirical evidence supporting the provision of consultation recordings in oncology, the uptake of this intervention into practice has been limited. Knowledge translation theories are useful for understanding why the uptake of promising psychosocial interventions is slower than might be expected, given the strong evidence base. These theories suggest that successful widespread dissemination requires that obstacles which impede uptake be identified and addressed.

While translation of healthcare knowledge is not successful if the knowledge itself is not relevant, unbiased, and based on all available evidence (Boissel *et al.* 2004), translation is also not possible if the knowledge is not adequately transferred. Knowledge transfer is a component of knowledge translation and refers to the technical process that brings information from the empirical literature to practitioners and caregivers. One of the more common findings from health service research is a failure to routinely translate research findings into daily clinical practice (Grimshaw *et al.* 2004). Simple diffusion and passive dissemination of research findings are largely ineffective at changing practice (Chilvers *et al.* 2002). Some practitioners have difficulty finding, assessing, interpreting, and applying the best evidence (Ely *et al.* 2002; Haynes and Haines 1998; Pearcey 1995).

One useful theoretical framework to consider when moving empirically promising communication interventions into mainstream clinical practice is the Promoting Action on Research Implementation in Health Services (PARIHS) Framework (Rycroft-Malone 2004). The PARIHS framework was conceived by colleagues at the Royal College of Nursing (RCN) Institute in the United Kingdom (Harvey *et al.* 2002; Kitson *et al.* 1998; McCormack *et al.* 2002). They posited that knowledge translation can be explained as a function of the relationship between *evidence* (research, clinical experience, and patient preferences), *context* (culture, leadership, and measurement), and *facilitation* (characteristics, role, and style), with these three elements having a dynamic, simultaneous relationship. The most successful implementation occurs when evidence is robust, the context is receptive to change, and the change process is appropriately facilitated (Kitson *et al.* 1998). Without a thorough understanding of the contextual factors that serve to stimulate, support, and reinforce the use of audio recordings in oncology, this

practice is likely to fail. Given the interrelationship between evidentiary, contextual, and facilitative factors, it is necessary to examine the complexities of these relationships if audio-recording practice is to be successfully adopted.

Evidence

Evidence (Rycroft-Malone *et al.* 2004) comes from four sources: research, clinical experience, patients, and the local context/ environment. Research organizations have traditionally focused on the generation of research evidence demonstrating effectiveness. This is certainly the case for consultation audio recordings. Systematic reviews of the empirical literature, such as the Cochrane review of consultation recording studies, quicken the rate at which research findings are understood but provide no promise of integration of clinical practice and research findings. This lack of integration may be a function of well-intentioned clinicians trying their best to work in healthcare settings that are busy and complex (Grimshaw *et al.* 2004). When research is successfully translated, this is often after considerable, unacceptable delay (Pearcey 1995). Rycroft-Malone (2004) calls for an enhanced understanding of the ways in which research evidence interacts with the evidence of clinical practice, the needs and experiences of patients, and the feedback mechanisms of the social and professional networks that comprise the organizational history and culture. By this definition, evidence in support of consultation audio-recording use is broader than published empirical reports of effectiveness, and efforts to transfer consultation audio-recording knowledge become multifaceted. Little research, for example, has been conducted to understand the experiences and perceptions of oncologists with respect to consultation audio-recording (Fig. 10.1).

While the empirical literature unequivocally demonstrates benefits for patients associated with having a consultation audio recording, we do not understand the mechanism(s) by which these benefits are derived. The benefit of recall is clearly associated with listening to the recorded consultation. However, it is not known why and how anxiety is reduced, and why patients are satisfied with the intervention. While it may be inferentially argued that more informed patients are consequently more satisfied, little is known about how patients derive benefit from listening to the audio

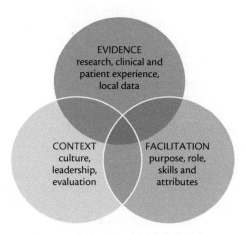

Fig. 10.1 PARIHS framework: knowledge translation as interrelationship of evidence, context, and facilitation.

recording. For example, what information on the audio recording is most helpful to patients and families? Does the audio recording inform treatment decision-making? Is there a more intangible benefit to having a recording, such as being more positively disposed towards the oncologist, or feeling more 'connected' to family members who listen to the audio-recording? If the factors that contribute to the derivation of patient benefit can be systematically identified, then we can better facilitate the uptake of consultation audio-recording use to maximize patient benefit.

Context

Context is characterized as having three themes: culture, leadership, and measurement or evaluation (McCormack *et al*. 2002). The culture of a practice context needs to be understood if meaningful and lasting change is to be achieved. By examining the context of consultation audio-recording use in cancer centres, the cultural, leadership, and measurement factors that shape the uptake of consultation recording use can be identified. With respect to organizational climate, few cancer centres have established policies governing consultation recording use.

Although many important barriers to knowledge translation exist at the level of the healthcare professional (Rycroft-Malone 2004), there are structural and organizational barriers to integrating research evidence into practice which operate at levels beyond the control of the individual clinician. Structural barriers are those environmental factors that impede knowledge translation. In oncology settings, a frequently occurring structural barrier to adoption of psychosocial interventions is a lack of financial resources; consultation recording equipment must be purchased and staff resources may be necessary to enable implementation. A potential organizational barrier is the absence of institutional or collegial peer pressures to use this intervention. The likelihood of uptake of consultation recordings may be enhanced through the support of 'champions' at all levels of the organization, including senior administrators and clinical staff.

Facilitation

Facilitation (Harvey *et al*. 2002) refers to the process of enabling the implementation of evidence into practice; 'enabling others' rather than 'doing for others'. In the context of knowledge translation, 'enabling' may have a greater impact than 'doing', because practitioners need time to consider and assimilate research findings. If oncologists tend to only use consultation recordings within the context of a research study, then we may be merely obtaining time-limited 'buy-in', 'doing for others' or, more precisely, 'guiding the hands of others' rather than enabling oncologists to become self-motivated and self-directed in using this intervention.

Motivation is a critical behaviour change factor that underlies the use of consultation audio recordings by oncology professionals. Lack of exposure to the benefits of consultation audio recordings may result in clinicians who believe there is a lack of positive, consensus evidence for their use. Where unfounded negative attitudes towards this intervention exist, such as the risk of litigation, these attitudes may serve as strong barriers for implementation. For this reason, efforts to educate oncologists about the benefits of consultation audio recordings may be a fundamental component of oncologist acceptance of the intervention and successful implementation.

Continued positive reinforcement will sustain positive oncologist attitudes towards consultation audio-recording use.

Social barriers to knowledge translation are often critical when groups of individuals are encouraged to adopt an intervention. The successful uptake of consultation audio-recording use relies on a substantial proportion or 'critical mass' of oncologists integrating the intervention into clinical practice. Social network theory is useful for examining ideas about the best ways to overcome the social barriers that impede the transfer and uptake of consultation audio-recording use. Social network theory predicts that an intervention is more likely to be adopted, the greater the number of interconnected individuals who use it, and if an integrated social structure can be established to support adoption (West *et al*. 1999). By deliberate rewiring of the interactions between oncologists, nurses, patients, and families through the provision and explanation of evidence, support in the use of consultation audio recordings, and the application of policies guiding consultation audio-recording use within the organization, we may potentially increase the density of the cancer patient–professional social network (Buchanan 2002). West *et al*. (1999) argued that a dense social network has advantages for knowledge translation: 'The multiplicity of ties gives members the opportunity to persuade, cajole, and monitor the performance of others' (p. 635). An objective for promoting consultation audio-recording use is to utilize the professional hierarchy of oncology practice to 'cascade' consultation audio-recording evidence, increasing the density of the social context of consultation audio-recording use, and thereby facilitating uptake into clinical practice. Social network theory also suggests that those individuals with the most influence or power in using the intervention and promoting its use among others should be identified as change agents. Among oncologists, disease site leaders might be identified and approached, particularly if these oncologists can instruct other oncologists and nurse specialists within their disease specialty to adopt consultation audio-recording use.

An implicit assumption in much of the writing on social barriers is that most knowledge translation activities should be directed towards the health professional. There are proportionately fewer studies that identify selected patient groups as the target for change. This is perhaps not surprising given that the goal of most knowledge transfer activities is to change the treating clinicians' practice style. However, there may be evidence that is sufficiently compelling to cause a significant proportion of cancer patients or the general public to mobilize in an effort to change clinical practice. The significance of cancer patients and their advocacy organizations in promoting interventions that may enhance their psychosocial well-being should not be underestimated. Indeed, advances in computer technology have made it easier for cancer patients to audio-record consultations on their mobile phones, and this key technological development is associated with an increase in the proportion of patients who are recording their consultations with or without the expressed permission of health professionals. Many local, legal jurisdictions allow for patients to record their consultations as 'co-owners' of their consultation. In these jurisdictions, cancer patient advocacy groups can play a significant role in encouraging cancer centres to audio-record pivotal consultations. Studies are needed to identify and address the role of cancer patients and their advocacy groups as change agents in the consultation audio-recording transfer process.

Case study: Assessment of receptiveness to consultation audio recordings

By way of example, we will use respective consultation recording research programmes in Australia, Canada, and the United Kingdom to illustrate the application of the PARIHS framework for enhancing the transfer and uptake of the consultation audio-recording intervention. Consistent with the functions of knowledge 'brokering', if the translation goal is to see more clinicians using a new intervention, then the probability of success will be enhanced if clinicians are included as co-investigators of the research and if they are involved in an advisory capacity throughout the research process (Lomas 2007). We sought out oncologists who have used consultation audio recordings in clinical practice and who hold senior positions within their respective cancer disease sites. We identified health professionals who are well suited by their practice history and power status to serve as local champions for the use of consultation audio recordings, and invited them to join the research team as co-investigators.

In the development phase of a recent project, the principal investigator travelled to each participating centre to interview oncologists, nurses, and other frontline staff about consultation recording use, asking them to share their opinions on the relative merits, perceived barriers, and facilitative facets of this intervention. Given that an understanding and acceptance of the best empirical evidence in support of consultation recording use is fundamental to successful uptake, the principal investigator arrived at each interview with evidence in hand: a copy of the Cochrane Collaboration systematic review of consultation recording use (Pikethly *et al.* 2008), copies of publications of the consultation recording studies conducted by the research team, and a copy of a recent newspaper article speaking to the value of consultation audio recordings for newly diagnosed oncology patients. These materials were offered to the interviewee, if appropriate. Nearing the end of each interview, the interviewer explained that a detailed proposal to examine the transfer and uptake of the consultation audio-recording intervention would be developed only if there was sufficient interest among the oncologists and nurses being interviewed. It was encouraging that all of the interviewees supported the idea and expressed their willingness to participate. The interview transcripts showed that the oncologists and nurses were able to identify several barriers and contextual factors that inhibited consultation audio-recording use at their centre. The respondents frequently differed both in their assessment of the benefits to patients of receiving a consultation audio-recording, and in their identification of factors that were critical to enhancing the uptake of consultation audio-recording use. These and other considerations of evidence, context, and facilitation are presented in Box 10.1 as guidelines for use when designing a research study to examine the consultation audio-recording intervention within a knowledge translation framework.

Looking forward

For oncology professionals who want to integrate audio-recording of key consultations into their practice, we offer the following basic suggestions:

- Secure the availability of audio-recording equipment in all clinic rooms.
- Assign responsibility for recording the consultation to a specific staff member.

Box 10.1 Evidence, context, and facilitation considerations for consultation audio-recording studies

Knowledge of consultation recording evidence. Are patients, families, and oncology staff aware of the evidence?

Perceived quality of evidence. How do patients, families, and oncology staff rate the quality of the evidence?

Perceived value and benefit. What is the perceived value and benefit of consultation recordings?

Relative value and benefit. How does this intervention compare against other ways of providing information?

Perceived impact of consultation recording on oncologist behaviour. Will oncologist involvement possibly reduce spontaneity during consultation; or improve the quality of communication?

Leadership. Is there an individual or group to champion the intervention?

Legal concerns. Who owns the recording—the patient, oncologist, or cancer centre? Can oncology staff or the cancer care organization be successfully sued for what is said on the recording? Is there a need to consult legal counsel?

Time constraints. Is there sufficient time for oncology staff to record consultations?

Privacy. What protective measures need to be taken to minimize patient risk?

Data storage. Where and how will recordings be stored, if at all?

Infrastructure. Is there a sufficient number of recording devices and associated materials available in clinic?

Intervention cost. What is the cost to sustain the intervention?

Resource cost. What is the staff cost to implement *and* sustain the intervention?

Motivation. Will oncology staff be compensated or reinforced for participating? Will oncology staff performance be evaluated?

Technology type. What options are available for recording the consultation—USB key (memory stick)? Mobile phone? Web address? Should the digital recording be converted to a text file? Should one type of technology be used for all patients or should options be available?

Availability of technology. Are all patients able to access the chosen technology? Do older patients have access to mobile phones or computers? Is there a need to accommodate different computer operating systems?

Delivery mode. Will the patient or cancer centre supply the recording equipment? Will the intervention be patient or provider driven? Who will press the 'record' button? How will the recording be accessed by patients and family members?

Staff support. Who will identify eligible patients—clerks, nurses?

Message. Will the entire consultation be recorded or only a portion thereof? Will the medical history be recorded? Will the physical examination be recorded? Which healthcare professionals will be recorded?

- Introduce to patients the topic of consultation recordings. For example: 'Today I will provide you with important information about your disease and treatment that you may want to remember. To make it easier to remember what we talk about, many patients find it helpful to receive an audio recording of the discussion. I would like to offer you an audio recording of our discussion. You can then take the recording home with you to listen to on your own or with family and friends.'

♦ Obtain, from the patient, informed written consent to be recorded. Consider including a disclaimer statement to protect the recorded professional from medico-legal liability associated with patient use of the recording.

♦ As an expression of respect for patient privacy, do not record the physical examination portion of the consultation.

♦ Retain a copy of the recorded consultation within the oncology department.

While recent reviews provide a compelling, evidence-based case for consultation audio-recording use, additional studies are warranted. Studies are needed to examine the process of implementing consultation audio-recording use into oncology practice. We need to address the factors that impede the transfer and uptake of consultation audio-recording use and test ideas about the best ways to transfer intervention knowledge and support intervention uptake. These studies should be guided by theoretical frameworks relevant to knowledge transfer and uptake, such as the PARIHS Framework and Social Network Theory. The field of knowledge translation is growing rapidly, and new theoretical frameworks are being developed, while existing ones are being adapted for use as knowledge translation frameworks. Further research is needed to examine the suitability or heuristic value of these theories to examinations of the transfer and uptake of the consultation audio-recording intervention.

While the empirical evidence base demonstrates the value of furnishing patients with consultation audio recordings, greater attention needs to be paid to the benefits that family members receive from listening to the audio recording, the manner by which patients and families derive benefit and value, and the benefits to clinicians of having their consultations recorded for use by patients and family members. We need to identify and describe any subgroups of patients and families for whom consultation audio recordings are most beneficial. Last, we need to document the types of consultations that are most valuable to patients and families. While most of the empirical literature has focused on the initial treatment consultation, there may be unique benefits associated with providing patients with audio recordings of any consultations in which a change of treatment or care is indicated, such as consultations following disease recurrence or a switch to palliative care.

References

Boissel JP, Amsallem E, Cucherat M, Nony P, Haugh MC (2004). Bridging the gap between therapeutic research results and physician prescribing decisions: knowledge transfer, a prerequisite to knowledge translation. *Euro J Clin Pharmacol* **60**, 609–16.

Buchanan M (2002). *Nexus: Small Worlds and the Groundbreaking Theory of Networks*. W.W. Norton & Company, New York, NY.

Chilvers R, Harrison G, Sipos A, Barley M (2002). Evidence into practice: Application of Psychological Models of Change in Evidence-based Implementation. *Br J Psychiatry* **181**, 99–101.

Ely JW, Osheroff JA, Ebell MH, *et al.* (2002). Obstacles to answering doctors' questions about patient care with evidence: qualitative study. *BMJ* **324**, 1–7.

Grimshaw JM, Eccles M, Tetroe J (2004). Implementing clinical guidelines: current evidence and future implications. *J Contin Ed Health Prof* **24** (Suppl 1), S31–7.

Hack TF, Degner LF, Watson P, Sinha L (2006). Do patients benefit from participating in medical decision making? longitudinal follow-up of women with breast cancer. *Psychooncology* **15**, 9–19.

Hack TF, Ruether JD, Weir LM, Grenier D, Degner LM (2013). Promoting consultation recording practice in oncology: identification of critical implementation factors and determination of patient benefit. *Psychooncology* **22**, 1273–82.

Harvey G, Loftus-Hills A, Rycroft-Malone J, *et al.* (2002). Getting evidence into practice: the role and function of facilitation. *J Adv Nurs* **37**, 577–88.

Haynes B, Haines A (1998). Barriers and bridges to evidence based clinical practice. *BMJ* **317**, 273–6.

Kitson A, Harvey G, McCormack B (1998). Enabling the implementation of evidence based practice: a conceptual framework. *Qual Health Care* **7**, 149–58.

Lomas J (2007). The in-between world of knowledge brokering. *BMJ* **334**, 129–32.

McCormack B, Kitson A, Rycroft-Malone J, Titchen A, Seers K (2002). Getting evidence into practice: the meaning of 'context'. *J Adv Nurs* **38**, 94–104.

Pearcey PA (1995). Achieving research-based nursing practice. *J Adv Nurs* **22**, 33–9.

Pitkethly M, MacGillivray S, Ryan R (2008). Recording or summaries of consultations for people with cancer (review). *Cochrane Database Syst Rev* **16**, CD001539.

Rycroft-Malone J (2004). The PARIHS framework—a framework for guiding the implementation of evidence-based practice. *J Nurs Care Qual* **19**, 297–304.

Rycroft-Malone J, Seers K, Titchen A, Harvey G, Kitson A, McCormack B (2004). What counts as evidence in evidence-based practice? *J Adv Nurs* **47**, 81–90.

West E, Barron DN, Dowsett J, Newton JN (1999). Hierarchies and cliques in the social networks of healthcare professionals: implications for the design of dissemination strategies. *Soc Sci Med* **48**, 633–46.

CHAPTER 11

Learner-centred communication training

Suzanne M. Kurtz and Lara J. Cooke

Introduction to learner-centred communication training

In the last 20 years, medical education and the broad profession that it serves have taken on communication education and training as an important component of the curriculum. In many countries, substantive communication training has become a requirement for accreditation of undergraduate schools and residency programmes across all specialties. Continuing education (CE) offerings on communication are widespread. Undergraduate, residency, and CE programmes have developed a variety of approaches for enhancing communication in healthcare. These advances notwithstanding, formal communication training is still a relatively recent development in medical education.

The overarching purpose of this chapter is to explore ways of implementing learner-centred, experiential communication teaching in palliative care and oncology. Drawing parallels between effective physician–patient communication and effective communication teaching, we discuss building on the learner-centred approach as a means for moving towards the emerging paradigm of relationship-centred education and care. The chapter offers evidence-based best practices regarding what to teach in clinical communication curricula and how to teach it. In the process, we consider how communication teaching can enhance accuracy and efficiency, as well as the 'culture of compassion' that is so significant to the practice of medicine in palliative care and oncology.

Because how we think about communication has a major impact on how we communicate in medical and educational contexts, this chapter begins by examining assumptions and (mis)perceptions that students, residents, physicians, and medical educators frequently hold about communication. Next, we look at the goals, approaches, paradigms, and first principles that inform decisions about what is worth teaching in communication education and training. Finally, we offer specific strategies and techniques for teaching communication effectively in medicine. We combine these elements into an organizational structure around which to develop more comprehensive, systematic, and coherent communication programmes from undergraduate, through residency, and on to continuing education. This structure is a crucial foundation for experiential learner-centred education.

How we think about communication influences what we do

The process of initiating a communication programme at any level in medical education inevitably prompts certain questions from learners and faculty alike. Three of the most persistent of these questions reflect underlying assumptions that have a major impact on how we teach communication and the degree to which learners will engage in such training.

Question A: Isn't communication in medicine just an optional add-on in an overcrowded curriculum, a social skill in which learners are already adept? One learner's succinct comment on this is representative: 'Hey, I'm good to go socially—I don't need communication training'. However, an extensive body of research supports an alternative point of view (Silverman *et al.* 2005; Kurtz *et al.* 2005). Literature indicates that there are major problems with communication in medicine and that more effective communication improves medical consultations substantively by increasing accuracy and efficiency; enhancing supportiveness, trust, collaboration, and partnership between physician and patient; and reducing conflicts, complaints, and malpractice litigation. Research also shows that more effective communication improves outcomes of care, including understanding and recall, follow-through and adherence to treatment plans, symptom relief, physiological and psychological outcomes, patient satisfaction, and physician satisfaction. More effective communication enhances coordination of care and reduces costs. Communication in medicine is not the same as social skill—it is a crucial component of clinical skill that should be taught as rigorously and intentionally as medical technical knowledge, physical examination, and medical problem solving.

Question B: Can communication skills really be taught? The literature provides an unequivocally positive response to this question. Several comprehensive reviews outline models of communication training that have resulted in specific, measurable improvements in physicians', residents', and medical students' communication performance (Aspergren 1999; Kurtz *et al.* 2005; Fallowfield and Jenkins 2006). Communication is not an innate talent; it is a learned skill or, more accurately, a series of learned skills.

Question C: Is it really necessary to teach communication—won't physicians and other caregivers get it through experience anyway? Unfortunately, when it comes to communication in medicine, experience may be a poor substitute for formal education. While experience is often an excellent reinforcer of habit, it tends not to discern between good and bad habits. Consider, for example, a series of studies showing that without ongoing reinforcement, communication skills may deteriorate from the time students enter medical school to when they begin practice (Helfer 1970; Maguire *et al.* 1986*a*, 1986*b*). On measures of empathy, medical students who have been trained, perform better; however, empathy skills have been shown to decline over time and are measurably lower at the end of medical training than at the beginning (Poole and Fisher 1979). Furthermore, it appears that communication skills may be relatively entrenched by the time residents complete their training—that is, more experience probably does not improve communication skills (Maguire *et al.* 1986*b*; Ridsdale *et al.* 1992). Deficiencies in communication skills have been delineated across the continuum of medical education, including at the level of residency and practising clinicians. Physicians interrupt their patients' opening statements within the first 30 seconds, on average, despite the fact that 'spontaneous speaking times' for complex medical patients average less than two minutes (Beckman and Frankel 1984; Marvel *et al.* 1999; Langewitz *et al.* 2002; Dysch and Swiderski 2005). Physicians use closed-ended questions in an effort to structure and expedite interviews, but unfortunately this results in as little as 50% of the relevant patient concerns being elicited during some interviews (Stewart *et al.* 1979; Roter and Hall 1987). The result is a failure to discuss key patient concerns, perspectives, and agendas during the medical interview. This in turn has a negative impact on both patient and clinician satisfaction with medical interviews (Roter *et al.* 1997). Studies measuring the use of patient-centred communication behaviours in primary care senior residents showed that these behaviours (e.g. checking for patient understanding, responding to patients' emotional cues) occur in only 58% of recorded interviews (Campion *et al.* 2002). Experience alone is not sufficient; explicit communication training is necessary.

Acknowledging these questions and responding to the underlying assumptions they reflect, puts communication skills teachers in a position to initiate programmes with strong credibility that have an essential element needed to motivate adult learners and even reluctant participants. That element is relevance.

Deciding what is worth teaching

A number of factors affect how we conceptualize communication teaching and make decisions about what is worth teaching in communication education.

Goals of communication teaching

At the most basic level, what we decide to teach depends on the outcomes we are trying to achieve through communication education. We draw our goals directly from research evidence and have applied them to communication programmes at all levels of medical education, and in a variety of contexts. At more senior levels, we expect deeper mastery of skills and more mature development of attitudes and capacities (compassion, integrity, mindfulness, etc.). Contexts and problems become more complex as learners advance, but the goals of training remain constant. Regardless of whether the learners are medical students, residents, or practising physicians or surgeons with years of experience, the outcomes we are aiming for invariably include (Kurtz *et al.* 2005):

◆ promoting relationships of collaboration and partnership;

◆ increasing:

- accuracy
- efficiency
- supportiveness

◆ enhancing patient and physician satisfaction; and

◆ improving health outcomes.

The ultimate goal of ensuring that we improve every physician's communication skills in practice to a professional level of competence dictates that communication curricula focus not only on what learners understand cognitively (knowledge), but also on their communication skills and behaviours (competence), what they choose to do in practice (performance), and what happens to patients as a result (outcomes) (Miller 1990).

While the above goals fit all learners, different educational levels do lend themselves to different emphases. Medical students spend less time on explanation and planning than on history-taking, presumably due to the paucity of their medical expertise and their lack of confidence regarding information giving (Kauffman *et al.* 2000). In contrast, residents' responsibilities give them the opportunity to reinforce effective information-gathering skills and to add an emphasis on explanation and planning skills. Despite this shift, residents often receive little training in the communication skills related to explanation and planning (Kaufman *et al.* 2000). If this gap is not addressed during residency or medical school, difficulties with explanation and planning are likely to persist into medical practice and in many cases go unchecked (6, 17). Underscoring this gap, one study demonstrated that 70% of malpractice cases include four problems related to explanation and planning: deserting the patient; failure to understand the patient's perspective; devaluing the patient's views; and delivering information poorly (Beckman *et al.* 1994). We suggest that residency training is the time and place to add a focus, not only on explanation and planning, but also on communication between colleagues or with other members of the healthcare team.

In oncology and palliative care—where long-term care, high stakes, and a bewildering array of serious issues are the norm—there can be no doubt that it is important to develop communication skills. The relationship between the physician, healthcare team, patient, and patient's significant others will determine, to a large extent, the degree to which patients comprehend and adhere to complex medical treatment regimes. The effectiveness of oncologists' and palliative care specialists' communication will also impact the extent of emotional suffering, anxiety, and uncertainty experienced by patients with cancer or those at the end of life.

Given what we know about the importance of communication in healthcare generally, and in oncology and palliative care in particular, we need to make communication professionals out of everyone who goes into clinical practice. We can achieve this goal, but only if we extend communication education from the early years of medical school, through clerkship, into residency and beyond.

Skills vs. attitudes and capacities vs. issues

The debate is ongoing about how best to bridge the gap between doctors' communication behaviours during consultations and the behaviours that research has shown to make a positive difference in the outcomes of care for each of the players. Three primary views on how to structure communication training and education have emerged from the debate:

1. The skills perspective structures learning around three types of communication skills: what doctors say (content skills); how they say it (process skills); and what they are thinking and feeling (perceptual skills). These skill sets are interdependent; a weakness in any of them results in a weakness in all. Skills-based programmes give primary attention to the development of process skills, since they are the least emphasized in most medical curricula, and secondary attention to content and perceptual skills, since they are the focus of other parts of the medical curriculum.

2. The attitude perspective focuses teaching on preparation of the inner ground; that is, on enhancing attitudes, capacities, intentions, assumptions, and psychological factors that influence how doctors communicate. Here the rationale is that these underlying factors block effective communication and attending to these factors will improve communication.

3. The issues perspective suggests that we structure learning around specific communication issues, such as delivering bad news, death and dying, obtaining informed consent, communicating treatment risks and benefits, and reducing error, as well as issues related to gender or culture and to communication with children, geriatric patients, neurologically compromised patient, etc.

Without preparation and development of the 'inner ground' of intentions and capacities, the masterful use of skills becomes manipulation. On the other hand, the best of intentions and the most well-developed capacities are essentially useless if we do not have well-developed skills to demonstrate or apply them in practice. The dilemma in using issues as the primary focus is inefficiency. This perspective can promote the mistaken notion that each issue requires a different set of skills, when in fact the same communication process skills are useful in responding to each of these issues. The context changes from issue to issue, the content of the communication changes, the skills may need to be applied with greater intentionality, intensity or mastery, but the skills themselves remain the same.

The historical perspective: The shot put vs. the frisbee approach

Another take on what to teach comes from a brief look at the long history of communication training in academe. From this vantage point, what we end up teaching in communication programmes (and how we teach it) boils down to two basic perspectives that Alton Barbour (2000) has metaphorically dubbed the 'shot put approach' and the 'frisbee approach'. The first was in vogue literally from the time of the ancient Greeks to the middle of the twentieth century. It defined communication as the well-conceived, well-delivered message. Effective communication consisted of content, delivery, and persuasion. As when throwing a shot put, all the speaker had to do was put together a message, deliver it, and his job was done.

In the 1940s, the focus began to shift towards interpersonal communication and the frisbee approach. As Barbour suggests, two new concepts are central to this approach; both are significant to medicine and especially relevant to palliative care and oncology. The first concept is confirmation, which RD Laing (1961) defined as recognizing, acknowledging, and endorsing the other person. The second concept is mutually understood common ground.

This common ground, of which both parties in the interaction are aware, is a necessary foundation for trust, which is in turn the basis for authentic relationships. Decades ago, SJ Baker (1955) called this idea 'reciprocal identification' and pointed out that people reach mutual understanding of common ground primarily by talking with each other about it. His model offers an excellent remedy for moments of discomfort, defensiveness, or conflict: simply (re)establish some sort of mutually understood common ground. Establishing mutually understood common ground does not mean that people agree, but that they understand each other. In medicine, this can be as straightforward as a mutual understanding of the reasons for the patient's visit or of the next steps physician and patient will take. In the frisbee approach the message is still important, but the emphasis shifts to interaction, feedback, and relationship.

Shifting paradigms in medical (and educational) practice

Shifts in the predominant paradigms for conceptualizing healthcare (including physician–patient interaction) and those that help us conceptualize education (including teacher–student interaction) have followed a similar pattern. In education, a shift has occurred from teacher-centred education, wherein teachers held control and told essentially passive students what to think and do, to learner-centred education. The latter places emphasis on the learner's perspectives and learners take a much more active, participatory role; learners assist in setting their own objectives and experiential activities, which demand high levels of learner participation. Both teachers' and learners' agendas and contributions are important.

Similarly, in healthcare, we have moved from doctor-centred care, wherein the physician held most of the control hierarchically and told essentially passive patients what to do, to patient-centred care (Stewart et al. 2003). The latter has required that doctors understand their patients, as well as their patients' disease. Patient-centred care placed new emphasis on eliciting and responding to the patient's perspective regarding the patient's thoughts, beliefs, feelings, and expectations, as well as the effects of illness on their lives. Building on patient-centred care, a third paradigm shift is in progress. Called relationship-centred care (Beach et al. 2006), it sees relationship as central to all healthcare and healing, including the clinician's relationship with patients, self, colleagues, and communities.

Principles of effective communication and teaching

The 'first principles' of communication provide another way to frame the content of communication curricula. Not surprisingly, the 'first principles' of effective communication are identical to the first principles that characterize effective teaching.

Effective communication and teaching:

◆ Ensure interaction, not just transmission of a message.

◆ Reduce unnecessary uncertainty, e.g. about roles and responsibilities, a patient's prognosis, the patient's expectations for the visit, etc.

◆ Require planning and thinking in terms of outcomes. Effectiveness can only be determined in the context of the outcomes you and the other(s) are working towards.

◆ Demonstrate dynamism by engaging authentically with the other and also remaining flexible, developing a deep enough repertoire of skills to allow different approaches with different people or contexts.

♦ Follow a helical rather than a linear model. Once and done is never enough. Effective communication, like effective teaching and learning, requires reiteration, coming back around the helix at a little higher level, taking feedback to your communication (or efforts at teaching or learning) into account at each turn. The helix serves as an excellent model for curriculum development.

Special considerations regarding communication issues in oncology

A recent survey of 394 oncology patients (Cox *et al.* 2006) sought to determine the information needs and experiences of cancer patients in the United Kingdom. The vast majority of patients wished for complete disclosure of information in the cancer setting. In addition, while most patients indicated that they received adequate information about their diagnosis, initial tests, and prognosis, fewer patients reported having discussions about clinical trials and psychosocial issues. In a field where delivering bad news is an essential skill, and in some cases, where clinical trials may represent the only hope for medical treatment, it is essential that addressing these shortfalls be a part of any new communication curriculum.

Another recent study investigated oncologists' communication patterns in relation to patient characteristics. Siminoff *et al.* (2006) showed that physicians' communication style was more likely to be oriented towards establishing rapport and relationship building when interacting with patients who were younger, white, affluent, and had more education. Similarly, patients who were younger, had higher educational levels, and were more affluent, were more likely to engage in relationship-building conversation with their oncologists, and were more likely to ask questions. While it is doubtful that these findings are unique to the area of cancer care, this study underscores the need to build in activities that attune residents and practising clinicians to the possibility of differences in the quality of communication between oncologists and patients with varying demographics.

Choosing effective strategies for teaching communication in medicine

The comprehensive reviews of communication education referred to earlier in this chapter (Aspergen 1999; Kurtz *et al.* 2005; Fallowfield and Jenkins 2006) identify experiential, learner-centred education as a best practices approach to teaching and learning communication in medicine. This approach is the most efficacious way to teach communication, if what you are looking for is engaged learners who effectively enhance or change their behaviour, deepen their understanding, are able to apply both skills and understandings in real interactions with patients or others, and sustain their learning over time.

Learner-centred, experiential education

Experiential, learner-centred education follows the premise that learning is at its best when the following criteria are met:

♦ the learner sees the relevance of the content;

♦ the content is presented in a goal or task-oriented light;

♦ there is opportunity for considerable autonomy and self-direction on the part of the learner; and

♦ the individual learner's prior knowledge and level of experience are recognized and acknowledged as legitimate (Knowles 1984).

As is the case in patient and relationship-centred care, learners are active and interactive participants in their own learning process and in that of their peers. Couple this with problem or inquiry-based learning, in which learners have the opportunity to apply theoretical understanding to real-life situations and problems, and you have participatory, learner-centred, experiential education. The agendas of both learner and facilitator are important. The facilitator has considerable responsibility in structuring the learning sessions and guiding learners to stretch their comfort zones, experiment, and move beyond what they already know how to do. Learners have the responsibility to prepare for, and participate in, experiences and discussions. Feedback in this kind of learning is interactive: a conversation between all the participants, rather than a lecture.

What it takes to enhance communication skills and change behaviour

Research indicates that knowledge about communication skills and capacities, and about their relative importance in caring for patients is very useful, but generally not sufficient to change behaviour effectively. Several other elements emerge from the research that are essential if we want to enhance communication skills, change behaviour in practice, and sustain that learning over time (Kurtz *et al.* 2005):

♦ systematic delineation and definition of skills;

♦ observation of learners communicating with simulated and actual patients;

♦ video (or at least audio) recording of the interaction for later review;

♦ well-intentioned and detailed descriptive feedback;

♦ repeated practice and rehearsal of skills in a safe setting;

♦ active small group or one-to-one formats for learning.

Given this list of essentials, and the responsibilities and time pressures in clinical practice, it becomes clear that some dedicated time for communication training away from the clinic or ward is essential. Fallowfield *et al.* (2002) provide one example of a dedicated programme that incorporates many of the essential elements. The authors conducted a controlled, randomized trial of an intensive, three-day, experiential communication workshop for 160 oncologists in the United Kingdom. Participants in the programme were directly observed, videotaped, and given feedback on their consultative skills. Participants showed between 30 and 50% improvement in specific, measurable communication skills, such as use of open-ended questions, summarizing, and use of empathetic statements. Not only did the authors demonstrate that their programme was efficacious, in a one-year follow-up study, they were able to demonstrate that the effects were also enduring (Fallowfield *et al.* 2003).

Identifying the communication skills to teach and learn

A quick reread of the bulleted list above reveals that all of the essential elements depend for implementation on our ability to delineate and

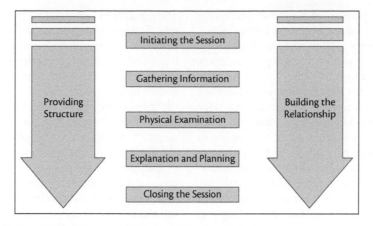

Fig. 11.1 Framework for medical consultations and the Calgary–Cambridge guides (Kurtz *et al.* 2003).
Reproduced with permission from Wolters Kluwer Health: Kurtz S *et al.* 'Marrying Content and Process in Clinical Method Teaching: Enhancing the Calgary-Cambridge Guides', *Academic Medicine*, Volume 78, Number 8, pp. 802–809, Copyright © 2003 Association of American Medical Colleges.

define the skills. Numerous models have been developed to identify the skills that are the focus of many communication programmes. For example, the Maastricht's Maas Global (the Netherlands), the Segue Model (USA), Patient-Centered Care (Canada), the Model of the Macy Initiative in Health Communication (USA), and the Calgary–Cambridge guides (Canada and England). The most effective programmes are based upon models such as these.

Skills models and the feedback instruments through which they are presented constitute a particularly important part of the organizational structure. They summarize the communication skills curriculum and allow us to deconstruct communication. Used as guides to structure observation and feedback, the instruments help us identify individual learner's specific strengths and weaknesses and enable more systematic, concrete learning. As Faldon *et al.* (2004) indicate, comprehensive models overcome two problems: overconfident learners are introduced formally to unique aspects of medical interviewing; and learners who lack confidence are offered a lifeline.

So, what specific communication skills are worth teaching? As an example, we will examine more closely our own highly evidence-based Calgary–Cambridge guides (C–C guides) (Silverman *et al.* 2005; Kurtz *et al.* 2003, 2005). As is true of most instruments, the C–C guides have gone through numerous iterations (in this case over the last 30 years) that drew on the work of medical colleagues in Australia, Canada, England, the Netherlands, the United States, and elsewhere. Riccardi and Kurtz (1983) published an earlier version. Many students, faculty, and patients have added their feedback and suggestions. The C–C guides have enjoyed widespread international recognition and have, to our surprise, been translated into numerous languages. The guides and the Calgary–Cambridge approach to teaching communication apply equally well to a variety of disciplines and levels. Communication programmes in nursing and allied health professions, teacher education, and veterinary medicine are employing the guides with minor modification. In fact, we use the exact same guides with learners at every level of medical education because there are no 'basic' or 'advanced' skills. There are only varying degrees of mastery and sophistication in applying the skills, and varying expectations for how far learners at different levels will take a given case.

The C–C guides form the backbone of the curriculum. The 71 items on the process guides provide a usable summary of the

research literature on what makes a difference in doctor–patient communication. To make this comprehensive list more manageable and memorable, the skills are organized around the framework in Figure 11.1, plus subheadings in each section that represent the aims clinicians need to accomplish within each task. This framework corresponds directly to the tasks that are undertaken in any consultation: initiating the session; gathering information (including communication skills associated with physical examination); providing structure; building the relationship; explanation and planning; and closing the session. With the exception of relationship building and providing structure, which occur throughout the consultation, all the tasks occur more or less sequentially in any given interaction. In essence, the guides comprise a four-page summary of the content of the communication programme.

Although only a few pages in length, the guides have several advantages. They delineate and define the skills that make up effective doctor–patient communication, offering guidance with considerable flexibility for personal style and varied contexts. They provide an accessible summary of the evidence regarding doctor–patient communication and present a common language for labelling and referring to specific behaviours. The guides make transparent the skills content of the course; since the same instrument is used for both feedback during learning sessions and summative assessment, the guides also help to make evaluation transparent. They provide a basis for consistent teaching and feedback, and form a common foundation for communication programmes at all levels of medical education.

Putting the other essential elements into play

As other chapters in this book demonstrate, consultations that provide the experiential basis for communication training can include interactions with various 'patients'. Simulated patients are trained to portray specific situations (ideally based on real cases) that course organizers select or that learners bring to the table, based on situations they have encountered. Learners role play situations they have experienced. Volunteer patients replay their real medical problems. Actual patients participate through their ongoing care. Learners can work with live consultations or use videotapes of consultations. Video-taping is an invaluable part of the programme that offers learners a check and balance for their own perception and self-assessment, a feedback and teaching tool for the group, and a way to focus on specific points of strength or weakness.

Pairs or small groups of learners, guided by an expert facilitator or coach, work especially well because they offer the opportunity for individual practice, as well as the benefits of gaining feedback from the perspective of others. With trained, simulated patients (or in some cases with volunteers and during video review) where the facilitator or a fellow learner takes on the role of the patient in the interview, learners can 'rewind' parts of the interview to give the original interviewer a chance to try an alternate communication approach or to see how a colleague would handle the situation. Small groups that meet regularly are best able to develop a place of trust that enables the experimentation and mistake-making that are hallmarks of experiential learning. One-to-one formats are also useful, but these have the disadvantage of potential power struggles and fewer points of view.

Agenda-led outcome-based analysis (ALOBA): A protocol for feedback and facilitation

Teaching and learning communication skills are substantively different from other clinical skills. Communication is more complex than simpler procedural skills; so many more variables influence it. Although it is not a personality trait, communication is closely bound to self-concept. To put it another way; no one is invested in how they palpate a liver before they learn how to do it, but we are often heavily invested in our communication skills and the connection we perceive those skills to have with our personal style. Unlike procedural skills, which have an achievement ceiling, you can always improve on communication skills. Even if you are exemplary one day, the next a variety of distractions—or the variety of people you get to communicate with—can make you feel awkward and inept.

The idea of communication training is to enhance what learners already do well, expand each learner's repertoire of skills, work with applying comfortable skills in more complex circumstances, and break habits that serve neither clinician nor patient well. While focusing on communication process skills, and the content and perceptual skills that interact with them, learners and facilitators also need to keep the ongoing development of right capacities and attitudes in mind. Perfecting skills without developing the inner ground of capacities, such as respect, integrity, and compassion, amounts to manipulation. Capacities are relatively useless without refinement of the skills that are needed to demonstrate those capacities.

Agenda-led outcome-based analysis (ALOBA) is a protocol developed for giving feedback and facilitating experiential, learner-centred, problem-based sessions (Kurtz *et al.* 2005); it maximizes participation and learning of the entire group, reduces defensiveness, and enhances learning. ALOBA begins by greeting the group and, in the initial meeting, getting to know each other briefly and agreeing on rules of conduct (confidentiality, participation, attendance, experimentation, etc.). Next the facilitator prepares the group to observe an interaction that will be the basis for individual feedback, as well as a gift of 'raw' material for the entire group's learning. Before the interaction begins, the facilitator asks for the agenda of the learner who is about to interact with a patient, engage in a simulation, or share a video. For example, the facilitator might ask: 'What do you want us to watch for?' or 'What do you want feedback on?'.

The group then observes the interaction and makes concrete and specific notes on the interaction using the C–C guides. The learner or the coach may call 'time-outs' during the interaction to get ideas if problems arise or try something over, but these are generally kept to a minimum. Once the observation is complete, the facilitator, in true learner-centred fashion, again requests information about the learner's perspectives and insights before allowing others to weigh in with their ideas on the interaction: 'How do you think that went?', 'What are your feelings about the interaction?', 'Anything else you'd like us to look at now regarding the interaction?'.

Spotting skills and discussing feedback is the next step. After the group and the patient (if present) respond to the learner's agenda, others may point out things the learner may not have thought to ask about. By offering well-intentioned, descriptive feedback that is as concrete and specific as possible, the group is essentially holding up a mirror to reflect what they saw or heard. The facilitator and all group members are responsible for ensuring that the feedback is balanced; between reinforcing what worked and discussing problem areas, and the next steps to make the interaction even better. The group offers alternative approaches and participates in 'rewinds' to try them out.

The outcome-based part of ALOBA comes into play when trying to determine what communication skills and approaches would be most effective. Instead of trying to evaluate what is good or bad, or attempting to reach consensus about the 'best' approach, ALOBA urges consideration of the outcomes the learner was trying to accomplish at a given moment, as well as the outcomes the patient was trying to work on. The facilitator or a group member might ask: 'What were you trying to accomplish just then?', 'And what was the patient needing or working on?', 'Was what you were doing getting at both sets of outcomes?', 'What else would be an effective way to work towards those outcomes?'. With communication skills, effectiveness can only be determined in the context of the outcomes sought by the various players in an interaction.

Figure 11.2 offers a graphic representation that facilitators have found useful as a quick reference guide for how to run a session using the ALOBA approach (Kurtz *et al.* 2005). The protocol is not cast in stone; it is intended as a flexible guide, a framework that facilitators can adapt to their learning groups' changing needs and purpose. Note how closely the ALOBA protocol resembles the tasks on the C–C guides (Fig. 11.2). Not surprisingly, the skills required to effectively facilitate a session using ALOBA are the same as those listed in the C–C guides, but are here applied to the learner group.

Modelling and the informal curriculum

In communication training and education, as in the teaching of other clinical skills, there is most definitely a place for the traditional apprenticeship strategy of modelling on the part of more experienced practitioners. Modelling can have a profound effect on attitudes, as well as communication skills. It can influence behaviour in extremely valuable ways and sometimes, inadvertently, in adverse ways. Obviously clinicians model communication skills and attitudes whenever they interact with a patient. They may be less aware of what they are inadvertently modelling as they interact with colleagues or other staff, and of what learners pick up from how experienced clinicians treat the learners themselves. The point here is that those of us whom learners observe or who interact with learners, either as teachers or as role models, need to become more

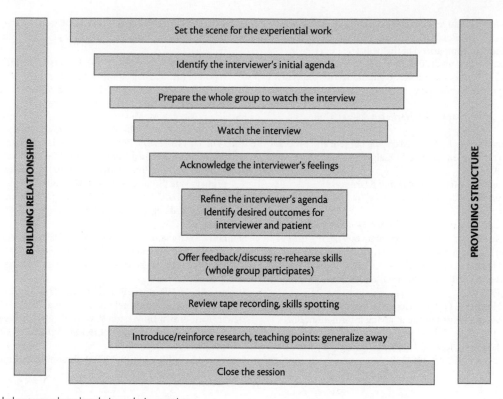

Fig. 11.2 How agenda-led outcome-based analysis works in practice.
Reproduced with permission from Kurtz SM, Silverman JD, and Draper J, *Teaching and Learning Communication Skills in Medicine, Second Edition*, Radcliffe Publishing, Oxford, UK, Copyright © 2004.

aware of what we are contributing to this informal, hidden curriculum (Suchman and Williamson 2003).

Optimal learning occurs when the formal curriculum, consisting of experiential learning opportunities, structured around a strong organizational framework, and a model that delineates communication skills, combines forces with informal curricular interventions during daily practice that are associated with modelling to advantage. Such interventions include cueing, observation, guided reflection, explicit commentary, and questions regarding what we are modelling—the very same interventions that we bring to bear when teaching other clinical skills.

Summary

Quality communication training enhances accuracy, efficiency, and relationships—three elements that are essential to the delivery of quality healthcare. Effective communication training also facilitates the creation and maintenance of the 'culture of compassion' that is so important to the practice of medicine in oncology and palliative care. To accomplish these ends, we have set forth evidence-based foundations and best practices for teaching and learning clinical communication skills and capacities. In addition to enhancing the implementation of individual programmes, this chapter calls for the development of more comprehensive, systematic, and coherent communication training in oncology and palliative care that extends from undergraduate, through residency, and on to continuing education.

Acknowledgements

We wish to acknowledge Drs Jonathan Silverman and Julie Draper, who are co-authors with Dr Kurtz of two companion books that discuss in greater detail many of the concepts, approaches, and research findings offered here. Listed as the first two references in this chapter, the books are a primary source for these materials.

References

Aspergren K (1999). Teaching and learning communication skills in medicine: a review with quality grading of articles. *Med Teach* **21**, 563–70.

Baker SJ (1955). The theory of silences. *J Gen Psychology* **53**, 145.

Barbour A (2000). Making contact or making sense: functional and dysfunctional ways of relating. Paper presented for Humanities Institute Lecture 1999–2000 Series, University of Denver, CO.

Beach MC, Inui T and the Relationship-Centered Care Research Network (2006). Relationship-centred care: a constructive reframing, *J Gen Intern Med* **21**, S3–8.

Beckman HB, Frankel RM (1984). The effect of physician behaviour on the collection of data. *Ann Intern Med* **101**, 692–6.

Beckman HB, Markakis KM, Suchman AL, *et al.* (1994). The doctor-patient relationship and malpractice. *Arch Int Med* **154**, 1365–70.

Campion P, Foulkes J, Neighbour R, *et al.* (2002). Patient centredness in the MRCGP video examination: analysis of large cohort. *BMJ* **325**, 691–2.

Cox A, Jenkins V, Catt S, *et al.* (2006). Information needs and experiences: an audit of UK cancer patients. *Eur J Onc Nurs* **10**, 263–72.

Dysch L, Swiderski D (2005). The effect of physician solicitation approaches on ability to identify patient concerns. *J Gen Intern Med* **10**, 267–70.

Faldon J, Pessach I, Toker A (2004). Teaching medical students what they think they already know. *Ed for Health* **17**, 35–41.

Fallowfield L, Jenkins V, Farewell V, *et al.* (2002). Efficacy of a Cancer Research UK communication skills training model for oncologists: a randomized controlled trial. *Lancet* **359**, 650–6.

Fallowfield L, Jenkins V, Farewell V, *et al.* (2003). Enduring impact of communication skills training: results of a 12-month follow-up. *Br J Cancer* **89**, 1445–9.

Fallowfield L, Jenkins V (2006). Current concepts of communication skills training in oncology. *Recent Results Cancer Res* **168**, 105–12.

Helfer RE (1970). An objective comparison of the pediatric interviewing skills of freshman and senior medical students. *Pediatrics* **45**, 623–7.

Kauffman DM, Laidlaw TA, Macleod H (2000). Communication skills in medical school: Exposure, confidence, and performance. *Acad Med* **75** (Suppl 10), S90–2.

Knowles MS (1984). *The Adult Learner—A Neglected Species*. Gulf, Houston, TX.

Kurtz S, Silverman J, Benson J, *et al.* (2003). Marrying content and process in clinical method teaching: enhancing the Calgary–Cambridge guides. *Acad Med* **78**, 802–9.

Kurtz S, Silverman J, Draper J (2005). *Teaching and Learning Communication Skills in Medicine*, 2nd edition. Radcliffe Publishing, Oxford and San Francisco, CA.

Laing R (1961). *The Self and Others*. Pantheon Books, New York, NY.

Langewitz W, Denz M, Keller A, *et al.* (2002). Spontaneous talking time at start of consultation in outpatient clinic: cohort study. *BMJ* **325**, 682–3.

Maguire P, Fairbairn S, Fletcher C (1986*a*). Consultation skills of young doctors: 1—benefits of feedback training in interviewing as students persists. *BMJ* **292**, 1573–6.

Maguire P, Fairbairn S, Fletcher C (1986*b*). Consultation skills of young doctor: II—most young doctors are bad at giving information. *BMJ* **292**, 1576–8.

Marvel MK, Epstein RM, Flowers K, *et al.* (1999). Soliciting the patient's agenda: have we improved? *JAMA* **281**, 283–7.

Miller GE (1990). Commentary on clinical skills assessment: a specific review. National Board of Medical Examiners' 75th Anniversary. Philadelphia, PA, 48–51.

Poole AD, Sanson Fisher RW (1979). Understanding the patient: a neglected aspect of medical education. *Soc Sci Med* **13A**, 37–43.

Riccardi VM, Kurtz SM (1983). *Communication and Counseling in Healthcare*. Charles C. Thomas, Springfield, IL.

Ridsdale L, Morgan M, Morris R (1992). Doctors' interviewing technique and its response to different booking time. *Family Pract* **9**, 57–60.

Roter DL, Hall JA (1987). Physicians' interview styles and medical information obtained from patients. *J Gen Int Med* **2**, 325–49.

Roter DL, Stewart M, Punam M, *et al.* (1997). Communication patterns in primary care physicians. *JAMA* **277**, 350–6.

Silverman J, Kurtz S, Draper J (2005). *Skills for Communicating with Patients*, 2nd edition. Radcliffe Publishing, Oxford and San Francisco, CA.

Siminoff LA, Graham GC, Gordon NH (2006). Cancer communication patterns and the influence of patient characteristics: Disparities in information-giving and affective behaviours. *Patient Educ Couns* **62**, 355–60.

Stewart MA, McWhinney IR, Buck CW (1979). The doctor patient relationship and its effect upon outcome. *J R Coll Gen Pract* **29**, 77–82.

Stewart MA, Brown JB, Weston WW, *et al.* (2003) *Patient-Centred Medicine: Transforming the Clinical Method*, 2nd edition. Radcliffe Medical Press, Oxford, UK.

Suchman AL, Williamson PR (2003). Personal communication.

SECTION B

A core curriculum for communication skills training for oncology and palliative care

Section editor: David W. Kissane

CHAPTER 12

Breaking bad news

Walter F. Baile and Patricia A. Parker

Introduction to breaking bad news

The cancer clinician is likely to give bad news many thousands of times during the course of his or her career (Baile *et al.* 2000). The goal of this chapter is to review the concept of breaking bad news, highlighting salient points and controversies in the literature, and make training recommendations. It will consider a definition of bad news, why the topic is so important, the challenges to clinicians in breaking bad news, protocols for giving bad news, research on bad news disclosure, and directions for the future.

Definition of 'bad news'

Bad news in the oncology context has been defined in many different ways. One common definition is 'any news that seriously and adversely affects the patient's view of her future' (Buckman 1984). In other words, the 'badness' of the news is the gap between the patient's expectations of the future and the medical reality. It cannot be determined a priori, but is dependent on an individual's subjective evaluation. This is a key point because it distinguishes bad news from other types of more emotionally neutral information about cancer, such as information about chemotherapy. It also cautions the practitioner that what s/he might think is good news to one patient ('I'm glad this tumour can definitely be removed') might be perceived as troubling to another ('Oh my god … I just can't handle another surgery'). Thus, it is essential to discover the recipient's expectations and understanding of their medical situation as part of the discussion.

Breaking bad news is a complex communication task and involves a verbal component (giving the news), as well as recognizing and responding to patients' emotions, involving the patient in decision-making, and finding ways to frame 'hope' and provide support (Baile *et al.* 2000). Ideally, bad news disclosure is a dynamic interaction between the clinician and patient, in which information is not only transmitted to the patient, but the patient's reactions provide cues to the clinician regarding how the information has been received and what concerns the patient may have (Baile and Blatner 2014).

Why skills in breaking bad news are important

Breaking bad news is a key aspect of communicating with cancer patients

Patients may experience bad news at several points during the course of the illness, including initial diagnosis, recurrence, disease progression, and transitioning to palliative care, as well as end-of-life discussions. Bad news not only includes medical setbacks but also events that could be life-changing, such as the occurrence of irreversible side effects of cancer (e.g. peripheral neuropathy), or the discussion of resuscitation. Including these events acknowledges the fact that protocols for giving bad news are widely applicable. Box 12.1 lists key events along the cancer trajectory that are likely to involve bad news discussions. Furthermore, as genetic testing becomes more available, patients are told about additional risks for many common malignancies.

Giving bad news sensitively is a prime concern of patients, who can be traumatized when bad news is given bluntly or matter-of-factly (Hanratty *et al.* 2012). Giving bad news is the 'gateway' to many important aspects of patient care, such as discussing a treatment plan, shared decision-making, obtaining informed consent, and involving the family in the patient's care. Receiving the news in a direct but sensitive and well-planned manner has been reported as being best received; additionally, receiving the news with a family member or other support person present (Hanratty *et al.* 2012). If bad news is given poorly, it can increase patients' distress and suffering, resulting in dissatisfaction with medical care and can negatively impact patients' perceptions of their condition and their relationship with their healthcare team. Poor communication has also been found to be associated with medical malpractice suits.

Patients have a right to information about their health status

In Western societies, ethical guidelines and the lack of available cancer treatments have influenced bad news disclosure since the 1950s. At one time, the principle of beneficence took precedence over that of autonomy, and physicians made the decision as to how much and what kind of information to give patients. Many patients were not told about their cancer due to the fear that it would send them into a deep depression. Since the 1970s, as better treatments became available, the principle of autonomy has prevailed to allow patients to make important healthcare decisions. Safeguards have been implemented to protect individuals from medical experimentation against their will. After World War II, the Nuremberg trials established that the physician's judgement that a treatment would help a patient (beneficence) was insufficient to protect individuals from abuse. Every patient needs to consent before receiving a medical procedure. This agreement has established principles for codes of ethics and rules for informed consent, both for treatments and clinical trials. However, controversies still exist over application of these standards. These include whether or not a doctor's claim of therapeutic exception (that bad news will harm a patient) is valid,

Box 12.1 Cancer events warranting 'bad news' discussions and key communication challenges at these points on the cancer trajectory

- **The cancer diagnosis.** Most patients want as much information as is available on treatment. Patients may not hear the information conveyed because of an emotional response to their diagnosis. In some countries, the diagnosis is withheld because of culture, family, and other issues.

- **Prognosis of the illness.** Discussing prognosis can be tricky and a major concern of clinicians is not to destroy hope. Checking with the patient may provide information as to what information the patient wants about the likelihood of success of treatment.

- **Prescription of harsh treatments.** Patients may have preconceived ideas about treatments or side effects. Others may underplay potential side effects. Asking them what they know and expect can help clarify misconceptions.

- **Disease recurrence.** Patients may want less detailed information than at the time of diagnosis. Demoralization is a common psychological response.

- **Unexpected or severe side effects.** Even when patients are cured, side effects may diminish quality of life. Patients may feel angry or cheated when their disease is cured but they are left with disabilities.

- **Treatment failure.** Discussing the possibility of cancer treatments not working while 'hoping for the best' may be a useful strategy to use when first and second-line treatments fail.

- **End of anti-cancer treatment/DNR.** Transitioning patients to palliative care is one of the most difficult tasks for cancer clinicians. The doctor's own emotions, lack of communication skills, and fear of destroying patient hope are significant barriers to overcome in not unnecessarily continuing anti-cancer therapy.

- **Discussion of discontinuation of ventilation.** Goal setting with families early on in an intensive care unit (ICU) stay can reduce unrealistic expectations and shorten ICU stay when the prognosis is grim. Family meetings are an important way of accomplishing this.

- **Sudden unexpected death.** The physician should be prepared to handle very strong emotions in the patient and family and often him/herself.

- **Genetic test results.** It helps to be familiar with current protocols for disclosure since this is a highly specialized discussion.

whether these codes cover discussion of prognosis or the probability of a specific treatment working, and the complex interactions when families seek to have the information disclosed to them first. However, the overarching position of many patients is that decisions made about them should not be made without them.

Patients wish to receive as much information as possible about their health

This is true, even in countries where traditionally bad news (especially that with a dire prognosis) has been withheld from patients. Not all patients, however, desire complete information. Thus, an important first step may be to ask patients about their information preferences.

Parker and colleagues asked 351 patients with varied cancers at different stages about their communication preferences when given bad news about diagnosis or recurrence (Parker *et al.* 2001). The highest rated concerns included: the doctor being up-to-date with the latest research, informing the patients about the best treatment options, taking time to answer all questions, being honest about the disease severity, using simple language, giving the news directly, and giving full attention to the patient. Differences were noted in patients' preferences based on gender, age and level of education, underlying the importance of tailoring the discussion to each individual. Cancer type did not predict patients' preferences. Through elicitation of each patient's perspective, many incorrect beliefs can be clarified beneficially (Parker *et al.* 2001). The amount and type of information patients prefer may also differ based on where in the cancer trajectory and other disease related characteristics. For example, in the metastatic setting, patients may be especially interested in information regarding prognosis and symptom control (Danesh *et al.* 2014). Another factor that may influence patients' preference is their health locus of control. In a study in which cancer patients watched videotaped scenarios of physicians breaking bad news, patients with higher internal locus of control and lower in powerful others prefer having the 'empathic professional' breaking bad news, whereas those with lower internal locus of control and higher in powerful others preferred a more distant or a more emotional professional (Martins and Carvalho 2013).

Patients can be traumatized by the way that bad news is given

A patient reported that when she went to the doctor for a lump in her neck and was found to have metastatic cancer of the tongue, she was told 'If I were you I'd go home and make my will and get my affairs in order'. She subsequently became panicky and suicidal.

When patients receive bad news, they may be shocked or demoralized. Women who experienced less emotional support are at significantly increased risk for feeling traumatized. These psychological states are worsened by the bad news being given abruptly or insensitively. On the other hand, physicians are a vital source of support for patients who are receiving bad news (Parker *et al.* 2001).

The stigma of cancer

There continues to be stigma surrounding a cancer diagnosis (Else-Quest *et al.* 2009). Many patients fear cancer more than any other catastrophe. Many still believe that stress causes cancer; perceived stigma is commonly behind this (Phelan *et al.* 2013).

These health beliefs are analogous to the primitive fears of children of the dark or a 'boogeyman'—a monster popularized by folklore. The boogeyman metaphor denotes something that is feared irrationally. The concept is portrayed in titles like 'Beating the boogeyman. A cancer patient's diary' (Sikes 1984). Here Sikes writes '… emotions associated with this disease do not easily lend themselves to logic. Because cancer is still mysterious, insidious and life-threatening, it calls forth feelings that few other diseases can inspire. That is enough to rupture any protective membrane of intellectualization' (Sikes 1984). The notion that cancer grows by stealth invokes deep fear.

The diagnosis is an essential prelude to treatment planning

Giving bad news is imperative to 'patient-centred' care. In many Western countries, there are administrative sanctions associated with non-disclosure, including malpractice suits and censure. Patients cannot be given treatments against their will. Without disclosure, the criteria for informed consent or shared decision-making cannot be fulfilled. Better perceived communication about cancer treatment and management (e.g. treatment goals and options while maintaining empathy) may be associated with patients receiving disease-directed, stage appropriate treatment (Lin *et al.* 2014).

Disclosure can promote psychosocial adjustment

Although honest disclosure can have a negative emotional impact in the short term, most patients adjust well over time. Gratitude and peace of mind, positive attitudes, reduced anxiety, and better adaptation are some of the benefits arising from sharing the truth. Relief from uncertainty can also be therapeutic. An increased understanding of illness promotes a sense of order. Bad news should be delivered tactfully, honestly, and in a supportive fashion. Not being told the severity of their condition, or being denied the opportunity to express their worries and concerns, may limit understanding, and even lead some to believe that nothing can be done to help them. Transmission of bad news bluntly or too quickly can exacerbate distress. Being told 'there is nothing more we can do' tends to engender feelings of abandonment (Sep *et al.* 2014). Predictors of patient satisfaction include perceiving the physician as personally interested, being able to understand the information, being informed in a private setting (doctor's office), and having more time to discuss the situation. Although the majority wish to receive complete and accurate information, many still feel the news is forced upon them. This could be protected against by allowing the patient to declare their preferences for how much they want to hear ('Are you the type of person who wants to know all the details about your condition?'). Empathic communication during bad news consultations may decrease physiological arousal in breaking bad news consultations. In a study with analogue patients who viewed two scenarios, one which included empathic communication and another a standard condition, breaking bad news evoked physiological arousal in the individuals watching both scenarios. However, those who watched the empathic communication had a decrease in physiological arousal and had greater recall of the details of the consultation than those who viewed the standard condition (Sep *et al.* 2014).

Current practices in disclosing bad news

There are significant geographic and cultural differences in the information given to cancer patients about their diagnosis and prognosis. In North America, attitudes towards disclosure about cancer have evolved considerably. Prior to the 1970s, most physicians did not inform their patients of the diagnosis. The discussion of diagnosis matured during the 1960s and 1970s. Improved treatment modalities, changing societal attitudes, and legislation enforcing the patient's right to informed decision-making drove physician–patient communication in a more open direction. Consequently, today in many Western countries, there is total open disclosure of cancer. Physicians report various types of bad news discussions in a typical month: amid an average of 36 discussions, they had

12.8 about a new cancer diagnosis; 7.6 about recurrent disease; and 7.4 about treatment failure (Baile *et al.* 2002). If actively encouraged to ask questions, prognosis is the one area in which patients desire information and actually increase their question asking. Patients often want to know the probability of cure, disease stage, chance of curative treatment, and 10-year survival figures comparing receipt and non-receipt of adjuvant therapy. However, patients vary in their desire for such information; those with more advanced cancer may be more ambivalent. Partial and non-disclosure is more prevalent in areas where medical paternalism predominates, where families play a major role in decision-making, where cultural beliefs influence non-disclosure, and where clear ethical and legal guidelines do not exist. In countries where healthcare costs are substantially assumed by the consumer, the consequences of withholding information about health status can have serious repercussions. Lack of discussion can result in unnecessary treatment, prolonged stays in the intensive care unit, or burdensome and unreimbursed hospital costs (Institute of Medicine 2015). Although conversations about prognosis and disease progression are common, clinicians may fail to tell patients that treatment may not cure their disease (Robinson *et al.* 2008), or communicate in a way that patients do not understand them (Weeks *et al.* 2012).

Influences of ethnicity and cultural factors on disclosure

In non-Western cultures, and some European countries, the diagnosis of cancer is often revealed to the family first. The main argument for not telling the patient is one of non-malfeasance, the concept that it would do irreparable harm to the patient. The counter to this argument is that most patients want to know and already suspect, so that telling the family without a discussion with the patient violates the patient's autonomy. In some cultures, patients may prefer that the family be told first. However, when families insist that the news not be given to the patient, an ethical and care dilemma is created for the doctor, who enters into a conspiracy of misinformation, which can undermine trust and the therapeutic alliance, not to mention thwart the notion of informed consent and shared decision-making. In such circumstances, the contemporary 'patient-centred' model of practice is voided.

Patients from many countries believe in a culturally-determined value inherent in non-disclosure of diagnosis and terminal prognosis. In this family-centred model of decision-making, autonomy is seen as isolating. Patients may believe that dignity, identity, and security are conferred by belonging to a family; illness is managed by the family. A recent review of attitudes and beliefs regarding truth disclosure about cancer throughout the Middle East revealed that social stigma and misperceptions about curability are pervasive (Khalil 2013). Physicians typically tell family members the truth about the diagnosis and may conceal it from the patient. At the same time, however, there is an acknowledgement about the patient's right to know (Khalil 2013). Giving patients an unfavourable diagnosis and prognosis can be seen as a curse. Sometimes, the negative stigma associated with the word 'cancer' is so strong that its use is perceived as rude, disrespectful, and even causal. A recent study used a questionnaire based on the SPIKES subscales in German cancer patients (Siefart *et al.* 2014). Forty-six per cent of patients were satisfied with how bad news had been broken to them and their preferences for how they would have liked the news were significantly different from how they were told news of their cancer.

Having clarity about disease progress in assessing patients' comprehension, having enough time and being able to ask questions were the highest rated preferences when breaking bad news (Siefart *et al.* 2014). While sensitivity to culture is crucial, it is difficult to tease apart the various ethnic, family, economic, and related issues from the stigma of giving bad news.

Barriers to bad news disclosure

Physicians frequently have difficulty in delivering bad news and many doctors find it stressful and demanding (Friedrichsen and Milberg 2006). Moreover, many are concerned that they may be perceived as less compassionate and caring by patients and families (Tanco *et al.* 2015). Bad news disclosure is made difficult by several other factors. Giving bad news has not been conceptualized as an acquirable skill, but seen rather as an innate ability that doctors should have. Additionally, oncologists have rarely been trained in techniques for giving bad news, with only about 5% of oncology training programmes historically teaching communication skills (Baile *et al.* 2002). Certification exams have not demanded proficiency in communication skills and there has been a lack of qualified teachers among oncology faculties. Additionally, when physicians have to tell a patient that treatment has not worked, they can experience negative emotions, such as anxiety, fear being blamed, or of losing control (Friedrichsen and Milberg 2006).

Giving bad news evokes strong emotions in both the deliverer and the recipient

Dealing with emotions is one of the most important aspects of giving bad news. Physicians may experience anticipatory anxiety when preparing to give the news, subject to the type of news and the physician's perceptions about their ability to convey it effectively (Buckman 1984). While physicians may be more stressed prior to delivery of unwelcome news, the height of patient stress is after the news has been given. Because of their 'technical-scientific' orientation, many physicians do not typically see themselves as a source of support for the patient, whereas patients are often acutely tuned into the supportive elements of oncologists' behaviour (Zachariae *et al.* 2003). Patients assess a supportive style as highly desirable in their clinicians. Supportive processes include expressions of concern, provision of comfort, if the patient is distressed, and encouragement to talk about feelings (Parker *et al.* 2001).

Communicating with dying patients readily generates anxiety, sadness, and frustration in clinicians, combined with the historic tendency of Western medicine to focus on cure. Shaw *et al.* reported that about one third of physicians experienced a sustained and significant stress response when they had to break bad news, even when it involved simulated encounters (Shaw *et al.* 2013). They may react to reduce stress by offering false hope, premature reassurance, or they may omit salient information. Moreover, patients may process information through a repertoire of coping styles including denial, 'blunting', or dumbing down. They may avoid asking questions, be overly optimistic about the outcome, and distort information to put it in a better light.

Concerns about destroying hope

Physicians strive to achieve a delicate balance between providing honest information sensitively and not discouraging hope (Shockney and Back 2013). Consistent with the assumption that one needs hope to battle cancer, physicians fear that the revelation of a grim prognosis may dash hope and take away patients' will to survive. Physicians avoid putting odds on longevity, recurrence, and cure, since they do not know how each individual patient will fare. Patients may not measure hope solely in terms of cure, but their hope may represent achieving goals, having family and clinician support, and receiving the best treatment available. Protective features to preserve hope include the physician being up-to-date on all treatment options and stating that s/he will not abandon the patient. Research suggests that being truthful does not rob patients and families of hope or lead to depression and that being truthful does not hasten death (Shockney and Back 2013). Adopting a 'hope for the best prepare for the worst approach' can allow clinicians to preserve patient expectations for a positive outcome while preparing them for the future.

Guidelines for giving bad news

Learning to give bad news is a complex task, which involves major communication skills such as establishing rapport, obtaining information from the patient, providing information in understandable language without jargon, responding to patient emotions, and providing a treatment plan to guide the patient through cancer therapy. Insight into how drastically bad news may alter a person's perception of their reality is helpful. Thus the dictum 'ask, before you tell' becomes relevant. If an individual is prepared for bad news, their reaction will be different to a person who is oblivious to the danger. Secondly, awareness of what type of crisis the news will precipitate will also help the clinician to prepare.

Historically, physicians did not form a consistent plan when they broke bad news. At an annual meeting of the American Society of Clinical Oncology, 22% of clinicians reported that they did not have a consistent approach to breaking bad news, while 51.9% used several techniques or tactics, but not an overall plan. Determining what patients believe to be important helps refine guidelines to create evidence-based recommendations for this task (Baile *et al.* 2000).

Many guidelines can be recommended for giving bad news. The news should be broken in an appropriate setting (quiet place, with uninterrupted time), assessing the patient's understanding of their illness, providing information the patient wants, allowing the patient to express their emotions and responding empathically, before summarizing the information provided and coming up with a plan for the next step(s).

Both the structure and content of the consultation influence the patient's ability to remember what has been said in several ways:

1. Patients usually recall facts provided at the start of a consultation more readily than those given later;

2. Topics deemed most relevant and important to the patient (which might not be those considered most pertinent to the doctor) are recalled most accurately;

3. The greater the number of statements made by a doctor, the smaller the mean percentage recalled by the patient; and

4. Items that patients do manage to recall do not decay over time as do other memories.

One protocol for disclosing bad news is represented by SPIKES (Baile *et al.* 2000), a six-step approach shown in Table 12.1. The schema of strategies is short, easily understandable, and leads to

Table 12.1 Strategies to discuss bad news using the SPIKES protocol

Strategies using the SPIKES anagram	Key skills and tasks	Examples of the clinician's comments
1. **Set up** the interview	Use a private space with uninterrupted time; seated; tissues available; consider who should be there Review the agenda with the aim of building rapport and settling the patient into the process	'We're here today to discuss the results of your pathology.' 'Before we turn to the results, do you have any issues or concerns that you'd like to put on our agenda?'
2. Review the patient's **Perception** of the illness	Check understanding Determine information gaps and expectations Correct misunderstanding and define your current role and goal	'I'd like to make sure you understand the reasons for the tests.' 'Do you remember that we sent the tissue from your operation to the pathologist for examination?' 'Most patients have some ideas about what's causing their symptoms. What do you suspect?'
3. Get an **Invitation** from the patient to deliver the news	Determine what type and how much information the patient wants Acknowledge that information needs change over time	'Are you the type of person who wants every bit of detail, or do you prefer an overview of what we found?'
4. Give the patient **Knowledge** and information	Forecast what will come Share the information in chunks, avoiding jargon Draw diagrams and write down details Check understanding	'I'm afraid I've got some bad news for you.' 'The pathology shows that the cancer has spread through the wall of the bowel into a nearby lymph gland.'
5. Respond to the patient's **Emotions**	Explore emotions Acknowledge empathically Validate the emotions Promote a sense of support	'I can see how upsetting this is for you.' 'Can you tell me what you are feeling right now?' 'It is very common for patients to feel this way.'
6. **Summarize** the treatment plan and review all that has been communicated	Discuss future treatment options Check understanding and future needs Review next steps	'We have good treatments using chemotherapy and radiation for your situation. I can tell you about these in due course.' 'Can you summarize for me what you've learned so that I can see how much you've been able to take in.' Note: Video examples of Breaking Bad News using the SPIKES protocol can be found at https://www.mdanderson.org/ICARE

Source: data from Walter F. Baile et al., 'SPIKES—A Six-Step Protocol for Delivering Bad News: Application to the Patient with Cancer,' *The Oncologist*, Volume 5, Number 4, pp. 302–311, Copyright © 2000 AlphaMed Press.

specific skills that can be practised. Moreover, it can be applied to most breaking bad news situations including diagnosis, recurrence, transition to palliative care, and even error disclosure. Its reflective style helps the physician deal with his/her own distress as the 'messenger of bad news'. It incorporates many of the historical recommendations for giving bad news. A recent article proposing an enhancement of SPIKES by focusing on the emotional component provides specific words that clinicians can use in responding to patient emotions, an approach which clinicians training in SPIKES may find useful (van Vilet and Epstein 2014).

When threatened, individuals mobilize different types of coping responses including denial, reframing the threat as a challenge, or mobilizing family support. For most people, the diagnosis of cancer is an immediate threat and elicits strong emotional reactions. These can include shock, helplessness, fear of dying, uncertainty, loss of control/vulnerability, and lowered self-esteem. The clinician needs to recognize the patient's response to be able to empathize appropriately with them.

Teaching breaking bad news

Guidelines provide a useful roadmap for key steps or issues to focus on in giving bad news (see previous section). However, as with any

other skill development, giving bad news is best learned through practice. One training model is described in the programme 'Oncotalk' (see Chapter 56), where oncology fellows were given a didactic lesson in how to give bad news and then afforded practice with standardized patients (Back et al. 2007). Each fellow was given the opportunity to practice across a spectrum of giving bad news, including discussing abnormal laboratory findings, disclosing the diagnosis of cancer, discussing disease recurrence, transitioning to palliative care and end-of-life conversations, including how to say goodbye to patients. Compared with standardized patient assessment (SPA) before the workshops, post-workshop SPAs showed that participants acquired significantly more skills in breaking bad news (Back et al. 2007).

Other studies have confirmed the value and validity of communication skills training using standardized patients in simulated breaking bad news encounters (Kissane et al. 2012; Fujimori et al. 2014). Recently, Baile and Walters (2013) have adopted methods derived from psychodrama and sociodrama to enhance role play and simulations used in bad news discussions. These techniques are particularly useful when small group training is not feasible, or when standardized patients are not able to be used. They are based upon learners developing an empathic understanding of the plight of the patient and family, so that communication effectively addresses anxieties and other emotions, which often opens the door to a further understanding of patient concerns (Epner and Baile 2014). Although many of the skills associated with giving bad news are verbal, serious attention should be given to emotional self-regulation and helping those who give bad news to regulate their anxiety and discuss their negative emotions.

Conclusion

Communicating in ways that address patients' information needs and provide emotional support increases the likelihood of trust, hope, respect, and a willingness to partner with the doctor to achieve the best possible outcome. Communication skills training has been shown to produce significant patient outcomes. Nothing less than a commitment on the part of oncology programmes to regard training in improving communication to be as equally important as other skills associated with care provision will propel this forward. Multiple opportunities exist to teach skills in clinics, hospital inpatient rounds, seminars, and case-based conferences. A major barrier to training is a narrow biomedical approach, often characteristic of academic cancer centres, where a focus on research is to the exclusion of preparing well-rounded trainees. The addition of core competency requirements in communication skills is a bright light for an improved future.

References

Back A, Arnold R, Baile W, et al. (2007). Efficacy of communication skills training for giving bad news and discussing transitions to palliative care. *Arch Intern Med* **167**, 453–60.

Baile W, Blatner A (2014). Teaching communications skills: using action methods to enhance role-play in problem-based learning. *Simul Healthc* **9**, 220–7.

Baile WF, Buckman R, Lenzi R, et al. (2000). SPIKES A six-step protocol for delivery bad news: Application to the patient with cancer. *Oncologist* **5**, 302–11.

Baile WF, Lenzi R, Parker PA, Buckman R, Cohen L (2002). Oncologists' attitudes toward and practices in giving bad news: an exploratory study. *J Clin Oncol* **20**, 2189–96.

Baile W, Walters R (2013). Applying sociodramatic methods in teaching transition to palliative care. *J Pain Symptom Manage* **45**, 606–19.

Buckman R (1984). Breaking bad news: why is it still so difficult? *Br Med J (Clin Res Ed)* **288**, 1597–9.

Danesh M, Belkora J, Volz S, Rugo H (2014). Informational needs of patients with metastatic breast cancer: what questions do they ask, and are physicians answering them?. *J Cancer Educ* **29**, 175–80.

Else-Quest N, Loconte N, Schiller J (2009). Perceived stigma, self-blame, and adjustment among lung, breast and prostrate cancer patients. *Pyschol Health* **24**, 949–64.

Epner D, Baile W (2014). Difficult conversations: teaching medical oncology trainees communications skills one hour at a time. *Acad Med* **89**, 578–84.

Friedrichsen M, Milberg A (2006). Concerns about losing control when breaking bad news to terminally ill patients with cancer: Physicians' perspective. *J Palliat Med* **9**, 637–82.

Fujimori M, Shirai Y, Asai M, Kubota K, Katsumata N, Uchitomi Y (2014). Effect of communication skills training program for oncologists based on patient preferences for communication when receiving bad news: a randomzied controlled trial. *J Clin Oncol* **32**, 2166–72.

Hanratty B, Lowson E, Holmes L, et al. (2012). Breaking bad news sensitively: what is important to patients in their last year of life? *BMJ Support Palliat Care* **2**, 24–8.

Institute of Medicine (2015). *Dying in America: Improving Quality and Honoring Individual Preferences Near the End of Life*. The National Academies Press, Washington DC, WA.

Khalil R (2013). Attitudes, beliefs and perceptions regarding truth disclose of cancer-related information in the Middle East: A review. *Palliat Support Care* **11**, 69–78.

Kissane DW, Bylund CL, Banerjee SC, et al. (2012). Communication skills training for oncology professionals. *J Clin Oncol* **30**, 1242–7.

Lin J, Lake J, Wall M, Berman A, et al. (2014). Association of patient-provider communication domains with lung cancer treatment. *J Thorac Oncol* **9**, 1249–54.

Martins R, Carvalho I (2013). Breaking bad news: patients' preferences and health locus of control. *Patient Educ Couns* **92**, 67–73.

Parker PA, Baile WF, de Moor C, et al. (2001). Breaking bad news about cancer: patients' preferences for communication. *J Clin Oncol* **19**, 2049–56.

Phelan S, Griffin J, Jackson G, et al. (2013). Stigma, perceived blame, self-blame, and depressive symptoms in men with colorectal cancer. *Psychooncology* **22**, 65–73.

Robinson T, Alexander S, Hays M (2008). Patient-oncologist communication in advanced cancer: predictors of patient perception of prognosis. *Support Care Cancer* **16**, 1049–57.

Sep M, Van Osch M, Van Vliet L (2014). The power of clinicians' affective communication: how reassurance about non-abandonment can reduce patients' physiological arousal and increase information recall in bad news consultations. An experimental study using analogue patients. *Patient Educ Couns* **95**, 45–52.

Shaw J, Brown R, Heinrich P (2013). Doctor's experience of stress during simulated bad news consultations. *Patient Educ Couns* **93**, 203–8.

Shockney L, Back A (2013). Communicating with patients on treatment options for advanced disease. *J Nat Compr Canc Netw* **11**, 684–6.

Siefart C, Hofmann M, Bär T, Riera Knorrenschild J, Seifart U, Rief W (2014). Breaking bad news-what patients want and what they get: evaluating the SPIKES protocol in Germany, *Ann Oncol* **25**, 707–11.

Sikes S (1984). Beating the boogeyman. A cancer patient's diary. *Bull Menninger Clin* **48**, 293–317.

Tanco K, Rhondali W, Perez-Cruz P (2015). Patient perception of physician compassion after a more optimistic vs a less optimistic message: a randomized clinical trial. *JAMA Oncol* **1**, 176–83.

Van Vilet L, Epstein A (2014). Current state of the art and science of patient-clinician communication in progressive disease: patients' need to know and need to feel known. *J Clin Oncol* **32**, 3474–8.

Weeks J, Caalano P, Croninc A, et al. (2012). Patients' expectations about effects of chemotherapy for advanced cancer. *N Engl J Med* **367**, 1616–25.

Zachariae R, Pederson C, Jensen A (2003). Association of perceived physician communication style with patient satisfaction, distress, cancer-related self-efficacy, and perceived locus of control over the disease. *Br J Cancer* **10**, 658–65.

CHAPTER 13

Discussing prognosis and communicating risk

Phyllis N. Butow, Martin H.N. Tattersall, and Martin Stockler

Introduction to discussing prognosis

'Prognosis' and 'risk' are terms used to refer to the chances of a health state occurring, including the development of an illness or disability, symptoms of the illness, benefits and side effects of treatment, and the likelihood of, or likely time to death. Estimating how long people diagnosed with cancer have to live, and the likely outcomes of treatment, is not easy. Communicating these concepts to patients in a way that is both clear and supportive is even harder. Many health professionals are uncertain how much risk information to give and in what format. In this chapter we aim to help health professionals better communicate prognosis and risk to people who have cancer. We discuss legal perspectives, patients' and doctors' views, patients' understanding of prognosis, and the impact of discussing prognosis on patient outcomes. Finally, summary guidelines and strategies for training are provided.

Background and evidence from the literature

The legal position

There has been a shift towards more open disclosure of cancer diagnosis and prognosis over the past 20 years, due to better treatments and improved outcomes, reduced stigmatization of cancer, the development of the medical consumer movement and increasing medico-legal concerns. The legal view pertaining to information provision is that the patient has a basic human right of self-determination. This is protected by the written constitutions of many countries, in which the standard of disclosure focuses on the informational needs of the *reasonable patient*, in the particular patient's position (Giesen 1993) This approach may, however, fail to protect those whose religious or cultural beliefs and information needs lie outside the mainstream of society.

Many health councils publish guidelines that, while not legally binding, may be consulted in disciplinary or civil proceedings. These attempt flexibility, but as a result leave considerable latitude on the part of the doctor. For example, the relevant document produced by the National Health and Medical Research Council (NHMRC) of Australia states that information provided to patients should cover such aspects as: known severe risks of treatment, even when occurrence is rare; the degree of uncertainty of any diagnosis or therapeutic outcome; and any significant long-term physical, emotional, mental, social, sexual, or other outcome which may be associated with a proposed intervention. However, the information should be 'appropriate to the patient's circumstances, personality, expectations, fears, beliefs, values and cultural background' and may be influenced by 'current accepted medical practice' (NHMRC 2004).

What do patients want?

Two systematic reviews encompassing over 100 studies concluded that most patients want specific information about their prognosis, including chance of cure, life expectancy, best and worst case scenarios, and the possible effects of cancer and treatment on their life (Hagerty *et al.* 2005; Hancock *et al.* 2007). However, a small minority (2–10%) consistently reports a preference for not knowing their prognosis and for never discussing it (Hagerty *et al.* 2004), while in palliative care, a larger proportion prefer not to discuss survival time for fear of bad news (Kutner *et al.* 1999). Many patients would like the physician to check first to see if they want prognostic information (Hancock *et al.* 2007).

Patients have strong views on the format for receiving prognostic information (Hancock *et al.* 2007). For example, in one study more patients (80%) wanted a qualitative than quantitative (50%) prognosis (Kaplowitz *et al.* 2002). More metastatic patients surveyed preferred words (47%) or percentages (42%) to graphical presentations (21%), which they described as 'too cold, clinical, and confronting' and difficult to understand (Hagerty *et al.* 2004).

There is, however, diversity in preferences. For instance, more educated patients prefer graphical presentations, probably because they find them easier to process and understand (Hagerty *et al.* 2004). Many Anglo-Saxon patients prefer words, while those without good English better understand numbers. Furthermore, patients' views change, with less information desired as disease progresses (Butow *et al.* 1997). Conversely caregivers may need more information at the end of life (Hancock *et al.* 2007) to enable them to prepare mentally and feel confident they can provide appropriate physical and emotional care.

Who wants prognostic information?

In early stage cancer, younger, female patients, those with a better prognosis and those who are less anxious are more likely to want prognosis disclosure (Hagerty *et al.* 2005). Patients who are offered intensive treatment want to know more about treatment side effects and the chance of cure (Meredith *et al.* 1996), perhaps to assist them to make an informed choice about an arduous treatment.

In advanced cancer, patients whose prognosis is better are more likely to want to discuss prognosis at the first consultation (Hagerty *et al.* 2004). Patients who are more open to discussing a bad prognosis are more likely to be depressed (Hagerty *et al.* 2004); this association between openness to a poor prognosis and low mood has led to calls for provision of better support alongside disclosure (El-Jawahri *et al.* 2014). Patients without children and those with strong religious faith are more willing to discuss death and dying, perhaps because they can face dying more readily (Steinhauser *et al.* 2000).

Expectations for prognostic disclosure do differ in different cultures. In some communities, the doctor should not disclose prognosis to the patient or involve them in decision-making. These cultures prefer the family to have a high level of involvement and for the family to be informed first, so that the patient is either told gradually or not at all (Iconomou *et al.* 2002; Yoshida *et al.* 2013). However, within cultures there are diverse expectations, and over time an international shift towards open disclosure is evident. Recent studies emerging from Asia and surveying Asian people who have immigrated to other countries have shown an increased interested in full information and involvement in decision-making among patients. Doctors need to avoid stereotypes when discussing diagnosis and prognosis (Moore and Butow 2005). Both patients and caregivers indicate that doctors should clarify individual information needs and tailor information provision accordingly (Hagerty *et al.* 2005; Hancock *et al.* 2007). And preferences need to be renegotiated over time.

Patients' understanding of prognostic information

In most studies of patients' understanding, wide discrepancies exist between doctor prognostication and patient report (Chochinov *et al.* 2000), with both patient optimism and poor health professional communication contributing to this misunderstanding. As Jackson *et al.* (2013) have noted, patients fluctuate in their ability to assimilate approaching death and will often disclose contradictory understandings that vary over time.

Doctors' views regarding prognostic discussions

Medical views about discussing prognosis have been influenced by the struggle between different ethical principles: beneficence (acting for the good of others); paternalism (the doctor takes responsibility for the patients' presumed best interests); and autonomy (the patient's integrity and right to self-determination are respected). Some have called this struggle: 'the sacred lie principle' versus 'the justified medical truth' (Gramma *et al.* 2013). Reticence to disclose prognosis is often based on a concern that disclosure may cause psychological distress, and take away the benefits afforded by denial and hope (Hancock *et al.* 2007). Conversely, as embodied in the principles of informed consent and shared decision-making, it is argued that patients have a right to control what is done to

their body, be provided with full information, and make their own decisions.

In practice, most doctors combine these positions, suggesting that honest disclosure is only effective when given compassionately, while sustaining hope (Butow *et al.* 2002). However, a delicate balance exists between fostering realistic hope and creating false expectations of longevity (Clayton *et al.* 2005).

How do doctors and patients discuss prognosis?

Unlike diagnosis, prognosis is still commonly not discussed, with some clinicians frankly admitting to not divulging or overestimating prognosis with patients. Audiotape audits of consultations also reveal little discussion of prognosis. In one analysis of 142 consultations, representing the first one or two consultations after diagnosis with metastatic disease of 31 Anglo-Australian and 24 Chinese, 11 Arabic and 12 Greek immigrant patients and 115 of their relatives with one of 10 oncologists, life expectancy was not discussed with ¼ of Anglo-Australians and ½ of immigrants who needed an interpreter, while fears and concerns about prognosis were discussed in less than 16% of consultations (Butow *et al.* 2013). In another study of patients with metastatic breast cancer, patients' questions were most often about prognosis, but these were answered in only ⅓ of instances (Danesh *et al.* 2014). If a prognostic discussion has occurred in the metastatic setting, it is more likely between the doctor and someone other than the patient (Bradley *et al.* 2001). Both doctors and patients tend to avoid discussing prognosis by focusing on the treatment plan. Health professionals and patients may fall into a 'conspiracy of silence' where both are too frightened to raise the issue of prognosis (The *et al.* 2001).

Communication of risk and prognosis by the multidisciplinary team

The management of persons with cancer is increasingly conducted within a multidisciplinary team. Inevitably there is the potential for inconsistent information to be presented to the patient by different members of the team, with resulting confusion. The patient's family doctor is rarely informed of what prognostic information has been communicated (McConnell *et al.* 1999). Nor is prognostic discussion usually documented in the patient's medical record.

Outcomes of discussing prognosis and risk

Evidence suggests that increased question asking about, and discussion of, prognosis does not increase anxiety, but rather leads to greater patient satisfaction, lower anxiety, and less likelihood of using alternative therapies (Hagerty *et al.* 2004). Longer discussion of prognosis leads to greater uptake of treatments offering long-term benefits, suggesting that additional explanation does assist understanding. Discussion about prognosis takes on special importance during treatment decision-making. Here clear, balanced presentation of facts is imperative, with sufficient time and explanation to assist patients to understand and adjust to the facts being presented.

Suggestions for discussing prognosis

Determining what and how people want to know

Since people vary in whether they want to know their prognosis, and how they want to hear it, it is important to directly negotiate the approach to this discussion. *Stepwise disclosure* is a process

Box 13.1 Discussion between patient and doctor about prognosis

Dr: Most patients in your situation do very well, but in a small proportion the cancer will come back. Having chemotherapy reduces the chances of the cancer coming back. Unfortunately we don't know upfront who will do well and who won't. Therefore, we have to give chemotherapy to everyone to achieve that reduction in risk. So we would normally recommend chemotherapy to someone like you.

Now, are you the sort of person who likes numbers? Some people like to know what their risk is in numbers, other people don't like that degree of preciseness.

Pt: Well, will it make a difference to the treatment I get?

Dr: It won't change my recommendation, but this is a trade-off between reducing risk and putting up with the side effects of chemotherapy for a few months. You may feel differently to me about that trade-off.

Pt: Oh, I see. Well yes, I would like to know what we are dealing with here.

Dr: OK. About three in ten people in your situation would have their cancer come back without treatment. If they have treatment, only 2 in 10 will have the cancer come back. How do you feel about that? Was it what you expected?

Pt: Well, actually, I guess I was hoping for better odds than that. Even a 2 in 10 chance still sounds awfully high to me. Is there nothing else we can do to reduce that risk down further?

Dr: Not that we know of today, but there is always research going on trying to improve outcomes for people, so other treatments may become available in the future. I'm sorry I can't offer you better odds. But remember a 2 in 10 chance of the cancer coming back also means you have an 8/10 chance of everything going well.

Pt: Thanks, I appreciate that. It does sound a bit better that way!

Dr: Please feel free to ask me questions about this, or anything else about your cancer and the treatment, at any time. If you feel you would like some support, because you are worrying a lot about the cancer coming back, we can arrange for you to see our social worker or psychologist, who are great to talk to.

wherein specific prognostic data is only offered after patients first understand the nature of the information and then indicate their interest in receiving it. Box 13.1 depicts a short negotiation between a doctor and patient on this topic. If a patient chooses not to discuss prognosis, the doctor can clarify that they may raise this again in case the patient changes their mind. Depending on the urgency of the situation, the doctor may also raise concerns about the potential impact on the patient and family if prognosis is not discussed (Jackson *et al.* 2013).

Patients will often raise prognosis themselves, not necessarily in a straightforward manner. For example, they may comment that they are thinking of travelling overseas in about six months. Exploration of what the question really means is helpful. For example, the doctor might say: *'So this is what you are thinking about. Do you want advice on how well you are likely to be in six months, and whether you are likely to be able to travel?'*

One method proven to facilitate prognostic communication is a question prompt list (see Chapter 14). Question prompt lists endorse question asking and contain lists of questions in categories that patients can ask if and when they wish. The questions are devised by asking patients, carers, and health professionals in focus groups what questions they asked, were asked, should ask, or wish they had asked. Question prompt lists increase question asking in oncology and palliative care settings, particularly about prognosis (Brown *et al.* 2001).

Accurately conveying prognosis and uncertainty

Prognostic estimates are typically derived from key prognostic indicators linked to large databases of patient outcomes, usually collected as part of clinical trials. A number of computer programs and phone apps are now available to help clinicians prognosticate, the most well known of which is Adjuvant Online (Ravdin *et al.* 2001), accessible at https://www.adjuvantonline.com. Adjuvant Online is a US-developed tool which provides a tailored risk profile of developing recurrent disease and/or dying within 10 years, taking into account individual prognostic factors and the treatment received. Currently it is available for early stage breast, colorectal, and lung cancer, and has been shown to be valid and reliable for US patients under 70, although recent work suggests it consistently overestimates the survival of older patients, and may require adjustment in different cultures.

Any estimate of survival should always be accompanied by a clear explanation of the inherent uncertainty in forecasting. If the data required to calculate prognosis are available, median survival and the interquartile range are probably the best statistics to convey prognosis (West *et al.* 2014). Best and worst case scenarios can also be given, using the tenth and ninetieth percentiles. Recent research in breast cancer patients found that most judged presentation of best case, worst case, and typical scenarios for advanced cancer prognosis preferable, more reassuring, and helpful than presentation of just median survival time (Kiely *et al.* 2013). Thus the recommended answer to the question 'How long have I got?' might be something like: *'This is a hard question. The typical person with your kind and stage of cancer lives about 12 months. This means that half the people live longer than 12 months and half live shorter than 12 months. If we had 100 people exactly like you, then we'd expect that the 10 who did worst might only live a few (2) months, but the 10 who did best might still be around in a few (3-4) years, and that most (about half) would live somewhere between six months and two years.'*

Formats for presenting prognosis

Prognosis can be presented in a variety of formats, including words, numbers, and graphs (see Figs 13.1 and 13.2). Most people find numbers and 100-person diagrams the easiest to understand, although some find the latter confronting (Davey *et al.* 2003). Pie charts and survival graphs are harder to take in, and some find them too clinical and cold when discussing life and death (Kiely *et al.* 2013). The bar graphs generated by Adjuvant Online for breast, colon, and lung cancers appear to be well understood by patients.

The way prognosis is discussed is just as important as what is said about it. Stop often and check that people have understood what has been said, invite questions, explore whether the information was as they expected, what this means to them in the context of their lives (e.g. its impact on holiday, home, and work plans) and how they are coping with the news. If they are upset, the oncology team's support and reassurance that they will be working with them to maximize their chances and quality of life will be very important. Write down important messages for them to take home.

Words: **You have a good chance of being alive in five years time. Most people in your situation are alive five years after they are diagnosed and some people live much longer than that.**

Numbers: **You have a 50:50 chance of being alive in five years. In other words, half of the people with your sort of cancer are alive five years on. This means that half the people like you live more than five years and half live less than five years. About 10%, or 1 in 10, live for less than one year, but another 10 % live for 15 years or more.**

100 person diagram

Of 100 women who have metastatic (type) cancer like you, about 50 will be alive in five years.

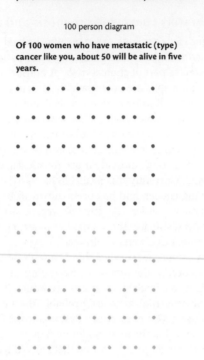

Survival graph

The percentage of people alive over time.

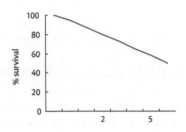

Fig. 13.1 Ways to present prognosis.

Maintaining hope

Communication strategies found to increase patient hope (Hagerty *et al.* 2004) include:

◆ Talking about psychosocial issues and providing emotional support;

◆ Answering questions and providing information honestly and openly;

◆ Offering the most up-to-date treatment and demonstrating expertise;

◆ Discussing outliers;

◆ Focusing on positive and achievable goals;

◆ Couching the patient's prognosis in terms of reaching goals or 'landmarks', or overcoming 'hurdles';

◆ Normalizing preparations for death, as something that everyone needs to do.

◆ Reassuring the patient that discussing death does not make it an inevitable event.

Summarizing, recording, and communicating to others

Documentation in letters to referring doctors about what has been said to patients in oncologist consultations is important, so that the potential for multiple and differing estimates being conveyed to patients is reduced (McConnell *et al.* 1999).

Guidelines

The Australian National Breast Cancer Centre has produced a set of evidence-based guidelines for clinicians on communicating prognosis. Consensus-based guidelines for discussing prognosis and end-of-life issues have also been published (Clayton *et al.* 2007). Recommended steps for discussing prognosis, based on these guidelines, are shown in Box 13.2.

Learning to discuss prognosis

Role play practice of how to discuss prognosis is invaluable to try out and develop new skills. Note that all health professionals, such as nurses and allied health workers, can contribute to and are impacted by prognostic discussions (McLennon *et al.* 2013), and need training in managing these discussions.

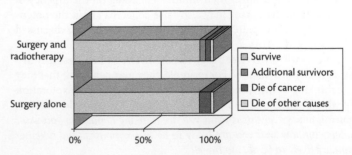

Fig. 13.2 A bar graph can be useful for communicating relative prognosis with and without therapy.

Box 13.2 Recommended steps for discussing prognosis with people with cancer

Prior to discussing prognosis:

◆ Ensure that the discussion will take place in privacy.

◆ Ensure as much as possible that there will be no interruptions (e.g. switch off mobile phones and pagers; inform staff).

◆ Check if the patient would like to have a friend or relative present.

◆ Check if the patient would like another medical person present (if applicable).

Negotiating the agenda:

◆ Ask first if the person wants to be given information about prognosis (e.g. 'I can tell you what happens to most people in your situation. Would you like me to do that?') and explore what he or she currently understands and expects.

◆ Explore and negotiate with the patient the *type* (e.g. staging details; the chances of being cured; short and long-term side effects of treatment; survival estimates) and *format* (e.g. words, numbers, graphs) of prognostic information desired, and adhere to these preferences.

Aspects of prognosis to discuss:

◆ Adhere to the person's stated preference for information about prognosis. If/when desired, the following can be provided:

 • staging details and their implications for prognosis

 • chances of being cured or that cancer will never return

 • likely benefits and risks of treatment

 • chances of the cancer shortening the individual's life compared to other life events, e.g. heart disease

 • average and longest survival times, emphasizing a range rather than a single time point

How to discuss prognosis:

◆ Adopt an honest and straightforward, yet sensitive approach.

◆ Encourage a collaborative relationship with the patient (e.g. provide opportunity to ask questions).

◆ Use the most up-to-date information, and if desired, explain its source. Explain how this may be revised by additional information. Suggest a time frame for when additional prognostic information is likely to be available.

◆ Preface any statement of prognostic estimates with the limitations of prognostic formulations. Explain that you can't predict how the person as an individual will respond to the illness and its treatment.

◆ If giving a time frame, emphasize a range, and not specific endpoints.

◆ Use mixed framing, i.e. give the chances of cure first, then chances of relapse.

◆ Present information in a variety of ways (e.g. words, graphs, statistics).

◆ Present absolute risks with and without treatment.

◆ Broaden discussion of the prognosis to include the effect of the cancer on the individual's lifestyle.

◆ Emphasize hope-giving aspects of the information, e.g. extraordinary survivors.

◆ Repeat negotiation of information preferences and needs over time.

◆ When explaining relative risk reduction, provide several examples of the calculations.

◆ Only use statistical terminology (e.g. median, hazard risk ratio) if a person is familiar with these concepts.

Concluding the discussion:

◆ Summarize main points of the consultation and reassess the person's understanding.

◆ Emphasize hope-giving aspects of the information.

◆ Check the patient's emotional reaction to the information and offer support or referral if needed.

◆ Indicate your availability for contact to address any questions or concerns and arrange a further appointment to review the situation within a stated time period.

Adapted with permission from National Breast Cancer and National Cancer Control Initiative, *Clinical Practice Guidelines for the Psychosocial Care of Adults with Cancer*, National Breast Cancer Centre, Camperdown, New South Wales, Australia, Copyright © National Breast Cancer Centre 2003, http://www.nhmrc. gov.au/_files_nhmrc/file/publications/synopses/cp90.pdf

The scenario illustrating a breast cancer patient with possible variations for different health professionals is provided below:

Mary Green, aged 57, has early stage breast cancer. Mary has had a lumpectomy. The axillary dissection showed three positive lymph nodes. Mary is married, with three adult children, two of whom are married with children of their own. Mary is a home-maker; her husband is a dentist. Mary wants a lot of information. She has searched the internet and has found a range of numbers concerning her chance of cure. She wants to know facts and figures, and what this means for her as an individual. She will not be fobbed off with words or reassurance.

Surgeons: Mary is meeting you for the post-surgical consultation.

Oncologists: Mary is meeting you to discuss radiotherapy or chemotherapy. The surgeon has told her that she has an excellent chance of cure.

Nurses: Mary tells you that the surgeon said she is almost certainly cured, while the oncologist told her she has a 50% chance that the cancer will return, and she is now confused and upset.

Social workers/psychologists: Mary says she cannot make a decision about whether or not to have chemotherapy. She cannot make sense of the figures she has been given, and what they mean for her as an individual.

Conclusion

The discussion of prognosis and risk is revisited frequently in cancer care, and needs to be tailored to each individual and considered in every treatment plan. Adept communication of prognosis contributes greatly to supportive care provision.

References

Bradley E, Hallemeier A, Fried T (2001). Documentation of discussions about prognosis with terminally ill patients. *Am J Med* **111**, 218–23.

Brown R, Butow P, Dunn S, Tattersall M (2001). Promoting patient participation and shortening cancer consultations: a randomised trial. *Br J Cancer* **85**, 1273–9.

Butow P, Dowsett S, Hagerty R, Tattersall M (2002). Communicating prognosis to patients with metastatic disease: what do they really want to know? *Support Care Cancer* **10**, 161–8.

Butow P, Mclean M, Dunn S (1997). The dynamics of change: Cancer patients' preferences for information, involvement and support. *Ann Oncol* **8**, 857–63.

Butow P, Sze M, Eisenbruch M, et al. (2013). Should culture affect practice? A comparison of prognostic discussions in consultations with immigrant versus native-born cancer patients. *Patient Educ Couns* **92**, 246–52.

Chochinov H, Tatartyn D, Wilson K, Enns M, Lander S (2000). Prognostic awareness and the terminally ill. *Psychosomatics* **41**, 500–4.

Clayton J, Butow P, Arnold R (2005). Fostering coping and nuturing hope when discussing the future with terminally ill cancer patients and their caregivers. *Cancer* **10**, 161–8.

Clayton J, Hancock K, Butow P (2007). Clinical practice guidelines for communicating prognosis and end-of-life issues with adults in the advanced stages of a life-limiting illness, and their caregivers. *Med J Aust* **186** S77, S79, S83–S108.

Danesh M, Belkora J, Volz S, Rugo H (2014). Informational needs of patients with metastatic breast cancer: what questions do they ask, and are physicians answering them? *J Cancer Educ* **29**, 175–80.

Davey H, Butow P, Armstrong B (2003). Patient preferences for written prognostic information. *Br J Cancer* **89**, 1450–6.

El-Jawahri A, Traeger L, Park E, et al. (2014). Associations among prognostic understanding, quality of life and mood in patients with advanced cancer. *Cancer* **120**, 278–85.

Giesen D (1993). Legal accountability for the provision of medical care: a comparative view. *J R Soc Med* **86**, 648–52.

Gramma R, Parvu A, Enache A, Roman G, Ioan B (2013). Truth or lie—some ethical dilemmas in the communication of a severe diagnosis. *Rev Med Chir Soc Med Nat Iasi* **117**, 172–82.

Hagerty R, Butow P, Ellis P (2004). Cancer patient preferences for communication of prognosis in the metastatic setting. *J Clin Oncol* **22**, 1721–30.

Hagerty R, Butow P, Ellis P (2005). Communicating prognosis in cancer: A systematic review of the literature. *Ann Oncol* **16**, 1005–53.

Hancock K, Clayton J, Parker S (2007). Discrepant perceptions about end-of-life communications: as systematic review. *J Pain Symptom Manage* **34**, 190–200.

Iconomou G, Viha A, Koutras A, Vagenakis A, Kalofonos HP (2002). Information needs and awareness of diagnosis in patients with cancer receiving chemotherapy: a report from Greece. *Palliat Med* **16**, 315–21.

Jackson V, Jacobsen J, Greer J, Pirl W, Temel J (2013). The cultivation of prognostic awareness through the provision of early palliative care in the ambulatory setting: a communication guide. *J Palliat Med* **16**, 894–900.

Kaplowitz S, Campo S, Chui W (2002). Cancer patients' desire for communication of prognosis information. *Health Commun* **14**, 221–41.

Kiely B, Mccaughan G, Christodoulou S, et al. (2013). Using scenarios to explain life expectancy in advanced cancer: attitudes of people with a cancer experience. *Support Care Cancer* **21**, 369–76.

Kutner J, Steiner J, Corbett K, Jahnigen D, Barton P (1999). Information needs in terminal illness. *Soc Sci Med* **48**, 1341–52.

McConnell D, Butow P, Tattersall M (1999). Improving the letters we write: An exploration of doctor-doctor communication in cancer care. *Br J Cancer* **80**, 427–37.

McLennon S, Lasiter S, Miller W, Amlin K, Chamness A, Helft P (2013). Oncology nurses' experiences with prognosis-related communication with patients who have advanced cancer. *Nurs Outlook* **61**, 427–36.

Meredith C, Symonds P, Webster L (1996). Information needs of cancer patients in west Scotland: cross sectional survey of patients' views. *BMJ* **313**, 724–6.

Moore R, Butow P (2005). Culture and oncology: impact of context effects. In: *Cancer, Communication and Culture*. Spiegel D (ed.). Kluwer Academic/Plenum Publishers, New York, NY.

National Health and Medical Research Council, Australia (2004). General guidelines for medical practitioners on providing information to patients. *National Health and Medical Research Council, Commonwealth of Australia*. Australian Government Publishing Service, Canberra, Australia.

Ravdin P, Siminoff L, Davis G, Mercer M, Hewlett J, Gerson N (2001). Computer program to assist in making decisions about ajuvant therapy for women with early breast cancer. *J Clin Oncol* **19**, 980–91.

Steinhauser K, Christakis N, Clipp E, Mcneilly M, Mcintyre L, Tulsky J (2000). Factors considered important at the end of life by patients, family, physicians, and other care providers. *J Am Med Assoc* **284**, 2476–82.

The A, Hak T, Koeter G, Van Der Wal G (2001). Collusion in doctor-patient communication about imminent death: an ethnographic study. *West J Med* **174**, 247–53.

West T, Kiely B, Stockler M (2014). Estimating scenarios for survival time in men starting systemic therapies for castration-resistant prostrate cancer: a systematic review of randomised trials *Eur J Cancer* **50**, 1916–24.

Yoshida S, Shiozaki M, Sanjo M, et al. (2013). Practices and evaluations of prognostic disclosure for Japanese cancer patients and their families from the family's point of view. *Palliat Support Care* **11**, 383–8.

CHAPTER 14

Achieving shared treatment decisions

Martin H.N. Tattersall and David W. Kissane

Introduction to achieving shared treatment decisions

Reaching treatment decisions in oncology often involves trade-offs between quality of life and quantity of life. Decisions are best informed by evidence and patients need to understand that that their engagement in decision-making is desirable because frequently there is not one best treatment and their values, preferences, and goals are important in reaching shared treatment decisions.

In the screening context, screening may identify abnormality that is not cancer but still merits surgery. Some cancers detected by screening may have already metastasized, and the consequence of 'early detection' is extended survival with incurable disease, rather than a normal life expectancy. In the adjuvant setting, not every person recommended treatment experiences disease recurrence even if they choose not to receive chemotherapy. Adjuvant treatment may be the standard of care, but patients need to understand that disease recurrence is possible, and the outcome may be extension of disease-free survival, and not disease elimination. In patients with metastatic cancer, systemic treatments at the best may cause tumour shrinkage and prolongation of survival, but some patients will derive no benefit and experience the side effects of chemotherapy.

The Institute of Medicine defined patient-centred care as 'care that is respectful of and responsive to individual patient preferences, needs and values' (Barry and Edgman-Levitan 2012, p. 780). Involving patients in discussions about treatment options and reaching a shared treatment decision highlights the importance of doctors and patients working together to produce the best outcomes possible. Shared decision-making is applicable to most clinical consultations. It is especially important in circumstances where the evidence does not strongly support a single clearly superior option or where a preference-sensitive decision is involved, that is, the decision is likely to be strongly influenced by patient's preferences and values (Hoffmann et al. 2014). Shared decision-making enables research evidence to be incorporated into discussions with the patient, with their preferences explored and considered in reaching a treatment recommendation.

Shared decision-making

Models of shared decision-making advocate discussions of information and involvement preferences and discussion of treatment options for all. Patients vary in the extent to which they wish to participate in decisions and in the decisions in which they wish to participate. A survey of 8,119 European adults reported that over 50% preferred to share decisions with their healthcare provider and the highest rate (74%) was found in the age group less than 35 years (Coulter and Jenkinson 2005). Older patients are less likely to prefer involvement in decision-making, and meeting older patients' needs for information and decision support can be challenging. Many patients are also unfamiliar with being invited to share decision-making. Outlining that they have some choices, which the doctor would like to go through with them, before deciding together about the next steps may reassure patients who might otherwise feel overwhelmed and uncertain.

This process may be enabled by prompting patients to ask a small number of questions (Shepherd et al. 2011b; Hoffmann et al. 2014). Three questions are: 'What are my options?', 'What are the benefits and harms?', and 'How likely are these?' Data show that these three questions increased family physician consideration of patient preferences about treatment options, thus facilitating patient involvement. Patients received higher quality information about therapeutic options and their benefits and harms, without increasing consultation length. By promoting a patient-centred approach and shared decision-making, these three questions may facilitate evidence-based practice, helping physicians to make better decisions with patients, strengthen patient–physician communication, and improve safety and quality of care. An alternative five-question series amended to the clinicians' perspective are: 'What will happen if we wait and watch?', 'What are your test or treatment options?', 'What are the benefits and harms of these options?', 'How do the benefits and harms weigh up for you?', and 'Do you have enough information to make a choice?'

Patients' perspectives about treatment choices

Cancer patients' expectations of information and involvement in decision-making have changed rapidly. Now most cancer patients in the Western world are told the diagnosis, and expect to be informed about the disease and its management. Cancer patients report wanting to be involved in treatment decision-making. If patients are to be active partners in decisions about their care, the information they are given must accord with the available evidence and be presented in a form that is acceptable and useful. However, many patient information materials currently in use do not meet these standards (Coulter *et al.* 1999). Van der Weijden and colleagues (2013) explored how clinical practice guidelines can be adapted to foster shared decision-making. One scenario concerned the options of mastectomy or lumpectomy followed by radiotherapy in operable breast cancer. They found that guidelines could be adapted to inform shared decision-making based on generic and specific strategies. Specific strategies were related to a single recommendation, and included three types: increasing the clinicians' awareness of options; improving deliberation of patients' preferences; and providing patient support tools.

Unfortunately patients often do not appreciate that when a treatment decision is to be reached, the decision likely depends on their input including their values, preferences and goals, and that they are entitled to participate in the decision-making process. Oncologists often assume they know patients' preferences and do not engage patients in reaching a treatment decision by communicating options, risks, and benefits. Patients who participate in reaching treatment decisions experience better quality of life and are more compliant with the treatment. Surveys of patients with cancer have revealed that their desire for information and involvement in decisions is high, unless their quality of life has recently deteriorated, when they may want progressively less involvement (Butow *et al.* 1997). Another survey of oncologists involved in Ontario (Charles *et al.* 2004) reported that patient involvement in decision-making was less than the oncologist would like. These findings indicate that oncologists should ask patients how much they want to know, and how involved they prefer to be in decision-making.

Patients may also need to be prepared for their potential role in the consultation. In one study, we aimed to determine whether a successful tailoring of patient participation conferred benefits to patients, and whether patients who jointly decided on treatment with their oncologist experienced better outcomes. A match between preferred and perceived roles in decision-making was found for just over one third of patients, with 29% more active than preferred, and 37% participating to a lesser degree then preferred. Patients whose level of participation was less than desired wanted more information about treatment options and side effects, and expressed a greater need for assurance, as well as the chance to talk about their fears. Patients less active in decision-making than desired were also significantly less satisfied. Irrespective of preference, patients who reported a shared role in decision-making were most satisfied with the consultation, and with information about treatments and emotional support. Importantly, patient reports of the level of participation in decision-making were correlated with oncologists' behaviours. This finding suggests that the consultation itself, and the oncologist's behaviour in particular, may be pivotal in generating the discrepancy between preferred and actual roles in reaching treatment decisions. Oncologist training to promote increased compatibility between patient information needs and participation expectations may be useful.

Setting the agenda for shared decision-making

Consultations that are focused on developing a treatment plan often follow ones that have generated investigations aimed at confirming the diagnosis or the disease extent. Sometimes the previous consultations will have been conducted by another physician,

in which case the 'management consultation' must ensure that the clinician is aware of the patient's understanding of their situation and the purposes of this consultation. A frequent opening may be 'What is your understanding of the situation and why we are meeting today?' The patient's response to this question may enable the physician to clarify any misunderstanding and to provide an overview of the treatment goals and options.

Clinicians and patients bring differing values and preferences to each clinical predicament that necessitates a treatment choice. The objective of a shared decision-making consultation is to ensure that the patient achieves a fully informed treatment choice based upon a comprehensive understanding of the disease and the available treatment options to manage. Shepherd *et al.* (2008) concluded that cancer physicians experience difficulties when reaching treatment decisions with their patients. Interventions and strategies that physicians support are required to enhance patient involvement in reaching a treatment decision.

Physicians' perspectives on shared decision-making

Shepherd and colleagues (2011*a*) conducted 22 telephone interviews with doctors treating a range of cancers. These interviews probed for physicians' attitudes to shared decision-making, views of when patient involvement is appropriate, and what motivated them to encourage involvement. These doctors described disease, patient, physician, and societal influences on their support for patient participation in treatment decisions.

Involvement of patients in decision-making was considered important where evidence for one treatment option compared to another was not conclusive. Treatments that were not based on evidence, or no treatment when treatment offered a significant advantage, were not considered real options. The influence of treatment options on decision-making was mitigated when patients' individual circumstances made some options inappropriate. Treatment recommendations were described as 'clear cut' or 'grey'. When treatment options were 'clear cut', the impact of treatment on patients' quality of life and self-image, and the influence of consumer groups motivated doctors' support of patient involvement (Shepherd *et al.* 2008). Some doctors mentioned that established protocols or guidelines could prohibit discussion of some treatment options, whereas scenarios that considered clinical trial participation added to the options, and the need for discussion. The notion of uncertainty about which treatment option was optimal in breast, prostate cancer, and lymphoma was often contrasted with the situation in colorectal or gynaecological surgery, where contention was ruled out. Uncertainty surrounding the optimal prostate cancer treatment option was viewed as mandating doctors to involve patients in treatment discussions, a context with which doctors were comfortable.

Physician's characteristics and the culture of particular specialties (the norms and expectations of these specialties) were thought to influence attitudes to sharing decision-making with patients (Shepherd *et al.* 2008). Surgeons, in general, were thought to be less likely to support patient involvement, but breast surgeons and gynaecologists were often stated to be exceptions because of the multidisciplinary approach to breast cancer care and the expectations of female patients.

Doctors identified seven key characteristics which influenced whether or not they involved their patients in treatment decisions: anxiety, age, gender, cultural background, personality, occupation, and involvement preferences. Older patients, particularly males, are less likely to prefer shared decision-making, but younger females were usually motivated to share decision-making with their oncologist.

Advocating and promoting shared decision-making as the preferred way of discussing treatment options presents some challenges and contradictions for many cancer doctors. Most believe shared decision-making is only necessary or desirable when there are varied treatment options. This is especially true in breast cancer, where consumer groups have encouraged patients to take an active role in all treatment consultations.

Eliciting the patient's preference for involvement in decision-making

Little is known about variation in oncologists' consultation behaviours with regard to patients' preferences for information or involvement in decision-making. In Australia, one audit of oncologists' consultations discussing consent for clinical trials reported that patients' preferences and concerns were elicited in only 39% of the consultations, and ongoing decisional support was offered in 34% (Brown *et al.* 2004). This finding revealed the low levels of preference elicitation in a situation where one had hoped it would be high.

Cancer doctors' consultations need to elicit and discuss patient information and involvement preferences, and to acknowledge that a reliance on doctors' expertise and their treatment recommendations is not an adequate reason to omit discussion of other possible treatment options. The Dutch initiative to modify clinical practice guidelines to foster shared decision-making is welcome (Van der Weijden *et al.* 2013).

The importance of healthcare team members reaching shared treatment decisions

The growth of multidisciplinary team (MDT) meetings in the decision-making and delivery of cancer care is an opportunity as well as an obstacle to shared decision-making. On the one hand, the outcome of MDT meetings is rarely presented as a patient choice between options. On the other hand, the MDT report may include a recommendation of suitability for recruitment to a clinical trial. The need for a summary document of the MDT meeting discussions to inform the patient and the family practitioner and other health professionals involved in future care is obvious, but a suitable template needs to be developed and evaluated from the perspective of shared decision-making.

The presence of a second health professional at consultations where shared (between oncologist and patient plus family members) treatment decisions are considered (and sometimes reached) is not routine practice. Nevertheless, patients may benefit from the presence of a second health professional to support question asking and to assist in clarifying issues and options. Moreover, the second health professional may meet after the oncologist has withdrawn to review the information presented and to further explore the patient's values and preferences, thus helping him or her reach a final decision.

Audio-recording consultations about treatment decisions

The role of audio-recording the consultation and providing a copy for the patient is a cheap and valued addition. Recordings may also be used to monitor (i) the information provided on treatment options; (ii) the participation of the patient and their family; and (iii) to explore the quality of health professional's consultation skills. This approach has been supported by evidence (Tattersall and Butow 2002), but is rarely adopted in practice. Patients appreciate listening again to these recordings and integrating a deeper understanding of what the doctor said.

Decision aids

Encouraging cancer patients to actively participate and ask questions in the consultation is one approach to helping them achieve a greater understanding of their medical care. Most cancer patients express a desire for full information about their illness and are often uncertain about what they should ask their oncologist. Communication interventions help patients to identify concerns and questions they may have about their diagnosis and treatment, and by encouraging them to seek information and answers. How best to implement shared decision-making remains an unresolved challenge (Legare *et al.* 2010; Stiggelbout *et al.* 2012). Patient decision aids either used within or outside the medical consultation have been shown to improve patient's knowledge regarding options and risk perceptions, to reduce their decisional conflict related to feeling uninformed and uncertain about their personal values, and improve congruence between the chosen option and the patient's values. They stimulate people to take a more active role in decision-making and improve patient–practitioner communication. However, decision aids are not commonly implemented in daily practice.

Companions sometimes accompany cancer patients into the consultation, to provide emotional or practical support, and share decision-making. Companions can increase the complexity of the consultation. A systematic review of triadic medical consultations led to recommended preliminary strategies for health professional behaviours (Laidsaar-Powell *et al.* 2013). These include encouraging the attendance of companions, highlighting helpful companion behaviours, and clarifying patients' preferences for companions. Further research is needed to empirically develop and evaluate specific strategies optimizing triadic consultations.

Option grids are a systematic way of presenting information to patients. Option grids are one-page summaries of the evidence in tabular format to enable rapid comparison of options using questions that patients frequently ask. They are tables in which a set of options, with related pros and cons, are depicted. Judgements have to be made about the number of questions that can be posed, and which options are summarized. It is usually possible to list six to eight frequently asked questions. Comparing options using a small number of attributes is helpful, because making a choice often rests on a small number of important assumptions, sometimes even just the single most important reason. Option grids work best when they show a maximum of two or three options. Achieving this degree of brevity requires the following: (i) decisions have to be made about the relevance of information, which leads to a selection based on what matters most to most patients when making decisions; and (ii) meticulous editing is needed to ensure that the language is concise, accessible, and clear. The option grid can be read in a few minutes by an individual with a reading age of 10 to 12 years, or read aloud by the health professional when preferred. Option grids have not yet been evaluated for effectiveness.

Question prompt lists (QPLs) given to patients before their consultation have been used extensively in the oncology setting to enhance patient question asking and to improve communication. Patients can select the questions that are relevant to them and ask those questions during their consultation (Dimoska et al. 2012). QPLs have been tested for different cancer types (Bruera et al. 2003), and with the goal of enhancing questions on topics such as surgery (Smets et al. 2011) or palliative care (Clayton et al. 2007). The effectiveness of using QPLs in cancer has been assessed in several reviews (Dimoska et al. 2008; Dimoska et al. 2012; Henselmans et al. 2012). QPL interventions are effective in enhancing patient question asking, reducing anxiety at follow-up, and enhancing recall of information. QPLs are easy-to-implement tools with the potential to improve informed decision-making.

Eleven out of 20 oncology studies of QPLs reported the number of questions listed. These ranged from 10 to 112 questions, with a mean of 31.8. In most of the studies, QPLs used 10 to 35 questions. Providing patients with too many potential questions may overwhelm them. Six out of the 20 studies were found to be of high quality. In four studies, oncologists or palliative care physicians were asked to actively endorse the QPL. After conducting the best evidence synthesis, it was concluded that there is evidence that QPL interventions are effective in increasing the number of questions that patients ask, moderately enhancing recall of information, and increasing patients' satisfaction.

Barriers and facilitators to shared decision-making

A systematic review and thematic synthesis of patient-reported barriers and facilitators to shared decision-making concluded that patients need knowledge and power to become engaged in shared decision-making—knowledge alone is insufficient, and power is more difficult to attain (Joseph-Williams et al. 2014). Patient-reported barriers and facilitators to shared decision-making relate to how the healthcare system is organized and to what happens in the consultation. Inadequate information provision is one of the most significant barriers and inadequate preparation for the consultation, including perceiving the opportunity and personal ability to be involved, is another major problem. Most patient-reported barriers and facilitators are potentially modifiable and many could be addressed by attitudinal changes at the level of the patient, clinician, or healthcare team, including organizational change.

Oncologists are broadly supportive of shared decision-making, with only the minority advocating a paternalistic approach. Physicians treating breast or gynaecological cancer are supportive of shared decision-making, more so than physicians managing haematological cancer or children with cancer. Reasons for this discrepancy could be linked to the existence of treatment options and the acknowledgement of clear treatment choices with similar survival outcomes (e.g. mastectomy versus lumpectomy for breast cancer). Physician-identified barriers to sharing insufficient information include the timing of the initial consultation and insufficient time. Facilitators of sharing decisions included patient trust and position, providing written information about treatment options, and the presence of a third person during the consultation. Box 14.1 summarizes potential barriers to shared decision-making,

---

Box 14.1 Potential barriers to shared decision-making

Doctor factors

- I have insufficient information to make a decision about treatment at the first consultation.
- There is insufficient time to spend with the patient.
- I experience difficulty knowing how to frame the treatment options for the patient.

Patient factors

- The patient has other health problems (e.g. heart disease).
- The patient has difficulty accepting s/he has cancer.
- The patient has misconceptions about the disease or treatment.
- The patient does not understand the information I have given.
- The patient is indecisive.
- The patient is too anxious to listen to what I have to say.
- The patient does not want to participate as much as I would like him/her to.
- The patient wants to make a decision before receiving the information from me.
- The patient wants to participate more than I would like him/her to.
- The patient comes expecting a certain treatment rather than a consultation.
- The patient brings too much information to discuss.
- The patient has received conflicting recommendations from various specialists.
- The patient requests a treatment not known to be beneficial.
- The patient refuses a treatment that may benefit him/her.
- There are cultural differences between the patient and me.
- The patient's family overrides the decision-making process.

---

grouped as doctor factors, patient factors, and a mismatch between patient preferences for involvement and the doctors' perspective.

Teaching shared decision-making

In a communication skills training module about shared decision-making, the following goal would apply: to make sure that the patient achieves a fully informed treatment choice, based upon a comprehensive understanding of:

1. the disease or clinical predicament and the available treatment options to deal with this;

2. the benefits and risks of each treatment choice; and

3. the capacity to appreciate the significance of each outcome for the lifestyle and values of the person, so that the choice can be made to optimally suit them.

Table 14.1 Exemplary statements made by clinicians to achieve the desired communication strategies in shared treatment decision-making

Communication strategies	Exemplary comments by clinicians
1. Establish the consultation framework	'We're here today to talk about the treatment options for your cancer.' 'Before we begin, are there particular agenda items that you want to ensure we cover today? Making me aware of these will help me to cover them at the appropriate time in our conversation.'
2. Establish the physician–patient team	'People differ in the amount of information they like to receive from their doctor. Help me to understand whether you are the sort of person who only likes to hear overviews, or sufficient detail to inform your choice, or all possible information about the issue.' 'People also differ in their decision-making style. Some are very independent and make the decision completely on their own, some consult in a shared manner with their physician, family, and friends; others want to follow precisely what their doctor recommends. Do you know which style suits you best?' 'Well, let us now work together to understand your treatment options and consider which choice may be best for you.'
3. Develop an accurate, shared understanding of the patient's situation: (a) disease features; (b) prognosis without treatment; (c) psychosocial needs and concerns; (d) other factors influencing the treatment decision	'Let me check on what sense you've been making of this diagnosis? What is it called? How serious do you perceive this illness to be?' 'What have you discovered already about your treatment options?' 'Have you known other family members or friends to receive treatment for this illness?' To a relative, 'Are there any issues or concerns that you think will influence X's decision about this treatment?'
4. Present established treatment options	'Let me first of all summarize each of the three treatments that are possible for you. Then we'll discuss each in turn.' 'Are there questions that you want to ask?' 'Let me clarify what you've understood about each of these treatment options. Can you summarize the key points for me please?' 'Remember that you don't have to reach a final choice about your treatment today. It will be fine to think it over, talk more with your family, and let me know when you feel confident about your choice.'
5. Discuss patient's values and lifestyle factors that may impact on the standard treatment decision	'Let me check if you carry any concerns about the impact of this treatment on your employment, lifestyle, fertility, or sexuality?' 'Help me to understand if a treatment preference is emerging for you and why?'
6. Present a clear statement of the recommended treatment option and invite patient choice	'Now that you understand the range of treatment options, I want to make sure that you understand what I recommend for you. If you were my father/wife, I'd …' 'Are you in a position to make a treatment choice today, or would you prefer to think about it for a few days?'
7. Close the consultation	'Let me tell you what the next steps are. You'll need to sign an informed consent form, see our booking officer, and get an appointment to see the anaesthetist.' 'If further queries come up for you, please don't hesitate to give me a call.'

This objective would be achieved through the sequence of seven strategies laid out in Table 14.1. Having established the consultation framework, which is dependent on reaching agreement about an agenda for this conversation, a sense of partnership is initially developed through an exploration of the patient's preferences for receipt of information and involvement in decision-making. There can be no better way than to ask a patient directly how much detail they like in the descriptions of treatment approaches—a simple overview, moderate attention to major benefits and side effects, or considerable detail about all potential risks and benefits. In a similar manner, asking the patient about their preferred role in making decisions proves to be useful in engaging them in the process. Do they generally like to make their own decision about what happens to their body, or are they guided by the views of their physician and family? Table 14.1 illustrates some of the comments that clinicians make to achieve each strategy in this clinical encounter.

It is wise to clarify the patient's and any companions' understanding of the illness, its seriousness or prognosis, and what they expect the treatment will need to be. This approach ensures that everyone is on the same page before commencing the discussion. Establishing pre-existing concerns empowers the clinician to address them as the conversation unfolds, while any misunderstandings can be corrected early.

Offering a preview of the range of treatment options proves helpful first, with data being categorized into portions large enough to digest readily. Be clear about the benefits of each treatment option, alongside its risks and side effects, including early, long-term, and late effects. Present the strength of evidence for each treatment modality to optimize understanding. Use of diagrams, lists, and take-home literature will usually be appreciated.

At this stage, clarification of any potential impact on lifestyle, employment, relationships, or family life is worthwhile. The concept of shared decision-making does not mean that physicians should be passive about recommending their preferred mode of treatment for each patient. Their insight is governed by their training and experience; a clear treatment recommendation helps uncertain and anxious patients. In working towards a consensus, clinicians retain a responsibility to avoid endorsement of futile treatments and to provide a strong rationale for what they recommend. Offering a decision delay can helpfully provide time for more deliberative persons.

Communication training to achieve a shared treatment decision

Range of tumour-specific patient scenarios to guide role play exercises

◆ **Breast cancer.** A 38-year-old actor and divorced mother of one is about to see you with a diagnosis of ductal carcinoma-*in-situ*, with unclear margins following a recent initial lumpectomy. Radiation therapy, mastectomy with implant, or mastectomy with free flap reconstruction are potential treatment options. Her new partner, accompanying her, is a corporate lawyer and lifestyle factors will likely impact upon her treatment choice.

◆ **Prostate cancer.** A 58-year-old physician comes to you for a second opinion about treatment of his recently diagnosed prostate cancer. After a serial rise in his prostate specific antigen titres, biopsy has revealed a moderately undifferentiated carcinoma with a Gleason score of 7. MRI imaging suggests localized disease. He has expressed interest in brachytherapy, but wonders what the Da Vinci Robotic approach to radical prostatectomy surgery may have to offer him. His wife from his third marriage will accompany him.

◆ **Rectal cancer.** A 62-year-old married stockbroker has been referred with a quite low-lying rectal cancer. One surgeon has offered him an abdominoperineal resection with a permanent stoma, but he has heard about the development of neorectal pouches. He declares that he has become confused about the side effects of these different approaches and wants to discuss the potential benefits versus risks of each treatment option. His wife suffers from chronic anxiety and is known to be a very fussy woman.

◆ **Lung cancer.** This 55-year-old woman has suffered from chronic obstructive pulmonary disease and emphysema, consequent upon many years of smoking. Her biopsy was recently positive for non-small cell lung cancer in her right upper lobe, but her respiratory reserve makes uncertain her suitability for attempting lung resection. She wants to discuss both surgical and non-surgical approaches to management and comes to you as an oncologist to learn about recent advances in the chemotherapeutic treatment of lung cancer.

Scenario for simulated female patient with breast cancer for discussion of adjuvant chemotherapy

Nadia is a 38-year-old woman who developed awareness of a lump in her left breast. She had an ultrasound and mammography/MRI of the breast. Imaging-guided biopsy was obtained and the report suggested a 2.4 cm main lesion consistent with malignancy and with smaller surrounding areas of calcification. The core biopsies confirmed a grade III invasive ductal carcinoma of the breast from the main lesion, and invasive ductal carcinoma plus adjacent ductal carcinoma-*in-situ* (DCIS) from the larger of the adjacent satellite areas.

Nadia is a married mother of two children aged 10 and 8 years; she works as a molecular biologist at a local university. Her husband is an engineer.

Her surgeon performed a left mastectomy with sentinel node biopsy. A tissue expander was inserted as a first step towards reconstruction. The pathology report confirmed grade III invasive ductal carcinoma, with clear margins, and two lymph nodes were positive out of five eventually sampled. The tumour was oestrogen receptor strongly positive and progesterone receptor strongly positive, but HER2 was not amplified. Thus Nadia has stage 2 breast cancer with positive hormone receptors. After this surgery, she is referred to a medical oncologist to discuss adjuvant chemotherapy. Her surgeon has told her that her disease is curable and she should anticipate a long life.

Discussing further treatment using a shared decision-making process

As a medical oncologist, you see Nadia for consideration of adjuvant treatments with chemotherapy and later hormone receptor modulation therapy. She wants to understand more precisely how many additional patients out of every hundred will survive if she embarks on adjuvant chemotherapy. She worries about premature menopause and wants to discuss the impact that your proposed treatment might have on her sexuality and femininity. You realize that there are several regimens of chemotherapy that you could recommend, and want to select your recommendation based on what impact it might have on several lifestyle factors that appear important to her. She will similarly question you about the choice between tamoxifen and aromatase inhibitors in your recommendation of any selective oestrogen receptor modulation therapies.

Scenario for simulated male patient with colon cancer for discussion of adjuvant chemotherapy

Anatoly is a 42-year-old man who first presented with some blood mixed with his bowel motion. He underwent a colonoscopy, which revealed a bleeding mass in the sigmoid colon. This was biopsied. A CT-scan of his abdomen was also requested, which showed both the mass and two 1 cm-sized lymph nodes adjacent to this area. His liver and other organs were normal. The biopsy of his mass returned a pathology report of grade III adenocarcinoma of the bowel.

Anatoly is a married father of two children aged 10 and 8; he works as a civil engineer. His wife is a molecular biologist.

His surgeon performed a hemicolectomy to remove his tumour. It was possible to do this without needing a colostomy. His pathology report showed the adenocarcinoma just reaching through the muscularis layer of the colon's wall, and two lymph nodes were indeed positive for tumour. The overall surgical margins were reported as clear. He has a Duke's stage C cancer of the colon. His surgeon told him that his outlook was good and would be further improved by adjuvant chemotherapy.

Discussing further treatment using a shared decision-making process

As a medical oncologist, you see Anatoly for consideration of adjuvant treatment with chemotherapy. You realize that there are several options that you could offer and want to find out whether he has a preference for a particular treatment regimen. He has been studying the internet and wonders about the length of treatment and which combination of drugs might offer him the best chance. He wants to ask about the potential side effects of treatment and whether these might impact in any way upon his lifestyle.

Table 14.2 Communication strategies, process tasks, and communication skills required by clincians for shared treatment decision-making

Communication strategies	Process tasks	Communication skills
1. Establish the consultation framework	Greet patient appropriately Make introductions of third parties Ensure patient is clothed Sit at eye-level	Declare your agenda items Invite patient's agenda items Negotiate agenda
2. Establish the physician–patient team	Introduce the approach to shared decision-making, offering choices to the patient and the goal of reaching a mutual understanding of which is preferred	Check patient preferences for information and decision-making style Endorse question asking Make partnership statements
3. Develop an accurate, shared understanding of the patient's situation: (a) disease features; (b) prognosis without treatment; (c) psychosocial needs and concerns; (d) other factors influencing the treatment decision	Begin with patient's understanding, including any third party's understanding when others are present Correct misunderstandings	Check patient understanding Clarify Invite patient concerns
4. Present established treatment options	Categorize into chunks Present treatment benefits Present treatment side effects and potential inconveniences Present the source and strength of evidence for each treatment Avoid jargon Draw diagrams	Preview the information Summarize the information Check patient understanding Endorse question asking Offer decision delay
5. Discuss patient's values and lifestyle factors that may impact on the standard treatment decision	Consider the impact of treatment on employment, lifestyle, and relationships Explore patient views and feelings about treatment options Avoid interruptions or blocking	Ask open questions Clarify Empathically acknowledge, validate, or normalize emotional responses Reinforce value of joint decision-making Make a partnership statement
6. Present a clear statement of the recommended treatment option and invite patient choice	It is generally helpful for the clinician to state their treatment recommendation clearly Work towards consensus and confidence with the treatment choice	Summarize Ask open questions Offer decision delay
7. Close the consultation	Arrange for signing of consent forms as needed Arrange for any additional consultations or referrals Create plan for next steps	Affirm value of the discussion Bid goodbye

Guide to training actors for decision-making role plays

The actor can be directed to play a well-educated, confident, and somewhat narcissistic individual, who likes always to make his/her own choices or, alternatively, an uncertain and timid person, who worries constantly, and is unsure about what is best to choose. Irrespective of the role selected by the facilitator, the actor should strive to ask questions about the potential advantages and disadvantages of each treatment option, and consider the impact of these on their workplace, relationships, and family life. The actor will value the opinion of the clinician and seek the views of any accompanying third party, ask about reliable websites for further consideration, indicating that they would like to learn a lot about the disease and its possible treatment. The worth of a second opinion should be queried routinely.

Modular blueprint for shared decision-making role play

Regarding shared decision-making about treatment options, the goal here is to ensure the patient makes a fully informed decision based upon (i) a thorough understanding of the clinical condition and its available treatment options; (ii) a dialogue about the implications of treatment on the patient's life, and (iii) the capacity to integrate the key aspects of the information into the decision-making process. This objective is best achieved within a partnership between the clinician and patient (see Table 14.2).

References

Barry MJ, Edgman-Levitan PA (2012). Shared decision making: the pinnacle of patient-centered care. *N Engl J Med* **366**, 780–1.

Brown RF, Butow PN, Ellis P, *et al.* (2004). Seeking informed consent to cancer clinical trials: describing current practice. *Soc Sci Med* **58**, 2445–57.

Bruera E, Sweeney C, Willey J, *et al.* 2003. Breast cancer perception of the helpfulness of a prompt sheet versus a general information sheet during outpatient consultations: a randomized trial. *J Pain Symptom Manage* **25**, 412–19.

Butow PN, Maclean M, Dunn SM, *et al.* (1997). The dynamics of change: cancer patients' preferences for information, involvement and support. *Ann Oncol* 8, 857–63.

Clayton JM, Butow PN, Tattersall MHN, *et al.* (2007). Randomized controlled trial of a prompt list to help advanced cancer patients and their care givers to ask questions about prognosis and end of life care. *J Clin Oncol* 25, 715–23.

Charles C, Gafni A, Whelan T, *et al.* (2004). Self-reported use of shared decision-making among breast cancer specialists and perceived barriers and facilitators to implementing this approach. *Health Expect* 7, 338–48.

Coulter A, Entwistle V, Gilbert D (1999). Sharing decisions with patients: is the information good enough? *BMJ* 318, 318–22.

Coulter A, Jenkinson C (2005). European patients' views on the responsiveness of the health systems and healthcare providers. *Eur J Public Health* 15, 355–60.

Dimoska A, Tattersall MHN, Butow PN, Shepherd H, Kinnersley P (2008). Can a "prompt list" empower cancer patients to ask relevant questions? *Cancer* 113, 225–37.

Dimoska A, Buttow PN, Lynch J, *et al.* (2012). Implementing patient question-prompt lists into routine cancer care. *Patient Educ Couns* 86, 252–8.

Henselmans I, Haes HCJM, Smets E (2012). Enhancing patient participation in oncology consultations: a best evidence synthesis of patient-targeted interventions. *Psychooncology* 22, 961–77.

Hoffmann TC, Legare F, Simmons MB, *et al.* (2014). Shared decision-making: what do clinicians need to know and why should they bother? *Med J Aust* 201, 35–8.

Joseph-Williams N, Elwyn G, Edwards A (2014). Knowledge is not power for patients: A systematic review and thematic synthesis of patient-reported barriers and facilitators to shared decision making. *Patient Educ Couns* 94, 291–309.

Laidsaar-Powell RC, Butow PN, Bu S, *et al.* (2013). Physician-patient-companion communication and decision-making: A systematic review of triadic medical consultations. *Patient Educ Couns* 91, 3–13.

Legare F, Ratte S, Stacey D, *et al.* (2010). Interventions for improving the adoption of shared decision-making by healthcare professionals. *Cochrane Database Syst Rev* May 12950, CD006732.

Shepherd HL, Tattersall MHN, Butow PN (2008). Physician-identified factors affecting patient participation in reaching treatment decisions. *J Clin Oncol* 26, 1724–31.

Shepherd HL, Butow PN, Tattersall MHN (2011a). Factors which motivate cancer doctors to involve their patients in reaching treatment decisions. *Patient Educ Couns* 84, 229–35.

Shepherd HL, Barratt A, Trevena LJ *et al.* (2011b). Three questions that patients can ask to improve the quality of information physicians give about treatment options: A cross-over trial. *Patient Educ Counsel* 84, 379–85.

Smets EMA, Van Heijl M, Van Wijngaarden AKS, *et al.* (2011). Addressing patients' information needs: a first evaluation of a question prompt-sheet in the pre-treatment consultation for patients with oesophageal cancer. *Dieases of the Oesophagus* 25, 512–18.

Stiggelbout AM, Van der Weijden T, De Wit MP, *et al.* (2012). Shared decision making: really putting patients at the centre of healthcare. *Br Med J* 344, e256.

Tattersall MHN, Butow PN (2002). Consultation audio tapes: an underused cancer patient information aid and clinical research tool. *Lancet Oncol* 3, 431–7.

Van der Weijden T, Pieterse AH, Koelewijn-van Loon MS, *et al.* (2013). How can clinical practice guidelines be adapted to facilitate shared decision making? *BMJ Qual Saf* 22, 855–63.

CHAPTER 15

Responding to difficult emotions

Jennifer Philip and David W. Kissane

Introduction to responding to difficult emotions

Clinicians must be prepared to allow the expression of a variety of emotions in cancer care. There are times during the illness when emotional responses may be anticipated, such as when a patient is first diagnosed with cancer, when a recurrence occurs, or when the disease is progressing despite anti-cancer treatments. There will be other times when the physician is unaware of the particular stimulus for distress. A seemingly benign discussion can result in an unexpected response due to vulnerabilities in the lives of patients, not directly related to the cancer care. To be supportive, physicians must be skilled in the delivery of empathic responses. There is a substantial body of evidence demonstrating that these are teachable skills (Moore *et al.* 2004; Liénard *et al.* 2010; Heyn *et al.* 2013).

The assessments of physicians and their responses will vary according to the acuity or chronicity of the emotions expressed. We will divide this chapter accordingly. We take the angry patient as one example of an emotionally difficult encounter and offer a model of how the clinician can respond. This approach can be applied to a range of other challenging interactions.

Acute emotional distress

The implications of a cancer diagnosis, its treatment and prognosis inevitably evoke emotional expression. For many patients, these reactions are private, or confined to home and family. Indeed, it is surprising that physicians are witness to relatively few intense emotional outbursts in view of the losses incurred.

Patients exhibit a range of emotions post-diagnosis including, but not limited to, mood changes such as sadness, fear, worry, anger and frustration (Alexander *et al.* 2011); existential concerns around fear of recurrence and living with uncertainty; concerns about body image, sexuality, changing roles, employment and finances; and relational issues including the family's emotional response (Andersen *et al.* 2005; Reddick *et al.* 2006; Knobf 2007). The prevalence of anxiety in cancer patients is between 25 and 48% (Stark *et al.* 2002; Kangas *et al.* 2007; Mehnert and Koch 2007), while for those with advanced cancer, depression affects between 5 and 28% of patients (Miovic and Block 2007).

While the form of expression of emotions may vary, there are some commonalities in the approaches taken by physicians that patients find helpful. These are outlined in Box 15.1. Physicians will be discomforted by extreme emotions, but quiet acknowledgement of the discomfort to oneself may be sufficient to remain aware of the patients' needs and avoid the use of defensive behaviours.

Box 15.1 Responses of the physician to the emotional distress of patients

- ◆ Be prepared to 'be present' with the distress as one human being to another.

- ◆ Listen, ask open-ended questions, and show care, compassion, and interest.

- ◆ Allow time to understand the experience and gain insight into what may have prompted this response, and at this time.

- ◆ Take care not to use distancing techniques or strategies that indicate the emotional response is unwelcome. For example, do not focus only on physical questions when emotional cues are offered by the patient.

- ◆ Show empathy by acknowledging the emotional distress you see.

- ◆ Provide support: this may be from the clinician, but also recruited from the patient's own networks. Therefore, determine who the patient's usual supports are, and consider ways, with the patient's permission, to mobilize their supportive role.

- ◆ Follow-up: this should be formally organized.

'Difficult emotions'

Not infrequently, there will be consultations where the patient's particular acute emotional expressions make communication more difficult. The patient (or their family) may be extremely distressed, demanding, unable to make decisions, or may challenge the physician. Hahn and colleagues suggest that one-sixth of all outpatient consultations are 'difficult' (Hahn *et al.* 1996). The presence of co-morbid psychiatric conditions increases the likelihood of this: depression and alcohol use create a threefold increase; anxiety disorders a sevenfold increase; and somatoform disorders a twelvefold increase (Hahn *et al.* 1996).

An approach to the difficult consultation

The construct of patients being considered 'difficult' should be treated with caution, as it suggests a punitive situation where the patient is not adopting the proper role or expected response. The notion of 'difficult' is usually determined by the physician and usually reflects his or her own reaction to an encounter. As such, in this moment of reflection when a sense of 'difficult' is raised, an opportunity exists to use the physician's personal response as a 'diagnostic barometer' to enable deeper consideration of the patient's emotional experience and the consultation dynamics. The problem may not lie with the patient (or the physician), but instead the difficulty may exist within the communication between the patient and physician (Kagawa-Singer and Kassim-Lakha 2003). Within this framework, the challenges are more appropriately located in the space between those present in the encounter. It is within this space that a shared understanding and partnership may be formed, leading to a constructive clinical relationship. Equally, however, when there is misunderstanding or reluctance to engage, difficulties arise.

Such misunderstanding may result from different expectations. In clinical interactions, people bring their cultural understanding of the body. These explanatory models of illness will influence how they consider health, including how it is defined, and the means by which it is maintained or regained (Feldman-Stewart et al. 2005). Even within the same culture, there can be variation in the adherence to certain practices. And then, in addition to their formal cultural background, people bring other influences—their role as mother, occupation, or family expectations, to name just some. Meanwhile, the health professional will represent her discipline and bring its language and expectations as well as her personal qualities, expectations, and roles.

Misunderstandings arising from different expectations may be conferred by roles, beliefs, values, basic understandings of disease and well-being, ethnicity, and many other parameters in life, not all linked with the medical concerns at hand (Feldman-Stewart et al. 2005). Shimoji and Miyakawa have noted that '[i]n the gap, loophole, between the two epistemological systems [of the doctor and patient] is the space where clinical dialog is pursued at its deepest level' (Shimoji and Miyakawa 2000). The approach to negotiating this interpersonal space is common to each 'difficult' clinical encounter, with the same strategies being helpful in a number of situations. We use anger as an illustration.

Anger

Anger is common in clinical oncology, said to be evident in 9–18%, even up to 53% of consultations (Stefanek et al. 1987; Kissane et al. 1994; Alexander et al. 2011). For patients with cancer, there are many possible sources of anger. They are forced to deal with many potential and real losses, and the resulting anger may be stated directly or be expressed as another complaint, such as discontent at a perceived or real neglect, and sometimes abandonment (Kissane 1994). At times, physicians will feel that anger is being voiced despite appropriate care.

Among suffering patients, Cohen and colleagues suggest that angry outbursts may be linked to episodes of increased pain (Cohen et al. 2004). In this study, anger resulted from an awareness of dying and was expressed more openly than complaints of pain.

Anger may be regarded as an opportunity for more creative channelling of energy (Philip et al. 2007). By encouraging emotional expression, health professionals assist with the emergence of these constructive emotional responses. Attempts to 'deal with' anger may occur at some personal cost to the health professionals involved. Such impact is little discussed, yet most physicians will readily recall a clinical encounter where they were the object of anger, and express discomfort despite the incident having occurred several years earlier.

Clinicians meeting anger may feel threatened, become defensive or, indeed, angry in response. These reactions are generally considered unhelpful as they are likely to result in an escalation of the patient's anger (Kissane 1994; Philip et al. 2007).

Longer term results from angry encounters have included absenteeism, substandard patient care, and reduced job satisfaction in health professionals (Rowe and Sherlock 2005). Taylor and colleagues reported that among hospital physicians in the United Kingdom, 32% had psychiatric morbidity and 41% suffered from emotional exhaustion (Taylor et al. 2005). Among those in cancer care, this stress and burnout was attributed, among other things, to dealing with distressed, angry, and blaming relatives.

Response to anger

For the majority of patients expressing anger, due attention to their concerns, allowing them to feel heard and facilitating some shift in perspective will result in a useful outcome for all concerned (Kissane 1994; Philip et al. 2007). This ideal outcome is nevertheless challenging to achieve and often dependent upon careful attention to a sequence of strategies that help ameliorate the distress. A practical approach to this is summarized in Box 15.2.

Step 1: Preparation

It is useful to be forewarned if a patient is angry so that some personal preparation can be made before the encounter, especially if the clinician concerned is the focus of the anger. Care should be taken to be well acquainted with the medical details available. If the patient is in a hospital ward, move the conversation from a shared room or corridor to a quiet room, showing a willingness to provide uninterrupted attention, 'making space' both physically and metaphorically.

Step 2: Listen

The angry patient needs to be heard and understood. Ventilation alone, however, is unlikely to lead to improved interpersonal

---

Box 15.2 Sequence of strategies for the difficult communication encounter

1. Preparation. Be clear about clinical details and investigation results prior to meeting the patient. Make time.

2. Listen. Using open-ended questions, allow the narrative to unfold. Develop a shared understanding of the experience, and develop shared goals from this point.

3. Offer an empathic acknowledgement of the emotions expressed.

4. Provide symptom relief.

5. Involve experienced clinicians.

6. If anger persists, reconsider your approach.

   A. Important early role for senior staff to recognize, to guide junior staff, and to model appropriate behaviour.

   B. Ensure team unity and support.

   C. Consider limit-setting to the expression of emotion, where behaviours present danger, or disruption to care.

   D. Consider a second opinion or the involvement of an independent broker.

communication in the clinical encounter (Kissane 1994). Instead, the approach must attempt to establish a shared understanding of the patient's experience and emotion, and may ultimately involve encouragement to direct the energy as constructively as possible (Kissane 1994; Philip *et al.* 2007).

A practical way of facilitating these psychotherapeutic tasks is to invite the angry patient or family member to tell her story. 'I can see you are upset. I wonder if you could tell me what has been happening. Perhaps you could take me back to the beginning of this'. The patient's story should be allowed to unfold. The clinician must take care to avoid interruptions or defensiveness, and, in the first instance, should not attempt to correct misunderstandings. Instead, the story should be heard in its entirety. Throughout this narrative, there will be opportunities for clarification and reflection on occasions of triumph and disappointment. Questions that may facilitate the recounting of grievances and allow insights into the patient's experience are listed in Box 15.3.

As the narrative nears the present, the doctor and patient reach a common understanding of what happened, which creates a connection within the consultation. This should be followed by an exploration of the patient's understanding of the present predicament and then, after careful clinical assessment, with the physician's understanding of the reality. Differences of perception should be examined and, if possible, a common position reached. Finally, some goals of care need to be negotiated and agreed upon. When taking this approach, it is almost always possible to agree to some common goals. Though anger may still be present, this usually allows the patient and family to direct the energy of anger into another avenue.

Step 3: Offer empathic acknowledgement

While hearing the story, simple strategies such as repeating phrases or stating, as appropriate, 'that must have been very upsetting' may be useful. Such phrases used in the context of empathetic listening serve not only to acknowledge the distress, but also to rename the anger as an alternative emotion. These psychotherapeutic strategies may be encapsulated as: allowing the patient to recount grievances; working towards a shared understanding of the patient's emotion and experience; and showing empathy (Philip *et al.* 2007).

If anger is justified, then validation of its expression frequently results in its amelioration. Even if anger is seemingly incomprehensible, its non-judgemental acknowledgement can be helpful for many patients. 'I can see you are very angry and upset by this'. Unhelpful responses, including indifference, lack of empathy, rushing consultations, blocking questions with premature reassurance, and failure to conduct a deeper enquiry, may all result in anger escalating. Clinicians need self-awareness about such behaviours.

Box 15.3 Questions to prompt the patient narrative

◆ Help me to understand what has been happening.

◆ Tell me what you thought went wrong, and the events leading up to this.

◆ What do you think caused the problem?

◆ Can you take me back to when all this began: when was this, and what was the first thing you noticed?

◆ What is your sense of what is happening?

The narrative approach described in this section is effective for many and frequently results in improvement of the patient–physician relationship. Anger may be considered to be a symptom requiring exploration, expression, and understanding (Philip *et al.* 2007) and its expression is viewed as an opportunity to facilitate the emergence of alternative and more creative emotional responses to the illness. When anger is transformed into more mature emotions, relationships are enriched both within and beyond the clinic.

Step 4: Provide symptom relief

The approach to anger should also include careful attention to, and relief of, symptoms that may be exacerbating the complexity of the emotional experience. The reduction of pain, for example, will allow the space for a distressed patient to consider alternative emotional responses.

Step 5: Involve experienced clinicians

The capacity of physicians to interact constructively with angry patients and families increases with experience. Meanwhile, the skilled physician has an educational responsibility to model constructive responses to anger for junior staff.

On occasion, anger may persist unabated, despite intensive and conscientious efforts by the physician (Kissane 1994). For some, anger may persist because the initial grievances have not been adequately addressed, but for a few, anger may represent a lifelong pattern of response to a challenge or crisis. When anger is persistent, there are frequently unfortunate consequences for patient care. If the competence or effort of staff is continually questioned, confidence will be undermined. Staff may be reluctant to engage with the patient, thereby protecting themselves, but also reducing the opportunities for therapeutic relationships. Ultimately, care may become fragmented and adversarial positions between the patient (or family) and staff become fixed, further limiting the opportunities for discourse and negotiation. In such a challenging situation, staff should be supported, but efforts must also be made to prevent intransigent positions being adopted.

Step 6: If anger persists, reconsider the approach

When anger persists despite the thoughtful efforts of experienced staff, then the approach should be reconsidered. In such a situation, the aims should change from attempting to resolve the anger to supporting the healthcare team. Early recognition of a patient or family who appear to be persistently angry is important. When anger is not abating, junior staff need guidance to cease making themselves vulnerable to the expression of such anger, and senior staff should be actively involved. Junior staff should feel comfortable to defer complaints to their senior colleagues, who in turn must be willing to show leadership and model adaptive behaviours.

In the presence of resolute anger, support of the health professional team is critical, and the reinforcement of team unity is vital (a separate but related task). All staff should be actively informed of the goals of care through regular meetings and through the development of a detailed care plan for the patient concerned. Involve all disciplines as appropriate, including medical, nursing, allied health, security, and food services, since all may be subject to the anger expressed. This will both support staff and reduce the ambiguity of 'mixed messages', thus providing certainty to patients. On occasion, a single member of staff and a single member of the family concerned may be nominated as persons through which communication best occurs. Staff should actively facilitate the collegiate support of all within the care team.

On occasion, anger is so extreme that limits on behaviour and interactions are required. Staff have responsibilities to a number of patients, and they must be confident that they can conduct their duties in a safe, non-threatening (verbally and physically) environment. The use of limit-setting can be a constructive way of containing anxieties and enable the best use of the time available. A family meeting may be helpful (see Chapter 18). Take care that senior staff are involved, more than one staff member is present, and use the formality of the process to achieve containment. Senior staff should always be involved in the negotiation of such limits, and it may be helpful to involve non-clinical staff (such as the director of nursing). In this way, limits that initially appear unpalatable may be negotiated without compromising what remains of the therapeutic relationship.

In the presence of continued dissatisfaction and questioning of competence, offer a second medical opinion. Another approach is the involvement of an outside independent broker. Such mediation may take the form of a clinical ethics consultation or a patient's representative or advocate. This independent opinion may be particularly helpful in an extreme situation, where seemingly intransigent positions between staff and the patient are set.

In effect, the model delineated here for anger is useful in its application to a number of difficult clinical encounters, including patients who are anxious, resentful, distressed, or fearful. In each scenario, a response from the empathetic physician, which involves listening, hearing the illness narrative and, as necessary, involving senior clinicians, will contain distress.

Prolonged emotional distress

Suffering

The lay press might consider suffering as synonymous with pain, but in clinical care, the two are not so easily equated. One person may feel pain but not be suffering. Another may suffer when they lose something central to their life, such as losing employment, yet they have no physical injury. Instead, a richer understanding of suffering stems from the notion that human beings exist with a sense of their wholeness, identity, and embodiment. Suffering results when this integrity is threatened.

> Suffering is experienced by persons not merely by bodies, and it has its source in challenges that threaten the intactness of the person as a complex social and psychological entity (Cassel 1982, p. 639).

In this sense, suffering is understood as a disintegration of the self. Suffering is not universal in terminal illness. Its causes are intensely personal, cannot be predicted, and we must enquire directly as to their nature (Cassel 1982). An approach to suffering, therefore, requires not only an understanding of the disease and its symptoms, but also the nature of what it is to be human in all its complexity.

If suffering is understood as a disintegration, then the approach to assisting the person who is suffering should be aimed at reintegration. The use of open-ended questions, attentive listening, and encouraging personal narratives may all assist some form of reintegration. The phrase 'tell me what you were like at the top of your game' may be useful. Hearing each person's description of him or herself when they were at their best not only reminds them that they live and exist as an entity distinct from the current illness, but it

Box 15.4 Phrases that may be useful in the presence of someone suffering

- Take me back to before this cancer started or to when you last felt really well in yourself. Tell me when this was, how you were, how you spent your time, your interests.
- Now can you describe to me what first made you go to the doctor, and then … How were you getting on then, how did the treatments go from your point of view?
- You seem to be having a very difficult time at the moment.
- Are you suffering? Can you help me understand what you are feeling and what is making you suffer?
- Can you take me back to when you were 'at the top of your game', when you were feeling absolutely at your peak. When was that? What were you doing? Tell me about your life at that time.

also recalls a time when they were fully integrated. Aspects of this approach have been formally developed in an intervention for terminally ill patients termed Dignity Therapy (Chochinov et al. 2005). Such an approach not only helps patients redevelop a sense of meaning in their lives, but also assists their families during bereavement (Chochinov et al. 2005). Some phrases that may be useful when caring for a patient who is suffering are outlined in Box 15.4.

Demoralization

Demoralization may be understood as a particular reaction to threat experienced by patients with significant illness, which is characterized by poor coping, lowered morale and an inability to determine the way forward (Clarke and Kissane 2002). This helplessness may progress to a more generalized hopelessness, where the patient feels a loss of direction and pointlessness to his or her life. If help is not forthcoming, the patient feels isolated and, if coupled with reduced self-esteem, a severe form of demoralization may result. This mental state can be equivalent to the existential distress of suffering discussed previously.

The patient who is demoralized may be able to laugh and enjoy the moment, but is unable to anticipate the future with any pleasure, while the depressed patient cannot experience pleasure at any level. The demoralized patient does not know how to act or what to do, with a pervasive helplessness about their state, but for the patient with depression, even though the path to act may be evident, s/he has lost the motivation to pursue that course (Kissane 2014; Robinson et al. 2015).

Once again the approach to the demoralized patient is not significantly different to other 'difficult' clinical encounters. Such an approach should include:

- The relief of symptoms.
- The use of open-ended questioning, empathic listening to encourage connectedness, valuing, and relationships.
- An exploration of life's meaning, including views on relationships, beliefs, and roles. The patient should be encouraged to consider his or her life as a whole, including times when they were connected and integrated.

Conclusion

A number of emotions will be expressed in the journey with cancer. Some will occur at times when bad news is delivered; others will be unexpected, and may take the physician by surprise. Skills that help acute distress include listening with empathy, using open-ended questions to allow gentle exploration of the related feelings, avoiding strategies that tend to distance patients, and providing the information and appropriate reassurances to enable a person to recruit their own coping responses.

It is both surprising and humbling that most patients negotiate this journey with little or no significant assistance from their physician, but instead draw upon their personal resources and those of their immediate family and community.

The difficult clinical encounter is one characterized by essential differences between the patient and their clinician. This difference lies in the expectations of the participants, their beliefs, cultures, understanding of illness, approach and roles, and results in a mismatch in communication. Our model of negotiating this difference has utility across a number of different clinical scenarios and settings.

Finally, when emotional responses have become more chronic, a state of demoralization may result. Here the helplessness becomes overwhelming and, if help is not offered or proves ineffective, a state of existential distress may develop. When severe, this represents a form of suffering. The approach to care for such patients must include a careful and gentle exploration of the source of distress in the context of a caring clinical relationship. For some patients, telling their story to a physician who is truly listening will be of great benefit. For others, an exploration and improved understanding of his or her beliefs, values and sense of meaning may allow some mobilization of personal resources to assist the intensely personal task of reintegration. The care of a clinician who is willing to be open and to spend time in the space occupied by the suffering patient will enable some patients to emerge, even in some small way, from a state of suffering. In turn, there may be rich rewards, which flow to the clinician himself. Michael Kearney suggests that the physician who is prepared to accompany 'another as he journeys into the depths of his experience' (Kearney 1992) may himself be enriched. For '... the healing on offer may be there not just for the patient and his family but also for us as people who are physicians, and in some small way for western medicine itself'(Kearney 1992, p. 46).

Clinical scenarios for use in role play in communication skills training

Scenario for simulated female patient with breast cancer

Nadia is a 38-year-old woman who developed awareness of a lump in her left breast. You sent her for ultrasound and mammography/MRI of the breast, and requested biopsy if the radiologist deemed it suspicious. Imaging-guided biopsy was obtained and the report suggested a 2.4 cm main lesion consistent with malignancy and with smaller surrounding areas of calcification. The core biopsies confirmed a grade III invasive ductal carcinoma of the breast from the main lesion, and invasive ductal carcinoma plus adjacent ductal carcinoma-*in-situ* (DCIS) from the larger of the adjacent satellite areas.

Nadia is a married mother of two children aged 10 and 8 years; she works as a molecular biologist at a local university. Her husband is an engineer.

Nadia as an angry patient

Nadia had a lumpectomy and sentinel node biopsy performed by her surgeon. The pathology report was returned with unclear margins. Her surgeon went back to perform a wider excision, leaving a noticeable distortion and asymmetry in her remaining breast. Wound infection then developed, necessitating several weeks of dressings and courses of antibiotics. This delayed Nadia's suitability to commence chemotherapy. Nadia's frustration developed with this experience and she began to blame her surgeon for the complications that had developed.

Nadia presents to you (select choice of discipline, e.g. medical oncology, plastic surgery) to discuss chemotherapy (or reconstructive surgery or other ongoing care provision). She is irritable and distressed about her predicament and angry at her surgeon. She questions the surgeon's skill and appears quick to blame.

Nadia as an emotionally distraught patient

You meet Nadia two years later as her medical oncologist when she has been found to have both multiple bone and liver metastases. Her two children are now aged 12 and 10. She is devastated at the possibility that she might die before they fully grow up. She cries intensely before you, expressing fear of dying, and of leaving her children. She is emotionally distraught. You find it hard to get her to focus on any positive ideas you have about being able to control her cancer for a time. She simply seems to be too distressed in her grief that this cancer has recurred.

Simulated male patient with colon cancer

Anatoly is a 42-year-old man who first presented with some blood mixed with his bowel motion. You referred him for a colonoscopy, which revealed a bleeding mass in the sigmoid colon, which was biopsied. A CT scan of his abdomen was also requested, which showed both the mass and two 1 cm-sized lymph nodes adjacent to this area. His liver and other organs were normal. The biopsy of his mass has returned a pathology report of grade III adenocarcinoma of the bowel.

Anatoly is a married father of two children aged 10 and 8; he works as a civil engineer. His wife is a molecular biologist.

Anatoly is managed with left hemicolectomy and a successful immediate re-anastomosis of his colon. His surgery is followed for adjuvant chemotherapy for a six-month period.

Anatoly as an angry patient

You meet Anatoly three years later after he developed some abdominal pain. A CT scan was performed, which showed mild bilateral hydronephrosis associated with several enlarged retroperitoneal lymph nodes, and several large metastases in his liver. Anatoly is angry that his previous chemotherapy didn't cure him. He feels cheated. His two children are now aged 13 and 11. He is very annoyed at the possibility that he might die before they fully grow up. He wonders how his family will survive financially without him. You find it hard to get him to focus on any positive ideas you have about being able to control his cancer for a time. He simply seems to be too aggravated and upset that this cancer has recurred.

References

Alexander SC, Pollak KI, Morgan PA, *et al.* (2011). How do non-physician clinicians respond to advanced cancer patients' negative expressions of emotions? *Support Care Cancer,* **19**, 155–9.

Andersen BL, Shapiro CL, Farrar WB, *et al.* (2005). Psychological responses to cancer recurrence. *Cancer* **104**, 1540–7.

Cassel EJ (1982). The nature of suffering and the goals of medicine. *N Engl J Med* **306**, 639–45.

Chochinov HM, Hack T, Hassard T, *et al.* (2005). Dignity therapy: a novel psychotherapeutic intervention for patients near the end of life. *J Clin Oncol* **23**, 5520–5.

Clarke DM, Kissane DW (2002). Demoralization: its phenomenology and importance. *Aust N Z J Psychiatry* **36**, 733–42.

Cohen MZ, Williams L, Knight P, *et al.* (2004). Symptom masquerade: understanding the meaning of symptoms. *Support Care Cancer* **12**, 184–90.

Feldman-Stewart D, Brundage M, Tishelman C (2005). A conceptual framework for patient–professional communication: an application to the cancer context. *Psychooncology* **14**, 801–9.

Hahn SR, Kroenke K, Spitzer RL, *et al.* (1996). The difficult patient. *J Gen Intern Med* **11**, 1–8.

Heyn L, Finset A, Ruland CM (2013). Talking about feelings and worries in cancer consultations: the effects of an interactive tailored symptom assessment on source, explicitness, and timing of emotional cues and concerns. *Cancer Nurs* **36**, E20–E30.

Kagawa-Singer M, Kassim-Lakha S (2003). A strategy to reduce cross-cultural miscommunication and increase the likelihood of improving health outcomes. *Acad Med* **78**, 577–87.

Kangas M, Henry JL, Bryant RA (2007). Correlates of acute stress disorder in cancer patients. *J Trauma Stress* **20**, 325–34.

Kearney M (1992). Palliative medicine-just another specialty? *Palliat Med* **6**, 39–46.

Kissane D (1994). Managing anger in palliative care. *Aust Fam Physician* **23**, 1257–9.

Kissane D (2014). Demoralization—A life-preserving diagnosis to make in the severely medically ill. *J Palliat Care* **30**, 255–8.

Kissane DW, Bloch S, Burns WI, *et al.* (1994). Psychological morbidity in the families of patients with cancer. *Psychooncology* **3**, 47–56.

Knobf M (2007). Psychosocial responses in breast cancer survivors. *Semin Oncol Nurs* **23**, 71–83.

Liénard A, Merckaert I, Libert Y, *et al.* (2010). Is it possible to improve residents breaking bad news skills? A randomised study assessing the efficacy of a communication skills training program. *Br J Cancer* **103**, 171–7.

Mehnert A, Koch U (2007). Prevalence of acute and post-traumatic stress disorder and comorbid mental disorders in breast cancer patients during primary cancer care: a prospective study. *Psychooncology* **16**, 181–8.

Miovic M, Block S (2007). Psychiatric disorders in advanced cancer. *Cancer* **110**, 1665–76.

Moore PM, Wilkinson SS, Rivera Mercado S (2004). Communication skills training for health care professionals working with cancer patients, their families and/or carers. *Cochrane Database Syst Rev* **2**, 1–20.

Philip J, Gold M, Schwarz M, *et al.* (2007). Anger in palliative care: a clinical approach. *Intern Med J* **37**, 49–55.

Reddick BK, Nanda JP, Campbell L, *et al.* (2006). Examining the influence of coping with pain on depression, anxiety, and fatigue among women with breast cancer. *J Psychosoc Oncol* **23**, 137–57.

Robinson S, Kissane D, Brooker J, *et al.* (2015). A systematic review of the demoralization syndrome in individuals with progressive disease and cancer: a decade of research. *J Pain Symptom Manage* **49**, 595–610.

Rowe M, Sherlock H (2005). Stress and verbal abuse in nursing: Do burned out nurses eat their young? *J Nurs Manag* **13**, 242–8.

Shimoji A, Miyakawa T (2000). Culture-bound syndrome and a culturally sensitive approach: From a viewpoint of medical anthropology. *Psychiatry Clin Neurosci* **54**, 461–6.

Stark D, Kiely M, Smith A, *et al.* (2002). Anxiety disorders in cancer patients: their nature, associations, and relation to quality of life. *J Clin Oncol* **20**, 3137–48.

Stefanek ME, Derogatis LP, Shaw A (1987). Psychological distress among oncology outpatients: prevalence and severity as measured with the Brief Symptom Inventory. *Psychosomatics* **28**, 530–9.

Taylor C, Graham J, Potts HW, *et al.* (2005). Changes in mental health of UK hospital consultants since the mid-1990s. *Lancet* **366**, 742–4.

CHAPTER 16

Denial and communication

Linda Sheahan and David W. Kissane

'And once again his thoughts dwelt on his childhood, and once again that was painful for Ivan Ilyich, and he tried to banish those thoughts and think of something else' (p. 204).

Reproduced from Leo Tolstoy, *The Death of Ivan Ilyich and Other Stories*, Translated by Nicolas Pasternak Slater and Edited by Andrew Kahn, Oxford World's Classic, Oxford University Press, Oxford, UK, Copyright © 2015, with permission from Oxford University Press.

Introduction to denial and communication

Patients who appear not to acknowledge the diagnosis of an illness, or its gravity, are said to be 'in denial'. A patient's history readily illustrates this in Box 16.1.

Denial is considered a common reaction, especially when an illness is life-threatening. After being told of the diagnosis of terminal cancer, approximately 20% of patients deny they have cancer, 26% partially suppress awareness of impending death, and 8% demonstrate complete denial (Greer 1992). A meta-analysis suggested that the prevalence of denial of the cancer diagnosis ranged from 4 to 47%, and denial of negative affect from 18 to 42% (Vos and De Haes 2007).

Although the term 'denial' is an accepted part of the medical vernacular, it is used in a variety of clinical circumstances, with varying definitions and little consensus. Furthermore, as with all of the body's defences—physiological, immunological, psychological—denial can become maladaptive.

This chapter will establish a pragmatic view of denial, explore how it functions within the clinician–patient relationship, and then demonstrate when intervention is appropriate and how that intervention is best undertaken. Specific attention will be given to the communication skills required for an effective clinical response to denial.

Definition

The term *denial* has not acquired a monolithic meaning—that is, there is no common agreement as to when and how to use the word. Psychoanalysts describe it as one of several cognitive defence mechanisms, which serve to protect a person against anxiety. A patient demonstrates denial by refusing (self-aware) or being unable (unaware) to acknowledge some painful aspect of reality or emotion that would ordinarily be apparent to self or others. The term *psychotic denial* is used when there is, in addition, gross impairment in reality testing (see Box 16.2).

Throughout the medical literature, the construct of denial has been used to describe anything from illogical behaviour and non-compliance, to the patient's pretence to family that all is well, to non-integration of medical information into the patient's worldview (Vos and De Haus 2007). To make matters more complicated, there is also denial as a specific clinical sign associated with neurological damage (Ellis and Small 1993). This can lead to confusion and uncertainty as to how to manage denial. The importance of defining denial, or at least setting functional parameters, is to enable management. The key to management of denial is thoughtful communication.

How should we define denial? The term 'denial' is applied to patients who, consciously or unconsciously, alleviate their anxiety (primarily directed at death or pain) by portraying a serious health situation as either exaggerated or non-existent (Cousins 1982). Why do people deny? One answer is that the human brain is designed to enable it to accommodate practically any trauma that it confronts. When an event is too difficult or painful to integrate immediately, denial is used as a coping mechanism, as a self-protective buffer. Sometimes this defence mechanism is adaptive, and sometimes maladaptive. An analogy for how it becomes a morbid process might be drawn to the body's immune system, to

---

Box 16.1 Denial leading to morbid consequences

TC was a 36-year-old man with recently diagnosed metastatic colorectal cancer. Clearly told it was incurable, he received palliative chemotherapy. TC was admitted to hospital for pain management and multiple medical complications related to progressive disease. He was cooperative with staff and treatment plans, but remained convinced that his disease was curable. The treating team sensed his reluctance to discuss prognosis, and subsequently avoided speaking directly about the cancer and his deterioration. His family and his nine-year-old son were not informed about the extent of his illness. TC wanted to go home. His mood deteriorated and the psycho-oncologist diagnosed depression with denial, complicated by collusion of the treating team. A family meeting, including the patient, discussed the overall goals of care, gradually achieving a realistic consensus.

Box 16.2 Psychotic denial associated with late presentation of advanced cancer

JN was a 71-year-old retired oncology nurse, who presented to the emergency department with abdominal pain. She was found to have a large fungating chest wall lesion, consistent with advanced breast cancer. Investigations confirmed malignancy, with chest wall invasion and liver metastasis. On questioning, she insisted that she had extensive experience with cancer in her work, and that this was not cancer. She also claimed that the mass had been there for over 20 years, and was due to severe dermatitis. On being asked why she had not sought a medical opinion, she simply said that she thought it was nothing to worry about. On further questioning, JN admitted that it had changed slightly over the last few months. Gradually, after a number of consultations with the medical staff, she began to exhibit inconsistencies in her belief that it was dermatitis, and began to accept the possibility that it might be cancer.

diseases that fail to distinguish self from non-self. Furthermore, denial is dynamic—it comes and goes 'at will', as needed. Factors that influence the presentation of denial include level of anxiety (primarily of death), the passage of time (Zimmermann 2004), professional relationships, and stage of disease. The clinician's job is to assess whether denial is adaptive or not, and avoid harm to the patient whenever possible.

We propose conceptualizing denial as a spectrum (see Fig. 16.1). The key variables are:

1. the degree to which the patient is aware of their denial; and

2. how effectively the denial functions in striking a balance between subjective fear and the threat of illness.

At one end of the spectrum, when a person consciously avoids discussion of an upsetting experience, his or her active avoidance can facilitate an adaptive outcome by minimizing the seriousness of a concern so that the focus is sustained on hopeful optimism. However, when anxious procrastination leads to delayed investigation or treatment of any condition, the potential for a morbid outcome increases. At the other end of the spectrum, disavowal involves disclaiming knowledge about or understanding of the existence of a condition or its seriousness. In the psychoanalytic use of the word 'disavowal', the splitting off of an unwelcome trauma is

employed to unconsciously deny that it ever existed. At the heart of this process of subconscious disavowal is the potential for maladaptive outcomes, because of the primitive blocking of awareness that occurs.

Denial in the clinical environment

To help us understand the clinical application of denial, we will examine four clinical contexts in which denial is seen:

1. beneficial;

2. detrimental;

3. clinician's complicity; and

4. familial and cultural.

Denial as beneficial

Denial functions as a form of self-protection, and there is some evidence that it may be beneficial in patients with life-limiting illness. Longitudinal studies of breast cancer patients showed that those patients who denied the seriousness of the cancer diagnosis experienced significantly less mood disturbance than those with 'acceptance' coping styles (Watson *et al.* 1984). Denial was negatively correlated with anxiety in adult cancer patients (Vos and De Haes 2007), and positively correlated with good adjustment in survivors of childhood cancers (Greer 1992). Denial may also lead to patients experiencing fewer physical complaints, and it may have a positive effect on function (Vos and De Haes 2007). Longitudinal studies of a cohort of patients with lung cancer suggested that denial facilitated better social outcomes and less anxiety and depression (Vos *et al.* 2011), better overall perception of health, improved physical function, and lower symptom burden (Vos *et al.* 2010).

Furthermore, the use of denial as a coping strategy may be predictive of a more favourable disease trajectory (Garssen 2003). In a 15-year prospective study of adjustment styles in breast cancer, Greer and colleagues (1990; 1992) followed a group of non-metastatic breast cancer patients at 5, 10, and 15 years following surgical intervention. Women who used fighting spirit or denial as coping strategies survived longer than those who reacted with stoic acceptance or helplessness. An overall trend in meta-analysis suggested a positive relationship between denial and survival (Garssen 2003), although it is possible that a negative survival outcome from hopelessness-helplessness underlies this finding. Active minimization has also been associated with longer survival (Brown *et al.* 2000).

Then there is the question of denial in the service of hope. Druss and Douglas (1988) correlated healthy denial with optimism and resilience, where what was being denied was not the disease or infirmity itself, but rather the fearful implications and emotional impact. Patients may interpret what they are told about their condition according to the fear they experience or the hope they wish to maintain. In studies of hospital patients interviewed with a diagnosed but undisclosed malignancy, 88% suspected they had cancer on admission, but 68% had no wish to augment that knowledge (McIntosh 1976). Patients used denial to both maintain uncertainty and to support hope. This relationship to hope has also been explored in the coping strategies used by family members and loved ones (Benkel 2010).

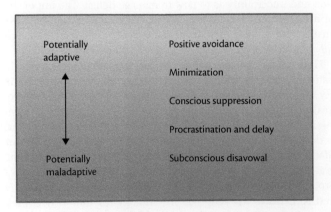

Potentially adaptive

Positive avoidance

Minimization

Conscious suppression

Procrastination and delay

Subconscious disavowal

Potentially maladaptive

Fig. 16.1 Spectrum model of denial.

Box 16.3 Denial leading to non-adherence to recommended treatment

LD was a 26-year-old man with acute leukaemia whose mother worked as a natural therapist, promoting herbal medicine. She designed a comprehensive nutritional programme, bringing the ancient wisdom of Chinese herbal medicine to an exercise regimen and other homeopathic remedies. LD was greatly influenced by his mother and declined the chemotherapy recommended by his haematologist in favour of treatment by these natural therapies. A second opinion was obtained from an overseas naturopath, who added additional herbs to the regimen. Although he was encouraged to take both treatment approaches in parallel, LD expressed concern that chemotherapy would interfere with his natural therapy regimen.

Box 16.4 Denial as a pathway towards futile medical care

AH was a 19-year-old girl with metastatic osteosarcoma refractory to chemotherapy. AH and her family were from the Middle East and held strong religious beliefs that she would be cured, despite multiple discussions with her oncologist regarding the palliative nature of her treatment. They were adamant that every modality of treatment should be trialled since 'where there is life, there is hope'. Staff became increasingly concerned that the family were 'living in denial', which resulted in an almost daily discussion regarding prognosis and the futility of chemotherapy. AH then developed spinal cord compression. She and her family remained steadfast in their insistence on attempting further treatment, and her physician acquiesced by giving her a dose of 'emergency' chemotherapy in the early hours of the morning. There was no effect, and she died a couple of days later in hospital.

Denial as detrimental

However, denial can also be detrimental. In spite of the success of public screening for certain cancers, denial still contributes to late clinical presentation (Zervas *et al.* 1993). Denial creates a barrier between clinician and patient, which can reduce effective communication (see Box 16.3). This in turn effects the patient's ability to make informed health choices and, in extreme cases, to poor compliance with treatment. Denial may prevent patients from preparing for death, both pragmatically and psychologically; and lead to complicated grief in the bereaved (Watson *et al.* 1984). It can appear as an obstacle to open discussion of death, dying at home, stopping 'futile' treatments, advanced care planning, and symptom control (Zimmerman 2007).

Clinician's complicity with denial

Traditionally, the term denial has been applied to patients; however, the clinician is not immune from denial as part of the therapeutic relationship (Helft 2005). A physician may deny prognostic information to patient or family, thereby encouraging hope (Cousins 1982). The continuation of ineffectual chemotherapy, use of subtherapeutic dosing, or the exaggeration of the length of survival are three examples of clinicians employing denial. For instance, rather than promote acceptance of natural processes of dying in the face of terminal frailty from advanced cancer, a clinician's suggestion that cardiopulmonary resuscitation may be beneficial can precipitate intubation and ventilatory support in the intensive care unit, in place of the more emotionally demanding conversation about the reality of impending death.

Denial by physicians may be employed as part of their defences against the difficult feelings evoked by their work, including any sense of mortal vulnerability. While these defences are protective, they can seriously hamper communication. This can be characterized by emotional distancing, detachment, intellectualization, nihilism, or even aggression. In turn, this may affect the patient's adherence to treatment, pain control, information recall, preparation for dying, and overall satisfaction with care (Favre 2007).

Family's complicity and cultural context

Some families use denial to cope with the patient's illness. Tacit agreement between family members to 'deny' illness can appear as 'mutual pretence awareness'. At times it can be distressing or

detrimental for the patient, particularly when communication patterns are disturbed, leading to anxiety, isolation, and suspicion. Cultural and religious variance has a significant impact on the use of denial as a psychological mechanism of coping (Gall 2004; Chan *et al.* 2005; Travado *et al.* 2005). Many societies—Japanese, Chinese, and Indian—are evolving from a past avoidance of prognostic discussions to more open and direct communication about the clinical reality. To what extent should clinicians respect these variances, and 'allow' ongoing denial? Box 16.4 illustrates the potential for futile medical care to be administered through collusion with a family's process of denial. At its most extreme, futile care could lead to extended suffering and prolonged dying from advanced cancer in the intensive care unit.

A 'functional' or clinical approach to denial

When should denial be broached? Only when it is causing self-harm? Or when it is judged that denial is blocking acceptance? What role do cultural or individual values play?

Clinicians need a functional definition of denial. Denial scales have been trialled in various studies without much success, but perhaps the most effective way to view denial is dimensionally, as displayed in Figure 16.1. At one extreme is completely subconscious disavowal, and at the other, active forgetting. Elements of denial are evident within each of the labelled domains in this spectrum. Patients' level of denial may fluctuate and move from one domain to the other, depending on the patient's perceived—conscious or not—level of threat. However, only certain domains in certain circumstances require active intervention.

Role of patient's self-awareness

Denial is often assumed to be by definition unconscious, in contradistinction to more 'healthy' coping mechanisms, such as minimization or positive avoidance, in which there may be some self-awareness. Nevertheless, elements of denial in minimization and avoidance are recognizable and these coping mechanisms should be integrated into the dimensional nature of denial. Active forgetting involves consciously setting aside, suppressing, or pushing into the background information that is too painful, as in the

Table 16.1 Strategies and communication skills to use in response to denial

Strategies	Skills	Process tasks	Model statements
1. Recognize the presence of denial, and exclude misunderstanding, neuropathology, or misinformation	Ask open questions Check patient understanding	Find out how much the patient knows about their disease Correct any misunderstandings Identify denial in self or team, and ensure it is not impacting adversely on management; gather collaborative history from family and supportive others	'Could you describe for me in your own words what you have been told about your illness?' 'Just to ensure that I understand you correctly, you think …' 'Is it clear to you why you had treatment?' 'Have you asked any of the hospital staff for information regarding your treatment? Was the information they gave to you clear?'
2. Determine whether it is maladaptive or adaptive for the given circumstance	Declare your agenda items (explore patient coping style and its effect) Determine and normalize past psychological coping style	Determine if denial is evident in the patient's previous response to stress Evaluate the effect of denial on treatment compliance Determine if it is causing difficulties within the patient's support group/family Decide whether it is obstructing the patient's treatment	'Would it be ok if I explore how you are coping with your illness?' 'How have you coped with difficult things in the past?' 'How are you managing at home or at work?' 'What is difficult for you living with the illness?'
3. Provide information tailored to the needs of the patient	Clarify Acknowledge Normalize	Clarify the patient's preference for information and decision-making, including goals of care	'Different patients request different levels of information from their clinician. Are you someone who likes to be given a lot of information and detail, or are you someone who prefers an overview?' 'Have you talked to your family about this health problem? Would you like me to arrange a family meeting?'
4. Explore emotional reactions and respond with empathy	Ask open questions regarding emotional response and coping Empathize Validate Acknowledge Normalize Simplify Praise the patient's efforts Express a willingness to help	Ask about and acknowledge their emotional response Demonstrate empathy for the difficulty they are having confronting the threatening aspect of their illness Validate this difficulty Divide the emotional issues into smaller more manageable packets	'How are you feeling at this stage in your illness? I can see that you are afraid/uncertain, and I know that must be extremely difficult for you.' 'Difficulty coping is normal and understandable.' 'If we can put names to our emotions, it is sometimes easier to deal with them. Let's try that for you and see if it is helpful?' 'If something I am saying makes you too uncomfortable, please let me know.'
5. Where denial is maladaptive, identify and gently challenge inconsistencies in the patient's narrative. Maintain an open dialogue, particularly so that shifts in denial can be addressed, if required	Clarify Endorse question-asking Summarize Review next steps	Ask the patient to identify their disease status and phases of management Explore the factors which support a more realistic understanding of the situation Confront ambivalence sensitively Be wary of abrupt interventions that may precipitate overwhelming anxiety Confrontation often requires repeated visits Encourage optimism Work with family and treating team re collusion. Involve psychosocial services if required	'Could you explain to me why you think this lesion is severe dermatitis?' 'Is there a time, even just for a moment, when you consider that it might not be as simple as dermatitis?' 'Does the fact that it has changed over the last few months make you suspicious that it could be more serious?' 'How do you explain the recent changes?' 'It looks as though part of you prefers to believe that it is not serious, but another part of you is willing to consider that it is more serious?'
6. Follow up and monitor denial in context as disease progresses	Reinforce joint decision steps	Monitor for gradual adjustment to the stressor, and acceptance of next steps as context changes Monitor adaptive denial for signs that it is becoming maladaptive	'I understand that this is how you feel about your illness currently. I would like us to meet again in … just to check how things are going, and discuss things a little further.'

epigram from Tolstoy. Clinicians do well, for example, to promote active avoidance of any fear of recurrence when patients are about to undertake routine re-staging imaging. Adaptive coping is the desirable outcome here.

Role of context

The central question is whether denial is functioning in a beneficial or a maladaptive way. Adaptiveness is judged by how well a person can cope with the practicalities of the illness (and its implications) despite anxieties and fears. Thus, if the denial is accompanied by self-harm or neglect, it could reasonably be labelled as maladaptive and require healthcare intervention. The definition of 'self-harm' is relative and requires the prudent judgement of the healthcare team. Broad parameters include: non-compliance; unrealistic expectations by patient or family regarding goals of care; damage to relationships with family and loved ones (Helft 2005); and inability to find 'closure'.

'Acceptance' is not always necessary. Patients may die without ever acknowledging the full extent of their illness or the imminence of death. In these cases, the priority is symptom control—physical, emotional, and spiritual—notwithstanding denial. There is no rationale for intervening in cases of benign or adaptive denial by forcing acceptance upon patients, as this may only serve to increase distress and, indeed, may not be ethically prudent.

The insightful clinical response

Denial is a response to fear, typically of death. The expression of denial depends on personality, coping styles, degree of self-awareness ('I'm not going to think about it any more') and the extent to which the patient can manoeuvre their illness pathway through the healthcare system. It ranges on a spectrum from beneficial coping to maladaptive self-harm. The best approach is to develop a 'feel' for their coping style, support the patient, and note the balance between fear and adaptation. Generally, a trusting relationship and good communication will be all that is required to allow the patient to open up and 'let go' of denial.

Communication with patients using denial

Although there are no empirical studies exploring the best way for a physician to challenge denial in their patient, physicians are not always confident of their communication skills in dealing with denial (Travado et al. 2005). When 'breaching' the defence of denial, often an indirect approach is best. Given that denial functions as a response to a fear (of death), then by shoring up a person's self-esteem, dignity, morale, and life's meaning, the fear will likely recede and denial will commensurately cease to have a function. The following recommendations are a compilation of findings based on case study reviews and expert opinion (Maguire and Pitceathly 2003; Schofield et al. 2003; Hudson et al. 2006; Owen and Jeffrey 2008) about communication in the face of denial:

◆ Exclude neuropathology, misunderstanding, or inadequate information.

◆ Determine whether denial is maladaptive or adaptive.

◆ Determine whether denial requires management.

◆ Explore emotional background to fears.

◆ Provide information tailored to the needs of the patient and clarify goals of care.

◆ Be aware of cultural and religious issues and respond sensitively.

◆ Monitor the shifting sand of denial as the disease progresses.

These strategies, together with their related communication skills and process tasks, are outlined in Table 16.1.

Conclusion

Denial can be a temporary, adaptive coping mechanism to help a person deal with a difficult and usually frightening new circumstance. Generally, it is best to support the patient's method of coping with their illness. Where denial is seen to function in a maladaptive way, however, it may be necessary to tackle and expose the denial, albeit with care and wisdom.

References

Benkel I, Wijk H, Molander U (2010). Using coping strategies is not denial: helping loved ones adjust to living with a patient with a palliative diagnosis. *J Palliat Med* **13**, 1119–23.

Brown JE, Butow PN, Culjak G, Coates AS, Dunn SM (2000). Psychosocial predictors: time to relapse and survival in patients with early stage melanoma. *Br J Cancer* **83**, 1448–53.

Chan CLW, Perry D, Wiersgalla D, Schlinger JM, Reese DJ (2005). Beliefs, death, anxiety, denial, and treatment preferences in end-of-life care. *J Soc Work End Life Palliat Care* **1**, 23–47.

Cousins N (1982). Denial. *J Am Med Assoc* **24**, 210–12.

Druss RG, Douglas CJ (1988). Adaptive responses to illness and disability. *Gen Hosp Psychiatry* **10**, 163–8.

Ellis SJ, Small M (1993). Denial of illness in stroke. *Stroke* **24**, 757–9.

Favre N, Despland JN, De Roten Y, Drapeau M, Bernard M (2007). Psychodynamic aspects of communication skills training. *Support Care Cancer* **15**, 333–7.

Gall TL (2004). The role of religious coping in adjustment to prostate cancer. *Cancer Nurs* **27**, 454–61.

Garssen B (2003). Psychological factors and cancer development: evidence after 30 years of research. *Clin Psychol Rev* **24**, 315–38.

Greer S, Morris T, Pettingale KW, Haybittle JL (1990). Psychological response to breast cancer and 15-year outcome. *Lancet* **335**, 49–50.

Greer S (1992). The management of denial in cancer patients. *Oncology* **6**, 33–6.

Helft PR (2005). Necessary collusion: Prognostic communication with advanced cancer patients. *J Clin Oncol* **23**, 3146–50.

Hudson PL, Schofield P, Kelly B, et al. (2006). Responding to desire to die statements from patients with advanced disease: recommendations for health professionals. *Palliat Med* **20**, 703–10.

McIntosh J (1976). Patients' awareness and desire for information about diagnosed but undisclosed malignant disease. *Lancet* **2**, 300–3.

Maguire P, Pitceathly C (2003). Managing the difficult consultation. *Clin Med J* **36**, 532–7.

Owen R, Jeffrey D. 2008. Communication: common challenging scenarios in cancer care. *Eur J Cancer* **44**, 1163–8.

Schofield PE, Butow PN, Thompson JF, Tatersall MHN, Beeney LJ, Dunn SM (2003). Psychological responses of patients receiving a diagnosis of cancer. *Ann Oncol* **14**, 48–56.

Travado L, Grassi L, Gil F, Ventura C, Martins C (2005). Physician-patient communication among southern European cancer physicians: the influence of psychological orientation and burnout. *Psychooncology* **14**, 661–70.

Vos MS, De Haes JCJM (2007). Denial in cancer patients, an explorative review. *Psychooncology* **16**, 12–25.

Vos MS, Putter H, Van Houwelingen HC, De Haes HCJM (2011). Denial and social and emotional outcomes in lung cancer patients: the protective effect of denial. *Lung Cancer* **72**, 119–24.

Vos MS, Putter H, Van Houwelingen HC, De Haes HCJM (2010). Denial and physical outcomes in lung cancer patients, a longitudinal study. *Lung Cancer* **67**, 237–43.

Watson M, Greer S, Blake S, Shrapnell K (1984). Reaction to a diagnosis of breast cancer: Relationship between denial, delay and rates of psychological morbidity. *Cancer* **53**, 2008–12.

Zervas IM, Augustine A, Fricchione GL (1993). Patient delay in cancer. *Gen Hosp Psychiatry* **15**, 9–13.

Zimmerman C (2004). Denial of impending death: a discourse analysis of the palliative care literature. *Soc Sci Med* **59**, 1769–80.

Zimmermann C (2007). Death denial: obstacle of instrument for palliative care? An analysis of clinical literature. *Socio Health Illn* **29**, 297–314.

CHAPTER 17

Communicating with relatives in cancer care

Isabelle Merckaert, Yves Libert, Aurore Liénard, and Darius Razavi

Introduction to communicating with relatives in cancer care

Due to the evolution of medicine and the organization of care, partners, parents, children, and other family members have become key supports for cancer patients throughout the disease. As a result, relatives are omnipresent throughout the cancer trajectory, starting with the cancer diagnosis consultation. Despite all this, little is known about how to communicate with relatives in cancer care. The aim of this chapter is to underline the difficulties encountered by relatives when they accompany patients during the illness trajectory and the role that they often play as a complementary source of information as regards patients' psychological and physical well-being. This chapter will then discuss relatives' place in the consultation in general and in breaking bad news consultations in particular, and the consequences of this presence on healthcare professionals' communication. A three-phase model of breaking bad news while integrating the relatives in the exchanges will be described. Finally, the chapter will discuss how to interact with a relative who is trying to protect the patient while asking for collusion.

Relatives' adaptation to their caregiver role

Starting with patient's diagnosis, relatives of cancer patients are confronted with a dual role: on the one hand, they have to deal with their emotional responses to the patient's diagnosis and prognosis and with their own difficulties; and, on the other hand, they have to deal with the high demands of the caregiver role. Although most relatives cope well with this dual role, studies have reported that 10 to 50% experience high levels of distress (Pitceathly and Maguire 2003; Vanderwerker et al. 2005; Merckaert et al. 2013a) and that they suffer from levels of distress comparable to those found in a cancer patient population (Mitchell et al. 2013), and higher than those found in the general population (Wittchen et al. 2002; Djernes 2006). Importantly, relatives are likely to become more distressed as the disease progresses and treatment becomes palliative (Pitceathly and Maguire 2003) and they receive less social support than patients (Mellon et al. 2006). Relatives' distress has been linked to a decrease in their own physical well-being (Bevans and Sternberg 2012), reduced family and marital functioning (Northouse et al. 2000), and with patients' poor social

rehabilitation (Northouse et al. 2000), poor treatment adherence (Given and Sherwood 2006), and increased emotional distress (Hodges et al. 2005). Despite these stresses, relatives are as reluctant to seek professional help for their psychological difficulties as patients (Vanderwerker et al. 2005; Merckaert et al. 2013a). When healthcare professionals communicate with relatives, they should be aware that they face individuals who may be as distressed as patients, whose needs are less likely to be met, and who are unlikely to seek professional psychological help.

Relatives' role in cancer care as a source of complementary information

Beyond their supportive role towards patients, relatives often play another important role in cancer care, in that their report of patients' difficulties are often a key source of complementary information for health professionals. Meanwhile, there are few data regarding the accuracy of relatives' perceptions about a patient's experience. In theory, relatives' reports could be influenced by patients' self-perception, as well as by relatives' feelings about what to disclose. Relatives' feedback could also be impacted by their own perception of difficulties, as well as their feeling about what is relevant to share in order to provide patients with appropriate support.

Consequently, a relative's collaborative history of a patient's difficulties may be impaired by two types of inaccuracies: not reporting difficulties that the patient experiences, and falsely reporting difficulties not experienced by the patient. Non-report errors could lead health professionals to miss or underestimate important patient difficulties, while misperceptions could lead health professionals to focus their attention, and interventions, on difficulties not actually experienced by the patient.

When they interact with relatives, healthcare professionals should be aware that relatives under-report a significant amount of patient difficulties, especially social difficulties. In contrast, primary informal caregivers often over-report other difficulties, such as psychological struggles (Libert et al. 2013). One explanation for the discrepancy in reports may be that both patients and relatives often have negative outcome expectancy beliefs regarding communication with each other about cancer and its consequences. As a result, they often prefer to display a fighting spirit. Moreover, patients may be reluctant to disclose their difficulties to their relatives in order to protect relationships. Likewise, many relatives may be reluctant to question patients about their experiences, as they do not want to add additional stress to the patient's condition. Unfortunately, protective concern for the patient may decrease a relative's wish to actively address a patient's suffering. In addition, it is paramount that relatives maintain a supportive role, which can be difficult since they have to manage both proximity and distance with the patient in order to avoid unnecessary distress. As a result of this relationship, an accurate perception of the patient's difficulties may not be the priority for a relative.

Healthcare professionals should therefore, above all else, consider relatives' reports of patient difficulties as a way to obtain appropriate help from health professionals. Health professionals should affirmatively acknowledge this role and relatives' willingness to support patients. Second, before deciding to take the needed actions to help patients as requested by caregivers, health professionals should recommend to caregivers to check with patients their perceptions and make sure that they are right. When the patient is present, health professionals may check the validity of the caregiver's report using the skill of circular questions.

Circular questions are a useful communication strategy when a patient is accompanied by a relative in an interview (Dumont and Kissane 2009). Circular questions may be used to assess patients' and relatives' concerns, to support, or to gain a deeper understanding. Circular questions establish both connections, but also distinctions between the different members of a family. This style of questioning stimulates the emergence of information in a manner that encourages new ways of seeing the problem. The purpose of circular questioning is to optimize understanding of the difference in point of views and also establish connections, pathways to open up communication, and therefore to consider the problem from a different angle.

There are two different types of circular questions. As displayed in Table 17.1, type 1 circular questions aim to directly assess the impact of the situation and the level of emotional distress of each protagonist. They are used to recognize and clarify things said by one of the protagonists and summarize what has been said in order to assess its impact on the other protagonist and on the dyad they constitute. Type 2 circular questions are used to indirectly assess the impact of the situation and the level of distress of one of the

Table 17.1 Examples of circular questions

Type 1 circular questions	
HCP:	*Madam, how do you feel emotionally about what I just told you?*
Comment:	The professional clarifies the patient's feelings in response to the bad news.
HCP:	*Madam, are there other things you feel as a result of what I just told you?*
Comment:	The professional verifies whether there are other feelings that the patient still has not disclosed.
HCP:	*Madam, may I ask your partner how he feels?*
Comment:	The professional asks for the patients' agreement to discuss his/her relative's feelings. If the patient agrees:
HCP:	*Sir, how do you feel exactly about what I just said?*
Comment:	The professional clarifies the relative's feelings in response to the bad news.
HCP:	*Sir, are there other things that you feel as a result of what I just told you?*
Comment:	The professional verifies whether there are other feelings that the relative still has not disclosed.
Type 2 circular questions	
HCP:	*Madam, how do you feel emotionally about what I just told you?*
Comment:	The professional clarifies the patient's feelings in responses to the bad news.
HCP:	*Sir, what do you think of this feeling of despair experienced by your wife?*
Comment:	The professional asks the relative about his perception concerning the patient's emotional response to the bad news.
HCP:	*Madam, are there other things you feel about what I just told you?*
Comment:	The professional verifies whether there are other feelings that the patient still has not disclosed.
HCP:	*Sir, what do you think of this feeling of anger experienced by your wife?*
HCP:	*Madam, may I ask your partner how he feels?*
Comment:	The professional asks for the patient's agreement to discuss his/her relative's feelings. If the patient agrees:
HCP:	*Sir, how do you feel exactly about what I just said?*
Comment:	The professional clarifies the relative's feelings in responses to the bad news.
HCP:	*Madam, what do you think of this feeling experienced by your husband?*
Comment:	The professional asks the patient about her perception concerning her partner's emotional response to the bad news.

Abbreviation: HCP—Healthcare professional.

protagonists starting from the other's point of view. Circular questions help each partner to think the issue through from the other person's perspective. As shown in Table 17.1, type 2 circular questions are therefore used after recognizing a predicament from one of the protagonist's points of view and summarizing the discussed elements in order to investigate the perception of the other protagonist about what has just been said.

Caution should however be exercised in the use of circular questions, in order to respect the choice of the patient in terms of sharing his/her feelings about the situation in the presence of his/her companion. A professional may be insensitive and intrusive if he or she forces the patient (or the relative) to talk about anxieties when the other is present, while they have a habitual relational dynamic that excludes this type of emotional sharing. Before using circular questions, healthcare professionals should first clarify patients' and their relatives' habits and desire in terms of sharing their feelings and fears as regards cancer. Second, they should negotiate with them, starting with the patient, asking permission to explore coping in the consultation. Starting with the patient allows healthcare professionals to underline implicitly that the patient is the central focus of care, while acknowledging the importance of the relative's integration in the process of care.

Relatives' place in cancer consultations

Although studies investigating the presence of a relative in cancer consultations are scarce, some have shown that approximately 20% of medical interviews in cancer care occur in the presence of a relative (Beisecker and Moore 1994) and that this rate increases to 86% in breaking bad news consultations (Eggly et al. 2006). A recent review indicated that accompanying relatives are predominantly spouses, followed indeterminately by children, parents or siblings, and that relatives are often present in 'difficult' situations, especially when patients are 'vulnerable' (Laidsaar-Powell et al. 2013). Relatives are more likely to be present when (i) the patient is older and has a poorer performance status; and (ii) at specific time points in the course of the disease: (a) for initial visits, (b) immediately after cancer recurrence, and (c) in the terminal phase of the disease, rather than in a routine follow-up visit. They mainly accompany the patient to provide support, to serve as the patient's advocate, or to participate in decision-making (Laidsaar-Powell et al. 2013).

Despite the importance of the accompanying relative for optimal cancer care, few studies have compared physicians' communication when a patient is alone and when a patient is accompanied by a relative. One study showed that when a relative was present, interactions were slightly longer (three minutes) and physicians were likely to provide more information (Labrecque et al. 1991). One recent study reported that accompanied and unaccompanied breast cancer patients were equally active in asking questions (Del Piccolo et al. 2014). Another study showed that the combined 'companion plus patient' participation did not differ from the participation of unaccompanied patients. Street and Gordon noted that patterns of companion participation varied greatly across consultations. Almost half the interactions had a relatively passive companion (contributed to less than 40% of the 'patient plus companion' active participation) while 33% of the consultations had an active companion and passive patient (Street and Gordon 2008). Overall, physicians appear able to only slightly adjust their communication style to the presence of a third party. The third party seems either to take the patient's place in the interview, or to remain somewhat unacknowledged.

Although several authors have recognized the need to adjust communication skills to accommodate the concerns of both patients and relatives during breaking bad news consultations, guidelines and recommendations have mainly focused on providing effective individual consultations, that is, consultations that include only the patient. Our team developed a three-phase model of the breaking bad news process that was adapted to breaking bad news in a triadic consultation (Liénard et al. 2010; Merckaert et al. 2013b). As shown in Box 17.1, this adapted model includes the following three phases. The first phase would be devoted to preparing the patient and his/her relative for the delivery of bad news by assessing what they know, understand, and feel about the current situation. This would be referred to as the 'pre-delivery phase'. The second phase, the 'delivery phase', would be devoted to delivering the bad news precisely and concisely. Finally, the third phase, the 'post-delivery' phase, would be devoted to providing emotional support and additional information to both the patient and their relatives. Completing these three phases represents a complex task that requires the use of specific communication skills for which physicians in general, and residents in particular, have not been sufficiently trained.

Relatives' desire to protect their loved ones and collusion

Relatives may also desire to protect their loved ones from what they judge to be unnecessary hardships. They may ask healthcare professionals not to disclose some pieces of information to the patient, such as diagnosis or transition to palliative care. A patient may also want to protect his or her relatives from terrible news. Collusion can be defined as a 'secret' or implied understanding between two or more people to delay or avoid certain topics among themselves, or with third parties.

Who does not want to protect his family and reduce the burden of terrible news about the disease? The desire behind this attitude is common and is rooted in a strong relationship between two people. In the medical context, health professionals need to have methods to respond to collusion demands. Two objectives must be pursued together: first, respecting the patient's right to know; and second, identifying and validating the feelings and motivations of the family. The professional can achieve both goals by emphasizing the obligation to inform the patient if he so requests, while formulating an empathic response acknowledging the relative's desire to protect the patient that is implicitly expressed in this request.

Five steps can be helpful in the management of collusion with a relative wishing to protect his or her loved one from difficult information (see Table 17.2 for an example). First, it is important to explore his/her motivations; second, to validate his/her attitude; third, to evaluate the psychological costs for that person of having to manage the situation alone; fourth, to request permission to assess the perception of the patient about the situation; and finally, to negotiate the contract, that is to say, what steps you will take together. It is important to underline that it is impossible to break the collusion without feeling the sorrow of the couple. Promoting communication between them can however have great benefits.

Training healthcare professionals in communicating with relatives

Although many studies have reported the usefulness of communication skills training programmes addressed at physicians working

Box 17.1 Core elements of the three phases of the breaking bad news process in the presence of a relative

Phase 1: Pre-delivery phase

- Welcoming both the patient and the relative.
- Negotiating the relative's presence in the interview.
- Acknowledging the importance of relative's presence.
- Clarifying the relative's intended role in the consultation.
- Assessing the patient's and the relative's concerns using circular questions.
  - Assessing first the patient's concerns and needs
  - Assessing the relative's reactions towards what the patient just said
- Asking for the patient's agreement to assess the relative's concerns.
  - Assessing of the relative's concerns and needs
  - Assessing the patient's reactions towards what the relative just said
- Acknowledging the importance of what has been said and summarizing.
- Defining the consultation agenda.

Phase 2: Delivery phase

- Delivering the bad news precisely and concisely while including the relative in the non-verbal exchanges (e.g. eye contact, nods of the head).

Phase 3: Post-delivery phase

- Clarifying the patient's reactions to the bad news and need for further information.
- Providing empathic support.
- Asking for the patient's agreement to assess the relative's reactions to the bad news and needs for further information.
- Delivering information about treatment.
- Assessing the patient's and the relative's level of understanding of the information and ability to receive further information.
- Delivering and/or clarifying information if needed.
- Assessing the patient's and the relative's concerns, starting with the patient and using circular questions.
- Acknowledging the difficulty of the situation and offering support.
- Organizing the agenda of care.
- Closing the consultation.

Table 17.2 Examples of the five strategies that form a sequence for managing collusion with a relative

Strategy 1: Exploring the relative's motivations	
HCP:	*I know it is a terrible ordeal for you. You told me that your husband could not bear to know what happens. Could you tell me what worries you most?*
Relative:	*If he finds out, he will collapse. And that I do not, I could not stand that.*

Strategy 2: Validating the relative's attitude	
HCP:	*You know your husband better than me and you may be right. Are there reasons why you think that?*
Relative:	*He will collapse, withdraw into himself, and let go.*
HCP:	*Do you have other reasons to think that?*
Relative:	*No.*

Strategy 3: Assessing the costs of collusion for the spouse	
HCP:	*I understand that you do not want him to be informed. I share your desire to save your husband from greater distress. But tell me, what effect does this have on you to carry alone that secret?*
Relative:	*It's terrible. I am tense, I sleep badly, I have nightmares.*
HCP:	*Can you tell me a little more about these nightmares?*
Relative:	*I dream he dies.*
HCP:	*Hmm, this may indeed happen.*
Relative:	*This concerns me greatly.*
HCP:	*Are there other consequences of this tension in your everyday life?*
Relative:	*Sometimes I'm about to crack, and I unburden myself on the children. I do not know how to tell him without demolishing him.*
HCP:	*Do you still have other problems because of not telling him?*
Relative:	*Yes, we are less and less close. I want to be more kind to him, but I'm afraid he would guess why. He says I keep my distance, but I cannot explain why. It's horrible. I want to be closer, but there is a widening gap between us.*

Strategy 4: Requesting permission to assess patient's perception of the situation	
HCP:	*So this silence has for you a lot of consequences. This makes you tense and drives you away from him. Can you tell me what could be done about it?*

Strategy 5: Negotiating the contract	
Relative:	*You're not going to tell him?*
HCP:	*Not necessarily, but I want to know what he thinks about his current situation. Perhaps he will tell me he knows he has cancer and in this case, there is no reason to say otherwise.*
Relative:	*You're not going to tell him?*
HCP:	*No, I just want to know what he knows. If, as you think, he knows nothing, or if he doesn't want to know anything, I will leave it at that and I will not tell him.*
Relative:	*(Hesitantly) Okay, okay.*

Abbreviation: HCP—Healthcare professional.

in cancer care, few studies have specifically assessed their usefulness on physicians' communication skills when a third party is present. Our group designed and assessed two communication skills training programmes, which included a focus on the three-person interview.

The aim of the first study was to assess improvements in physicians' communication skills and the transfer into clinical practice of newly acquired communication skills in three-person interviews, resulting from participation in six 3-hour consolidation workshops following a 2.5-days basic training programme (Delvaux *et al.* 2005). Consolidation workshops focused on different issues, including how to communicate with relatives in three-person interviews. Results showed a transfer of skills acquisition to clinical practice. We also underline that changes towards relatives are more modest in actual interviews than in simulated interviews. Patients who interacted with physicians who were randomized to the consolidation workshops reported higher scores concerning their perception of physicians' assessment of their concerns, and a higher degree of satisfaction with physicians' performance. This higher degree of satisfaction with physicians' performance was not found for relatives, however. This may be related to the modest changes that were observed in physicians' use of communication skills when they addressed relatives. Our study showed that the transfer of skills addressing relatives' concerns and needs remains limited. Another interesting outcome was that although physicians who were randomized to the consolidation workshop failed to show an improvement in their ability to better assess patients' distress in two-person interviews (Merckaert *et al.* 2005), they showed an improvement in their detection of patients' distress when a third party was present (Merckaert *et al.* 2008). This contrast in the effectiveness of a communication skills training programme on physicians' detection in two- and three-person interviews could be explained by the added value of a relative's presence in a consultation. This added value may, on the one hand, be linked to the fact that patients may be more prone to express their concerns when a relative is present because they may feel supported when disclosing their concerns. On the other hand, relatives may volunteer information to the physician that the patient would not have spontaneously disclosed, and may thus help physicians in having a better perception of the patient's concerns. When an accompanying relative is present in an interview, there may be a higher likelihood that concerns will be disclosed.

The second study aimed at assessing the efficacy of a 40-hour dyadic and triadic communication skills training programme on residents' breaking bad news when a relative is present and was associated with a training in stress management skills (Merckaert *et al.* 2013*b*). Results of the study in simulated three-person consultations showed that, after training, (i) the duration of the pre-delivery phase was longer for the trained residents; (ii) the simulated relative's first turn of speech about the bad news more often came during the pre-delivery phase; (iii) third party communication was more often initiated by the trained residents; and (iv) trained residents also used more assessment and supportive utterances. This study showed that the pre-delivery phase lasted approximately one minute before training, and approximately two minutes after training. Moreover, assessments of the relative's concerns about cancer by residents also increased following training, with approximately 90% of trained residents addressing the simulated relative's concerns regarding the bad news in a consultation, compared with only 40% of residents before training. In addition, residents also addressed the concerns of the simulated relative more often in the 'pre-delivery phase' following training.

Conclusion

Physicians should be aware that communicating with a patient and a relative is a complex task that requires the use of specific communication skills, for which healthcare professionals have not been sufficiently trained. The specificity of three-person interviews met so frequently in cancer care should be recognized (patient's and relative's respective agendas, adequate interview duration, and specific communication skills). The practice of three-person interviews should thus ideally start during medical school and should be consolidated further by specific training modules targeting barriers towards addressing relatives. Skills transfer into the clinic may be facilitated by asking physicians to choose to practice specific skills related to the core elements of a three-person consultation in between training sessions. Finally, the need to devote more consultation time for three-person interviews should be recognized, in order to allow physicians to address the relatives' concerns and needs.

There are four lessons to be taken away. First, communicating with a patient and a relative requires a motivation to include the relative in the process of care. Second, the inclusion of the relative requires the acquisition of specific skills. Third, the acquisition of these skills requires appropriate training. Fourth, the use of these skills would probably be facilitated by devoting a longer consultation time for this purpose.

References

Beisecker AE, Moore WP (1994). Oncologists' perceptions of the effects of cancer patients' companions on physician-patient interactions. *J Psychosoc Oncol* **12**, 23–39.

Bevans M, Sternberg EM (2012). Caregiving burden, stress, and health effects among family caregivers of adult cancer patients. *JAMA* **307**, 398–403.

Del Piccolo L, Goss C, Bottacini A, *et al.* (2014). Asking questions during breast cancer consultations: does being alone or being accompanied make a difference? *Eur J Oncol Nurs* **18**, 299–304.

Delvaux N, Merckaert I, Marchal S, *et al.* (2005). Physicians' communication with a cancer patient and a relative: a randomized study assessing the efficacy of consolidation workshops. *Cancer* **103**, 2397–411.

Djernes JK (2006). Prevalence and predictors of depression in populations of elderly: a review. *Acta Psychiatr Scand* **113**, 372–87.

Dumont I, Kissane DW (2009). Techniques for framing questions in conducting family meetings in palliative care. *Palliat Support Care* **7**, 163–70.

Eggly S, Penner LA, Greene M, Harper FW, Ruckdeschel JC, Albrecht TL (2006). Information seeking during "bad news" oncology interactions: Question asking by patients and their companions. *Soc Sci Med* **63**, 2974–85.

Given B, Sherwood PR (2006). Family care for the older person with cancer. *Semin Oncol Nurs* **22**, 43–50.

Hodges LJ, Humphris GM, Macfarlane G (2005). A meta-analytic investigation of the relationship between the psychological distress of cancer patients and their carers. *Soc Sci Med* **60**, 1–12.

Labrecque MS, Blanchard CG, Ruckdeschel JC, Blanchard EB (1991). The impact of family presence on the physician cancer-patient interaction. *Soc Sci Med* **33**, 1253–61.

Laidsaar-Powell RC, Butow PN, Bu S, *et al.* (2013). Physician-patient-companion communication and decision-making: a systematic review of triadic medical consultations. *Patient Educ Couns* **91**, 3–13.

Libert Y, Merckaert I, Slachmuylder JL, Razavi D (2013). The ability of informal primary caregivers to accurately report cancer patients' difficulties. *Psychooncology* **22**, 2840–7.

Liénard A, Merckaert I, Libert Y, *et al.* (2010). Is it possible to improve residents breaking bad news skills? A randomised study assessing the efficacy of a communication skills training program. *Br J Cancer* **103**, 171–7.

Mellon S, Northouse LL, Weiss LK (2006). A population-based study of the quality of life of cancer survivors and their family caregivers. *Cancer Nurs* **29**, 120–31.

Merckaert I, Libert Y, Delvaux N, *et al.* (2005). Factors that influence physicians' detection of distress in patients with cancer: can a communication skills training program improve physicians' detection? *Cancer* **104**, 411–21.

Merckaert I, Libert Y, Delvaux N, *et al.* (2008). Factors influencing physicians' detection of cancer patients' and relatives' distress: can a communication skills training program improve physicians' detection? *Psychooncology* **17**, 260–9.

Merckaert I, Libert Y, Lieutenant F, *et al.* (2013*a*). Desire for formal psychological support among caregivers of patients with cancer: prevalence and implications for screening their needs. *Psychooncology* **22**, 1389–95.

Merckaert I, Liénard A, Libert Y, *et al.* (2013*b*). Is it possible to improve the breaking bad news skills of residents when a relative is present? A randomised study. *Br J Cancer* **109**, 2507–14.

Mitchell AJ, Ferguson DW, Gill J, Paul J, Symonds P (2013). Depression and anxiety in long-term cancer survivors compared with spouses and healthy controls: a systematic review and meta-analysis. *Lancet Oncol* **14**, 721–32.

Northouse LL, Mood D, Templin T, Mellon S, George T (2000). Couples' patterns of adjustment to colon cancer. *Soc Sci Med* **50**, 271–84.

Pitceathly C, Maguire P (2003). The psychological impact of cancer on patients' partners and other key relatives: a review. *Eur J Cancer* **39**, 1517–24.

Street RL, Gordon HS (2008). Companion participation in cancer consultations. *Psychooncology* **17**, 244–51.

Vanderwerker LC, Laff RE, Kadan-Lottick NS, McColl S, Prigerson HG (2005). Psychiatric disorders and mental health service use among caregivers of advanced cancer patients. *J Clin Oncol* **23**, 6899–907.

Wittchen HU, Kessler RC, Beesdo K, Krause P, Hofler M, Hoyer J (2002). Generalized anxiety and depression in primary care: prevalence, recognition, and management. *J Clin Psychiatry* **63**, 824–34.

CHAPTER 18

Conducting a family meeting

David W. Kissane and Courtney Hempton

Introduction to conducting a family meeting

Family meetings in oncology occur most commonly in four settings. The first is soon after diagnosis, when the patient and family are being oriented to the disease, potential treatment options, and the system of care with available supports. The second is in the setting of an inpatient admission, when goals of care need to be redefined and treatment options reviewed. The third is during palliative care, where the support of the family in planning ongoing care is essential to optimize such care. And the fourth is when there is conflict about the direction of care, sometimes in the setting of a patient with impaired capacity, when the medical staff and the patient's healthcare proxy disagree with goals of care and treatment. Family meetings are commonly held in paediatric oncology or genetic counselling settings. Some meetings are held 'impromptu'—the opportunity presents itself when staff and the family are available and the meeting is held.

Here we describe a model of conducting the basic, planned family meeting in the setting of a patient with advanced disease. The overall goals of such a meeting are to:

1. educate about the illness and its management;

2. assess caregiver needs regarding the cancer illness;

3. understand wishes about end-of-life care and views about place of death;

4. address the pragmatics of advance directives and who the decision-makers are within the family;

5. discuss discharge planning issues; and

6. assess family coping and identify high-risk families or members so that appropriate referrals can be made.

The principles we outline for conducting a family meeting in palliative care apply broadly to meetings in other settings. The family meeting is often co-facilitated by an oncologist or physician and a social worker, psychiatrist, or advance practice nurse. This co-facilitated approach is ideal to meet broader biopsychosocial goals and is dependent on mutual respect and collaboration.

Why a family meeting and who is the family?

The family is a crucial resource for patients living with cancer and facing life-threatening illness. Family members often serve as primary caregivers: they guide the provision of support for loved ones during their final days, actively participate in the decision-making processes, and serve as liaisons and proxy informants to healthcare practitioners. The journey of illness is thus a shared one. Distress reverberates through the family, leading to recognition that members are second-line patients through a model of family-centred care (Zaider and Kissane 2009). As a result, practitioners and researchers alike have taken an interest in understanding how the family accommodates the strain of serious illness, and in identifying ways to ensure optimal functioning.

Roles of family carers have become more pronounced (Kissane *et al.* 1996; Schuler *et al.* 2014). The principal caregiver is the spouse in 70% of cases, children (daughters and daughters-in-law predominate) in 20%, and approximately 10% comprise friends or more distant relatives (Zaider and Kissane 2009). The family is best defined as the 'psychological family'—people who share their lives and are recognized by the patient as belonging (Boss and Dahl 2014). Hence, visiting relatives from overseas, best friends, fellow workers, or neighbours of those without direct kin, could all be involved if they contribute to caregiving and support of the patient.

The resilient family

Resilience can be defined as a positive adaptation arising in a setting of significant adversity, so that the family is seen to strengthen its functioning to the benefit of its membership and community (Henry *et al.* 2015). Central family functions include: (a) cohesion, membership, and family formation (e.g. the family maintains a sense of belonging, including personal and social identity for its members); (b) economic support (e.g. the family provides for basic needs of food, shelter, and health resources); (c) nurturance, education, and socialization (e.g. the family affirms social values, and fosters productivity and compatibility with community norms); and (d) protection of vulnerable members (e.g. the family protects members who are young, ill, or disabled) (MacPhee *et al.* 2015).

The adaptive family is able to reorganize its roles, rules, and interaction patterns to ensure adequate care and protection of an ill member. Family assets empower growth and transformation via a style of functioning in which members communicate effectively, provide mutual support, and resolve differences of opinion through flexibility and buoyancy (Henry *et al.* 2015). Resilience is a likely outcome for those families who believe that strength is derived from teamwork, adversity is a shared challenge to be overcome together, and whose optimism and spirituality deliver new meaning and transcend suffering (Walsh 2014).

The family considered 'at risk'

Observational studies of families during palliative care and bereavement led Kissane and colleagues to develop a typology that defines families 'at risk' of morbid outcomes during bereavement (Kissane et al. 1996; Schuler et al. 2014). Poor family cohesion, communication, and conflict resolution were determinative of this classification which, in turn, was highly predictive of psychiatric disorder occurring during bereavement for the membership of these families. Dysfunctional families fell into two types: conflictual and uninvolved, while an intermediate type between well-functioning and dysfunctional families had low communication (Schuler et al. 2014).

When it is recognized during palliative care that these families are at greater risk for morbid outcome, commencing a preventive model of family therapy while the cancer patient is still alive has been shown in randomized controlled trials to ameliorate distress, and prevent development of prolonged grief disorder in bereavement (Kissane et al. 2006; Kissane et al. 2016). This may be an important approach, as Higginson and colleagues (2003) conducted a meta-analysis of 26 studies of palliative and hospice care teams and contrasted a slightly positive effect size on patient symptom outcomes (26 studies, weighted mean 0.33, SE 0.12 [95% CI 0.10, 0.56)]), with no proven benefit on caregiver and family outcomes (13 studies, weighted mean 0.17, SE 0.16 [95% CI 0.14, 0.48]). Palliative care as a discipline understands the need for family-centred care, but has struggled to find an effective model to accomplish this comprehensively.

How then do clinicians recognize those families in greatest need? While resilient families do well and are not in need of additional psychosocial resources, families with some limitation in their functioning as a group—reduced communication, limited teamwork, or prominent conflict—are worthwhile referring for prophylactic family therapy in the palliative care setting (Kissane and Bloch 2002; Kissane and Parnes 2014). Sometimes a basic family meeting clarifies these relational characteristics, and helps to have the family accept help through referral for ongoing work together. Additionally, families where members are already distressed, having suffered cumulative stress, loss and tragedy, benefit from early family therapy referral.

Range of family needs

Systematic reviews of family needs (Ventura et al. 2014) and of family meetings at the end of life (Sullivan et al. 2015) have identified the following challenges to optimally informing caregivers about their role:

- poor communication;
- conspiracies of silence about the prognosis;
- the timing and amount of information to be delivered;
- overcoming impaired concentration;
- avoidant responses;
- not wanting to bother; or
- outright rejection of the health provider's help.

Health systems, in their turn, need adequate staffing, skills training, educational materials, and a model of delivering carer training to achieve the desired goal.

Clarity about the content of carer educational sessions is derived from nursing research into key roles and tasks undertaken by carers in the home as they assist a dying relative (Hannon et al. 2012). These tasks include:

- symptom assessment and management;
- understanding the trajectory of illness;
- medication administration;
- help with ambulating, transferring the patient in and out of bed, or dressing the patient;
- liaising with doctors;
- instrumental care activities like meal preparation or transportation; and
- coordinating visits from volunteers and friends to achieve respite for the carer.

Information provision stands out as the key unmet need in assisting the carers' preparation for these roles, thus helping to minimize their burnout and exhaustion (Ventura et al. 2014).

Family education about caregiving is a fundamental service requirement that is applicable to families whose relative is at home, but also relevant to the family of an inpatient. A number of the latter families might be preparing for an eventual death at home. In addition to information about caregiving roles as described above, a number of other themes worthy of discussion with the family are listed in Box 18.1. Coverage of these has been shown to be immensely helpful to families (Hudson et al. 2008).

Families with special needs include those with young children, particularly those losing a key parent, or when a single parent is dying and will leave children orphaned (Muriel 2014); families caring for ageing parents; those with adult children living with disability or mental illness; and those isolated through migration, language barriers (Lubrano di Ciccone et al. 2010), or in some way disenfranchised from relatives and support. Listening to a family's story and assessment of its needs is a crucial clinical task.

Box 18.1 Themes often discussed in family meetings in the palliative care setting

1. The nature of the illness and its symptoms.
2. Prognosis and future predictions about the course of the illness.
3. Caregiving roles about symptom management, medications, and nursing care.
4. Liaison with the healthcare team.
5. Emotional demands of the caregiving role.
6. Importance of self-care and respite from caregiving.
7. What to expect as death approaches.
8. How to talk with the patient about death and dying.
9. The process of saying goodbye.
10. How to manage a death in the home.
11. Positive aspects of the caregiver role.
12. Teamwork and sharing the role of caregiver.
13. When to seek help and how.
14. Support from volunteers and other community resources.

Communication principles in conducting a family meeting

Facilitators of a family meeting do well to join initially with each person present through a round of introductions that identify names, ages (if appropriate), occupations, place of residence, and relationship to the ill person. Agendas and expectations of meeting together are also shared, so that all concerns are placed on the table at the beginning of the conversation. The unifying or common focus of the meeting is: 'What is best for the patient?' Linear questions tend to be used here as an exchange occurs between the facilitators and individuals speaking about their personal point of view. Facilitators wisely avoid taking sides with individuals expressing contentious issues, lest loss of neutrality damages the ability to guide the family as a whole to their preferred solution (Del Gaudio et al. 2012).

The use of circular questions is a communication skill through which the facilitator preserves this neutrality and promotes the family's search for a solution from among its members (Dumont and Kissane 2009). Using such circularity, each member can be invited to express an opinion about the needs, functioning, health, or interaction styles of other members of the family unit. Thus, 'Who talks to whom about the patient's illness?', 'Who provides transport, food, or material support?', 'Who is most stressed?', 'How will the family cope?'

As facilitators embed a potential solution into the wording of a question, it becomes strategic in style as a communication skill. Thus, 'Is it possible that sharing feelings together will help you grow closer?' Strategic questions can also harness a direction of change: 'What might help motivate your son to visit more often?'

Other questions might raise a hypothesis, inviting the family to reflect on a range of possible choices they could adopt, with such reflexive questions serving a catalytic function for the family. There is generally a better outcome for the family as a group when more problem solving is done by the family, rather than the clinician (see Box 18.2).

A useful communication skill to promote movement towards consensus, or at least accommodation of differing views among the family, is for facilitators to offer a summary that reflects the tension between two or more points of view aired by members (Dumont and Kissane 2009). The goal is not to necessarily offer a solution, but to make explicit the advantages and disadvantages of the options, while leaving the choice as the family's. Further problem solving with consensus-building or accommodation is then evoked from the family. In circumstances involving future treatment recommendations or avoidance of futile care, the clinician may wish to make a firm recommendation. Delaying delivery of this recommendation for a time, while searching for their point of view, may allow the family to reach that position readily and with greater acceptance than were the outcome imposed. Partnership statements that acknowledge shared deliberation also prove supportive.

The family meeting often falls into two distinct parts: a physician-led part and a psychosocial-led part. The physician-led part or first phase of the meeting discusses the medical illness, including the course of the disease, medical management along the way, and future treatment options. These can include inpatient palliative care, community-based hospice care, and site of care. The goal of this phase of the meeting is to educate, clarify, and plan for the patient's future care. Then the psychosocial-led part focuses on

---

> **Box 18.2** Communication skills used in family meeting facilitation
>
> ◆ **Circular questions.** Ask each family member to comment in turn on aspects of others to promote curiosity and reflection by the group as a whole. For example, *'How are your parents and sisters coping with Dad's illness? Who is most upset in your view?'* (Dumont and Kissane 2009).
>
> ◆ **Reflexive questions.** Invite the family to reflect on possibilities, hypotheses, and a range of outcomes to stimulate their internal efforts to improve family life. For example, *'What benefits might come from caring for Dad at home? In what ways might this be hard for you as a family group?'* (Dumont and Kissane 2009).
>
> ◆ **Strategic questions.** Here a solution might be incorporated into the wording of the question to more directly guide the family towards an outcome that is considered preferable. For example, *'What change in Dad's symptoms would need to occur for you to realize that admission to an inpatient hospice bed is necessary?'* (Dumont and Kissane 2009).
>
> ◆ **Summary of family focused concerns.** The family's views are reflected back to highlight levels of tension or discordance in different member's opinions, while maintaining professional neutrality, yet inviting further problem solving by the family. For example, *'As a family, you recognize your father's desire to die at home, your mother's commitment to meet his wishes, and yet your concern that his confusion is becoming unmanageable and a burden to your mother. There is no easy answer here, as whichever solution you adopt will appear to demand more of each of you for a time'* (Del Gaudio et al. 2012).
>
> Source: data from Dumont I and Kissane D, 'Techniques for framing questions in conducting family meetings in palliative care,' *Palliative and Supportive Care*, Volume 7, Issue 2, pp. 163–170, Copyright © Cambridge University Press 2009.

coping issues and the emotional response to the illness, including its impact on the patient and the life of each family member. Families often express their feelings through narrative—stories of life before the diagnosis, and through the lived experience of cancer.

During the process of this two-phase meeting, the family participants have the opportunity to learn exactly what is happening to their loved one and why. They may also come to understand in a different way the complexities and uncertainties of medical care. The healthcare team may deepen their understanding of who this patient and family are, their strengths and their vulnerabilities, and what the experience of cancer has been like for them. The importance of the family is acknowledged, the present situation and goals of care are clarified, problem solving and counselling occur, and role modelling takes place, demonstrating teamwork, mutual respect, and open and honest communication.

The family meeting offers an opportunity to introduce the family to members of the interdisciplinary team who will be helping to organize the patient's care. The family is brought into partnership in planning such care. They have the chance to express their fears and concerns, and be offered support. Radwany and colleagues (2009) identified that where relatives lack insight into the seriousness of the patient's illness, they may feel unready to make important decisions, wanting more time to consider these. Conversation while making arrangements for the meeting to occur can ensure that the prognosis is understood, helping the family prepare for the gravity of the themes to be discussed (Sullivan *et al.* 2015).

One objective is to harness the family's energy into joint meaningful action. Additionally, the team starts to get to know the patient and family as individuals and a social group. They learn what the family values, their styles of communication and decision-making, which members carry significant levels of distress, and how the family can best benefit from the team. Problems that have remained unaddressed and festering can be brought to the surface with good potential for resolution.

Key process tasks in conducting family meetings

Process tasks are both plans and actions that are fundamental to achieve the communication goals of the family meeting. Several are important and considered here:

♦ **Set up of the meeting.** This involves identifying the important family members or significant individuals in the patient's life who need to be present (Sullivan *et al.* 2015).

- Who are the influential relatives and significant others who may bring wisdom and value to the session?

- Will the patient contribute usefully to the meeting and be important to include?

- Will there be any barriers to meeting?

- Which clinical staff will be needed to address relevant medical, nursing, psychosocial, and spiritual issues?

♦ **Co-facilitation.** Here it is important to clarify whether there are key medical agendas that differentiate from psychosocial needs (Gueguen *et al.* 2009). Should these be separated as distinct agendas for different phases of the meeting? Co-facilitators need to talk about their respective roles and the order of approach before the meeting starts. Medical issues place a greater emphasis on education, planning, and clarifying; psychosocial issues require more focus on listening, empathic skills, and fostering a sense of support. The tenor of each meeting phase can be distinctly different and hence the wisdom, as reviewed earlier, of structuring the session to complete one domain before moving to an exploration of the other.

♦ **Cultural sensitivity while avoiding collusion.** Ethnicity and family background impact directly on a family's approach to coping with illness. Clarification of the family's detailed understanding of the illness and its treatment, its progression and seriousness, their values and religious beliefs, and the appropriate goals of care for this stage of illness is necessary. In addition, points of consensus and dissonance need to be identified.

♦ **Understanding the family's strengths and vulnerabilities.** Family traditions, norms, and values can be harnessed adaptively when they are recognized as strengths and balanced with the family's worries and concerns. Achieving understanding of the reality of their family life is vital to any pragmatic planning for their future.

♦ **Familiarity with resources that are available to the patient and family.** These include educational materials, DVD, or website

resources, other information sources, community nursing, and related support services.

♦ **Follow-up.** Explain details of where to go from here, what the next steps are, and who will coordinate these with the patient and family. Is there an identified family member through whom ongoing communication can be channelled?

Typical sequence of strategies in conducting a family meeting in oncology

The concept of a 'sequence of strategies' involves the *a priori* plans of an ordered method that experience teaches will generally facilitate the communication goals of the meeting (Bylund *et al.* 2011). The sequence need not be rigidly applied, but can be adapted to the family's needs (see Box 18.3). Nevertheless, there is considerable logic to this sequence, as the patient's medical reality directly impacts upon the emotional consequences that follow.

After welcoming the family, an agenda is created by stating the goals of meeting together:

♦ to review where the patient is in his/her illness trajectory;

♦ to consider the family's needs in providing care; and

♦ to aim at optimizing the journey ahead.

The facilitators check for any other agenda the family might have, clarify the family's understanding of the gravity of the illness, and explore their understanding of the current goals of care. Questions are then asked about any key symptoms that are of concern to the family and that need to be addressed. The family's views of what the future holds are clarified including, if appropriate, advance directives and whether the preferred place of death has been discussed. If the preference is for care to occur at home, who from the family will be the primary carer? If the preference is for care in an inpatient setting, will somebody sleep over with the patient? Once goals of care and methods for achieving these have been considered, the

---

Box 18.3 Typical sequence of strategies for the conduct of a family meeting in oncology and palliative care

1. Prior planning and set up to arrange the family meeting.

2. Welcome and orientation of the family to the goals of meeting; clarifying the family's agenda.

3. Check each family member's understanding of the illness and its prognosis.

4. Check for consensus about the current goals of care.

5. Identify family concerns about the management of key symptoms and care needs.

6. Clarify the family's view of what the future holds.

7. Clarify how family members are coping and feeling emotionally.

8. Identify family strengths and affirm their level of commitment and mutual support for each other.

9. Close the family meeting by final review of agreed goals of care and consensus about future care plans.

facilitators clarify how the family is doing emotionally. Are there any questions that have been left unanswered? Finally, the facilitators affirm the family's caring commitment to the patient and to each other, while also affirming the team's commitment to support them.

A blueprint summarizing the core communication components employed in conducting a family meeting are outlined in Table 18.1 (Gueguen *et al.* 2009). The communication skills listed in this schema have been defined in detail in Chapter 3 of this book

(Bylund *et al.* 2010). Skills that are listed against each strategy are not intended to be used exhaustively, but selected as appropriate for the family at hand. The combination of skills and process tasks outlined here help in the accomplishment of each communication strategy (Kissane *et al.* 2012). The family meeting follows the agreed agenda, until the themes are worked through and the communication goal is completed. A final step is documentation in the patient's chart of what happened.

Table 18.1 Core communication components in conducting a family meeting

Strategy	Skills	Process tasks
1. Prior planning and set up to arrange the family meeting	Clarify Invite questions Restate	Consider who should attend and extend invitations; explain rationale and benefits; acknowledge challenges in attending Will the patient be included? Who will facilitate? What disciplines will help? Co-facilitators? Plan seating, privacy, availability of tissues
2. Welcome and orient to the goals of the family meeting	Declare agenda items Invite family agenda Negotiate agenda Ask open questions Clarify Restate	Round of introductions and orientation Include all present at the meeting Identify who is missing Normalize anxiety
3. Check each family member's understanding of the illness and its prognosis	Ask open questions Ask circular questions Check understanding Acknowledge/legitimize	Clarify name of the illness Clarify seriousness of the illness Clarify reasons for admission Clarify each person's concerns Normalize both concordance and divergence of views among family members Respect culturally sensitive views Acknowledge protective urges and any expressed desire to help
4. Check for consensus regarding the current goals of care	Ask open and circular questions Clarify Restate Summarize	Compare and contrast oncological, nursing, social, psychological, and spiritual goals of care Reality test sensitively where needed Correct misunderstanding
5. Identify family concerns about their management of key symptoms or care needs	Ask open questions Preview information Check understanding Clarify Summarize Make partnership statements	Consider medication or treatment concerns? Any hygiene issues? Any concerns about walking, moving, transferring? Any concerns about nursing? Any concerns about assessing palliative care resources—extra help? Financial issues? Any need for respite? Any concern about a sense of helplessness? Promote problem solving Educate as appropriate
6. Clarify the family's view of what the future holds	Ask circular questions Clarify Restate Summarize Make partnership statements	Are there advanced care directives? Health proxy appointed? Has the place of death been discussed? Consider cultural or religious concerns. If at home, who from the family will be providing care? If in the hospital, who will accompany? Help? Support? Educate as appropriate

(continued)

Table 18.1 (continued)

Strategy	Skills	Process tasks
7. Clarify how family members are coping and feeling emotionally	Ask circular questions Ask strategic or reflexive questions Acknowledge, legitimize, or normalize	Review family functioning as a group, asking specifically about their communication, cohesion, and conflict resolution Identify any member considered to be 'at risk' or a concern to others Discuss future care needs of family or individual when concerns exist Avoid premature reassurance
8. Identify family strengths and affirm their level of commitment and mutual support for each other	Ask circular questions Ask strategic and reflexive questions Praise family efforts Acknowledge, legitimize	Review family traditions, spirituality, mottos, and cultural norms
9. Close the family meeting by final review of agreed goals of care and future plans	Summarize Invite questions Acknowledge Make partnership statements Express willingness to help Review steps	Provide educational resources Clarify future needs, funeral plans Refer those 'at risk' to psychosocial services for further care Consider feedback to the patient if they were not present

Reproduced from Jennifer A. Gueguen et al, 'Conducting family meetings in palliative care: Themes, techniques, and preliminary evaluation of a communication skills module,' *Palliative and Supportive Care*, Volume 7, Issue 2, pp. 171–179, Copyright © Cambridge University Press 2009, by permission of Cambridge University Press.

Documentation of the family meeting

Documentation is a necessary part of communication among care providers in any institution. The note is comprised of the following:

◆ Who was present at the meeting, including the various disciplines of the healthcare providers and the relationship of the family members present to the patient;

◆ Whether the patient was present and, if not, what was the reason;

◆ A brief medical and social history;

◆ A genogram that sketches out the genders, ages, names, and relationships within the family;

◆ A process summary of the meeting with the various issues outlined and options discussed;

◆ The outcome of the meeting, including agreed goals of care;

◆ The follow-up plan; and

◆ Whether the outcome of the meeting was shared with the patient if s/he was not able to be present.

Conclusion

Family meetings play an important role in comprehensive cancer care, especially in the setting of advanced disease and when palliative care is the primary focus. The importance of family is acknowledged and an environment of support is created therein. Information exchange often includes 'hard news'. The family's dynamics are assessed and the family is 'engaged' in the partnership of care provision. Both the goals of care and the next steps in management are suitably discussed. In addition, specific problems are defined, steps to resolve these are outlined, commitment is demonstrated, role modelling is illustrated about how to build consensus, and family problem-solving skills are promoted.

A resiliency focus guides the identification of family strengths alongside any concerns, empowering the members to work together to optimize their mutual support. Any distress created by the cancer experience is thus ameliorated, with the prospect of family harmony creating a peaceful environment for the ill family member. A model of shared family care and partnership with the medical team is promoted.

Clinical scenarios for simulated family meetings

In running a family role play, actors can be engaged and trained to play the characters making up the family, or participants in the training can be asked to take these roles. A more detailed scenario needs to be constructed (compared to individual role play encounters) because the family members need to interact in a consistent manner, and yet display sufficient differences at times to create interesting dynamics to work with. It becomes obvious that actors playing simulated patients in a family meeting need to be trained up to a much higher degree to interact with apparent spontaneity, to ensure that engaging family dynamics are experienced by those facilitating the meeting. At appropriate times, these actors need to be able to increase emotionality, express assertively their differences of opinion, and yet moderate these reactions when they feel contained and supported by the facilitators of the family meeting.

Family meeting in the setting of progressive disease with advanced colon cancer

Here the material can be divided up into an introductory sheet about the family that can be shared with all participants, and individual sheets for each family member, which are not seen by everybody, but used to guide each family member to play a unique role in the encounter. Each instruction sheet has some background information about the simulated person and a list of concerns or potential questions and comments that they will bring into the family meeting to represent their character. In this manner, the material guiding the role play is similar to a screenplay written for the performance of a play on stage.

Introduction to the family

Maria is a 65-year old, married Italian woman with two children, Flaviana (45 years) and Mario (43 years), each of whom has two children of their own. Maria's husband, Giuseppe, 70 years, has retired from his legal practice, is in good health, and maintains a small vineyard as his hobby. While Flaviana followed her father into the law, Mario became a physician, working as a rheumatologist. Mario always speaks to the oncologist about his mother's treatment, follows test results, and seeks to reassure his mother that she is getting the best cancer care.

The patient's disease

Maria has an advanced colon cancer, metastatic to liver and lung. She had a left-sided hemicolectomy performed four years before and pathology showed stage II disease, with a high grade cancer invading the muscle layer of the colon (T2), but 0/12 lymph nodes involved (N0, M0), not necessitating adjuvant chemotherapy. She was followed by her surgeon and thought to be disease free until two years ago, when right-sided discomfort led to a computed tomography (CT) scan, which revealed multiple liver metastases. A positron emission tomography (PET) scan confirmed multiple, dispersed liver metastases, not suitable for liver resection, and small bilateral lung nodules. She was treated initially with first line chemotherapy of FOLFOX4 (oxaliplatin, leucovorin, and 5-FU) plus bevacizumab, with disease containment for 12 months and reasonable quality of life. When progression was evident on imaging and rising carcinoembryonic antigen (CEA) levels, second-line chemotherapy was selected, with irinotecan and cetuximab (monoclonal antibody against the eGFR). This time there was six months of disease containment, before nausea, fatigue, and anorexia emerged as symptoms, and imaging again showed disease progression. Liver lesions are now quite large, liver enzymes are rising, and her clinicians feel that her symptoms are related to emergent liver failure. It has become time to review the goals of care.

The predicament

The oncologist spoke to Mario, who asked about continued treatment with capecitabine, and requested the oncologist not to tell his mother they thought she was dying. He feared that this would take away all her hope. In his opinion, continued chemotherapy would always remain important. The oncologist had the idea that Maria was not going to accept further chemotherapy, as she had hinted that she felt she had gone through enough. Rather than debate this situation with Maria's son, he thought he would call a family meeting to explore what was best to do.

The oncologist asked a member of the psychosocial team (social worker, psychologist, or psychiatrist—whoever is available) to join him for this family session as a way to introduce more support into the family.

Family meeting

The following people are about to attend this family meeting:

1. Maria, 65, patient with advanced colon cancer
2. Giuseppe, 70, husband, retired lawyer
3. Flaviana, 45, daughter and lawyer
4. Mario, 43, rheumatologist physician
5. Cancer doctor (can be oncologist, palliative care physician, primary care physician)
6. Psycho-oncologist (can be social worker, psychologist, psychiatrist, family therapist)

Particular instructions to the patient: Maria

You grew up in a comfortably off, middle-class family with two younger sisters, and you were a smart student, completing high school, and learning to play the violin quite superbly. Initially, you had planned to go to university, but you met Giuseppe, fell in love, and decided to marry him instead. The years have been very kind to you. It was an easy choice to stay home and care for your children. Your mother also looked for help caring for her father, who was dying from a bowel cancer. She needed quite a lot of support and it was an era when the word 'cancer' was not spoken.

You also cared for your own mother just over a decade ago, when she was treated for a rectal cancer. It was a distressing experience for the women of the family, for although your mother knew about the cancer, everyone remained very optimistic to protect your mother from worry. You thought it difficult, sensed your mother was courageous and could have easily talked about the situation, but the family maintained their tradition until the very end.

Maria's concerns for this role play:

1. You've always known that your family avoids talking about the cancer in front of you, but you can see their worry in their faces. You don't want to cause them distress. Giuseppe gets so sad. You want to find a way to let them all know that you are OK with whatever God wants for you.

2. You also worry that Mario thinks he can keep you alive forever. Modern medicine! You don't want him to be burdened by your illness, yet it is a help having a clever son who looks after you so well. You don't want him to blame himself for whatever happens.

3. You believe you understand life, the world, and the realities of our universe quite well. Through the years you've become quite wise. When you go to Mass, you feel more spiritual, and you wish the others in your family were better Catholics. Flaviana goes to church sometimes, but the grandchildren rarely do. You've wondered whether your illness will help the family to grow a bit closer to God.

4. Recently, with your appetite disappearing, and that sick feeling coming and going in your stomach, you've felt wearier. Your life has been blessed. But you don't feel afraid now. You wonder if the time is coming to stop this chemotherapy. You plan to ask your doctor about this when the time seems right. However, you don't want to upset Mario and Giuseppe. You wonder how can you get them to understand that you will be OK?

5. If asked about your family, you recall your mother's and grandfather's death from bowel cancers. You remember your mother becoming so weak and in so much pain. It seemed as if everyone was keeping her alive, instead of letting nature or God decide what is best. You hope they'll understand your perspective so that your death is not like your mother's. Given the chance, you'll tell them how much your mother suffered.

Particular instructions to the husband: Giuseppe

As a lawyer, you have seen your fair share of divorces and estate fights in families. You think it's becoming less common for families to stay together the way yours has. You feel blessed. Maria's faith has been a strength as she brought fine values to give to your children and grandchildren. You are less religious than she; after all the church is very wealthy, but you still believe in God.

Your son tells you that Maria's cancer is getting steadily worse. He wants her to have further chemotherapy. You sense that Mario is working hard to help his mother. He researches all the treatment options and wants to make sure that the doctors don't give up on Maria. Yet you know that Maria always makes up her own mind in the end.

Giuseppe's concerns for this role play:

1. You know that your son wants to make sure that Maria gets the best treatment. You also know that your wife likes to make her own choices. And she talks about God's will. You don't want any disagreements about what to do. You hope that Maria will follow the old traditions and just let the family decide what is best for her. You are not sure that meeting as a family is the right thing, but Maria seemed to want it when her oncologist suggested that you all meet.

2. You want Flaviana to take some more time off work to help care for her mother. There are other lawyers that can keep the office going. You will look for opportunities to encourage your daughter to spend more time at home helping you care for Maria.

3. You expect to be your wife's healthcare proxy. You have been married for 47 years and, as the family lawyer, you know what is wise and needs to be done.

4. You'll let your son try to do his best in guiding Maria's care, but if it is not what she wants, you know you'll have to step in and support your wife.

Particular instructions to the daughter: Flaviana

You work in family law and have helped many women through divorce, which has taught you much about the complexity of life. You have a fine husband, Sergio, 49 years, a banker, who has been an excellent provider. And you have two wonderful daughters, Anna (17 years), and Silvia (15 years). They are talented students, good musicians like your mother and very bright, enthusiastic, and good-looking. You enjoy your legal practice and are so glad that you chose a career.

Your mother has been sick this past year after her bowel cancer returned. You're lucky that your brother is a doctor and takes care of her. This takes some pressure off you. Italian families expect daughters to provide all the care. They don't understand the demands of a professional career on a woman's world.

Flaviana's concerns in this role play:

1. What is happening to your mother? What have the tests shown? Is your brother's suggested treatment with capecitabine the right thing to do to keep the cancer under control?

2. What will happen in the future? Should your mother be drawing up an advanced directive so that her wishes are known to all who care for her? You think to yourself that if the chance pops up in this family meeting, you'll suggest these things to your mother today.

3. Why is your brother so concerned about protecting mum? Does he seriously think that we can protect her from understanding the reality of her illness? Doesn't he see how brave she is? How much faith she has?

4. What can be done to help your father? He's been spoiled by mum for so many years that he'll be lost without her. Will he invite his sister or mum's sisters to come and stay? They would provide him with more help and lots of company.

Particular instructions to the son: Mario

You are a 43-year old rheumatologist, married to a dermatologist named Alessandra. She is 40 and together you have a son, Sam (14 years), and a daughter, Marieta (10 years), a small version of your mother. Medicine has been easy and good to you. You care for a lot of elderly people and know how to keep their spirits up and their pain well-controlled.

Unfortunately, your mother took ill again about a year ago, getting a recurrence of her colon cancer. She had been stage II, with a good prognosis. Adjuvant chemotherapy didn't seem indicated, as its benefit in reducing recurrence was only 2%. You had checked the National Cancer Institute (NCI) website in the United States and followed their treatment guidelines. You hoped your mother didn't blame you for not pushing for adjuvant chemotherapy.

Over the past year, her oncologist had seemed on top of it all, recommending the very latest in treatments. Alas, it appears to be an aggressive tumour. The NCI website lists capecitabine as another active chemotherapy that your mother hasn't had yet. Surely this will be the next regimen.

You reminded the oncologist that you don't want your mother to have hope taken away by telling her bad results. Your patients never seem to want to know very much about their tests. You wish this doctor had a similar style. His suggestion to set up a family meeting is a bit worrying. Why not just follow on to the next chemotherapy?

Mario's concerns in this role play:

1. To talk about the chronic disease model as appropriate for patients getting chemotherapy. With excellent symptom control and good pain management, the patient's quality of life will be preserved.

2. To ensure that hope is not taken away from your mother. She doesn't deserve to be told upsetting news.

3. To keep the family on the bright side, support your father, and encourage your sister to give more time to your mother. You realize that you may need to be assertive in the very beginning, putting the good news out about the progress in cancer treatments, and telling the family that the latest approach to chemotherapy has got easier with tablets, which your mother can now take— capecitabine tablets (pronounced 'cape-cita-been'). You reassure the oncologist that your family is strong. Your sister will work less and help your mother and father much more. You are always available.

4. Because you do love your mother and father, if they move in a different direction to these thoughts of yours, express surprise but be very respectful in following whatever wishes emerge. In this manner, allow family consensus to be achieved, rather than become conflictual.

References

Boss P, Dahl C (2014). Family therapy for ambiguous loss. In: Kissane DW, Parnes F (eds). *Bereavement Care for Families*. Routledge, New York, NY.

Bylund C, Brown R, Bialer P, et al. (2011). Developing and implementing an advanced communication training program at a comprehensive cancer center. *J Cancer Educ* **26**, 604–11.

Bylund C, Brown R, Gueguen J, et al. (2010). The implementation and assessment of a comprehensive communication skills training curriculum for oncologists. *Psychooncology* **19**, 583–93.

Del Gaudio F, Zaider T, Brier M, et al. (2012). Challenges in providing family-centred support to families in palliative care. *Palliat Med* **26**, 1025–33.

Dumont I, Kissane D (2009). Techniques for framing questions in conducting family meetings in palliative care. *Palliat Support Care* **7**, 163–70.

Gueguen J, Bylund C, Brown R, et al. (2009). Conducting family meetings in palliative care: Themes, techniques and preliminary evaluation of a communication skills module *Palliat Support Care* **7**, 171–9.

Hannon B, O' Reilly V, Bennett K, et al. (2012). Meeting the family: measuring effectiveness of family meetings in a specialist inpatient palliative care unit. *Palliat Support Care* **10**, 43–9.

Henry C, Sheffield MA, Harrist A (2015). Family resilience: moving into the third wave. *Family Relations* **64**, 22–43.

Higginson I, Finlay I, Goodwin D (2003). Is there evidence that palliative care teams alter end-of-life experiences of patients and their caregivers? *J Pain Symptom Manage* **25**, 150–68.

Hudson P, Quinn K, O' Hanlon B, et al. (2008). Family meetings in palliative care: multidisciplinary clinical practice guidelines. *BMC Palliat Care* **7**, 1–12.

Kissane D, Bloch S (2002). *Family Focused Grief Therapy: a Model of Family-Centred Care During Palliative Care and Bereavement*. Open University Press, Buckingham, UK.

Kissane D, Bloch S, Dowe D, et al. (1996). The Melbourne family grief study, 1: perceptions of family functioning in bereavement. *Am J Psychiatry* **153**, 650–8.

Kissane D, Bylund C, Banerjee S, et al. (2012). Communication skills training for oncology professionals. *J Clin Oncol* **30**, 1242–7.

Kissane D, McKenzie M, Bloch S (2006). Family focused grief therapy: a randomized controlled trial in palliative care and bereavement. *Am J Psychiatry* **163**, 1208–18.

Kissane D, Parnes F (2014). *Bereavement Care for Families*. Routledge, New York, NY.

Kissane D, Zaider T, Li Y, et al. (2016). Randomized controlled trial of family therapy in advanced cancer continued into bereavement. *J Clin Oncol* **34**, 1921–7.

Lubrano Di Ciccone B, Brown R, Gueguen J, et al. (2010). Interviewing patients using interpreters in an oncology setting: initial evaluation of a communication skills module. *Ann Oncol* **21**, 27–32.

MacPhee D, Lunkenheimer E, Riggs N (2015). Resilience as regulation of developmental and family processes. *Family Relations* **64**, 153–75.

Muriel A (2014). Care of families with children anticipating the death of a parent. In: Kissane DW, Parnes F (eds). *Bereavement Care for Families*. Routledge, New York, NY.

Schuler T, Zaider T, Li Y, et al. (2014). Typology of perceived family functioning in an American sample of patients with advanced cancer. *J Pain Symptom Manage* **48**, 281–8.

Sullivan S, Ferreira Da Rosa S, Meeker M (2015). Family meetings at end of life. A systematic review. *J Hosp Palliat Nurs* **17**, 196–205.

Ventura A, Burney S, Brooker J, et al. (2014). Home-based palliative care: A systematic literature review of the self-reported unmet needs of patients and carers. *Palliat Med* **28**, 391–402.

Walsh F (2014). Conceptual framework for family bereavement care: strengthening resilience. In: Kissane DW, Parnes F (eds). *Bereavement Care for Families*. Routledge, New York, NY.

Zaider T, Kissane D (2009). The assessment and management of family distress during palliative care. *Curr Opin Support Palliat Care*, **3**, 67–71.

CHAPTER 19

Communication about coping as a survivor

Linda E. Carlson, Janine Giese-Davis, and Barry D. Bultz

Introduction to communication about coping as a survivor

As medical cancer treatments become more successful, a growing cohort of cancer survivors is emerging. Maintaining communication with survivors poses new challenges to care providers as models of care shift towards greater survivor self-management and primary care providers (PCPs) increasingly take on follow-up maintenance. Development and implementation of communication strategies is crucial due to staggering numbers of survivors (over 14.5 million in 2014 in the United States). This chapter covers areas relevant to enhancing communication with survivors including: definitions of who is considered a cancer survivor; prevalence of survivors; key issues faced by cancer survivors; coping strategies, including the use of care plans and clinical practice guidelines; communication challenges with cancer survivors; models for survivorship care; and details about communication techniques in the survivorship consultation. Because the number of survivors is increasing, these communication strategies will be necessary for ongoing care for cancer survivors who will live with the biopsychosocial sequelae of cancer treatments, may experience recurrence or progression and consequent retreatment, and require continuity of care for many years to come.

Definition of survivorship

Though the term 'survivor' is commonly used, it has triggered debates and disagreements about who is included and when a cancer patient becomes a cancer survivor. The survivorship movement began in the United States in 1986 with the National Coalition for Cancer Survivorship (NCCS) (a grassroots organization of people living with cancer) adopting a broad definition of 'survivor'—anyone who has been diagnosed with cancer is a survivor—from the time of diagnosis and for the balance of life. Caregivers and family members are also cancer survivors.

The medical community typically defined 'survivor' as someone who had lived for at least five years; however, as people live longer with cancer it is now much clearer that for some cancers, living five years does not mean the cancer will not return. Clinical systems needing to segment care often define it as someone who has completed active treatment (surgery, chemotherapy, and radiation). Because the definition varies across professionals and agencies, clear communication about the definition of 'survivor' is important.

In this chapter, we have adopted the broader NCCS definition because for many people a cycle of diagnosis, treatment, remission, followed by a second diagnosis, retreatment, and remission

is becoming the norm. For many survivors, this definition of survivorship and a reconceptualization of the cancer continuum as circular resonates with their clinical experience (Rowland and Bellizzi 2008). This conceptualization sees the cancer care trajectory as moving through a variety of stages; from the time of diagnosis to treatment with either palliative or curative intent. After completion of curative treatment, people enter the realm of survivorship care, thought of as occurring at the juncture between the completion of active treatment and any return of disease. Survivorship care can follow any number of trajectories, interacting with other stages of care throughout the cancer journey. Regardless of the recurrence of cancer, survivorship care may last the duration of one's life and caregivers and family members also share in the survivorship journey.

Prevalence of cancer survivors

Because advances in effective biomedical screening for cancer and improvements in treatment have increasingly extended years of survival for most tumour groups, survivorship is an increasingly important aspect of patients' experience. The prevalence of American cancer survivors (those diagnosed and currently alive) has risen from 3 million in 1971 to nearly 14.5 million in 2014 (not including basal cell and squamous cell skin cancers). By 2024, this population of cancer survivors will increase to almost 19 million: 9.3 million males and 9.6 million females. The three most common cancers among male survivors are prostate (43%), colon and rectum (9%), and melanoma (8%) (American Cancer Society 2014). Among female survivors, the most common cancers are breast (41%), uterine (8%), and colon and rectum (8%). The majority of cancer survivors (64%) were diagnosed five or more years ago, and 15% were diagnosed 20 or more years ago. Almost half (46%) of cancer survivors are 70 years of age or older, while only 5% are younger than 40 years (American Cancer Society 2014). The most notable difference between incidence and survivorship figures is in lung cancers, which account for greater than 15% of the incidence of overall cancer but only 3% of survivors. This inconsistency is a testament to the poor prognosis for lung cancer cases, though early screening measures and advances in earlier and more effective treatments may change those statistics going forward.

While only 5% of all cancer survivors are under the age of 40 years, potential years of life lost (PYLL) better estimates the impact on these younger cancer survivors. For instance, in 2002, the incidence of cancer in young adults (age 15–39) was only 10% of the older age groups, but the PYLL was 28.3% of the total PYLL of all cancers (Canadian Cancer Society's Advisory Committee on

Cancer Statistics 2002). Over one-quarter of all years of life lost was in this younger group. This demographic must be borne in mind when considering all aspects of survivorship care.

With the formation of the Office of Cancer Survivorship (OCS) in the USA in 1996, survivorship research has increased over the past 20 years. Due to a high level of grassroots lobbying in the United States, survivorship activists have demanded better care, influenced treatment and service availability, and influenced politics. This politicization of cancer resulted in the creation of a number of comprehensive reports in the early 2000s, summarizing research and serving as excellent references for obtaining an overview of the state of the science in survivorship research and care. These included the President's Cancer Panel (2005) and an Institute of Medicine (2003) report on children's cancers.

One government report catalysed an international surge in research and practice change towards better survivorship care: *Improving Care and Quality of Life. From Cancer Patient to Cancer Survivor: Lost in Transition* (Committee on Cancer Survivorship 2006). It provided recommendations for care following primary treatment that could last until cancer recurrence or the end of life. Many of the detailed recommendations have become actionable since 2010, and motivated groups have begun to establish guidelines for survivorship care (Cancer Journey Survivorship Expert Panel *et al.* 2011; Cowens-Alvarado *et al.* 2013; Skolarus *et al.* 2014; Nekhlyudov *et al.* 2014). The American College of Surgeon's Commission on Cancer has mandated one of the key recommendations of the Institute of Medicine (IOM) report—delivering survivor care plans—and they propose using the IOM-recommended elements as standards of care (Cancer Program Standards 2012).

Key issues for survivors

The survivorship experience may touch individuals at every level, from the existential to the practical, patients as well as families and friends. Survivors of different types and stages of cancer report varied survivorship issues. These issues depend on the invasiveness of treatments that require specific follow-up and supportive-care regimens.

Though treatments are often difficult and disfiguring, many resilient survivors return to good health-related quality of life (Rowland and Bellizzi 2008). However, lingering biopsychosocial effects may compromise survivors' functional quality of life (Railton *et al.* 2015). Researchers distinguish between 'late effects' and 'long-term effects' of cancer treatment. Late effects are unrecognized toxicities that are absent or subclinical at the end of therapy, but manifest during later developmental processes, or due to the failure of compensatory mechanisms over time, or organ senescence. Long-term effects refer to side effects or complications of treatment for which patients must compensate that usually begin during treatment and continue beyond the end of treatment. Late effects, in contrast, appear months to years after the completion of treatment.

Long-term and late effects often include the following domains: physical and medical (e.g. early menopause, sexual impairment, infertility, secondary cancers, cardiac, lung, or liver dysfunction, osteoporosis, pain or lymphedema); psychological (e.g. depression, anxiety, uncertainty, isolation, fear of recurrence, altered body image, or cognitive impairments); social (e.g. changes in interpersonal relationships, concerns regarding health or life insurance, return to work, return to school, or financial burden); and existential and spiritual (e.g. sense of purpose or meaning, and appreciation of life). Cancer survivors often report as their top unmet needs: fears of cancer spread, feeling unsure the cancer has gone, fatigue, stress, and bad memory or lack of focus. In addition, psychosocial unmet needs are often higher in rural, minority, or aboriginal communities (Olson *et al.* 2014; Railton *et al.* 2015). Figure 19.1 illustrates the wide range of domains affected.

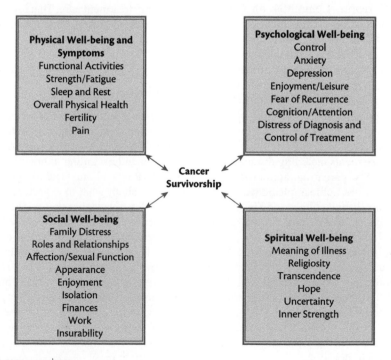

Fig. 19.1 Domains of quality of life in cancer survivors.
Adapted from City of Hope Beckman Research Institute, *Quality of Life Model*, Copyright © 2004 with permission from Betty Ferrell, Ph.D., M.A., F.A.A.N., F.P.C.N.

Cancer survivorship increases risk for secondary cancers; about 18% of all new cancer diagnoses are secondary cancers, three-quarters of them in different primary sites. Almost 60% of survivors—a number more than twice as high as in the general population—report one or more functional problems such as difficulties with self-care, completing household activities, or driving. Reasons for these and other late effects vary, but the common treatments for cancer often have long-term consequences. For example, surgical treatments often result in cosmetic side effects as well as pain related to scarring and wound healing. Treatments that affect the central nervous system including many forms of computed tomography (CT), cranial radiation therapy (RT), or brain and spinal cord surgery can result in impaired cognition, learning, memory, and motor function.

Treatment for cancers involving the gastrointestinal tract often result in the need for ostomies, which require a great deal of physical and psychosocial adjustment. Other treatments can result in urinary and sexual dysfunction, common after prostate cancer surgery. Another common side effect of lymph node resection is lymphedema, a painful swelling of the arms or legs that requires long-term management. These and many other late and long-term side effects are common and threaten to compromise the quality of life of many cancer survivors. Due to the psychological and medical late and long-term effects of cancer and its many treatments, it is important for survivors that access to care extends well beyond acute treatment, and that care is specific to the type of cancer, treatment regimen, and the patient's specific needs.

Coping strategies for survivors

Survivor care plans (SCPs) and clinical practice guidelines (CPGs)

Given the breadth of potential issues and persistent and late effects of cancer treatment as described above, a team of caregivers will likely provide best survivorship care, exacerbating the need to build mechanisms for communication among these providers and survivors. The IOM report, Committee on Cancer Survivorship: Improving Care and Quality of Life (2006), and later mandates by the American College of Surgeon's Commission on Cancer (Cancer Program Standards 2012) recommended that each patient and their PCP be given not only a treatment summary following discharge, but also an SCP moving forward that assures continuity of care. This summary should include a record of all care received and include a number of elements for a follow-up care plan (Stricker et al. 2011), described in Box 19.1. The SCP includes not only continued surveillance for late effects and potential cancer recurrence, but also psychosocial elements including discussion of relationship issues, sexuality, fertility, parenting, and social support, as well as legal and financial issues. Some implementations of SCPs also include distress screening, listing of upcoming follow-up appointments with dates and provider, lifestyle modification goals, and a plan to meet those goals (Hewitt and Ganz 2007).

Recommendations regarding implementation of health behaviours to enhance overall health and decrease the likelihood of contracting further cancers or chronic diseases are crucial aspects of any SCP (Hewitt and Ganz 2007). Important areas include weight management, nutrition and diet, exercise, smoking cessation, alcohol consumption, sunscreen use, complementary and alternative therapies, prevention of osteoporosis, and immunizations. Current lifestyle guidelines are summarized in Box 19.2.

While many CPGs exist for the treatment of different forms of cancer, tumour groups are now also working on consensus follow-up and surveillance guidelines for post-treatment care (Denlinger et al. 2014; National Comprehensive Cancer Network 2014; Skolarus et al. 2014), that can be provided outside cancer centres or by PCPs (Cowens-Alvarado et al. 2013; McCabe et al. 2013). Many of them echo the IOM report for survivorship and surveillance guidelines, which the IOM suggests cover the following domains:

1. Surveillance for recurrent disease
2. Monitoring/prevention of new primary and secondary cancers
3. Management of late sequelae of disease
4. Management of late complications of treatment
5. Management of psychological, social, and spiritual issues
6. Management of genetic issues
7. Management of sexuality and fertility issues
8. Locus of care

To this list, most survivorship guidelines now add exercise, nutrition, body mass index (BMI), and alcohol consumption; recent changes in National Comprehensive Cancer Network (NCCN) survivorship guidelines have added cognitive impairment and cancer pain (Kvale and Urba 2014).

Despite the need for comprehensive management of late and long-term effects and the existence of recommendations for care plans and healthy behaviours, very few comprehensive programmes of survivorship care yet exist beyond the eight Livestrong Survivorship Centers of Excellence (Shapiro et al. 2009). Even in those centres, uptake by clinicians of SCP implementation is inconsistent (Stricker et al. 2011; Forsythe et al. 2013). Additionally, culture change among clinicians in these innovative Livestrong Centers has taken time, primarily creating an awareness of the scope and need for cancer survivorship care, as opposed to traditional post-treatment care. There is some concern that the number of survivors is growing so rapidly that it will outpace our ability to provide this much-needed care.

Communication challenges in survivorship care

The previous section identified some barriers to the provision of survivorship care on the part of both patients and the care delivery system. Patient barriers often begin following their last treatment with little understanding of how to move forward to create a 'new normal' (Rowland and Bellizzi 2008), little direct information or education about what to expect, and little information about specific healthy behaviours that might improve their particular clinical course. They are often surprised by the level of distress they are experiencing at this time, and often have few resources available that provide adequate psychosocial care (Cancer Journey Survivorship Expert Panel et al. 2011) despite the efforts of national or international community-based organizations that have tried to reach out to them (e.g. Cancer Support Community, Wellspring, Gilda's Club). They often experience barriers returning to work, though some organizations have improved reintegration for employees of companies who pay to utilize these services (e.g. CAREpath™, Inc.).

Box 19.1 Survivorship care plan

Upon discharge from cancer treatment, including treatment of recurrences, every patient should be given a **record of all care received and important disease characteristics**. This should include, at a minimum:

1. Diagnostic tests performed and results.

2. Tumour characteristics (e.g. site(s), stage and grade, hormone receptor status, marker information).

3. Dates of treatment initiation and completion.

4. Surgery, chemotherapy, radiotherapy, transplant, hormonal therapy, or gene or other therapies provided, including agents used, treatment regimen, total dosage, identifying number and title of clinical trials (if any), indicators of treatment response, and toxicities experienced during treatment.

5. Psychosocial, nutritional, and other supportive services provided.

6. Full contact information on treating institutions and key individual providers.

7. Identification of a key point of contact and coordinator of continuing care. Upon discharge from cancer treatment, every patient and his/her primary healthcare provider should receive a written **follow-up care plan incorporating available evidence-based standards of care**. This should include, at a minimum:

   1. The likely course of recovery from treatment toxicities, as well as the need for ongoing health maintenance/adjuvant therapy.

   2. A description of recommended cancer screening and other periodic testing and examinations, and the schedule on which they should be performed (and who should provide them).

   3. Information on possible late and long-term effects of treatment and symptoms of such effects.

   4. Information on possible signs of recurrence and second tumours.

   5. Information on the possible effects of cancer on marital/partner relationship, sexual functioning, work, and parenting, and the potential future need for psychosocial support.

   6. Information on the potential insurance, employment, and financial consequences of cancer and, as necessary, referral to counselling, legal aid, and financial assistance.

   7. Specific recommendations for healthy behaviours (e.g. diet, exercise, healthy weight, sunscreen use, immunizations, smoking cessation, osteoporosis prevention). When appropriate, recommendations that first-degree relatives be informed about their increased risk and the need for cancer screening (e.g. breast cancer, colorectal cancer, prostate cancer).

   8. As appropriate, information on genetic counselling, and testing to identify high-risk individuals who could benefit from more comprehensive cancer surveillance, chemoprevention, or risk-reducing surgery.

   9. As appropriate, information on known effective chemoprevention strategies for secondary prevention (e.g. tamoxifen in women at high risk for breast cancer; aspirin for colorectal cancer prevention).

   10. Referrals to specific follow-up care providers (e.g. rehabilitation, fertility, psychology), support groups, and/or the patient's primary care provider.

   11. A listing of cancer-related resources and information (e.g. internet-based sources and telephone listings for major cancer support organizations).

Adapted from Suzanne H. Reuben, *Assessing Progress, Advancing Change 2005–2006 Annual Report*, President's Cancer Panel, National Cancer Institute, National Institutes of Health 2006.

Survivor barriers also include a lack of awareness of the late effects of cancer and its treatments (such as increased risk for osteoporosis or cardiovascular disease), resulting in less proactive care-seeking. In addition, only about half of men and women with cancer of childbearing age received timely information from their healthcare providers about their risk of infertility. Often options to preserve or restore fertility come too late to take any preventive measures. Similarly, breast cancer survivors often do not recall discussing the reproductive health impact of their treatment, and many report their concerns are not adequately addressed.

These examples highlight the importance of communication between care providers and patients regarding possible post-treatment survivorship issues. Survivors can also become confused about the aetiology of the symptoms they are experiencing, and their PCPs must learn to integrate care for the symptoms of other chronic diseases with the possible late effects of cancer treatment. Self-management programmes originally designed for other chronic illnesses, but recently adapted to cancer self-management may provide the needed understanding and coordinated symptom management (Risendal *et al.* 2014).

To add to these difficulties in communication, many patients may have literacy issues or not be comfortable conversing in specialized medical terminology, while others originate from different linguistic and cultural backgrounds. As such, communication barriers may arise that relate to sociocultural differences between survivors and their healthcare providers that may lead to higher

---

Box 19.2 Lifestyle guidelines for cancer survivors

Recommendations for cancer prevention (after treatment, cancer survivors should follow the recommendations for cancer prevention):

1. Be a healthy weight.

   Keep your weight as low as you can within the healthy range.

2. Move more.

   Be physically active for at least 30 minutes every day, and sit less.

3. Avoid high-calorie foods and sugary drinks.

   Limit high-calorie foods (particularly processed foods high in fat or added sugar, or low in fibre) and avoid sugary drinks.

4. Enjoy more grains, vegetables, fruit, and beans.

   Eat a wide variety of whole grains, vegetables, fruit, and pulses such as beans.

5. Limit red meat and avoid processed meat.

   Eat no more than 500 g (cooked weight) a week of red meat, such as beef, pork, and lamb. Eat little, if any, processed meat such as ham and bacon.

6. For cancer prevention, don't drink alcohol.

   For cancer prevention, it's best not to drink alcohol. If you do, limit alcoholic drinks to two for men and one for women a day.

7. Eat less salt and avoid mouldy grains and cereals.

   Limit your salt intake to less than 6 g (2.4 g sodium) a day by adding less salt and eating less food processed with salt.

   Avoid mouldy grains and cereals, as they may be contaminated by aflatoxins

8. For cancer prevention, don't rely on supplements.

   Eat a healthy diet rather than relying on supplements to protect against cancer

9. If you can, breastfeed your baby.

   If you can, breastfeed your baby for six months before adding other liquids and foods.

Adapted from *Food, Nutrition, Physical Activity, and the Prevention of Cancer: a Global Perspective*, World Cancer Research Fund/American Institute for Cancer Research, Copyright © 2007 World Cancer Research Fund International, with permission from the World Cancer Research Fund International.

---

first treatment; 26% reported not being given written information about what they should or shouldn't do following discharge; and 36% reported not being told about support or self-help groups.

In the United States, a poll of cancer survivors by the Lance Armstrong Foundation found nearly half felt their psychosocial needs were not being met by the healthcare system. Specifically, survivors expressed dissatisfaction with the provision of support for dealing with important issues such as depression, fear of recurrence, chronic pain, ongoing health challenges, infertility, sexual dysfunction, difficulty with relationships, and financial or job insecurity. Researchers are beginning to study the impact of communication interventions that engage survivors in monitoring their needs and symptoms, and coach them to communicate more effectively with their medical teams.

The fragmented care delivery system is another barrier which results in a loss of continuity of care (Forsythe *et al.* 2013; Cheung *et al.* 2013). With patients often seeing many different specialists (medical oncologist, surgeon, radiation oncologist, PCP) and potentially having care provided in more than one care setting, there are often multiple patient records in different non-compatible systems and no one provider has access to all medical information. This lack of continuity of care can result in sporadic follow-up care, and failure of any one care provider to take a leadership role in assuring proper survivorship care is provided can also prove detrimental. Hence, survivors can simply fall through the cracks as communication breaks down in transferring them from primary care, their 'medical home', to oncology and then back. Currently, the burden of responsibility is diffused through multiple practitioners who assume 'someone else' is taking care of the issues. Key strategies to improve the coordination of care include: providing educational supports; instituting patient-centred health records supported by modern information technology; ensuring accountability and defining roles for providers of care; and aligning financial incentives to ensure the delivery of coordinated care.

The model of the patient-centred medical home as the PCP's office may also be a key strategy moving forward. This is so that cancer survivors do not lose long-term relationships with their PCPs that may provide better integration and oversight. Much work is currently underway to evaluate models in which early-stage cancer survivors are transitioned back to PCP care (Railton *et al.* 2015) with adequate discharge letters to PCPs outlining survivorship follow-up guidelines. This movement follows randomized controlled trials demonstrating safety for early-stage breast cancer survivors with no differences in recurrence-related serious events and time to recurrence, better cost-effectiveness, and higher patient satisfaction and quality of life (Grunfeld *et al.* 2006).

Other issues complicating the delivery of coordinated survivorship care include lack of training of healthcare professionals across the full range of survivorship care needs; lack of communication between and among professionals, sites, as well as geographic locations and over long periods of time; lack of agreed-upon standards of follow-up care; and agreement about who is responsible for paying for such care. The Canadian Partnership Against Cancer, a government organization tasked to improve the lives of patients with cancer, has invested in a national team that will develop training modules for PCPs to facilitate communication with and knowledge of oncology, and develop a national strategy for SCPs. With the growing interest in survivorship care planning, there are clear guidelines for survivorship care; the issue now seems to be how to change behaviour and promote the uptake of these suggestions?

unmet survivorship needs (Olson *et al.* 2014). These may include differences in commonly held attitudes, norms, beliefs, expectations, and practices.

Other barriers to communication have been identified. At the most basic level, the expectations of survivors regarding follow-up care are quite disparate from what they typically receive. For example, a nationwide survey in England found 19% of survivors said doctors and nurses did not spend enough time, or none at all, telling them what to expect when they left the hospital after their

Models for survivorship care

Different models for survivorship care delivery include: (i) shared-care model of follow-up; (ii) nurse-led model; and (iii) survivorship follow-up clinics. Shared-care has been defined as care which applies when the responsibility for the healthcare of the patient is shared between individuals or teams who are part of separate organizations, or where substantial organizational boundaries exist. This is the model we have been discussing in the previous section, as it is the most commonly applied. In order for such a model to be successful, good communication between different providers, institutions, and the patient must be in place. Most of the onus in shared-care is placed on the PCP; their role is to ensure that all of the patient's health needs are addressed, both physical and emotional. The PCP assumes responsibility for all aspects of chronic disease care that are feasible in their setting; referral to specialists for periodic re-evaluations and to address issues that require focused expertise; surveillance for cancer detection and prevention; and consultation with specialists on areas of uncertainty. Studies document that PCPs often prefer this model, whereas oncologists prefer a model in which they direct survivors' care (Forsythe *et al.* 2013; Cheung *et al.* 2013).

For shared-care to be successful, specialists are required to communicate findings and recommendations back to PCPs so they can be carried out under PCP supervision. It is essential that each party understands his or her role, agrees to their responsibilities, and carries them out as necessary. Shared care is common in Europe, Canada, and Australia, but reimbursement models in the United States often interfere. Timely and comprehensive communication between providers is the key to the success of shared-care. Professional training of PCPs is imperative in this model, and risk-based models may improve PCP's management of survivors' needs (McCabe *et al.* 2013). In some countries this requirement becomes problematic due to a shortage of GPs and family physicians to act as the coordinating PCP.

The second proposed model of nurse-led follow-up care has been implemented for years in some childhood cancer centres. Ample evidence documents the success of nurse-led follow-up care in many settings, including rural and remote locations, research settings, and for the promotion of continuity of care (Committee on Cancer Survivorship 2006). Nurse-led follow-up services are acceptable, appropriate, effective, and can be an efficient means of maintaining contact with a large client group. Much like the PCP in a shared-care model, this model has nurses coordinating all aspects of survivorship care. However, a short supply of nurses in many countries and lack of community placement can limit this approach. This model also requires excellent cooperation and communication among care providers, as appropriate survivor referral to specialists is crucial. It would require adaptation on the part of specialists to receive referrals from nurses rather than physicians, and a willingness to work with nurses in a cooperative setting.

This nurse-led model has been applied successfully in Europe, but only recently piloted in the United States. Additionally, nurse-led survivor telephone clinics may offer an important link back to oncology centres in a shared-care model, where PCPs are primarily responsible for post-treatment care. These nurse-led telephone interventions offer specialized care, quick access, low costs, and may optimize survivors' experience (e.g. Kimman *et al.* 2011; Marcus *et al.* 2013).

The third proposed model of comprehensive survivorship care clinics gained momentum through the Livestrong Network in eight academic medical centres. These survivorship clinics integrate needed follow-up care expertise in one location. Such programmes can facilitate the application of a holistic and coordinated approach to medical and psychosocial problems. Livestrong clinics have led international understanding of how to meet the needs of cancer survivors (Shapiro *et al.* 2009; Forsythe *et al.* 2013; Tessaro *et al.* 2013). Additionally, paediatric oncology has been a leader in the development of survivorship care clinics, with as many as 35 clinics in the United States today. These clinics are usually run by oncology-trained nurse practitioners in collaboration with one or more paediatric oncologists. Additional personnel involved include social workers, psychologists, and other specialists such as cardiologists, fertility specialists, and genetic counsellors. Most specialists are involved on a case-by-case referral basis. The rehabilitation team recommended by the Association of Community Cancer Centers includes, but is not limited to, the following:

- Oncology nursing services;
- Psychosocial services;
- Physical, occupational, and recreational therapy services;
- Speech pathology services;
- Comprehensive, multidisciplinary lymphedema services;
- Enterostomal therapy services;
- Nutritional support services;
- Pharmacy services;
- Pastoral care services;
- A discharge planner to address home care and community and/or extended care facility services and needs;
- Qualified volunteers to provide support and advocacy for cancer patients and their families;
- Other complementary services, such as music/art therapy, relaxation, massage, and others, in conjunction with rehabilitation disciplines.

One potential disadvantage of such survivorship clinics, however, is the separation of survivorship care from other routine care, and again the difficulties of communication and coordination that may result. Hence, each model of survivorship care has liabilities and benefits; the key to success is communication among care providers and patients.

The survivorship consultation—an example of integrated care

Consider a typical consultation between a PCP and a patient who has recently completed cancer treatment in a shared-care model, currently the most common form of survivorship care. The PCP would ideally have a pre-existing relationship with the patient and have been following her progress through cancer treatment by requesting progress notes from her oncologists and other specialists. This consultation would be greatly facilitated by the provision of the treatment summary, SCP, and a discharge letter outlining surveillance schedules and guidelines for healthy behaviour from the treating oncologist, as outlined in Box 19.1.

If such a plan or discharge letter is not already available, the PCP should request it from the oncology team; if it is not forthcoming, the PCP and patient should reconstruct the summary and create a shared-care plan based on clinical practice guidelines that are acceptable to both. The first post-discharge consultation would consist of reviewing or creating the treatment summary and care plan with the cancer survivor, and if necessary reviewing relevant CPGs for their type of cancer. In preparation for the consultation, the PCP should do the following:

- Request the treatment summary from the treating oncologist;
- Request an SCP from the treating oncologist or cancer centre;
- Review relevant CPGs for the type of cancer and treatments the patient has received; and
- Obtain lists of referral options in the community for common survivorship issues.

During the consultation or over multiple visits, clinicians should discuss with patients the following:

- Current treatment toxicities, potential late effects and management strategies;
- Monitoring plans for signs of possible recurrence or second tumours (e.g. mammography, colonoscopy schedule);
- Education about what symptoms are worrisome and what symptoms are not;
- Effects of cancer/treatments on relationships, sexuality, fertility, parenting, finances;
- Effects of cancer or treatments on ability to work inside or outside of the home;
- Effects of cancer or treatments on mood, anxiety, quality of life, and referrals to reduce distress;
- Recommendations for specific healthy behaviours (diet, weight control, exercise, smoking cessation), with clear targets based on their cancer diagnosis;
- Risk to family members and any preventive measures they should be taking (e.g. screening, genetic counselling); and
- Referrals to specialists or programmes to help with any issues identified during the consultation.

Discussions and referrals should be summarized in PCP notes; referrals to other care providers should include a request for written care summaries to be sent back to the PCP. Placing PCPs' summaries periodically into oncology centre records, or seamless access between facilities would improve cross-communication among providers.

Summary, conclusions, and recommendations

Survivorship is an important phase in the cancer journey, potentially the longest phase that patients will experience. With the advent of increasingly successful acute care, more and more people are moving into this phase of cancer care, and many are finding themselves 'lost in transition'. Researchers and clinicians have devoted tremendous effort into developing ideas, programmes, and tools to help this growing cohort and researching their unique problems and needs. Government bodies and consumer groups have not only advocated for better care strategies and plans, but these have now also been mandated; the care system is at the cusp of implementing a variety of models of survivorship care. The key

issues vary across countries and regions; but what arises as essential is the need for agreement upon the components of survivorship care, and the determination of who is responsible for delivering and paying for each component.

Care providers have to be willing and able to communicate among one another and to see the value of trying to provide continuity of care between cancer specialists, the PCP, and other subspecialties involved in optimal cancer care. Patients need to become aware of their risks and care needs moving into the future, and be proactive in assuring their needs are met. The system, for its part, has to become more coordinated and receptive to a variety of models of care provision that are capable of meeting these needs. The future for cancer survivors is promising, and resources for treating cancer using models of chronic disease care and self-management interventions are becoming broadly accessible.

Acknowledgements

Dr Linda E Carlson holds the Enbridge Research Chair in Psychosocial Oncology co-funded by the Canadian Cancer Society Alberta/NWT Division and the Alberta Cancer Foundation. Her salary support is provided by Alberta Innovates—Health Solutions. Janine Giese-Davis' salary support is provided by the Enbridge Research Chair in Psychosocial Oncology. Thanks to Joshua Lounsberry for editing assistance.

References

American Cancer Society (2014). *Cancer Treatment and Survivorship Facts & Figures 2014-2015.* American Cancer Society, Atlanta, GA.

Canadian Cancer Society's Advisory Committee on Cancer Statistics (2002). *Canadian Cancer Statistics: Special Topic-Cancer incidence in young adults: Five-year relative cancer survival in Canada.* Canadian Cancer Society, Toronto, ONT.

Cancer Journey Survivorship Expert Panel, Howell D, Hack TF, Oliver TK, et al. (2011). Survivorship services for adult cancer populations: a pan-Canadian guideline. *Curr Oncol* **18**, 265–81.

Cancer Program Standards (2012). *Ensuring Patient-Centered Care.* American College of Surgeons Commission on Cancer. Posted online January 21, 2014.

Cheung WY, Aziz N, Noone AM, et al. (2013). Physician preferences and attitudes regarding different models of cancer survivorship care: a comparison of primary care providers and oncologists. *J Cancer Surviv* **7**, 343–54.

Committee on Cancer Survivorship (2006). *Improving Care and Quality of Life. From Cancer Patient to Cancer Survivor: Lost in Transition.* Hewitt M, Greenfield S, Stovall E (eds). Institute of Medicine and National Research Council, Washington DC, WA.

Cowens-Alvarado R, Sharpe K, Pratt-Chapman M, et al. (2013). Advancing survivorship care through the National Cancer Survivorship Resource Center: developing American Cancer Society guidelines for primary care providers. *CA Cancer J Clin* **63**, 147–50.

Denlinger CS, Carlson RW, Are M, et al. (2014). Survivorship: introduction and definition. Clinical practice guidelines in oncology. *J Natl Compr Canc Net* **12**, 34–45.

Forsythe LP, Parry C, Alfano CM, et al. (2013). Use of survivorship care plans in the United States: associations with survivorship care. *J Natl Cancer Inst* **105**, 1579–87.

Grunfeld E, Levine MN, Julian JA, et al. (2006). Randomized trial of long-term follow-up for early-stage breast cancer: a comparison of family physician versus specialist care. *J Clin Oncol* **24**, 848–55.

Hewitt M, Ganz PA (2007). *Implementing Cancer Survivorship Care Planning: Workshop Summary. A National Coalition for Cancer Survivorship and Institute of Medicine National Cancer Policy Forum*

Workshop in Partnership with The Lance Armstrong Foundation and The National Cancer Institute. National Academy of Sciences, Washington DC, WA.

Institute of Medicine (2003). *Childhood Cancer Survivorship: Improving Care and Quality of Life*. National Academy of Sciences, Washington DC, WA.

Kimman ML, Dirksen CD, Voogd AC, *et al.* (2011). Nurse-led telephone follow-up and an educational group programme after breast cancer treatment: Results of a 2x2 randomised controlled trial. *Eur J Cancer* **47**, 1027–36.

Kvale E, Urba SG (2014). NCCN guidelines for survivorship expanded to address two common conditions. *J Natl Compr Canc Net* **12**, Suppl, 825–7.

Marcus AC, Diefenbach MA, Stanton AL, *et al.* (2013). Cancer patient and survivor research from the cancer information service research consortium: a preview of three large randomized trials and initial lessons learned. *J Health Commun* **18**, 543–62.

McCabe MS, Partridge AH, Grunfeld E, Hudson MM (2013). Risk-based health care, the cancer survivor, the oncologist, and the primary care physician. *Semin Oncol* **40**, 804–12.

National Comprehensive Cancer Network (2014). *Survivorship*. National Comprehensive Cancer Network, vol. Version 2.2014. Washington DC, WA.

Nekhlyudov L, Levi, L., Hurria A, Ganz PA (2014). Patient-centered, evidence-based, and cost-conscious cancer care across the continuum: Translating the Institute of Medicine report into clinical practice. *Cancer* **64**, 408–21.

Olson RA, Howard F, Turnbull K, *et al.* (2014). Prospective evaluation of unmet needs of rural and aboriginal cancer survivors in Northern British Columbia. *Curr Oncol* **21**, e179–85.

President's Cancer Panel (2005). *Assessing Progress, Advancing Change*. National Cancer Institute, Bethesda, MD.

Railton C, Lupichuk S, McCormick J, *et al.* (2015). Discharge to primary care for survivorship follow-up: how are early-stage breast cancer patients faring? *J Natl Compr Canc Netw* **13**, 762–71.

Risendal B, Dwyer A, Seidel R, *et al.* (2014). Adaptation of the chronic disease self-management program for cancer survivors: feasibility, acceptability, and lessons for implementation. *J Cancer Educ* **29**, 762–71.

Rowland JH, Bellizzi KM (2008). Cancer survivors and survivorship research: a reflection on today's successes and tomorrow's challenges. *Hematol Oncol Clin North Am* **22**, 181–200.

Shapiro CL, McCabe MS, Syrjala KL, *et al.* (2009). The LIVESTRONG Survivorship Center of Excellence Network. *J Cancer Survi* **3**, 4–11.

Skolarus TA, Wolf AM, Erb NL, *et al.* (2014). American Cancer Society prostate cancer survivorship care guidelines. *CA Cancer J Clin* **64**, 225–49.

Stricker CT, Jacobs LA, Risendal, *et al.* (2011). Survivorship care planning after the institute of medicine recommendations: how are we faring? *J Cancer Surviv* **5**, 358–70.

Tessaro I, Campbell MK, Golden S, *et al.* (2013). Process of diffusing cancer survivorship care into oncology practice. *Transl Behav Med* **3**, 142–8.

World Cancer Research Fund/American Institute for Cancer Research (2007). *Food, Nutrition, Physical Activity, and the Prevention of Cancer: a Global Perspective*. AICR, Washington DC.

CHAPTER 20

Dealing with cancer recurrence

Lidia Schapira and Lauren Goldstein

Introduction to dealing with cancer recurrence

'The cancer is back' is the most unwelcome news, which typically signals an important and devastating change in prognosis. These are the words a clinician hopes he or she will not need to say and a patient never wants to hear. Shortly after first receiving a diagnosis of cancer, patients hear from expert cancer clinicians that therapies are geared towards preventing a relapse and it is the hope of cure that sustains them through the gruelling treatments.

Over one million individuals are diagnosed with a recurrence of cancer every year in the United States and more than half will die rapidly of their disease (Thornton *et al.* 2014). Not all cancer recurrences are fatal, however, and the prognosis depends on the type of cancer and availability of salvage or curative treatments. For example, a patient with recurrence of lymphoma can be treated again with curative intent, and a local recurrence of breast cancer could have an excellent outcome after appropriate therapy. However, the majority of cancer patients with disease progression or recurrence will need lifelong anti-cancer therapy and are likely to die from their disease. Disclosing the news of a cancer recurrence is especially tough for oncologists, because they, too, may experience a range of emotions, such as guilt, disappointment, frustration, or sadness (Buckman 2010; Granek *et al.* 2012). They are typically the first ones to receive the news of recurrence and need to process their own emotions before sharing the news with the patient and his or her family.

Fear of recurrence

Any patient living with cancer lives in fear of being diagnosed with recurrent disease. Predictably, fear of cancer recurrence is common and constitutes the most prevalent concern reported by cancer survivors (Allen *et al.* 2009). Patients often suffer from realistic fears stemming from the illness itself, the treatments utilized to fight the illness, and the associated or expected consequences of treatment (Dinkel *et al.* 2014). However, many patients also experience a heightened, even debilitating, degree of fear and anxiety stemming from living with uncertainty, and this generalized anxiety can be difficult to distinguish from fears about disease progression (Simard and Savard 2015).

Dinkel and colleagues (2014) investigated the relationship between fear of progression in patients with a chronic illness and clinical anxiety disorders. They found that patients who met criteria for clinical fear of progression did not differ meaningfully from patients who met criteria for a DSM-IV anxiety disorder, in regards to pathological worrying, generalized anxiety, symptoms of depression, and somatic complaints (Dinkel *et al.* 2014). Importantly, these intense fears of disease progression and recurrence are not always proportional to the real medical circumstances. Since clinicians are often singularly focused on prognostic estimates as they pertain to the medical reality, substantiated by scans and labs, they often fail to attend to patients' fears and anxieties that are borne out of the discomfort of living with uncertainty. For this reason, a cancer patient who is treated with curative intent and carries a very favourable prognosis may nonetheless feel paralysed by intrusive thoughts of recurrence that interfere with her daily function and ability to enjoy her life, and these feelings may go undetected or unexplored by her oncologist.

In recent years, there has been a considerable increase in research examining realistic illness-related fears among cancer patients. Thewes and colleagues (2013) examined the ways in which oncology team members manage patients' fear of recurrence, and they found a lack of consensus in approach: clinicians do not routinely assess patients' fear of recurrence, and may often miss the signals. Managing these fears through attentive listening, validation and, when appropriate, referral for psychological or behavioural therapies remains one of the most important clinical tasks of physicians and nurses engaged in the longitudinal care of cancer survivors (Simard and Savard 2015).

Discussing cancer recurrence

Pitfalls and strategies for effective communication

Throughout the treatment of cancer, death is considered the ultimate enemy and, as a consequence, broaching the topic of recurrence can be an extremely harrowing experience, not only for the patient but also for the physician, given that death due to cancer represents a fundamental clinical failure and can trigger considerable guilt and disappointment for the oncologist (Buckman 2010; Granek *et al.* 2012; Morgans and Schapira 2015). When physicians fail to broach this conversation in an empathic and informative manner, this misstep is generally attributable to one of two things: either (i) the physician is unclear with the patient, in an effort to protect the patient from the emotional impact of the news; or (ii) the physician addressed the medical reality, but failed to respond to the patient's consequent emotional needs.

Understandably, physicians seek to minimize the emotional burden of cancer for their patients, and news of a cancer recurrence is often a devastating blow. In attempts to protect their patients, physicians often utilize euphemisms and ambiguous language in order to communicate news more gently. For example, a physician might tell the patient that restaging scans showed 'little spots in the bone that could possibly be abnormal', rather than explicitly stating that these spots indicate secondary spread. Alternatively, s/he might communicate the news of recurrence clearly enough, but may then fail to clarify that the recurrence signifies that the disease is still *treatable*, but no longer *curable*. However well intentioned, ultimately this approach only obfuscates the reality and confuses the patient (Dunn *et al.* 1993).

In other cases, physicians will communicate the news of recurrence clearly to the patient but, either because the physician is highly anxious, or because he does not possess the skill set or confidence necessary to support the patient emotionally, will fail to respond to the patient's emotional reaction to the news. Some clinicians wish to minimize the time spent discussing disappointing and saddening news and, in so doing, block the patient's attempts to discuss the implications of recurrence. Gordon and Dougherty (2003) explored the language used to describe the news of advanced disease. Physicians frequently used troubling terms such as 'hitting over the head', 'pounding', 'hammering', 'bludgeoning', and 'dumping' to describe their practice of disclosing bad news. This finding reflected many physicians' underlying belief that the truth is injurious, the physician abusive, and the practice of disclosing bad news harmful (Gordon and Dougherty 2003). Physicians experience anxiety prior to giving bad news, as well as feelings of helplessness when confronted with extreme suffering (Ptacek *et al.* 1999; Panagopoulou *et al.* 2008; Back *et al.* 2015). Complex feelings associated with therapeutic failure, including feelings of personal failure, can blunt the clinician's ability to respond empathically and provide the emotional support that is so desperately sought by patients (Morgans and Schapira 2015).

Clinicians can improve communicating news of recurrence and helping patients cope in three main ways. First, clinicians ought to explain the recurrence in clear terms. Second, he or she should avoid formulaic approaches and tailor the conversation to the specific circumstances of each patient's illness, sense of urgency about prognosis, and consequent course of treatment. Finally, clinicians need to develop the self-awareness to understand their own preferred style of communication and then take steps to compensate for any of the patient's needs the clinician feels unable to meet. For example, clinicians who are uncomfortable showing affect can take a more cognitive approach to delivering the information and elect to have a social worker present during the conversation to provide emotional support.

How much to disclose?

Full disclosure of diagnostic and prognostic information, now standard practice in most Western countries, would have shocked our mentors and may even today be considered unnecessarily brutal in many cultures (Schapira 2004). Twenty-five years ago, anthropologists Delvecchio Good and colleagues (1990) wrote that in American oncology practice, hope is mainly conveyed through providing information; in contrast, in Europe and Asia, physicians conveyed hope primarily by fostering ambiguity. Practices have changed all over the world as a result of globalization and migration. Oncologists in the United States have become more sensitive to the challenges of cross-cultural communication and, in the course of a single day, may have conversations about cancer recurrence or goals of care with patients from many different cultures.

Many of these patients will not share the physician's orientation towards disclosure of information and may prefer to delegate the responsibility of making treatment decisions to family members or to the oncology team. Some patients and relatives do not wish to be briefed on every aspect of diagnosis and prognosis (Schneider 1998) and explicitly ask their physicians not to prognosticate; they find that articulating estimates of life expectancy is simply unhelpful and depressing, and they prefer their doctor to 'hope with them' for an improvement, an extension of life, or symptomatic relief. Patients' preferences for receiving medical news in European countries and Asia have also changed, reflecting greater acceptance of openness in communication, although many differences remain between countries and cultures. The practice of clarifying the level of detail any patient seeks is the only safe means to avoid causing harm through an automatic and unwarranted spiel of facts.

Often, patient preferences are incongruent with physicians' sense of humane medical practice. If physicians view withholding prognostic information as deceitful, they are likely to favour complete disclosure, but if they see withholding prognostic information as an important aspect of fostering hope, they may steer the conversation away from discussion of timelines and projections of future problems (Christakis 1999). As with any therapeutic option, the decision of how much to tell depends on the estimates of risk and benefit, but physicians need to balance their own moral imperatives with the patient's expressed preferences, and not forego one in favour of honouring the other (Schapira 2006). In situations where the physician's 'need to inform' conflicts with the individual's legitimate request and right not to receive information, physicians can perceive the delivery of bad news as abusive. In practice, we sometimes face competent, educated individuals, who simply do not wish to know detailed side effects, and prefer to skip the explanations of possible harm. They would rather sign the paperwork authorizing treatment without reading it. Case by case, physicians need to decide if the patient's unwillingness to listen invalidates or trivializes the process of obtaining consent for treatment (Schapira 2006). Some patients prefer not to take full ownership of their own treatment decisions, and in these cases, the oncologist must actively negotiate the locus of decision-making with the patient. One can ask a patient, 'if there is important news, would you like me to discuss this with you directly?'—and if the answer is no, then the patient needs to delegate this task to a designated individual who is empowered to make a decision about further treatment.

Coping with recurrence

Patients may experience the news of a recurrence with a sense of shock and disbelief, often despite their own attempts to prepare for bad news. Patients who have serial determinations of blood tumour markers or imaging studies, for example, know that the purpose of these tests is to detect early signs of recurrence and are, therefore, trained to expect important news at each visit. In some cases, this emotional preparation may mitigate the impact of hearing bad news; however, not all patients will fully grasp the prognostic significance of recurrence and will subsequently fail to understand that the disease is no longer curable. They may anticipate further treatments (e.g. chemotherapy, targeted therapy, or endocrine manipulations) without recognizing that the intention of treatment has evolved from cure to palliation. It may take repeated conversations for the patient to understand the implications of this grave news.

Hearing bad news spurs an emotional and cognitive reaction that needs to be acknowledged, addressed, and supported. In some instances, hearing the news of a cancer recurrence may simply confirm a person's pre-existing worries or suspicions. For others, suffering may impair the person's ability to imagine goals for the future, as well as his or her sense of control and self-efficacy (Halpern 2001). Since medical decisions can rest on rethinking or regenerating life goals, a process that involves coming to terms with grief as well as clear reasoning, it is best not to rush into discussions of treatment options (Halpern 2001). Salander's (2002) classic studies of patients who received bad news demonstrated the psychological meaning and importance of 'togetherness' at the time of diagnosis, a supportive atmosphere, and a personal touch. For the clinician, the challenge is to provide a calm and steady presence, to refrain from rushing to fix the problem, and to recognize that simply offering to share the burden of uncertainty carries tremendous therapeutic value (Schapira 2014). For many of us trained to act, this is often hard to do.

Many people, patients and physicians alike, find it difficult to cope with uncertainty, and some have more difficulty than others. Eisenberg and colleagues (2015) suggest a possible causal relationship or association between cognitive difficulties and the inability to handle uncertainty. They posit that individuals with little tolerance for uncertainty struggle to develop the cognitive flexibility necessary to process cancer survivorship and, consequently, those patients with low thresholds for tolerating uncertainty experience greater cancer-related distress long after active treatment has ended. These psychological and cognitive processes are not systematically explored during routine consultations and, unless they ask, physicians don't have any way to determine how distressed patients or relatives really are about the uncertain future. To that end, clinicians must strive to be as attentive as possible to the emotional and cognitive ripple effects of patients' medical realities. Paying particular attention to patients' overall quality of life, rather than focusing solely on their medical circumstances, is essential (Eisenberg *et al.* 2015).

Ultimately, uncertainty is unsettling, not only for patients but for their physicians as well. The best any physician can do is attempt to vocalize, and normalize, the difficulty of living with uncertainty, and make clear his or her willingness to share some of the burden of uncertainty with the patient, affirming a therapeutic alliance, and offering to share in the experience (Schapira 2014). Table 20.1 lists

Table 20.1 Practical checklist for discussing a cancer recurrence

Strategies	Skills and process tasks	Communication examples
Create setting	Provide a comfortable, safe, and private location, minimize interruptions	
Introductions	Introduce other team members if present and clarify their roles Observe the patient's body language, non-verbal, and verbal cues that indicate his or her level of ease or anxiety	
Perception of illness	Check the patient's present understanding	'What is your understanding of the reasons we did the MRI?'
Set the agenda	Inform the patient about the objectives of the meeting, time available, and how it will be spent	'Today we'll review further the results of these tests and work out what we need to do.'
Negotiate the exchange of information	Address the patient's need to receive and refuse information and clarify the level of detail preferred	'Help me understand your preferences for the level of detail you like in the information I'll give you.'
Provide information	Present facts that need to be conveyed so that a reasonable person can choose a treatment	Consider a warning first: 'I'm afraid the news is more serious than we suspected.' 'Unfortunately the PET scan showed that the cancer has spread to other organs.'
Use empathy	Words and gestures to convey the clinician feels or understands the patient's feelings	'I too am disappointed and had hoped for a better outcome ...' 'This must be very hard to hear ...'
Engage the patient and family in decision-making	Emphasize partnership	'I want to make it clear that we are here to support and help you. Don't worry alone.'
Share uncertainty	Recognizes uncertainty is unsettling	'Let's think about the next steps. Would it be helpful to talk about what can happen if the treatment does not work?'
Engage the patient and family in problem solving	Help the patient and family to think through available options Outline the big picture including standard treatment, clinical trials, and palliative measures	'Chemotherapy may stop the growth of this tumour.' 'There is a clinical trial you may wish to consider.' 'We have a terrific team and will work together to control your pain.'
Summary, including goals of future care	Check understanding—review medical facts and statistics, draw pictures, or graphs Summarize the action plan, including the time and place for next contact	'We need to bring this meeting to an end. Let me take a moment to go over the main points of our conversation ...' 'You have an appointment with my colleague in radiation oncology tomorrow at 3 o'clock.' 'I would also like you to call my nurse tomorrow morning to tell her if this medication helped with your pain.'

a series of steps and practical tips to help guide these conversations. These are based both on evidence and on consensus guidelines for best practice, and are not intended to script the dialogue between healthcare professionals and patients. Instead, these talking points can be viewed as aids or props to help sustain a meaningful connection between clinician and patient during times of high emotional stress.

Ideally, consultations involve the exchange of information in an atmosphere of mutual trust, followed by deliberation, and, finally, a recommendation from the physician based on the patient's goals and preferences. We recommend describing the standard treatment first (assuming one is available), and then guiding the patient to consider alternatives such as treatment on a clinical trial, supportive care without anti-cancer therapy, or complementary therapies. Doctors can help patients think through their options, verbalizing what could happen if s/he chose to forego anti-cancer treatments, or took a break to fulfil an important personal goal. In a non-judgemental exchange, the doctor can help his or her patients sort through various possibilities for treatment or observation, and imagine the consequences of each decision.

Provision of hope

Even when cure is no longer possible and the future is uncertain, patients need to feel hopeful, and the oncologist plays a major role in nurturing, shaping, and supporting patients' individual expressions of hope. Hope can take a variety of forms, ranging from miracle cure to peaceful death, and evolves over time as circumstances change for each individual patient. For some oncologists, it is easy to remain cheerful, even optimistic, and many do so by concentrating on diagnostic and therapeutic interventions, or simply by limiting their conversations to the present, avoiding 'big picture' talks. Others try to balance their therapeutic effect by offering treatment and symptom management and, at the same time, helping patients to recalibrate their expectations and hope for goals that are realistic and within reach.

Current guidelines recommend that the oncologist balance honest disclosure with sustaining hope (Clayton *et al.* 2005). In clinical scenarios, this can be accomplished through incremental steps designed to help the patient and his or her relatives to integrate new information over a period of time, and by anticipating the emotional repercussions. A few techniques that can help clinicians are (i) exploring the sources of meaning and hope; (ii) identifying potential problems, such as family members who may have difficulties coping and require support; and (iii) shifting the conversation to affirm the personal attributes and qualities that convey the value of the person. Encouraging patients to recall uplifting memories and shared experiences will also convey respect and foster a sense of connection that will serve both physician and patient well as they confront an uncertain future (Yellen and Cella 1995; Mount *et al.* 2007).

Recurrence of cancer role play and actor training

Breast cancer scenario

Mary is a 41-year-old married mother of three children, who was diagnosed with breast cancer one year ago. Her tumour did not express oestrogen nor progesterone receptors, but had spread to regional lymph nodes. She was treated with mastectomy, adjuvant chemotherapy, and radiation to her chest wall. She saw her oncologist for a six-month check-up, at which time she was asymptomatic, but still recovering from the sequelae of her lengthy treatments. Three months later, she developed a persistent cough, and after several weeks, a chest X-ray showed a vague peripheral nodule. Chest computed tomography (CT) scan showed pleural-based 'suspicious lesions', as well as two small peripheral pulmonary nodules, each measured at 4 mm. Mary returns to see you for her scan results.

Guide to training the actor

Mary is a well-informed and educated woman, who takes good care of herself and her family (three children, ages 11, 16, and 18). She has great confidence in her medical team. During her adjuvant therapy, she developed a strong working relationship with the nurses and oncologist. She suspects something is seriously wrong, but is not aware of the dismal prognosis associated with such an early relapse. She will come into the meeting with her husband and expects to hear that she will need more treatment. She may blurt out, 'I thought I was cured' or 'What are we going to do next?' and is not quite prepared for the devastating news she is likely to hear (i.e. that the tumour is incurable). Until this time, she was always eager to hear statistics and detailed information, but now she is really ambivalent. She is terrified, but tries to put on a brave front.

Colon cancer scenario

Barry is a 60-year-old, semi-retired CEO of a biochemical company, who is quite used to giving orders and having the final word. He has a bad marriage and grown-up children, who don't really like him very much. He has few close friends and maintains his distance from relatives. He has a passion for photography and often travels by himself to take pictures of wild animals in remote locations. He doesn't really trust the medical establishment and did not participate in routine colonoscopic screening for colon cancer. He was diagnosed three years ago with a node-positive colon cancer and was treated with surgery and adjuvant chemotherapy. His oncologist explained the rationale for periodic surveillance with tumour markers and CT scans in order to identify a possible 'early recurrence', which could still be treated with salvage surgery. Barry's carcinoembryonic antigen (CEA) began a slow and steady climb, but his CT scan did not show any disease. However, his positron emission tomography (PET) scan shows multiple liver metastases. Barry has a scheduled appointment to discuss results. Surgery is no longer an option.

Guide to training the actor

Barry is physically fit and in his sixties. He is gruff, smart, and does not particularly care for small talk. He has built a successful business and is used to giving orders. He is not close to his wife or his grown children, but he is not unpleasant. His hobby is wildlife photography and he did, on one occasion, invite his son to accompany him on a photo safari to Africa, where they had a good time together. Barry thinks doctors cannot really 'prevent' disease and only sees his internist (GP) when he does not feel well. Prior to his colon cancer, his only exposures to the medical establishment were quite brief and successful: arthroscopic surgery for a torn knee ligament and medical therapy for gastroesophageal reflux. Three years ago, he found blood in his stool and this led to a diagnosis of colon cancer. He was rebuked for having 'waited so long' and for not having ever had screening colonoscopies. He saw a brilliant, technical surgeon, who did not care for small talk either and was then referred to the oncologist for adjuvant chemotherapy. He 'endured' the treatments, although he never really had much faith that he would derive a personal benefit. He 'went along' with a plan to watch him carefully, because he understood that a local recurrence or solitary hepatic metastasis could still be treated (surgically) with curative intent. His oncologist explained that his tumour marker was rising and ordered CT and then PET scans. His CT 'showed nothing'. He thinks that the blood test is probably wrong. Living with this uncertainty does not suit him well. The only acceptable option with a recurrence of cancer would be more surgery with curative intent. He has no more patience for the chemotherapy and no interest in discussing his emotional life with nurses.

As he listens to the latest news, Barry could say: 'Why didn't we pick this up sooner?' 'How long do I have to live?' 'I'm a reasonable man, doctor. I know you keep talking about treatments and responses, but what chance do I have of getting a benefit from any of these drugs?'

Conclusion

Ultimately, consultations that deal with recurrence incorporate many of the strategies and skills involved with breaking bad news, discussing prognosis, the use of salvage treatments, providing a supportive framework, sustaining hope, and emphasizing, as appropriate, the chronicity of the illness. The clinician's goal is to tailor information based on knowledge of the patient's coping strengths and limitations, provide empathic support, and convey a commitment to the patient's care as the journey with cancer unfolds.

References

Allen JD, Savadatti S, Levy AG (2009). The transition from breast cancer "patient" to "survivor." *Psychooncology* **18**, 71–80.

Back AL, Rushton CH, Kaszniak AW, Halifax JS (2015). "Why are we doing this?" Clinician helplessness in the face of suffering. *J Palliat Med* **18**, 26–30.

Buckman R (2010). The invisible effects of therapeutic failure. *Oncologist* **15**, 1370–2.

Christakis NA (1999). *Death Foretold*. The University of Chicago Press, Chicago, IL.

Clayton JM, Butow PN, Arnold RM, *et al.* (2005). Fostering coping and nurturing hope when discussing the future with terminally ill cancer patients and their caregivers. *Cancer* **103**, 1965–75.

Delvecchio Good MJ, Good BJ, Schaffer C, Lind SE (1990). American oncology and the discourse on hope. *Cult Med Psychiatry* **14**, 59–79.

Dinkel A, Kremsteriter K, Marten-Mittag B, Lahmann C (2014). Comorbidity of fear of progression and anxiety disorders in cancer patients. *Gen Hosp Psychiatry* **36**, 613–19.

Dunn SM, Patterson PU, Butow PN, Smart HH, McCarthy WH, Tattersall MH (1993). Cancer by another name: a randomized trial of the effects of euphemisms and uncertainty in communication with cancer patients. *J Clin Oncol* **11**, 989–96.

Eisenberg SA, Kurita K, Taylor-Ford M, Agus DB, Gross ME, Meyerowitz BE (2015). Intolerance of uncertainty, cognitive complaints, and cancer-related distress in prostate cancer survivors. *Psychooncology* **24**, 228–35.

Gordon E, Dougherty CK (2003). Hitting you over the head: Oncologists' disclosure of prognosis to advanced cancer patients. *Bioethics* **17**, 142–68.

Granek L, Tozer R, Mazzotta P, Ramjaun A, Kryzanowska M (2012). Nature and impact of grief over patient loss on oncologists' personal and professional lives. *Arch Intern Med* **172**, 964–6.

Halpern J (2001). *From Detached Concern to Empathy: Humanizing Medical Practice*. Oxford University Press, Oxford, UK.

Morgans A, Schapira L (2015). Confronting therapeutic failure: A conversation guide. *Oncologist* **20**, 946–51.

Mount BM, Boston PH, Cohen RS (2007). Healing connections: on moving from suffering to a sense of well-being. *J Pain Symptom Manage* **33**, 372–88.

Panagopoulou E, Mintziori G, Montgomery A, Kapoukranidou D, Benos A (2008). Concealment of information in clinical practice: Is lying less stressful than telling the truth? *J Clin Oncol* **26**, 1175–7.

Ptacek JT, Fries EA, Eberhardt TL, Ptacek JJ (1999). Breaking bad news to patients: Physicians' perceptions of the process. *Support Care Cancer* **7**, 113–20.

Salander P (2002). Bad news from the patient's perspective: An analysis of the written narratives of newly diagnosed cancer patients. *Soc Sci Med* **55**, 721–32.

Schapira L (2004). Shared uncertainty. *J Support Oncol* **2**, 14–18.

Schapira L (2006). Breaking bad news to patients and families. In: *Tumours of the Chest: Biology, Diagnosis and Management*. pp. 597–605. Syrigos L, Nutting K, Roussos C (eds). Springer, New York, NY.

Schapira L (2014). Handling uncertainty. *Support Care Cancer* **22**, 859–61.

Schneider CE (1998). *The Practice of Autonomy: Patients, Doctors and Medical Decisions*. Oxford University Press, Oxford, UK.

Simard S, Savard J (2015). Screening and comorbidity of clinical levels of fear of cancer recurrence. *J Cancer Surviv* **9**, 481–91.

Thornton LM, Levin AO, Dorfman CS, Godiwala N, Heitzmann C, Anderson BL (2014). Emotions and social relationships for breast and gynecologic patients: a qualitative study of coping with recurrence. *Psychooncology* **23**, 382–9.

Yellen SB, Cella DF (1995). Someone to live for: social well-being, parenthood status, and decision-making in oncology. *J Clin Oncol* **13**, 1255–64.

CHAPTER 21

Introducing or transitioning patients to palliative care

A. Katalin Urban, Josephine M. Clayton, and David W. Kissane

Introduction to transitioning patients to palliative care

Despite advances in anti-cancer treatments, a large proportion of adult cancer patients still eventually die from their disease. Many other chronic illnesses such as cardiac or renal failure also result in a significantly reduced life expectancy. Patients with these life-limiting illnesses can have a large symptom burden and may benefit from palliative care support. Transition from active disease-modifying treatments to palliative management can be stressful for both patients and clinicians.

With cancer, the goals of care can change from curative to palliative, or they may be palliative from the moment of diagnosis in patients presenting with disseminated cancer. Palliative anti-cancer treatments aim to minimize the spread of cancer and disease progression, help control symptoms, and improve quality of life. Other palliative therapies include medications and interventions to relieve symptoms—including physical, psychosocial, and existential issues.

Transition to palliative care can be especially challenging with non-malignant diseases, where the point of change from disease control to symptom management is often difficult to define. Effective communication is essential in achieving an adaptive adjustment to disease progression and preparation for death.

The nature of palliative care

The 'palliative approach' is a model of care which focuses on improving quality of life by preventing and alleviating suffering in patients with a life-threatening illness and their families.

According to the World Palliative Care Alliance's policy, palliative care is not synonymous with end-of-life care and should not be offered only when disease-directed or life-prolonging therapy has failed (Gwyther and Krakauer 2009). Palliation is worthwhile at any point in a serious illness and can be provided simultaneously with treatments directed at disease control (Shin and Temel 2013).

Many principal national bodies, such as Australia's National Health and Medical Research Council (Clayton et al. 2007) and the American Society of Clinical Oncology (Smith et al. 2012), have recognized that palliative care is an integral component of best practice in the management of people with chronic, advanced, or terminal conditions. This involves 'primary' palliative care (referring to general communication about goals/advanced care planning, symptom assessment, and management provided by the primary provider), as well as 'specialist' palliative care. Specialist palliative care is administered by expert multidisciplinary healthcare services and may be reserved for more complex cases, but is not available everywhere. All healthcare professionals who care for patients with life-limiting illnesses should have skills in primary palliative care, as well as the ability to recognize when referral to specialist palliative care is required. For instance, patients with refractory symptoms or unusual difficulty with coping or decision-making can benefit from specialist input (Vergo and Cullinan 2013). As the patient's illness progresses, he or she may need referral to community or home-based palliative care services, or to an inpatient palliative care unit for terminal care.

Ideally, the palliative approach should be adopted over time as the person's disease progresses, involving a gradual transition/integration rather than a sharp demarcation. Early referral to specialist palliative care services, while the patient is still receiving disease-specific treatments such as chemotherapy and radiotherapy, may enhance symptom control, and reduce any sense of abandonment later, when chemotherapy is no longer appropriate. Along the way, clinicians can help patients to cultivate prognostic awareness at a less pressured pace through these different approaches (Jackson et al. 2013). In Boston, early referral of patients with metastatic lung cancer improved length of survival while also avoiding burdensome end-of-life interventions (Temel et al. 2010). Early referral can also reduce inappropriate hospitalizations and the use of high cost acute care (Haines 2011). Specialist palliative care can improve patient, carer, and clinician satisfaction, symptom control, quality of life, rate of home deaths, and can also reduce futile healthcare (Rabow et al. 2013).

Discussions about changing treatment goals (e.g. from curative to palliative, or from palliation with anti-cancer treatments to symptomatic care only) and referral to specialist palliative care can be challenging for patients, their families, and health professionals alike. An authentic dialogue that is tailored to each person and avoids platitudes is crucial. If not communicated sensitively and effectively by the healthcare team, these conversations can evoke fears of impending death, and a sense of helplessness or abandonment in the patient and their family. In this chapter, we conceptualize the process of transitioning patients to palliative care in four distinct ways:

1. transition to a palliative approach: when the goals of care change from curative to palliative;

2. introduction of specialist palliative care services;

3. when potentially life-prolonging treatments (including palliative anti-cancer treatments) are no longer effective and symptomatic care only is adopted; and

4. when the person approaches the terminal phase of their illness.

The timing of these transitions needs to be individualized depending on patient circumstances, and should be sensitive to patient and family psychosocial dynamics.

Communication about transitions in the goals of care

The general objectives for communicating transition to a palliative approach are to guide the patient collaboratively to understand that he or she has a life-limiting illness, and, through shared decision-making, establish appropriate goals of care that focus on quality of life, as well as emphasizing what can be done (symptom control, practical and emotional support, preservation of dignity), and fostering realistic hope (Evans et al. 2006).

Physicians are not good at predicting when and how much information patients want, and patients differ in their information needs and preferences (Innes and Payne 2009). Hitz et al. (2013) found that some patients prefer shared decision-making (45%), while others prefer the doctor to direct decisions (44%). These preferences should be elicited to ensure satisfactory communication consistent with a patient-centred approach. End-of-life conversations often occur during acute hospital admissions, not with the main provider and late in the course of illness (Mack et al. 2012). Ideally, discussions about transitioning to palliative care should occur gradually rather than as a single, one-off encounter. They are a central responsibility of the primary treatment team because they have an established relationship with the patient.

Identifying when to talk about shifting goals of care

A stereotypic trajectory of the journey with advanced cancer has been identified—slow and slight decline across many months, followed by a steep slope to death in the last two months (Lunney et al. 2003). In the past, referral to palliative care has often not occurred until this late stage, despite evidence that there may be negative consequences for patients who lack insight into their situation, such as unnecessary hospital admissions, higher proportion of hospital deaths, poorer symptom control, and less end-of-life planning (Innes and Payne 2009). With non-malignant illnesses, the trajectory is often different, with a gradual decline over time, with intermittent exacerbations needing acute care, which can make identifying the point of introduction even more difficult. There are predictable sentinel events which ought to trigger these discussions, such as diagnosis of central nervous system (CNS) disease, change in chemotherapy regimen, declining performance status, or hospital admission with disease exacerbation. We recommend that palliative care be gradually integrated early on in the disease course and delivered simultaneously with other active therapies, such as anti-cancer treatment, or medication for heart failure.

Patients identify several factors that culminate in the experience of a 'good death'. These include being in control and involved in decisions, having symptoms well-managed, adequate recognition of impending death permitting a sense of closure, affirmation of the self, trust in care providers, burden minimized and relationships optimized, death in the preferred place, having their affairs in order, prayer, or meditation, spiritual peace, and leaving a legacy (Khan et al. 2014). However, concordance between the physician's and patient's ratings of main concerns has been shown to be poor (Baile et al. 2011). Offering an open discussion about the transition to palliative and eventually end-of-life care is responsive to these patient preferences, and has not been associated with higher levels of depression or worry among terminally ill cancer patients (Wright et al. 2008).

Another important rationale for effective communication about the transition to palliative care is avoidance of futile care, potentially a major cost to society in times of scarcity of clinical resources and a burden to patients and their families, who often fail to appreciate the reality of the plight. Aggressive care at the end of life is associated with poorer patient quality of life and worse bereavement adjustment (Wright et al. 2008). A significant proportion of patients continue to receive chemotherapy in the final months of their life. Mack et al. (2012) reported that 16% received chemotherapy within 14 days of death, and 9% received intensive care within 30 days. Administering chemotherapy appears to be an easier option than discussing changing goals of care and may be felt to provide hope. However, this may deny patients and families the opportunity to prepare for death. Patients with other chronic, life-limiting illnesses often have aggressive treatments at the end of life, with higher rates of intensive treatments and lower uptake of hospice, as seen in dialysis compared to cancer patients (Wong et al. 2012).

The challenge of prognostication

Both patients and their physicians err commonly in being too optimistic about the prognosis, contributing to poor understanding of the clinical reality. Alarmingly, 69% of patients with metastatic lung cancer and 81% with metastatic colorectal cancer did not understand that chemotherapy would not cure them (Weeks et al. 2012). Although 98% of oncologists report telling patients when they have incurable cancer, 57% 'sometimes, rarely or never' give any prognostic estimate to their patients (Daugherty and Hlubocky 2008). Yet we know that in Western societies, the majority of patients want at least a broad indication of their prognosis (Innes and Payne 2009). There are consistent findings that clinicians who feel close to their patients overestimate survival by a five to sixfold error.

Given how challenging this appears to be, the question arises as to how a physician begins a conversation about dying. Usually this arises in conjunction with a set of investigational results revealing significant disease progression, despite active anti-cancer treatments, and often the presence of substantial tumour burden. Alternatively, admission to hospital with an exacerbation of the condition may be a trigger. Other strong markers of this time having arrived include symptoms such as anorexia, weight loss and cachexia, and changing performance status, with greater frailty, and increasing dependence on others. Questions from patients, with associated emotional cues indicating their concern, may indicate their readiness for this conversation. However, physicians should not wait for the patient to raise the issue; they have the responsibility to do this when appropriate, always proportionately to the information preferences of their patients.

Jackson *et al.* (2013) describe how patients may swing between more or less realistic understanding of prognosis. Guiding them towards prognostic awareness through a stepwise and partnered approach can help to set realistic goals and grieve unattainable ones. They suggest assessing illness understanding, followed by hypothetically asking the patient to imagine a poorer health state.

What to say to introduce the concept of transitioning to palliative care

Patients with advanced cancer have identified important skills they desire from their doctors to ease this type of communication. These include maintaining a calm and open manner, with respect for each person and sensitivity to their needs. They indicated that control of discussions should be given to the patient, but the doctor should take the initiative to raise complex or difficult topics (Walczak *et al.* 2011).

When treatment options have failed and at the end of life, it is important to check each patient's perception of their disease, understanding of recent investigations, and what the goals of treatment have been. This helps to achieve a uniform viewpoint or correct any misunderstandings and gaps in knowledge.

Warning patients that bad news is coming can help them to prepare. Similarly, prior to formally changing goals of care, a series of open-ended questions to elicit patients' concerns, personal goals, and values is worthwhile. This then enables the physician to negotiate new goals of care based upon attitudes that the patient reveals about their quality of life expectations. In doing this, clinicians should contrast 'cure' with 'care', introduce the concept of the palliative approach as 'always involving something that can be done to help' and acknowledge, where appropriate, that anti-cancer treatments may continue alongside symptomatic treatments. In contrast, if futile care is being sought, the concept that 'further chemotherapy may do more harm than good' is reasonable. In applying any of these options, great sensitivity to each patient's emotional response is called for, with empathic acknowledgement of the perceived outcome for the patient. Eliciting patient concerns, even when they can only be acknowledged but not necessarily solved, and responding with empathy can help to reduce emotional distress (Evans *et al.* 2006).

Grieving has been identified as an important part of dealing with transition to a palliative approach, necessitating a supportive and empathic response (Van Vliet *et al.* 2013). The clinician needs to normalize any tearfulness, tolerate the expression of emotion and not retract the information that has been provided. Avoidance of premature or false reassurance is necessary, while also finding sources of realistic hope before leaving the conversation (Jackson *et al.* 2013).

The maintenance of morale in the face of disease progression is challenging. The focus on living in the present, living life out fully, and maintaining a sense of normality, despite a life-limiting illness, may facilitate patients' well-being. Emphasizing what can be done, as well as discussing the availability of ongoing support and non-abandonment are essential (Van Vliet *et al.* 2013). One approach is

to refocus hope towards realistic goals, based on patient values, and preparation for death. This may involve not only social and legal acts (wills and advanced directives) but also life review, completion of unfinished business, leaving a legacy, talking about your children's future plans, expressing gratitude for the life you've shared, and beginning to say goodbye. Patients find value in taking care of their final responsibilities, and may want to make arrangements to support the lives of their future bereaved relatives. One way of opening such discussions is by using a hypothetical question to explore what would be most important to the patient should time be limited. Discussion of hospice care, preferred place of death, and wishes about one's funeral can all have a place. It proves helpful to emphasize that the process of farewell is not a final act, but rather can extend over several weeks or months, and bring many poignant moments to all concerned.

Many patients fear the process of dying. Therefore, to address this actively with medical information and reassurance, permission should be sought as to whether a discussion of this would be helpful. However, individual coping styles vary and not all patients want to discuss dying. Positive avoidance is a legitimate way of coping with life's greatest existential threat. In educating the patient and caregivers about the possible modes of dying, linkage to the goals of excellent symptom management promotes confidence in the care plan and peace. Many patients will cope with their dying by drawing upon religious beliefs, finding sources of spiritual peace, and using rituals long valued by their cultural or ethnic group. Clinicians do well to affirm each person's involvement with such traditions, inviting support from relevant chaplains or pastoral care workers, as available.

The family of the terminally ill provides fundamental support to their ill relative and they have needs of their own as well. Family acceptance of the status of the patient's illness and support for their choices have been shown to facilitate the patient's acceptance of life coming to a close (Walczak *et al.* 2011). Encourage their questions and examine any practical care needs that arise. They may have different information needs to the patient—gain consent from the patient before talking to the family and always give consistent information. Caregivers may want to know about what to expect as the disease progresses and what happens at the time of death. Affirm the importance of respite to avoid burnout and exhaustion in these carers. Recommend the use of home health aids, visiting nurses, or community volunteers, as available.

Early referral to a palliative care service enables key relationships to be established with the patient and their family, while this is still possible. Commitment to care and avoidance of abandonment are crucial. Many physicians understand these principles, but find the burden of end-of-life care challenging. Sharing such healthcare with physicians who choose to specialize in palliative care is entirely appropriate for those who have limited confidence with this aspect of medicine, and can reduce burnout (Vergo and Cullinan 2013). Parallel, shared-care over the latter months of a person's life helps to transition their care into an appropriate palliative care or hospice programme.

In closing any consultation that has covered this process of transitioning to palliative care, taking time to check understanding, answer queries, and affirm a focus on continued living is desirable. Expression of your commitment to care and availability, if needed, serves to reassure both patient and family. Informing the team of any agreement reached in the consultation (with appropriate documentation) helps all subsequent care providers to understand the agreed goals of care.

Strategies: Typical sequence of steps involved in communicating about the transition to palliative care

The communication goal is to guide the patient to understand the goals of care relevant to the palliative approach, focusing on maintaining quality of life. Based on clinical practice guidelines for communicating prognosis and end-of-life issues with adults in the advanced stages of life-limiting illness, and their caregivers, the strategies used to transition a patient from curative to palliative care, using the acronym PREPARED (Clayton *et al.* 2007), are shown in Table 21.1. There are a number of model statements

drawn from these guidelines and systematic reviews (e.g. Parker *et al.* 2007) that we can offer to also guide clinicians in their accomplishment of these strategies.

It is important to consider cultural needs during communication as, in some cultures, the risks of truth telling outweigh the benefits. In some Asian, European, and Middle Eastern cultures, direct statements such as 'you have incurable cancer' may be seen as insensitive and uncaring. Patients in these cultures may prefer indirect communication regarding their condition and prognosis. This can become more complex with variations within groups and immigrants, who take on characteristics of their new country. Recognizing cultural bias and negotiating with the patient and family about decision-making and information preferences offers respect for each patient. See Chapter 40 for more detail about working with interpreters and achieving culturally-competent communication.

Table 21.1 Core strategies when discussing the transition to palliative care

Strategies using the PREPARED acronym	Key skills and tasks	Examples of clinician's comments
Prepare for the discussion, where possible	Gather information about the patient's clinical circumstances and appropriate treatment options Liaise with other relevant healthcare providers Check if an interpreter is required Psychologically prepare yourself Ensure privacy wherever possible Minimize interruptions Negotiate who should be present	'Is there anyone else you would like to be here with you while we talk?' 'If there are things that you might prefer to discuss with me alone, I'd be happy to organize that.'
Relate to the person	Develop rapport Show empathy, care, and compassion during the entire consultation Sustain supportive environment	'This has been a tough time for you and your family, and you have faced the challenges of this illness with great courage.'
Elicit patient and caregiver understanding and preferences for information and involvement in medical decisions	Identify reason for consultation Elicit patient expectations Clarify understanding of their situation Correct misunderstandings Elicit information preferences Consider cultural factors	'What have you been told about your illness and what to expect?' 'What is your sense of how you are doing?' 'Do you have thoughts about where things are going with your illness?' 'What is your biggest concern at the moment?' 'Some people like to know everything that is going on with them and what may happen in the future, others prefer not to know too many details. What do you prefer?'
Provide information tailored to the individual needs of both patients and families	Offer to discuss what to expect in a sensitive manner Alert patient/family if bad news is coming Be honest without being blunt Pace information to the patient's preferences and understanding Explain the uncertainty of prognostic and end-of-life information Avoid being too exact with time frames (unless in the last few days) Avoid jargon Introduce palliative approach Commit to continuity of care	'I've looked at the test results and I'm afraid I have some bad news.' 'I want to talk about three things today: the test results, what this will mean for you; and the treatment that is possible. And you might have some things to discuss too. Is this ok?' 'Every person is different. I can only tell you what usually happens to people in your situation, not exactly what will happen to you.' 'The aim of treatment is changing more towards maximizing your function and comfort.' 'I cannot give you any specific treatment to make this illness go away, but there is a lot we can offer to help you cope with it.' 'Our team will do our best to support you throughout this illness.'

(continued)

Table 21.1 (continued)

Strategies using the PREPARED acronym	Key skills and tasks	Examples of clinician's comments
Acknowledge emotions and concerns	Explore and acknowledge patient's and caregiver's fears and concerns and their emotional reaction Normalize grief Allow some silence Respond empathically to distress	'How are you feeling about what we have discussed?' 'It sounds like this information is different from what you expected, and I think it would be upsetting for anyone.' 'Your tears are appropriate and completely normal.' 'I can't imagine how difficult this is for you.'
(Foster) Realistic hope	Do not give misleading information to positively influence hope Explore and facilitate quality of life goals Emphasize that something can always be done to help Describe elements of good symptom control Promote hope over grief or despair, but do not reassure prematurely Emphasize living over dying Affirm courage if evident	'What are your most important hopes/expectations about the future?' 'What are the things you want to do in the time you have?' 'We have a lot of ways to relieve pain, nausea, breathlessness, or other symptoms.' 'We will do everything we can to ensure that you are as comfortable as possible.' 'Many people find that it helps them to cope by trying to maintain some sense of normality or having a routine.' 'We can prepare for the worst while hoping for the best.'
Encourage questions	Endorse question asking Be prepared to repeat explanations Check understanding of what has been discussed and if the information meets the patient's and caregiver's needs Clarify caregiver's information needs (provided patient consents) Leave the door open for topics to be discussed again in the future	'Is there anything else you would like to discuss?' 'Don't hesitate to ask me again about any of the issues we have discussed today.' 'Have I given you the information you need so far?' 'To make sure we're on the same wavelength, I want to check your understanding of what we have discussed.' 'Is it ok if I tell your caregiver what I have discussed with you? Is there anything I should not discuss?'
Document	Write a summary of the discussion in the medical record Liaise with other key healthcare providers involved in the patient's care	

Adapted from Clayton JM, Hancock KM, Butow PN, et al. 'Clinical practice guidelines for communicating prognosis and end-of-life issues with adults in the advanced stages of a life-limiting illness, and their caregivers'. *Med J Aust* 2007 Suppl; 186(12):S77–S108 © Copyright 2007 The Medical Journal of Australia—reproduced with permission. The Medical Journal of Australia does not accept responsibility for any errors in translation.

Commencing or changing disease-specific, anti-cancer treatments

In the setting of an advanced cancer, the main aims of disease-specific, anti-cancer treatments, such as chemotherapy, are to improve the length and quality of life. Patients are helped by a realistic appraisal of the palliative intent of this treatment—that cure is not a treatment goal, but that the treatment can slow disease progression or ameliorate symptoms (see Table 21.2 for useful phrases for the clinician to use). For the patient to be fully informed and give consent as a result of this discussion, the clinician seeks to ensure that the patient understands the balance between the potential effectiveness of life-prolonging treatments and their side effects. Shared decision-making is an imperative here, with the clinician recognizing the patient's desire about their level of involvement (Hitz *et al.* 2013).

Ceasing disease-specific, anti-cancer treatments

When patients learn about disease progression or the lack of treatment response, clinicians should be ready for the patient to express emotional reactions, such as sadness, anger, or disheartenment. The use of silence, empathic touch, restatement of realistic hopes and

'I wish' statements can be helpful in sitting with the patient's emotion (Jackson *et al.* 2013). The continued availability of the clinical team and non-abandonment are also crucial (see Table 21.2 for useful phrases). An ongoing focus on expert symptomatic care is a means of sustaining the patient's and family's sense of continuing care.

Discussing referral to specialist palliative care teams

Referral to specialist palliative care services may not always be needed or feasible for a particular patient, depending on clinical issues, availability, and financial or insurance considerations. However, where available, referral may assist through provision of extra support for patients and their families. The expertise of the specialist service can improve quality of life through management of difficult physical, psychosocial, or spiritual concerns. Guidelines for making a referral to specialist palliative care services, with useful phrases to facilitate this, are shown in Table 21.2.

Conclusion

Communication skills training for health professionals has been shown to improve patient outcomes in decision-making with early stage disease. Further research is needed to show whether training

Table 21.2 Specific situations where the goals of care change and key strategies to manage them

Situation	Key skills and tasks	Examples of clinician's comments
Commencing or changing disease-specific treatments	Be clear regarding the goals of treatments and what outcomes may be improved, and how likely this is State whether or not survival will be improved by the treatment Give clear information about likely side effects, costs, and time involved Promote consideration of advantages and disadvantages of treatment choices and encourage the patient to share in decision-making according to their desired level of involvement	'There is about an X% chance that this treatment will shrink the tumour. That should make you feel better, but may only extend your life by a few (weeks/months/years).' 'The aim of this treatment is not to cure but to control the disease. This may improve your symptoms and make you feel better.' 'People vary in how they want to make medical decisions. Some people want to make the decision themselves, some people want to share the decision with the doctor, and some want the doctor to make/give a lot of help with the decision. What do you prefer?'
Cessation of disease-specific treatments	Sensitively explain that the disease in not responding to the treatment and that it is likely to cause more harm than benefit. Avoid conveying that nothing more can be done. Emphasize that treatments and support will be provided to help them cope with their illness	'Your disease is no longer responding to the treatment. More of this treatment would give you side effects without improving your disease. It is likely that you will have a better quality of life without it.' 'The aim of treatment is changing from trying to control the disease to minimizing the symptoms you might get.' 'As you get frailer with this illness, we will continue to be there to provide the best available treatments to help control the symptoms and support both you and your family.'
Introducing specialist palliative care services	Refer to palliative care professionals as part of the multidisciplinary team Clarify and correct misconceptions about palliative care services (especially that it is not only for those imminently dying) Discuss the role of the palliative care team, emphasizing expertise in symptom management and a wide range of support services Explain that disease-directed therapy can continue alongside referral to palliative care, and that the primary team will continue to care for the patient also	'I work closely with the palliative care team in looking after patients such as yourself (with COPD/cancer, etc.).' 'Many people have either not heard of palliative care or associate it with dying in the very near future.' 'The palliative care team has a lot to offer as support. This includes pain control and help with other symptoms resulting from your illness.' 'The palliative care team can help manage your symptoms while you continue to receive treatment for your cancer/lung disease/kidney failure.' 'I will still be your main doctor, but the palliative care team will provide extra support and advice about the best medicines for your symptoms.'

Adapted from Clayton JM, Hancock KM, Butow PN, et al. 'Clinical practice guidelines for communicating prognosis and end-of-life issues with adults in the advanced stages of a life-limiting illness, and their caregivers'. *Med J Aust* 2007 Suppl; 186(12):S77–S108 © Copyright 2007 The Medical Journal of Australia—reproduced with permission. The Medical Journal of Australia does not accept responsibility for any errors in translation. Source: data from Evans, W *et al.* 2006; Van Vliet, L *et al.* 2013; Hitz, F. *et al.* 2013; Parker, S *et al.* 2007; Jackson, V *et al.* 2013; Shin, J and Temel, J 2013; Temel, J *et al.* 2010; and Vergo, M and Cullinan, A 2013.

for health professionals will improve outcomes for patients and their families during the transition to palliative care. However, it is possible that communicating in the ways above may reduce patient anxiety, help patients to make appropriate decisions, and avoid overly burdensome and costly treatments at the end of life. Other objectives include the reduction of barriers to referral to specialist palliative care and the use of timely referrals. Achieving an adaptive adjustment to disease progression and preparation for death is a worthy goal of care.

Clinical scenarios for introducing or transitioning patients to palliative care

Here we offer two variations of role play scenarios; the first in the setting of advanced cancer, and the second when the patient is on dialysis with progressive non-malignant diseases. These are intended for experiential encounters with simulated patients, which permit rehearsal of the principles covered in this chapter.

Exemplar clinical scenario for advanced cancer

Emíly is 48-year-old nurse and mother of two teenage children. She has developed advanced ovarian cancer. Chemotherapy and

surgery to reduce tumour bulk have contained her disease over four years. A partial bowel obstruction has occurred recently, but settled with nasogastric drainage. Emíly knows at some level that her days are limited.

Instruction to the patient, Emíly

As a nurse, you remember seeing patients with ovarian cancer die. They seemed to have the worst deaths—feculent vomiting, such suffering. What will your death be like? You lie awake at night thinking about this. It is too hard to discuss with your husband. You fear that your death will be horrible. It can only get worse, can't it? And then you think of your children, two fun-loving girls, 13 and 15 years old. How sad to leave them! How unfair this wretched illness is! You sense a deep grief within you as you contemplate this reality. You must talk to someone about your fears. Who can help you with this terrible plight?

Instruction to her husband, Jorge

You are an accountant whose life was going beautifully until your wife took ill. Now, two surgeries and a batch of chemotherapy treatments later, you are deeply aware of her fear and sad demeanour. You admire her resilience and you do your best to protect her, to keep up a brave front. Yet you also worry about what will happen. How long does she have? She tells you that this cancer will kill her. What does the future hold?

Instruction to the oncologist/nurse

Emíly is a warm, religious, Latina woman. She has been a pleasure to treat and you sense there is great courage in her. Her recent bowel obstruction has brought some sadness to her demeanour. You want to discuss the role of a venting gastrostomy for drainage in place of her current nasogastric tube. You believe it is time to stop chemotherapy, as her disease has progressed through several regimens. You have a sense that she also wants to talk more about her illness.

Instruction to role play observers

Discussing the transition to palliative care is a challenging task, in which cultures differ enormously in their approaches, and each clinician approaches it differently. Your task is to add depth to the cultural sensitivity needed in this setting. Take careful note of the conversation, the phrases used in this role play, so that you can assist the discussion and help strategizing about how to communicate more effectively.

Key tips in training actors as simulated patients

In these simulations, be prepared to ask the clinician frank questions like, 'Am I going to die?' and 'Are you giving up on me, doctor?' The aim here is to confront the clinician with the inevitability of the cancer's progression and make sure there is potential for the discussion of palliative care. Other useful questions include, 'What is palliative care?', 'Will the drainage tube be permanent?', 'Does a referral to hospice mean that I'm dying, doctor?', and 'Can you promise a peaceful death, doctor?'

Clinical scenario for progressive renal and cardiac disease

Fred is a 61-year-old man with end-stage kidney failure due to IgA nephropathy. He has been on haemodialysis for five years. He has a history of ischaemic heart disease with previous bypass grafting and multiple stents. He recently had another heart attack and his heart specialist has told him that there is no further intervention possible. He often drops his blood pressure on dialysis. He has increasing angina, now happening every day. Fred is wondering how long the dialysis can keep him going for.

Instruction to the patient, Fred

Your cardiologist has told you that your heart will keep getting worse and worse, and that they cannot do anything else. He said you might die from a heart attack. You have pain in your chest several times every day and feel short of breath all the time. It is getting harder for you to do things for yourself. You are upset that you have lost your independence and feel like you are a burden to your caring wife and son, who is studying at university. Getting ready and going for dialysis three times a week feels like torture. You have heard that some people stop having dialysis, but you are not sure who to talk to about this and you don't want to let your doctors down. You wonder what would happen if you stopped, and what your family would think.

Instructions to his wife, Joanne

You can see that Fred is struggling and getting weaker every day. You want to help him but he is reluctant to accept it. He seems to be in a lot of pain, but doesn't complain. He dutifully gets up to go to dialysis three times a week, even though you can see it takes so much out of him. You are frightened that he could just have a big heart attack at home and die suddenly—what would you do? Who could you call on for help?

Instructions to the doctor/nurse

Fred is a down-to-earth, pragmatic sort of man. He has been very stoic and never really complained, but always complied with whatever treatment was recommended. You feel that his prognosis is poor, likely only weeks due to his heart, but you are not sure if he and his wife realize this. The dialysis nurse has told you that he asked her what would happen if he stopped having dialysis. You want to explore this, and let him know that things are not going so well so that he and his family have time to prepare. You also want to introduce palliative care so they can have extra support at home.

Instructions to role play observers

Discussing the transition to palliative care is a challenging task, and can be especially difficult with non-malignant illness. Take careful note of the conversation, the phrases used in this role play, so that you can assist the discussion and help strategizing about how to communicate more effectively.

Key tips in training actors as simulated patients

In these simulations, be prepared to ask the clinician frank questions like, 'How long do I have?' and 'Is it suicide to stop dialysis?' The aim here is to confront the clinician with the clinical deterioration and make sure there is potential for the discussion of palliative care. Other useful questions include, 'What is palliative care?', 'If I stop dialysis can I change my mind?' and 'What will happen to me if I stop dialysis?'

References

Baile W, Palmer J, Bruera E, Parker P (2011). Assessment of palliative care cancer patients' most important concerns. *Support Care Cancer* **19**, 475–81.

Clayton J, Hancock K, Butow P, *et al.* (2007). Clinical practice guidelines for communicating prognosis and end-of-life issues with adults in the advanced stages of a life-limiting illness, and their caregivers. *Med J Aust* **186**, S77–8.

Daugherty C, Hlubocky F (2008). Are terminally ill cancer patients told about their expected deaths? a study of cancer physicians' self-reports of prognosis disclosure. *J Clin Oncol* **26**, 5988–93.

Evans W, Tulsky J, Back A, Arnold R (2006). Communication at times of transitions: how to help patients cope with loss and re-define hope. *Cancer J* **12**, 417–24.

Gwyther L, Krakauer E (2009). WPCA Policy statement on defining palliative care. *Worldwide Palliative Care Alliance.*

Haines IJ (2011). Managing patients with advanced cancer: the benefits of early referral for palliative care *Med J Aust* **194**, 107–8.

Hitz F, Ribi K, Li Q, Klingbiel D, Cerny T, Koeberle D (2013). Predictors of satisfaction with treatment decision, decision-making preferences, and main treatments goals in patients with advanced cancer *Support Care Cancer* **21**, 3085–93.

Innes S, Payne S (2009). Advanced cancer patients' prognostic information preferences: a review. *Palliat Med* **23**, 29–39.

Jackson V, Jacobsen J, Greer J, Pirl W, Temel J, Back A (2013). The cultivation of prognostic awareness through the provision of early palliative care in the ambulatory setting: a communication guide. *J Palliat Med* **16**, 894–900.

Khan S, Gomes B, Higginson I (2014). End-of-life care—what do cancer patients want?. *Nature Rev Clin Oncol* **11**, 100–8.

Lunney J, Lynn J, Foley D, Lipson S, Guralnik J (2003). Patterns of functional decline at the end of life. *J Am Med Assoc* **289**, 2387–92.

Mack J, Cronin A, Keating N, *et al.* (2012). Associations between end-of-life discussion characteristics and care received near death: a prospective cohort study. *J Clin Oncol* **30**, 4387–95.

Parker S, Clayton J, Hancock K, *et al.* (2007). A systematic review of prognostic/end-of-life communication with adults in the advanced stages of a life-limiting illness: patient/caregiver preferences for the content, style, and timing of information. *J Pain Symptom Manage* **34**, 81–93.

Rabow M, Kvale E, Barbour L, *et al.* (2013). Moving upstream: a review of the evidence of the impact of outpatient palliative care. *J Palliat Med* **16**, 1540–9.

Shin J, Temel J (2013). Integrating palliative care: when and how? *Curr Opin Pulm Med* **19**, 344–9.

Smith T, Temin S, Alesi E, *et al.* (2012). American Society of Clinical Oncology provisional clinical opinion: the integration of palliative care into standard oncology care. *J Clin Oncol* **30**, 880–7.

Temel J, Greer J, Muzikansky A, *et al.* (2010). Early palliative care for patients with metastatic non-small cell lung cancer. *N Engl J Med* **363**, 733–42.

Van Vliet L, Francke A, Tomson S, Plum N, Van der Wall E, Bensing J (2013). When cure is no option: How explicit and hopeful can information be given? A qualitative study in breast cancer. *Patient Educ Couns* **90**, 315–22.

Vergo M, Cullinan A (2013). Joining together to improve outcomes: integrating specialty palliative care into the care of patients with cancer. *J Natl Compr Canc Netw* **11**, S38–46.

Walczak A, Butow P, Davidson P, *et al.* (2011). Patient perspectives regarding communication about prognosis and end-of-life issues: How can it be optimised? *Patient Educ Couns* **90**, 307–14.

Weeks J, Catalano P, Cronin A, *et al.* (2012). Patients' expectations about effect of chemotherapy for advanced cancer. *N Engl J Med* **367**, 1616–25.

Wong S, Kreuter W, O'Hare A (2012). Treatment intensity at the end of life in older adults receiving long-term dialysis. *Arch Intern Med* **172**, 661–3.

Wright A, Zhang B, Ray A, *et al.* (2008). Associations between end-of-life discussions, patient mental health, medical care near death, and caregiver bereavement adjustment. *J Am Med Assoc* **300**, 1665–73.

CHAPTER 22

Talking about dying: End-of-life communication training

Tomer T. Levin and Alison Wiesenthal

Introduction to end- of- life communication training

End-of-life communication skills training (CST) targets effective clinician–patient–family discussion at a vulnerable turning point in life. It aims to improve clinical outcomes, such as the sensitive and effective discussion of death and dying. This chapter discusses the core communication goals, strategies, and skills used to talk about dying. It considers the family meeting a portal for communication around decision-making, withdrawal of life-extending treatment, directives to Allow Natural Death (AND) (formerly called Do-Not-Resuscitate (DNR) directives) (Levin and Coyle 2015), and discussing prognosis. Common pitfalls of CST are identified.

The goal of end-of-life communication training: Sensitive implementation of palliative care

An important rate-limiting step for the implementation of palliative care is clear and empathic clinician–patient–family communication. End-of-life discussions with advanced cancer patients need to avoid futile medical care near death, and facilitate earlier hospice referrals (Wright *et al.* 2008). Additionally, cancer patients who die in a hospital or intensive care unit (ICU) have worse quality of life compared with those who die at home; therefore, it is crucial that these conversations take place in a timely manner.

Palliative care curricula (Weissman *et al.* 2007) alone are not enough. CST promoting effective communication is the vital link between emotional support and good decision-making.

It is burdensome to increase a dying person's suffering with invasive interventions that do not improve length or quality of life, such as ICU admissions or cardiopulmonary resuscitation (CPR). Minimal use of CPR during end-stage cancer is one proxy measure of effective communication, and the timeliness of discussions clarifying treatment goals near death is another. For example, the majority of DNR directives at a national cancer centre were completed the same day that the patient died, suggesting reduced attention to advance care planning (Levin *et al.* 2008). The National Comprehensive Cancer Network guidelines state that goals of care discussions should ideally be held when the prognosis is still years (Levy *et al.* 2014).

Discussion of death and dying in oncology should be a predictable process rather than an unexpected crisis. One in five Americans die in the ICU (Angus *et al.* 2004), and an estimated 90% of these involve withholding or withdrawing life-extending care. These data imply that CST can be applied to planning and training for these communication challenges.

One illustration of how the predictability of death can be harnessed in the ICU was seen when automatic ethics consultations occurred for mechanical ventilation >96 hours. It found significantly improved communication, more DNR directives, increased withdrawal of life-extending care, and reduced ICU length of stay (LOS) (Dowdy *et al.* 1998), and sits in contrast to the model where ethics consults are called only as a result of crisis.

Palliative care outcomes such as the quality of patient and family-centred decision-making, emotional, spiritual, and practical support, symptom management, LOS, family burden (caregiver burnout, depression, post-traumatic stress disorder), and the overall quality of, and satisfaction with, care can all be improved by CST (Curtis and Engelberg 2006).

Patient and family-centred communication in cancer care

Patient-centredness is achieved through six core functions of clinician–patient communication: 'fostering healing relationships, exchanging information, responding to emotions, managing uncertainty, making decisions and enabling patient self-management' (Epstein and Street 2007). Patients are embedded in the matrix of their families. Distress and decision-making reverberate through the family unit, and their burdens are often shared. Family can become second order patients, and this phenomenon is more common as death nears. One important opportunity for discussion of death and dying is the family meeting, a forum central to decision-making processes (Curtis 2004). It is generally desirable for a third party to be present for these significant conversations.

Sequence of strategies for end-of-life communication

Broadly accepted strategies for discussing dying are set out in Box 22.1 and detailed below. This sequence of strategies represents the approach that is taught in Memorial Sloan Kettering Cancer Center's Comskil laboratory.

Box 22.1 Sequence of strategies for the end-of-life patient and family conference

1. Pre-conference clinical team meeting

2. Opening: introductions and agenda

3. Explore the patient's and family's understanding of the illness, prognosis, and goals of care. Correct misperceptions. Educate about illness/prognosis:

   - Address emotions evoked by the discussion using empathic skills (see Table 22.2)

4. Explore plans, perceptions, and concerns regarding death and dying in one of three ways:

   - Ask directly

   - Ask about past experiences with death and dying among family or friends. Clarify how these might impact current end-of-life planning both positively and negatively. In the latter, explore potential improvements in care so that negative experiences of the dying are not repeated

   - Substituted decision-making: If the patient lacks capacity (e.g. unconscious), the family can be asked to reflect on, 'Who the patient is as a person?' with the medical team, and 'If the patient could speak to us right now, how might he or she guide us in our decision-making?'

   Following on from these questions, educate the patient/family about Allow Natural Death directives, CPR, prognosis, palliative care, and the dying process.

   Clinical Pearl: Use the words 'death', 'dying', and 'dying process'

5. Make guiding recommendations for end-of-life care (e.g. Allow Natural Death directives, withdrawal of life-extending care, or hospice care):

   - Use the shared decision-making approach to ease the burden of responsibility

   - Consider a time-limited decision delay to facilitate consultation with other family members or a trial of further treatment

   - Reassure the patient and family that they will be supported through the terminal process (non-abandonment), and that treating pain, suffering, and helping the family cope are priorities

   Clinical Pearl: Promote consensus for end-of-life decisions by asking family members and clinicians to weigh in; consider standards of reasonableness (e.g. how others in a similar situation might respond). Reinforce consensus by summarizing and asking for feedback.

6. Finalize the action plan:

   - Summarize the goals of care, and the utility of the Allow Natural Death directives within this context

   - Offer practical assistance and education; for example symptom management, spiritual needs, what to expect as death approaches

   - Set time for next meeting or update; elicit feedback

Pre-conference clinical team meeting

A multidisciplinary discussion is a prerequisite to reach consensus among team members about prognosis, the goals of care, 'Allow Natural Death' directives, and recommendations to remove ineffective life-extending interventions, so that the patient and family do not receive conflicting messages. A quiet room with seating for all helps to facilitate a supportive and open dialogue. If the meeting must be conducted at the bedside, protection of privacy is important. In multibed hospital rooms, the discussion could be upsetting to neighbours who cannot help but overhear. Clinicians should determine who constitutes the functional family and need to attend the meeting.

Opening: Introductions and agenda

The meeting, usually led by a senior clinician, and the seating arrangements set a tone of warmth and dialogue (rather than two opposing teams facing each other). Each family member and clinician should be introduced by name and role.

An opening empathic statement (see Table 22.1) helps to build trust: 'I know that this is a difficult time for your family …'

Next, set the agenda collaboratively: 'We would like to update you about your loved one's situation, and discuss the goals of our medical care. What would you like to put on our agenda?'

Clinical Pearl: For the clinician to refer to death in their introductory comments, s/he would need to know that earlier conversations about prognosis and palliative care have acknowledged the reality of death. If these have not yet occurred, the clinician should examine the goals of care first, then gradually and sensitively draw towards death talk.

Table 22.1 Ten skills for responding to emotions in end-of-life communication

Technique	Example
1. Normalizing/validation	'It is normal to be upset at difficult moments …' 'It is understandable that you are angry …'
2. Empathic observation	'You really have had a difficult time …'
3. Name/acknowledge emotion	'You seem sad …' 'I can see that you are upset …'
4. Encourage expression	'Tell me more about how you are feeling …'
5. Praise	'You are very brave …'
6. Paraphrase and repeat back	'If I understand you correctly, you are angry because you were told that your mother's pneumonia would respond to antibiotics …'
7. Express regret	'I am sorry that things have not turned out as we would have wished.'
8. Elicit feedback	'How did you feel about our meeting today? I know that it is not easy discussing death and the process of dying.'
9. Silence	A non-verbal way to say, 'I understand.'
10. Gesture or touch	Offering tissues; touching the patient's arm

Explore the patient and family understanding of the illness, prognosis, and goals of care

Ask open-ended questions, such as, 'How do you see the medical situation at the moment … Where do you see things heading?' Encourage narration: 'Tell me more …'.

When gathering information, listen empathically to improve rapport. More listening is correlated with higher family satisfaction (Curtis and Engelberg 2006) but can seem contrary to an action-oriented medical culture. A common communication error is for the clinician to embark on a medical monologue without first checking what is already understood. The patient and family may already know clinical, prognostic, and laboratory parameters from previous discussions with staff.

Having assessed understanding of the illness and prognosis, the clinician can correct misperceptions, and educate or update as necessary.

Clinical Pearl: Always respond to emotions before moving ahead with other agenda items. Reduction of emotional tension decreases the bracing for threat (fight, flight, freeze reaction) and promotes a learning mindset, which is essential for problem-solving. Ten common ways of addressing emotions are outlined in Table 22.1.

Explore plans, perceptions, and concerns regarding death and dying

a. Ask directly: The patient may already have well-developed thoughts about end-of-life goals of care (e.g. place of death, Allow Natural Death directives, hospice), which have evolved as the cancer worsened. Just ask! They may or may not have been articulated—cultural or family taboos about discussing death may have kept them covert. Nevertheless, most patients and families are grateful when they can share their thoughts about death and dying with a caring clinician.

Education about palliative care is vital at this juncture: 'What is your understanding of hospice care? … Correct, it is used when the cancer cannot be cured, to maximize quality of life, and allow a natural death …'

Clinical Pearl: It takes practice to discuss AND directives. Done empathically and with early recognition that the patient has entered their dying phase, we avoid the communication trap of mentioning it as an aside, at the end of the meeting, not allowing enough time to thoroughly process the concept cognitively and emotionally.

b. Ask about past experiences of death in family or friends: Useful exploratory questions include, 'Have you or anyone you know ever faced a similar circumstance in dealing with death? … What went well when your father had home hospice care? What could have gone better?' Past experience with a trustworthy hospice service may be reassuring. Negative experiences, such as a painful death, can be used to facilitate discussion of how the dying experience might be improved. The challenge here is the difficulty of talking about past losses at a time of imminent loss. Nevertheless, approaches that build on past experiences have an intrinsic strength.

c. Substituted decision-making: Where there is a lack of capacity to make medical decisions (e.g. the patient is unconscious), invite the family to describe who the patient is as a person, and how s/he might tackle the end of life. The substituted decision by a healthcare proxy serves ethically to (i) preserve the wishes of an incapacitated patient, and (ii) promote decisions that are in his or her best interests (Curtis 2004). If the patient has an advance directive, discussing it now is helpful.

Make guiding recommendations for end-of-life care

While respecting the spirit of shared decision-making, the physician should make a clear and guiding recommendation, so as to share the burden of decision-making near the end of life: 'Having weighed up all the alternatives, our recommendation is that it is reasonable at this time to stop the breathing machine, and let your loved one die as peacefully and naturally as possible. I know how difficult it is to hear this … [empathic silence].' Requiring that the family make the decision to 'pull the plug' can have a negative psychological impact on bereavement because they now feel complicit in the death of the patient at a moment when they feel most vulnerable (Wright *et al.* 2010).

Frequently, patients and families relate instances of an absence of a guiding voice, causing iatrogenic psychological trauma (Weiner and Roth 2006); at the other extreme, overly pessimistic physicians can demoralize their patients. Some physicians may prescribe more chemotherapy when asked to 'do something more', to the detriment of palliative and family care.

Done correctly, a guiding voice and clear end-of-life communication can produce effective outcomes. Lautrette and colleagues' randomized controlled communication training intervention had a mitigating effect on the traumatizing effect of an ICU death on families—90 days after the death, family members in the intervention group reported significantly lower post-traumatic symptoms and anxiety/depression scores (Lautrette *et al.* 2007). Better communication and more supportive decision-making can prevent unnecessary, later symptoms of bereavement-related distress.

Clinical Pearl: Inquire directly about death and dying, and the patient's view on their goals of care *before* recommending care transitions or an AND directive. It aids decision-making if the groundwork for the decision is already under active contemplation, rather than assuming a pre-contemplative stance: 'It sounds like an Allow Natural Death directive would be in keeping with your mother's wishes not to linger, and to die with the same dignity that she lived her life.'

Fear and doubt are ubiquitous, so consensus building is a vital step to consolidate support for any decision. This involves asking each family and clinical member to weigh in, summarize, or give feedback, and, in so doing, to address ambivalence.

Here, specific types of clinician reassurance are helpful: the patient will not be abandoned before death; staff will do everything to maximize patient comfort and minimize suffering; support for the family's decision to withdraw futile life-extending care will be provided (Stapleton *et al.* 2006). Praising the patient's and family's strengths in the face of adversity can be used to additionally bolster their sense of cohesion.

End-of-life decisions can also be framed by known standards to further garner consensus:

◆ Reasonableness: 'I think that *we* are making the most reasonable decision given the options.'

◆ How others in the same situation responded: 'The majority of people in your situation choose an Allow Natural Death directive as the most reasonable way to facilitate the process of natural death.' In one recent study, this type of phraseology resulted in more surrogates declining CPR likely to be futile (Barnato and Arnold 2013).

Where there is still uncertainty, a useful strategy is offering a time-limited empirical trial. Such careful reflection highlights the gravity of end-of-life decision-making (Rubenfeld and Crawford 2001): 'Let's see how your father does with another 24 hours on antibiotics, blood pressure support, and the breathing machine. If he does not respond, this will be helpful evidence that we should consider stopping the breathing machine, and let him die as peacefully and naturally as possible. Can we meet tomorrow morning to reassess Dad's situation and continue this discussion?'

Resistance to discussing dying is a cue for further exploration. For instance, a family may worry that they are killing their loved one by discussing end-of-life issues or be at a loss to imagine how they will cope alone, after the patient's death. An invitation such as 'Tell me more about why this conversation is so hard for you' can be revealing.

Additionally, contradictory wishes, such as both wanting to fight and desiring a peaceful death, can be adaptive (e.g. 'hope for the best and plan for the worst') or confusing; it is common for patients to express different wishes at different times in their illness trajectory (Hsieh *et al.* 2006).

Finalize the action plan

The end of the meeting is an opportunity to elicit feedback on the discussion, reinforcing a collaborative approach. The discussion should be summarized and the next steps specified. Problem solve specific practical issues (e.g. hospice, symptom management, spiritual needs). Parameters for the next meeting should be arranged to foster a sense of ongoing support.

Conflict over end-of-life communication

Good communication involves the better handling of end-of-life conflict and use of the consensus-promoting skills just described. Viewing end-of-life communication as a predictable and ongoing process, rather than an emergency, is an important frame of reference. This allows, for example, regular family meetings to be scheduled quite early on to promote a culture of palliative care. While conflict resolution can be aided by empathy and patience, ignoring disagreements can lead to festering wounds. We recommend more proactive approaches, such as early consultation with palliative care, psychiatry, the institution's ethics committee, social work, chaplaincy, patient representatives, and second opinions. Consultations promote dialogue which, in turn, fosters understanding and builds consensus.

Specific strategies for withdrawal of life-sustaining treatments

Withdrawal of life-extending treatment should be protocol-driven and carried out with the same meticulous care as any other medical procedure. A protocol buffers against the stuttering withdrawal of futile life-extending care. This can occur as a corollary of clinicians avoiding uncomfortable communication with the patient and family, or taking responsibility for guiding and facilitating the dying process.

Informed consent helps to promote communication and transparency, and an explicit plan for carrying out the procedure and dealing with complications promotes confidence in the medical decision.

Moving the patient to an appropriate setting for end-of-life care is helpful to the patient and family who are experiencing anticipatory grief. Typically this is a private room, or hospice setting with less medical technology. For patients who wish to die at home, setting up appropriate levels of home hospice services can facilitate the quality of the journey ahead.

Stopping electronic monitoring and routine blood tests enables focus on the whole person and family needs. However, it requires specific communication to patients and families to make this transition possible as technology may represent a symbol of 'trying' or maintaining life-extending treatment.

Clarification that 'the withholding of life-sustaining treatment' does not equate to 'withdrawal of care' is another helpful, pre-emptive communication strategy.

Finally, it is important that the process be evaluated in terms of outcomes with an eye to using these data for quality improvement. Care in the last hours of life is now seen as a core competency that includes attending to the grief and bereavement of the family (Ferris *et al.* 2003); the heart of this process is effective communication.

Specific strategies for discussing requests to die sooner

Patient requests to hasten death should not be blocked reflexively by saying that euthanasia is illegal or not your practice. Clinicians should instead explore these statements in an empathic manner: 'I'd like to hear more about your desire for me to help you die. Tell me what's on your mind.' More specific questions can elicit suffering: 'What is the hardest part about what you are going through?'

At one end of the spectrum, such requests for hastened death may represent fluctuating existential distress—an attempt to come to terms with an impending death. At the other end, they may reflect demoralization, depression, panic, suicidal ideation, or poorly controlled pain, all of which are potentially treatable (Hudson *et al.* 2006).

Requests to die sooner should be seen as a communication opportunity to engage the patient in their advance care planning (Back *et al.* 2002).

Use of video tools

Watching an educational video about the local hospice may help to demystify dying and facilitate decision-making. Volandes and colleagues have taken this a step further by creating brief videos to teach patients with late stage cancer about advance care planning, positing that we learn better by viewing images as opposed to hearing the doctor talking (Volandes *et al.* 2013). These videos (available at http://www.acpdecisions.org/) contain images of patients in the dying phase of their illness, with examples of ventilated patients, patients receiving hospice care, and simulated CPR.

Patients with advanced cancer who watched the video were more likely to decline CPR compared to patients who only heard the verbal narrative (Volandes *et al.* 2013). Additionally, low health literacy (but not race) was predictive of desiring more aggressive end-of-life (EOL) care, but the educational video helped both those with low and normal health literacy to make similar decisions (Volandes *et al.* 2008). These data are strong enough to suggest that such videos be routinely used to assist in discussions about advance care planning.

Clinician skill deficits and distortions in thinking

CST aims to correct skill deficits; approaches to common communication errors are presented in Table 22.2.

Another approach is to consider the clinician's emotional reaction to EOL discussions, traditionally called countertransference in psychiatric jargon, which can often present a barrier to palliative care. For example, physicians who sense that death talk will be upsetting to the patient, and who are uncomfortable managing the outpouring of emotion may continue giving ineffective chemotherapy to avoid discussing prognosis. CST can reframe the clinician's distorted belief by helping the learner to explore alternative ways of perceiving the dilemma: 'Would the patient or family be pleased to be given the chance to talk about their worst fears? Could end-of-life planning be helpful or meaningful for the family? Might the patient be grateful if you were able to guide them to achieve a better and more peaceful death for their father?'

A clinician's prior personal losses can be reactivated by discussions of death, but they can also fuel a desire to bring about better palliative care. In this context, CST can be a safe environment for personal reflection and growth. One illustrative programme was designed to improve end-of-life communication by focusing primarily on the clinician's emotional reaction to personal loss (Favre et al. 2007).

Table 22.2 Common pitfalls in end-of-life communication and alternative approaches

Approaches to avoid	Why this approach is problematic	Alternative approaches
1. There is nothing more that can be done	Although chemotherapy may no longer be helpful, symptomatic treatments can improve quality of life.	'We will strive to improve your quality of life, treat the pain, and support you and your family as best we can.'
2. If he gains more weight, we can give him more chemotherapy	EOL goals of care are deferred under the illusion that the cancer is curable. The patient is coerced to eat more, and may be blamed for not trying hard enough. Family focuses on eating rather than best supportive care.	'Your father's weight loss is because the cancer has spread. Chemotherapy may harm him more than help. We have many other ways of assisting him to be home and live as meaningful a life as possible.'
3. If your heart stops, would YOU want us to do everything?	Cardiac arrest is disconnected from multiorgan failure in a dying cancer patient, and is described as an isolated mechanical problem. Responsibility for the 'Allow Natural Death' directive is placed on the patient ('you'), rather than being a shared decision. The ineffectiveness of CPR at the end of life is not discussed, although in the physician's mind, implied; 'To do everything' is a euphemism for futile CPR, but the patient is unlikely to appreciate the illusion of this 'choice.'	'What do you know about CPR? Have you known anyone who required CPR?' This facilitates education about CPR at the EOL: 'Although CPR can help otherwise healthy people with heart attacks, it is usually ineffective when cancer is widespread, and would not be consistent with your goal of maximizing your quality of life ...' [empathic silence] 'May I share my thoughts on using CPR in your case? I don't think that CPR will help you. It will not reverse the cancer and you may die on a breathing machine in the ICU, which defeats your goal to make death as peaceful and natural as possible.'
4. If your heart was to stop, you would not want us to institute heroic measures, would you?	The opposite of heroism is cowardice. No one would want cowardly measures instituted, so this question has a coercive tone. 'Heroic measures' is a medical euphemism for ineffectual CPR at the end of life, but the patient may not understand this hidden meaning.	'What are your thoughts about the spread of your cancer? Do you worry about dying?' [Talk openly about death; use the term 'dying' rather than euphemisms]
5. His illness has progressed. His cancer is advanced	The words 'progressed' and 'advanced' have positive connotations in our society; however, in this context, progress, and advancement are euphemisms for dying.	'I am afraid that he has entered the dying phase of his illness.'
6. He has failed third-line treatment	The patient should not be blamed for the failure of treatment.	'The third-line chemo did not work. This cancer has spread despite our best efforts.'
7. If I talk about death, the patient will give up hope	There is no evidence that talking realistically about death results in loss of hope. On the contrary, a supportive EOL discussion helps the patient and family to prepare. Avoidance of death talk causes a 'conspiracy of silence' that worsens isolation and demoralization.	'While the cancer is not curable, there are still many things we can do to assist. Would it be helpful to talk together about the dying process, and plan together so that we can help you and your family to better deal with this challenge?'
8. CPR means pounding on your chest to restart your heart, likely cracking your ribs. Next they shove a big tube down your throat ...	This approach is coercive, traumatizing, and not in the spirit of shared decision-making or patient-centred care.	'CPR will not extend your life. It will more likely prolong your suffering and interfere with our goal of a natural death.'
9. This patient is in denial	Labelling patients as being 'in denial' sets them up as adversaries who must be convinced of imminent death. This erodes trust, making decision-making more complicated.	'How serious is the cancer? Where do you see things going? Have you given thought to what might happen in the future?' Decision-making is seen as a process of discovery that will evolve over time.

Using end-of-life discussions as a pathway to healing

The drive to heal is paramount to the human condition, even when facing death. Byock's book, *The Four Things that Matter Most*, describes four conversations that you should have before you die: 'Please forgive me. I forgive you. Thank you. I love you' (Byock 2004). Compassionate communication should lead to a healing and comforting discussion with the patient and family.

Kissane and colleagues' family-focused therapy uses the period leading up to death and the bereavement period to heal family conflict and rifts, improve cohesion and communication; so that death, almost paradoxically, strengthens the family rather than weakening it (Kissane *et al.* 2006).

Standardized role play scenarios

CST uses role plays to simulate and practice talk of death and dying. The best role play scenarios are constructed from actual cases, so that the challenges are tailored to disciplines (e.g. a surgical learner gets a surgical case) and the details are realistic.

Practising the ways to discuss modes of dying (see Table 22.3) lifts a learner's confidence, empowering them to share information that can be immensely reassuring to patients who fear what the future holds.

Conclusion

While CST focuses on improving communication to foster better end-of-life outcomes for patients and their families, these are among the most difficult conversations to conduct. Even a simulated CST session on talking about dying can be exhausting for learners. Clinicians are therefore assisted by a structured approach

that they can practise in the safety of a simulation laboratory, which promotes anticipation and planning for communication. While demonstrable competency in end-of-life communication should be a goal of the field, it should not detract from this being a personal and caring conversation between individuals at a time of crisis. The vulnerability of clinicians, patients, and families is often exposed in discussing death and dying; this should be acknowledged, and seen as an opportunity for growth, guidance, healing, and humanism.

Clinical scenarios for role play with simulated patients and family members

Here are some clinical scenarios that can be used for role plays discussing death and dying. One is located in the ICU, another is a patient with breast cancer, and the third involves colorectal cancer.

Planning for death in the ICU

Substituted decision-making about end-of-life care is not uncommon in the ICU, where communication occurs with the relative holding a medical power of attorney and their support persons. This case simulates an ICU family meeting to discuss end-of-life goals of care and an AND directive.

Mrs. Green is a 77-year-old retired widow with widely metastatic gastric cancer. She has continued to deteriorate despite several treatment regimens. She now has brain metastases. She underwent surgery three weeks ago for an ischaemic bowel, with multiple complications including sepsis and shock. Her MPM (mortality predicted model) prognostic score was 98% on admission to the ICU, which means that she was critically ill and, statistically, very likely to die during the admission. She has been on vasopressor support and ventilated in the ICU since surgery. She is now in anuric renal

Table 22.3 Ways to discuss modes of dying: the clinician is responsible for predicting clinical deterioration depending on each patient's circumstances

Anticipated mode of dying	Example of clinical communication
Always seek permission to do this before discussing any selected mode of dying	'Would it be helpful to learn more about what might happen when you die?'
Death from liver failure	'As your skin becomes yellower (what we call jaundice), you will gradually feel sleepier and will sleep more each day. If you develop nausea or itchy skin, we will give medication to lessen these. It can be a peaceful way to die.'
Death from respiratory failure	'We will help alleviate any breathlessness with medication to keep you calm. When the carbon dioxide level in your blood rises, you will become drowsy. It can be difficult for relatives to see your body breathing hard. We will reassure them and promise to keep you peaceful.'
Death from acute events	'Some 25% of cancer patients die suddenly from a cardiac event, sudden haemorrhage, severe infection, or from a clot travelling to the lungs. Sudden death limits suffering, yet it can still come unexpectedly.'
Death from a brain tumour	'The tumour can press on areas of your brain, and your arm or leg may become weakened. We will control any headache with medication. Eventually you will become drowsy and gradually drift off.'
Death from renal failure	'When your kidneys stop making urine, levels of minerals will build up in your bloodstream. They'll make you feel fatigued, and one day they may interrupt the normal rhythm of your heart. We will use medicine to keep you comfortable.'
Death from haemorrhage	'The location of your cancer creates some risk of bleeding. If this happens, we will apply pressure with towels to slow the bleeding and give you a sedative injection. We promise to keep you comfortable.'
Concluding comments	'Whatever way the dying process unfolds, our commitment is to look after you, maintain your comfort, and treat any symptoms that would otherwise upset you. We will aim for a very peaceful death. Let me check now ... do you have any questions?'

failure. It was decided that continuous renal replacement therapy (CRRT) would be incongruous with palliative care goals. You have conferred with your colleagues. It seems likely that she will die within days.

Your task is to now talk to her daughter, Henrietta, and her son-in-law, Bert, about the patient's condition, prognosis, goals of care, and in this context, the usefulness of an Allow Natural Death directive.

Advanced breast cancer at the end of life

Nadia is a 38-year-old married mother of two children aged 10 and 8; she works as a molecular biologist and her husband is an engineer.

You have used six different regimens of chemotherapy over four years in your efforts to palliate Nadia's cancer. You are running out of tumour-directed therapy options. The bone metastases have been helped by radiation therapy; pain is quite well controlled. However, the liver metastases have replaced most of her liver, her albumin has fallen, she has lost quite a lot of weight, and now some ascites has emerged. You had it drained by paracentesis this week. Her liver function enzymes have now become quite elevated, prothrombin has risen, and her bilirubin has just begun to rise. You perceive that Nadia is on the cusp of irreversible liver failure.

Talking to Nadia about her end-of-life care

When you saw her last week, you arranged for the hospice home care service to begin visiting her and to begin to transition her care to the palliative care service. There was much to talk about. Where might she prefer to die? Had she put her affairs in order?

Nadia now returns one week later because she has further questions that she wishes to ask you. You can see the icteric colour of her sclera, as her skin starts ever so faintly to turn yellow. She is weary and fatigued. But she wants to know what her dying will be like? Will she suffer? Will she be able to manage at home with her husband and the visiting nurse? Her mother is there each day and seems quite distressed. Will they all cope?

Her second question is about what to tell her children. She wants to say goodbye to them, but is unsure of what words to use. She asks, 'What would you tell them doctor?' What should she say?

Meeting with Nadia's family

You arrange to talk the next day with Nadia, her husband, mother, sister, and her two children. Nadia has asked you to tell them gently that she will die. She wants your help to say that she doesn't want to die, wishes she could be there for several years to see her children grow up, but feels that her body is much weaker. She doesn't know how long she can hang on for. She wants her children to know that she loves them, and for her husband and sister to promise to take good care of them. She wants her sister to look after her mother. From talking to her husband, you sense that the family has quite a lot of understanding about how sick Nadia is, but realize that she wants your help to be able to say more to them. You meet with a willingness to help as best you can.

Advanced colon cancer at the end of life

Anatoly is a 42-year-old married engineer who first presented with some blood mixed with his bowel motion. He was found to have a Duke's C cancer of his colon. He has two children aged 8 and 10 years, and his wife is a college administrator.

Shortly after his adjuvant chemotherapy was completed, he was found to have advanced disease in his liver. You have treated Anatoly for the past three years, containing the spread of his cancer with four different regimens of chemotherapy. Despite your best efforts, after some months of apparent control with each regimen, eventually disease progression broke through. You are running out of tumour-directed therapy options. Para-aortic lymphadenopathy caused ureteric blockage and hydronephrosis, necessitating stenting of his ureters. Although his kidney function improved, metastases have replaced most of his liver, his albumin has fallen, he has lost considerable weight, and ascites is worse. You had it drained by paracentesis this week. His liver function enzymes are elevated, prothrombin has risen, and his bilirubin is elevated.

You perceive that Anatoly is entering his dying phase. You arranged for the community-based palliative care service to begin visiting him at home. You know that you need to talk with him about his end-of-life care. There is much to talk about.

Discussing dying with Anatoly

Anatoly has indicated he has questions that he wishes to ask you. Where might he prefer to die? You can see the icteric colour of his sclera, as his skin starts ever so faintly to turn yellow. He is weary and fatigued. But he wants to know what his dying will be like? Will he suffer? Will he be able to manage at home with his wife and the visiting nurse? Will they all cope?

His second question is about what to tell his children? He wants to say goodbye to them, but is unsure of what words to use. He asks, 'What would you tell them doctor?' What should he say?

Meeting with Anatoly's family

You arrange to talk the next day with Anatoly, his wife, his sister, and his two children. Anatoly has told you that he wants to tell his children to take care of their mother. He knows she will be deeply distressed without him. He wished he could hang on, but feels that his body is much weaker. He doesn't know how much time is left. He wants his children to have successful lives, and he wants to also ask his sister to help his family. From talking to his wife, you sense that the family has quite a lot of understanding about how sick Anatoly is. They realize that he has been putting on a brave front, but may want to say more to them. You meet with a willingness to help as best you can.

References

Angus DC, Barnato AE, Linde-Zwirble WT, et al. (2004). Use of intensive care at the end of life in the United States: an epidemiologic study. Crit Care Med 32, 638–43.

Back AL, Starks H, Hsu C, Gordon JR, Bharucha A, Pearlman RA (2002). Clinician-patient interactions about requests for physician-assisted suicide: a patient and family view. Arch Intern Med 162, 1257–65.

Barnato AE, Arnold RM (2013). The effect of emotion and physician communication behaviors on surrogates' life-sustaining treatment decisions: a randomized simulation experiment. Crit Care Med 41, 1686–91.

Byock I (2004). The Four Things That Matter Most: A Book About Living, Free Press, New York, NY.

Curtis JR (2004). Communicating about end-of-life care with patients and families in the intensive care unit. Crit Care Clin 20, 363–80, viii.

Curtis JR, Engelberg RA (2006). Measuring success of interventions to improve the quality of end-of-life care in the intensive care unit. Crit Care Med 34, S341–7.

Dowdy MD, Robertson C, Bander JA (1998). A study of proactive ethics consultation for critically and terminally ill patients with extended lengths of stay. *Crit Care Med* **26**, 252–9.

Epstein R, Street RL (2007). *Patient-centered communication in cancer care: promoting healing and reducing suffering.* U.S. Dept. of Health and Human Services, National Institutes of Health, National Cancer Institute, Bethsda, MD.

Favre N, Despland JN, De Roten Y, Drapeau M, Bernard M, Stiefel F (2007). Psychodynamic aspects of communication skills training: a pilot study. *Support Care Cancer* **15**, 333–7.

Ferris FD, Von Gunten CF, Emanuel LL (2003). Competency in end-of-life care: last hours of life. *J Palliat Med* **6**, 605–13.

Hsieh HF, Shannon SE, Curtis JR (2006). Contradictions and communication strategies during end-of-life decision making in the intensive care unit. *J Crit Care* **21**, 294–304.

Hudson PL, Schofield P, Kelly B, *et al.* (2006). Responding to desire to die statements from patients with advanced disease: recommendations for health professionals. *Palliat Med* **20**, 703–10.

Kissane DW, McKenzie M, Bloch S, Moskowitz C, McKenzie DP, O'Neill I (2006). Family focused grief therapy: a randomized, controlled trial in palliative care and bereavement. *Am J Psychiatry* **163**, 1208–18.

Lautrette A, Darmon M, Megarbane B, *et al.* (2007). A communication strategy and brochure for relatives of patients dying in the ICU. *N Engl J Med* **356**, 469–78.

Levin TT, Coyle N (2015). A communication training perspective on AND versus DNR directives. *Palliat Support Care* **13**, 385–7.

Levin TT, Li Y, Weiner JS, *et al.* (2008). How do-not-resuscitate orders are utilized in cancer patients: timing relative to death and communication-training implications. *Palliat Support Care* **6**, 341–8.

Levy MH, Smith T, Alvarez-Perez A, *et al.* (2014). Palliative care, Version 1.2014. Featured updates to the NCCN Guidelines. *J Natl Compr Canc Netw* **12**, 1379–88.

Rubenfeld GD, Crawford SW (2001). Principles and practice of withdrawing life-sustaining treatment in the ICU. In: Curtis JR, Rubenfeld GD (eds). *Managing Death in the ICU : The Transition from Cure to Comfort.* Oxford University Press, New York, NY.

Stapleton RD, Engelberg RA, Wenrich MD, Goss CH, Curtis JR (2006). Clinician statements and family satisfaction with family conferences in the intensive care unit. *Crit Care Med* **34**, 1679–85.

Volandes AE, Mitchell Sl, El-Jawahri A, *et al.* (2013). Randomized controlled trial of a video decision support tool for cardiopulmonary resuscitation decision making in advanced cancer. *J Clin Oncol* **31**, 380–6.

Volandes AE, Paasche-Orlow M, Gillick MR, *et al.* (2008). Health literacy not race predicts end-of-life care preferences. *J Palliat Med* **11**, 754–62.

Weiner JS, Roth J (2006). Avoiding iatrogenic harm to patient and family while discussing goals of care near the end of life. *J Palliat Med* **9**, 451–63.

Weissman DE, Ambuel B, Von Gunten CF, *et al.* (2007). Outcomes from a national multispecialty palliative care curriculum development project. *J Palliat Med* **10**, 408–19.

Wright AA, Keating NL, Balboni TA, Matulonis UA, Block SD, Prigerson HG (2010). Place of death: correlations with quality of life of patients with cancer and predictors of bereaved caregivers' mental health. *J Clin Oncol* **28**, 4457–64.

Wright AA, Zhang B, Ray A, *et al.* (2008). Associations between end-of-life discussions, patient mental health, medical care near death, and caregiver bereavement adjustment. *JAMA* **300**, 1665–73.

SECTION C

Nursing

Section editor: Susie Wilkinson

CHAPTER 23

Communication skills education and training in pre-registration BSc Nursing

Deborah Lewis, Marie O'Boyle-Duggan, and Susan Poultney

Introduction to communication skills education and training in pre-registration BSc Nursing

Nursing degree students arrive with a variety of skills and while some students may have experience of caring, other students may have had limited exposure. Some younger students, although adept at negotiating social media, are often anxious about interacting with patients, clients, and carers for the first time particularly when dealing with sensitive issues such as end-of-life care or after a death (Poultney *et al.* 2014). All, however, need to develop their interpersonal skills to demonstrate compassion, empathy, and a person-centred approach to maintain patients' dignity alongside effective dialogue. Faculty students specializing in the fields of adult, mental health, learning disabilities, or children's nursing undertake a core clinical skills module including four hours of communication skills teaching in the first year.

This chapter will review the development of simulated learning in communication skills education in a large Faculty of Health, Education, and Life Sciences, highlighting the approach taken including the evaluation strategies and the challenges. Educational standards in the United Kingdom (UK), as specified by the Nursing and Midwifery Council (NMC) [Box 23.1] highlight the key competencies nursing students need to demonstrate proficiency in to become a Registered Nurse (NMC 2011). Additionally, particularly within mental health and learning disability nursing where it arises frequently, nurses have to be competent and confident in assessing mental capacity, as well as ensuring reasonable adjustments are made where needed to meet legislative requirements (Equality Act 2010). Such emphasis on communication is timely with an increasing focus on delivering empathetic, compassionate, and individualized care in a multicultural society in all fields of nursing (Atherton and Kyle 2014), especially at the end of life (Shannon *et al.* 2011).

Prior to the development of a new BSc (Hons.) Nursing programme in 2010, communications skills education was limited to lecture-style teaching. However, an opportunity arose to include high fidelity simulation (Aldridge 2012) with actors simulating patients and their carers using scenarios taken from clinical

> **Box 23.1** Pre-registration communication competency standards
>
> Nurses should be able to:
>
> - Communicate safely and effectively.
> - Build therapeutic relationships taking into account differences, capabilities, and needs.
> - Be able to engage in, maintain, and disengage from therapeutic relationships.
> - Use a range of communications skills and technologies.
> - Use verbal, non-verbal, and written communication.
> - Recognize the need for an interpreter.
> - Address communication in diversity.
> - Promote well-being and personal safety.
> - Identify ways to communicate and promote healthy behaviour.
> - Maintain accurate, clear, and complete written or electronic records.
> - Respect and protect confidential information.
>
> Reproduced with permission from Debbie Lewis *et al.*, 'Putting Words into Action project: using role play in skills training,' *British Journal of Nursing*, Volume 22, Issue 11, Copyright © 2013, MA Healthcare Limited. Source: data from Nursing and Midwifery Council (NMC), *Standards of Proficiency for Pre-registration Nursing Education*, Nursing and Midwifery Council, Copyright © 2013, MA Healthcare Limited, available from http://www.nmc.org.uk/standards/additional-standards/standards-for-pre-registration-nursing-education/

practice. After a systematic evaluation, this was supported by a Higher Education Academy Grant with local hospices as collaborators (Lewis *et al.* 2013). The BSc programme now aims to provide communication education throughout the pre-registration nursing programme alongside supported clinical experience, enabling students to develop more complex communication skills as they develop as practitioners.

Early challenges

Although there is conflicting evidence on the value of using simulated patients over other experiential learning, such as peer role play, using non-healthcare professionals enables constructive feedback for students from a lay perspective, which is recognized as invaluable (Bokken *et al.* 2009). In higher education, the realistic portrayal of a patient or carer may be undertaken by laypersons, clinical staff, lecturers, or other students as well as professional actors. In a BSc programme with over 700 new students annually however, professional actors are prohibitively expensive. Early work focused on increasing the faculty's pool of actors by training third year students from the Birmingham City University's School of Acting and clinical staff who already acted as simulated patients in the learning disability field of nursing (O'Boyle-Duggan 2010). This initial group, and later cohorts of drama students, participated in a two-day training programme to standardize practice and provide a common preparation level for all simulators. This included practising the scenarios and giving constructive feedback. The core elements of the faculty training programme are shown in Box 23.2.

Drama students are well-versed in aspects of communication such as observing non-verbal behaviours, listening for and delivering cues, and identifying linguistic issues related to pace, pitch, and tone—thus finding a common language to describe communication skills proved easier than anticipated (Lewis *et al.* 2013). Active feedback from lecturers who facilitate the teaching sessions is valued highly by the actors. Additional time spend on simulating learning disability scenarios helps them to portray a patient with a moderate or severe disability. Initially drama students also helped to improve the quality and depth of 12 field-specific scenarios, which are based on commonly occurring clinical situations (shown in Box 23.3).

New scenarios added recently include settling a distressed patient with Alzheimer's disease and assessing a teenager after a self-harming incidence. As nurses have a statutory responsibility to meet the care needs of all people to enhance the students' exposure to all nursing fields, each teaching session must

---

Box 23.2 Faculty simulator training

Facilitated by a lecturer and a professional actor:

- Introduction: What is expected of a professional simulator?
- Communication skills: What skills do we want to promote in healthcare professionals?
- Preparing for simulation sessions.
  - Using pre-written scenario.
  - Giving constructive feedback.
  - The value of delivering a lay person's perspective.
  - Establishing a suitable playing level.
  - Flexibility and improvisation.
- Practising scenarios and giving feedback.
- Simulating sensitive issues and the need for self-care strategies.

Box 23.3 BSc (Hons) simulation scenarios

Adult nursing

- Responding to a cancer patient's query: 'What does palliative mean?'
- Responding to a shocked and distressed patient in an outpatient clinic.
- Responding to an irritable and aggressive older patient unable to return home.
- Discussing options with a relative of an extended family staying beyond normal visiting hours.

Mental health

- Assessing a patient after finding a half-empty whisky bottle under their bed.
- Helping an aggressive, bed-bound patient who has been moved from another ward and is suffering nicotine withdrawal.
- Dealing with a patient's approach for a night out after their discharge from the ward.

Children's nursing

- Discussing the care of a baby with a cold with her anxious and socially isolated mother.
- Establishing conversation with a withdrawn adolescent patient with cystic fibrosis after the death of their close friend.
- Assessing a 15-year-old patient admitted to hospital after a self-harming episode.

Learning disabilities

- Assessing pain in a patient with moderate learning disabilities and limited speech who wants to return home.
- Managing a patient in casualty with autism and limited speech who wants to remove a head dressing.

Dementia care

- Settling a patient with Alzheimer's disease who is restless and distressed at evening visiting time.

Adapted with permission from Debbie Lewis *et al.*, 'Putting Words into Action project: using role play in skills training,' *British Journal of Nursing*, Volume 22, Issue 11, Copyright © 2013, MA Healthcare Limited.

---

include a scenario from each field. This has been particularly helpful in exposing not only the students, but also the lecturers to the communication challenges experienced in other fields of nursing.

Implementation and evaluation

Session facilitators are provided with written guidance including a lesson plan, suggested ground rules for negotiation, and a structured feedback strategy based on Pendleton's rules (Garala *et al.* 2007) (Box 23.4), originally developed in medical education, with

Box 23.4 Pendleton's rules for feedback (adapted)

The participating student has the opportunity to talk first and is encouraged to discuss positive points:

◆ The participating student has the opportunity to suggest alternative strategies to improve their performance.

◆ The observing group are invited to provide feedback with positive points given first.

◆ The facilitator and group provide constructive feedback with care taken to ensure comments are not given in a negative manner.

◆ An actor is invited to give a lay perspective.

Adapted with permission from Debbie Lewis et al., 'Putting Words into Action project: using role play in skills training,' British Journal of Nursing, Volume 22, Issue 11, Copyright © 2013, MA Healthcare Limited. Source: data from Garala M et al. 'Aid to learning', pp. 216–242, in Charlton R, (Ed.), Learning to Consult, Radcliffe Publishing Ltd, Abingdon, UK, Copyright © 2007.

recommendations to discuss ground rules prior to starting the session.

Grounds rules include allowing student volunteers and facilitators to halt a simulation at any time, to leave the room if distressed (although this happens rarely), to gather ideas from the group before commencing, and to highlight confidentiality issues. Prompt feedback and debriefing after simulated learning is acknowledged as particularly valuable (Aldridge 2012) and group discussion often broadens to include the effect of communication skills in developing or eroding relationships, power imbalances, the value of silence, and the use of touch as well as ethical issues. As recommended in all simulation work (Aldridge 2012), structured feedback during and after focuses on the student's positive achievements and helps to avoid humiliation, before constructive suggestions for improvement. It is also a cornerstone of generating a supportive environment, which is needed to encourage student participation. Using ice-breaker exercises that deliberately incorporate an element of surprise have been popular and useful in gaining active participation in quieter groups. A pre-session exercise encouraging students to self-record an interview with a friend on their mobile phone to gain insight into their normal speaking voice and to consider issues such as pitch, speed, and tone had a limited response, and may be incorporated into an earlier communication skills session. Linkage of the session content by facilitators to theoretical constructs covered in an earlier lecture-style session is encouraged. As suggested by Byland et al. (2009), workshop style training for lecturers was offered to promote competent facilitation of each teaching session. However, due to time pressures and the long standing experience of many lecturers, this had limited success and new facilitators are encouraged to 'see one' and 'do one' under supervision before embarking on solo facilitation. This has been successful in giving new facilitators some initial support and allowed others to decline this style of teaching if it is not their preferred option.

Quantitative and qualitative data analysis

Quantitative evaluation focused on 26 two-hour sessions delivered prior to the first year BSc (Hons.) students' first clinical placement, with a systematic approach to evaluation taken to determine the sessions' effectiveness regarding students' confidence, to support future bids for funding, and to highlight any cost benefits (Lewis et al. 2013). Attendees voluntarily completed an anonymized pre- and post-session survey using a 10-point Likert scale measuring confidences for a range of activities such as explaining the taking of a vital sign, responding to patients' verbal and non-verbal cues, explaining professional boundaries, dealing with strong emotions, and communicating with patients regarding specific issues such as dementia and learning disability. There are no standarised values for confidence levels in clinical skills training (Sook Yoo et al. 2010). This strategy was chosen however, as it is commonly used in simulation (Aldridge 2012) and communication skills training (Wlikinson et al. 2009).

A representative sample of 300 students, from the approximately 520 first year students who participated, completed the survey at the start and end of each session. There were 271 surveys returned with no missing data. Detailed statistical analysis has already been reported (Lewis et al. 2013) and will only be précised here; but of the 82 students who took part in a simulation (participants), 196 students observed and give feedback (observers) with 12 students not specifying their level of participation. Students also added their field of nursing, namely adult, mental health, learning disabilities, or children's nursing, and were given the opportunity to add free text comments. Calculation and tabulation of the response frequencies for pre- and post-session confidence scores demonstrated that students felt more confident immediately after the simulated learning. As the data was ordinal in nature, non-parametric inferential tests were used to demonstrate these differences were 'real' and unlikely to be due to mere chance, with a statistically significant increase in confidence following the teaching session for students in all nursing fields. Statistical analysis suggested all students benefited from the class. Splitting the data into the two groups of participants and observers also demonstrated that the amount of confidence improvement (the 'effect size') is unsurprisingly larger in the participant group compared to the observer group, possibly due to a greater sense of 'ownership' when students took part in the simulation. This information added to knowledge acquired in previous faculty research (O'Boyle Duggan et al., 2010).

Qualitative data collection in this project was limited, with students adding free text comments to the survey. Although the numbers of these were small, they were predominately positive, focusing on the value of simulated learning. As one student notes: 'This session taught me to concentrate solely on patients and relatives and them expressing their concerns.'

The value of structured reflection and debriefing of simulated scenarios with students may be particularly under-recognized, as reflectivity and the development of self-awareness may help to develop nurses who are emotionally-competent (Horton-Deutsch and Sherwood 2008). In post-registration degree level modules, student, peer, and facilitator feedback is enhanced by video-recording simulations (Garala et al. 2007), which nurses reflect on in assignment work Although initially self-conscious, this is a powerful tool for students, helping to raise self-awareness, and can be usefully employed provided the feedback is well-structured and delivered in a supportive environment. This may be particularly useful in oncology and palliative care where events are likely to have an emotional dimension, which can be a neglected area of healthcare education.

Facilitator and actor feedback

Explicating stating ground rules and a structured feedback strategy was helpful in protecting all participants, including facilitators, from unnecessary stress and emotional. A pack of written guidance was useful for facilitators. who also suggested the sessions might have improved the students' performance in a objective structured clinical examination (OSCEs) held after the sessions. This is unsurprising, as nursing practical procedures do require communication competence (Sook Yoo et al. 2010) and communications skills in medical education are recognized as a critical component of patient consultations.

Formal assessment of the facilitators' competence has not been undertaken, although evidence suggests this can be a key factor in ensuring effective simulated learning (Byland et al. 2009); regular open and honest peer review is also recommended. As noted earlier, a workshop for potential facilitators was poorly attended, but often advice is sought informally and care has been taken not to alienate colleagues. Some tasks within the session are more complex than others, such as resolving learning disability scenarios and gaining student participation in larger groups. Designing and negotiating facilitator competences and regular review by colleagues with individual feedback, perhaps as part of a faculty annual peer review process, may be a useful development for the future. The faculty also runs a Master's level module for simulated learning, which has provided a useful forum for discussing and promoting the need for effective facilitation skills.

Drama students from the School of Acting highlighted the satisfaction felt in using their expertise to help healthcare professionals develop key skills for clinical practice. It assisted their own development particularly in improvisation and other skills (Lewis et al. 2013). Although drama students found nursing students able and keen to learn, there are challenges. Drama students have a commitment to their own learning. Those who do participate however, are committed. They also often have experience as users of the health service which can be useful to nursing students. A University renumeration scheme and integrating the training into a BSc (Hons.) Applied Performance (Community and Education) module, has not increased the proportion of drama students able to undertake this role. Consequently, the faculty remains reliant on other actors for simulation work.

Learning disability

People with learning disabilities accessing mainstream healthcare face many challenges where health professionals continue to disregard the legal requirement to make reasonable adjustments (Equality Act 2010) for the communication difficulties experienced by many people with learning disabilities (Emerson et al. 2011). In general healthcare services, communication difficulties can hamper essential diagnostic and screening procedures such as taking an adequate history. Staff can lack confidence and, in busy clinical environments, consultation times are often inadequate to address concerns of the cognitively impaired. Even making an appointment can be a challenge. Education with a focus

on learning disabilities including communication can improve awareness, and demonstrates that discrimination can be tackled with positive changes in attitude and interpersonal skills (Webb and Stanton 2009).

With regard to end-of-life care, Read's work (2006) highlights that those individuals with a learning disability who have a life-limiting illness find it particularly difficult to access relevant end-of-life services, while Willner et al. (2011) has identified gaps in knowledge and training needs of healthcare professionals in relation to consent issues. Since 2010, nursing students have been exposed to live simulation to promote a person-centred approach to communication (O'Boyle-Duggan 2010), which is recognized as an important element in palliative care for people with learning disability (Morton-Nance and Schafer 2012). Pre-registration students from all nursing fields have an opportunity to interact with a simulated patient who exhibits a variety of learning and health needs related to the students' clinical field. Simulations take place in specifically designed skills rooms replicating the relevant clinical environment, such as a ward or a home environment, with students given extra time to assess a client's clinical needs using a range of strategies and clear, unambiguous language (Tuffrey-Wijne and McEnhill 2008).

Mixed methodology research (O'Boyle-Duggan et al. 2012) with 173 health students was conducted over a period of 18 months and involved students from the Operating Department Practitioners programme, and adult and children's nursing students. Students completed a standardized satisfaction and confidence survey, with focus groups conducted after a clinical placement experience to evaluate the benefits to the students in their clinical practice (O'Boyle-Duggan et al. 2012). Evaluation of responses indicated a confidence increase with students feeling involved and able to consider, from a personal perspective, how communication and behaviour affected service users. They also reporting feeling more competent in using skills related to theory when responding in real time to emotionally distressed simulated service users. This was particularly valued as students were able to make mistakes, which could then be safely explored and rectified. Debriefing and reflecting on performance were also an important component of the live simulation, which was highly valued by students who stated that this enhanced their learning (O'Boyle-Duggan 2010). Students felt observing simulations highlighted the issues and communication barriers that may be encountered in clinical placements as 'you saw it from the outside too', as well as learning how you would react in an unpredictable improvised situation; which as a simulation participant noted 'you can't get in a lecture'. Recommendations for practice and reflective statements from students as a result of this simulation work are shown in Box 23.5.

Such simulation work highlights that, when encouraged to do so, students will make reasonable adjustments in their nursing care, as per the Equality Act (2010), in a creative way to communicate with patients with learning disabilities—as illustrated by the following comments:

One gentleman, he'd like—I'd throw a ball at him and he'd throw it back, and he'd sit there for hours just playing ball. Another one was a piece of music and you put that on and instantly it's like, 'Yeah, I remember this,' and it'd make him happy, and you can talk to him. And it was really rewarding. Just finding something that they enjoyed and you could use (O'Boyle-Duggan et al. 2012).

Box 23.5 Student reflections and recommendations for practice

Recommendations for practice

◆ KISS: keep it short and simple.

◆ Talk more slowly.

◆ Talk to the child rather than parents.

◆ Take more time.

◆ Think about finding out the child's interests to initiate dialogue and to gain trust.

◆ Distraction techniques may be useful.

◆ Speaking to [the] patient without [his or her] parents.

Student reflections

◆ 'I didn't quite understand how difficult it can be to communicate with children who have learning disabilities.'

◆ 'Not all children with learning disabilities have challenging behaviour.'

◆ 'It is surprising how instinctive I can be when put into a scenario.'

◆ 'Even though each patient is an individual and should be treated the same, it is alright to make allowances and to take your time.'

◆ 'It reiterates that hands-on practice is the best way of learning and finding mistakes in our techniques.'

Adapted from O'Boyle-Duggan M et al. 'Effectiveness of live simulation of patients with intellectual disabilities.' *Journal of Nursing Education*, Volume 51, Issue 6, pp. 334–42, Copyright © 2012. Reproduced with permission of SLACK Incorporated.

Some comments also hint at a change in attitude:

I suppose it is the change in attitude, isn't it really? Instead of saying 'Oh I'm busy. I'm going to have to write all the notes up'. That really just takes two minutes, just to go and spend a bit of time with someone. And that can mean a lot to somebody (O'Boyle-Duggan et al. 2012).

The available literature however, suggests there is little evidence of outcome measures in terms of clinical impact when using simulation in nursing and other health education programmes. Work is developing in a variety of nursing and health and social programmes—such as social work and speech and language therapy—with a view to evaluating the clinical impact of improved communication in more depth. Live simulation, in collaboration with students, is also being developed for use in an end-of-life e-learning package for learning disability nursing.

Children's nursing

It may be under-recognized that communication dialogue in children's nursing often necessitates discussing topics of an intimate nature such as hopes and fears, developmental concerns, sexuality, drug use and abuse and, sadly, terminal illness. Communication may be very challenging, particularly within the context of oncology and palliative care (Potter et al. 2013). Nursing students must take account of the age, development, and any communication or learning disabilities a child may have while avoiding jargon or appearing patronizing (Chilman-Blair 2010). Qualitative research by Carson (2010) highlights the nurses' emotional insecurity in communication at the end of life, particularly with parents, coupled with feeling unsure of how much emotion to display themselves' after a death. Published work by Poultney et al. (2014) highlights students concerns such as 'What do I say if a patient asks am I dying?', 'How do I break news to a family?', 'What if I say the wrong thing?' (p. 347). Some of these issues are addressed in small group teaching entitled 'Perceptions of Dying', which leads on to the more detailed communication scenarios used in communication skills simulation sessions.

In addition, consultations in paediatrics are often 'triadic' with three participants involved at the same time such as a child, parent, and nurse, which presents special challenges. Parents have a key role and may act as an intermediary between the child and nurse clarifying questions and empowering the child or they may inhibit the child's role in the dialogue, answering on their behalf and disempowering the child (Lambert et al. 2012). In serious illness such as seen in oncology parents may attempt to block open and honest communication in the belief it will protect the child from emotional distress.

As seen in Box 23.3, three simulation scenarios have been developed for use in the first year of the BSc (Hons.) Nursing Child field, chosen for their transferability into a range of healthcare settings, their commonality, and the level of challenge for the students. They have also been filmed to allow the students access to the key communication skills via an online educational facility. These scenarios focus on reassuring an anxious parent of a one-week-old baby, taking with a distressed 15-year-old who has been self-harming, and communicating with an adolescent with cystic fibrosis, recently bereaved of a friend with the same condition. Guided by the facilitator examination of the specific skills and exploration of communication strategies encourages reflection in reluctant students. These discussions often broaden to include ethical and confidentiality issues alongside self-care and effective coping strategies. Simulations can include encouraging the students to write down information in a structured way, such as using the SBAR tool—Situation, Background, Assessment, and Recommendations—which may facilitate the safe handover of patient information between staff (Shannon et al. 2011). In some scenarios it is also pertinent to highlight technologies, which may be used to bridge communication gaps such as picture boards, synthesized voice recorders, and use of sign language, such as Makaton, among children with learning disabilities (Lambert et al. 2012). A video based around the family of a three-year-old child who has Down's syndrome has also been developed, illustrating how a family have overcome the challenges of communicating with their daughter who has little speech for her age by first using baby signing and then Signalong. Such strategies allow the whole family, including a two-year-old sibling to communicate together. Such electronic resources allow students to develop an understanding of some of the challenges faced in the communication with children with learning disabilities that will be transferable to clinical practice.

A clear barrier to communication training for children's nurses is the lack of 'children' to work as with. Within simulated communication training, it could be argued it is easier for adult, mental health, or learning disabilities nurses to accept an altered reality and 'buy in' to the simulation, because they are working with role players of a representative age and developmental level as their patients. Whenever possible, and to maximize the potential learning, actors employed in the children's nursing field are younger-looking actors able to portray an adolescent patient with realism—although the literature surrounding this issue is scarce. The importance of family-centred care within children's nursing is paramount and communicating with the child's parents within simulation is very realistic. Unfortunately, we may miss the essence of communicating with children, as well as assessing their levels of understanding, language acquisition, and using play as the avenue through which to build therapeutic relationships. Steps for the future include investigating how to explore these skills more fully, allowing the students to begin to embed such practice throughout the nursing programme, and increasing their confidence and competence for further development with children and families in clinical practice.

Conclusion

Integrating simulation into communication skills education and training in nursing education is a developing field and, in a large faculty, demanding in terms of staff time, effort, and financial cost. Systematic evaluation is always needed. Where it exists, it suggests that students derive an immediate benefit in terms of increasing confidence and developing self-awareness. It may aid their flexibility in using a range of communication skills and strategies to support dialogue with patients and clients. Useful in many situations, simulated learning may be valuable in addressing areas of sensitivity such as death and oncology and palliative care, to promote the need to make reasonable adjustments to communicate with people with a disability. Undertaking such work inevitability raises further areas for development. These include assessing the impact of such teaching on clinical practice. It does give educators however, a creative opportunities to link classroom learning to clinical practice.

Acknowledgements

Text extracts from O'Boyle-Duggan M *et al.* 'Effectiveness of live simulation of patients with intellectual disabilities,' *Journal of Nursing Education*, Volume 51, Issue 6, pp. 334-42, Copyright © 2012. Reproduced with permission of SLACK Incorporated.

References

Aldridge M (2012). Defining and exploring clinical skills and simulation-based education. In: Aldridge M, Wanless S (eds). *Developing Healthcare Skills Through Simulation.* Sage Publications, London, UK.

Atherton I, Kyle R (2014). How empathy skills can change nursing. *Nurs Stand* **29**, 24–5.

Bokken L, Linssen T, Scherpbier A, van der Vleuten C, Rethans JJ (2009). Feedback by simulated patients in undergraduate medical education: a systematic review of the literature. *Med Educ* **43**, 201–10.

Byland C, Brown R, Lubrano di Ciccone B, Diamond C, Eddington J, Kissane D (2009). Assessing facilitator competence in a comprehensive communication skills training programme. *Med Educ* **43**, 342–9.

Carson S (2010). Do student nurses within an undergraduate child health programme feel that the curriculum prepares them to deal with the death of a child? *J Child Health Care* **14**, 367–74.

Chilman-Blair K (2010). Communicating with children about illness. *Practice Nursing* **21**, 631–3.

Emerson E, Baines S, Allerton L, Welch VA (2011). *Health Inequalities & People with Learning Disabilities in the UK: Improving Health and Lives.* Public Health England. Available at: https://www.improvinghealthandlives.org.uk/ [Last accessed May 26, 2015].

Equality Act (2010). Crown Copyright. Available at: http://www.legislation.gov.uk/ukpga/2010/15/contents [Accessed May 14, 2015].

Garala M, Winborn L, Bhattacharyya A, *et al.* (2007). Aids to learning. In: Charlton R (ed.) *Learning to Consult.* Radcliffe Publishing Ltd, Abingdon, UK.

Horton-Deutsch S, Sherwood G (2008). Reflection: an educational strategy to develop emotionally-competent nurses leaders. *J Nurs Manag* **16**, 946–54.

Lambert V, Long T, Kelleher D (eds) (2012). *Communication Skills for Childrens' Nurses.* Open University Press, Berkshire, UK.

Lewis D, O'Boyle-Duggan M, Chapman J, *et al.* (2013). 'Putting Words into Action Project'—Integrating effective communication skills training using School of Acting students and role players from learning disabilities nursing into a BSc (Hons) Nursing programme. *B J Nurs* **22**, 638–44.

Morton-Nance S, Schafer T (2012). End of life care for people with a learning disability. *Nurs Stand* **27**, 40–7.

NMC (2011). *Standards of Proficiency for Pre-registration Nursing Education.* Nursing and Midwifery Council. Available at: http://www.nmc.org.uk/standards/additional-standards/standards-for-pre-registration-nursing-education/ [Last accessed May 17, 2015].

O'Boyle-Duggan M (2010). Developing a simulation model to explore challenging behaviour. *Learning Disability Practice* **13**, 35–8.

O'Boyle-Duggan M, Grech J, Brandt R (2012). Effectiveness of live simulation of patients with intellectual disabilities. *J Nurs Educ* **51**, 334–42.

Potter P, Deshields T, Berger J, Clarke M, Olsen S, Chen L (2013). Evaluation of a Compassion Fatigue Resiliency Program for Oncology Nurses. *Oncol Nurs Forum* **40** 180–7.

Poultney S, Berridge P, Malkin B (2014). Supporting pre-registration nursing students in their exploration of death and dying. *Nurse Educ Pract* **14**, 345–9.

Read S (ed.) (2006). *Palliative Care for People with Learning Disabilities.* Quay Books, London, UK.

Shannon S, Long-Sutehall T, Combs M (2011). Conversations in end-of-life care: communication tools for critical care practitioners. *Nurs Crit Care* **16**, 124–30.

Sook Yoo M, Young Yoo I, Lee H (2010). Nursing students' self-evaluation using a video recording of foley catheterization: effects on students' competence, communication skills, and learning motivation. *J Nurs Educ* **49**, 402–4.

Tuffrey-Wijne I, McEnhill L (2008). Communication difficulties and intellectual disability in end-of-life care. *Inter J Palliat Nurs* **14**, 192–7.

Webb J, Stanton M (2009). Better access to primary healthcare for adults with learning disabilities: Evaluation of a group programme to improve knowledge and skills. *Br J Learn Disabil* **3**, 116–22.

Wilkinson S, Linsell I, Perry R, Blanchard K (2008). Communication skills training for nurses working with patients with heart disease. *Br J Cardiac Nursing* **3**, 475–81.

Willner P, Bridle J, Price V, Dymond S, Lewis G (2011). What do NHS staff learn from training on the Mental Capacity Act? (2005) *Legal and Criminological Psychology.* Available at: http://onlinelibrary.wiley.com/doi/10.1111/j.2044-8333.2011.02035.x/full. [Last accessed May 17, 2015].

CHAPTER 24

SAGE & THYME

Michael Connolly

Introduction to SAGE & THYME

People with cancer have specific expectations of the nurses who care for them. They expect the nurses they meet to show concern; demonstrate caring behaviours; communicate effectively; be competent; and to be skilled (Oermann 1999). Patients value a form of communication with them which is therapeutic: where the relationship is part of the healing. Such therapeutic communication goes beyond the provision of advice and information; it includes discussions about emotions, thoughts, and worries (Choralalambous et al. 2008). As well as what the cancer nurse does, it seems that it matters how the cancer nurse interacts. Therapeutic cancer nursing, therefore, must value the experiences and knowledge of the patients and patients must become active partners in the own treatment and care (Oermann 1999). Such highly skilled nursing enables the empowerment of patients, and rejects 'paternalistic' relationships with them in which nurses assert an authoritative role (Saino et al. 2001).

Unfortunately, many nurses and other health workers simply lack the communication skills to assess the concerns and needs of the patients that they care for (Gysels et al. 2005). As a result, many patients are left feeling anxious, frustrated and dissatisfied: feelings which may impair their ability to comply with cancer treatments (Butow et al. 2002). Studies of qualified cancer nurses have described nurses distancing themselves from the emotional cues from patients, and adopting avoidance strategies or blocking behaviours to protect themselves from becoming involved in the patients' lives and suffering. Furthermore, the assessments by cancer nurses of their patients have been found to be lengthy, unfocused, and lacking in structure (Wilkinson et al. 2008). When observed, the nurses tended to move too quickly to solve the patients' problems and to give information before they had fully identified the patients' concerns. Far from valuing the experience and knowledge of patients, therefore, nurses have been observed interrupting by prematurely advising and informing patients (Booth et al. 1999). It appears, therefore, that nurses may believe that they establish therapeutic relationships with patients, but that their observed behaviours demonstrate otherwise.

It is clear from the evidence cited above that a gap exists between what cancer patients need and what nurses have been trained to provide. Years of clinical experience alone does not appear to fill this gap because senior clinical staff are known to display the same unhelpful communication behaviours as their more junior and inexperienced colleagues (Gysels et al. 2005). A second gap exists: between the existence of clinically helpful, research-based knowledge, and its implementation into clinical practice. Researchers have developed a considerable knowledge base about which communication skills are most helpful, but this same knowledge has not yet been exported from academic journals and text books into the clinical practice of most health workers (Fallowfield and Jenkins 1999; Maguire and Pitceathly 2002; Silverman et al. 2013). Teachers of communication skills in cancer care, therefore, stand in the gap between knowledge and practice, and the quality of communications skills teaching is pivotal. The challenge for teachers is to develop learning experiences for clinical nurses so that the research evidence becomes believable, usable, and memorable—and so that the helpful skills taught can be applied immediately in the nurses' clinical practice.

Helpful communication skills have been categorized into basic skills and advanced skills. European experts in cancer care recommend that basic or 'foundation level' communication skills training should be mandatory for all staff (Stiefel et al. 2010). Senior staff, who will need to discuss cancer treatment options or end of life issues with patients, require the advanced level communication skills training. Much of the focus of communication skills training programmes has been upon 'advanced skills training', in which senior clinicians in cancer care undertake two or three-day workshops in learner groups of less than ten people (Moore et al. 2013). Considering the recommendation that the 'foundation level' skills training should be mandatory for all staff in cancer care; basic or foundation level skills training have been relatively neglected.

This chapter describes foundation level communication skills, how those skills can be taught, and the impact of teaching such skills.

The research into communications skills in cancer care was pioneered in the 1980s and 1990s with observational studies (Fallowfield and Jenkins 1999; Maguire and Pitceathly 2002). This research identified the unhelpful and helpful communication behaviours of nurses and other health workers, mainly in cancer care. Some of the unhelpful behaviours are described in Box 24.1. These behaviours appear to be learned in practice from other health workers, or are the result of good intentions to be helpful. Alternatively, the unhelpful behaviours are a consequence of competing pressures of time and workload and unconscious attempts by nurses to protect themselves emotionally from the distress experienced by people with cancer (Gysels et al. 2005). These factors are powerful influences (Heaven et al. 2006). Teachers of communication skills, therefore, require sensitivity towards their learners as they guide them away from learned behaviours which feel protective, and towards new skills which open the nurses to the distress of the patients. The stress of nursing in cancer care is well recognized (Wilkinson et al. 2008) and many health and social care professionals do not feel adequately trained to handle the interpersonal issues

Box 24.1 Unhelpful communication behaviours

- Avoiding listening to the concerns of patients and their carers.

- Focusing on physical and practical issues.

- Changing the subject.

- Guessing what the concerns are.

- Blocking the exploration of concerns.

- Listening selectively for concerns that we can address.

- Focusing on the least threatening aspect of the conversation.

- Giving information or advice or reassurance too early.

- Dealing with the first concern before hearing all of the concerns.

Reproduced with kind permission of University Hospital of South Manchester NHS Foundation Trust. Source: data from Booth *et al.* 1999, Maguire and Pitceathly 2002, and Griffiths *et al.* 2015.

that arise in the care of patients with cancer (Gysels *et al.* 2005). Helping cancer nurses, therefore, to feel confident with the emotional distress of patients is thought to be vital to the alleviation of stress for nurses (Wilkinson *et al.* 2008).

What are foundation level communication skills?

Foundation level skills are described in Table 24.1. Nurses need to feel confident to notice and respond to the emotional cues of

patients. They need the listening skills that will allow the patients to describe their distress, and the nurses to prove that they can listen. Nurses need to understand empathy and its difference from sympathy, as well as the confidence to be patient-centred as they respond to the emotional distress of patients. For this confidence to exist, nurses need to be taught practical listening skills; they need to know precisely what is meant by 'patient-centred' responses, and which phrases display empathy.

The teaching of communications skills in cancer nursing

The way that communications skills have been taught is strongly influenced by the evidence relating to the teaching of advanced communication skills. This evidence favours relatively long courses of at least 20 hours provided by accredited trainers for relatively small groups of learners (no larger than six learners) (Gysels *et al.* 2005). The evidence also suggests that effective advanced communications skills training should involve a blend of learning styles including theoretical knowledge and experiential elements such as practical rehearsal (Gysels *et al.* 2005). Specifically, the evidence for advanced communication skills training favours workshops which provide the opportunity for each learner to practice or rehearse new skills and receive feedback from skilled facilitators and peers (Gysels *et al.* 2005). Basic or foundation level communication skills, however, have not been subjected to the same level of scrutiny and evaluation through randomized controlled trials. While such scrutiny is lacking, there remains the possibility that foundation level

Table 24.1 Foundation level skills

Foundation levels skills	Explanation
The skill to **notice cues and hints** about worries or concerns and to **ask about emotions**	Health workers have a tendency to focus on practical and physical issues. Skilled care requires a high level of sensitivity to the cues and hints that people give about their concerns and worries
The skill to **create the space, time**, and privacy for people to describe their concerns, worries	It is helpful to know what people are worried about. Creating the right environment for them to talk requires time and skill
The listening skill of **not interrupting**	This requires great self-control. Solutions and advice can be unhelpful if they interrupt the thoughts of the person who is describing their concerns. People who are upset need time to think. Silence allows them to think
The listening skill of **reflecting**	The only way to prove that you have heard the concerns, is to repeat them back
The listening skill of **clarifying**	It is helpful to check what you hear and to ask for clarification if you are unsure about what is being said
The listening skills of **summarizing**	Summarizing the concerns can prompt people to disclose other concerns
The listening of **screening** for other concerns	More concerns are likely to be disclosed if asked for. The first concern may not be the main concern
The skill of **holding back** with your own solutions, information, advice, and reassurances	Experienced health workers can struggle to hold back all of their ideas and solutions. The holding back, however, is a key skill: it allows the worried/upset person time to think for themselves. It is how people can become empowered
The ability to **show empathic responses**	Some health workers confuse empathy with sympathy or comforting
The **patient-centred skills** of using the patient's own support, ideas, and resources	Careful skills can help patients to think about who supports them and what further support or help they need
The skill to **explain** in ways that can be understood	The giving of information requires the exchange of knowledge if it is to be understood and retained. The advice, information and reassurances from health workers are valuable: the skill is hold back with this advice until the worried/concerned person has been able to think for themselves
The skill to **close a consultation**	A discussion about worries can be unfocused and circular unless the listener knows how to bring it to a close

Reproduced with kind permission of University Hospital of South Manchester NHS Foundation Trust.

communications skills training, with more modest teaching aims may not require so much time and such intense experiential elements (Connolly *et al.* 2010). Furthermore, it is possible that foundation level communication skills could be effectively taught with a new combination of teaching strategies that differ from those used in advanced skills training. The SAGE & THYME foundation level workshop has been developed and disseminated in the UK. It utilizes a structured and sequential guide to the interaction between patients' and health workers through which the skills taught can be retained in the memories of the learners (Connolly *et al.* 2010).

What is SAGE & THYME?

SAGE & THYME time is a reminder (a mnemonic), to use evidence-based, helpful communication skills in clinical practice. It has been constructed by placing a number of foundation level

skills together. Each step of the model is based upon published evidence. It suggests a sequence of questions and responses as a guide to nurses and other health workers when they encounter distressed or worried patients or carers. It shows health workers how to create an opportunity for patients to voice and explore their own concerns and solutions. SAGE & THYME is described in Table 24.2. It is designed to encourage nurses and other health workers to listen first to the concerns of patients without interrupting. It also discourages nurses from prematurely offering advice, information, or reassurance. It can be thought of as a toolbox to carry the helpful skills from the classroom to where they can be used in clinical practice. It is not intended to be an inflexible script for routine use in all situations, but as a comprehensive 'starter kit' for nurses and other health workers who wish to listen carefully and practice patient-centred care. The structure of SAGE & THYME, therefore, enables the work of listening and responding to concerns to

Table 24.2 SAGE & THYME

	Structure	Explanation and examples of language	Justification (Booth *et al.* 1999; Fallowfield and Jenkins 1999; Maguire and Pitceathly 2002; Wilkinson *et al.* 2008; Silverman *et al.* 2013)
S	SETTING	Notice when patients seem upset or worried Find or create a good time and place If you are busy, choose a time when you are less busy	People need privacy, time, and a clear opportunity if they are to disclose their concerns or worries
A	ASK	*'Can I ask what it is you are worried about?'*	Patients are sometimes unsure how or when to talk about their concerns **Just ask**
G	GATHER	Gather all concerns: *'Can I make notes so that I don't miss what you tell me?'* Reflect and summarize the concerns disclosed Listen for hints about other concerns Screen: *'Is something else worrying you?'*	The first concern may not be the only concern. It is helpful to hear all concerns, even those which have no solution. Simply **make a list** of concerns Resist the temptation to 'fix' or give advice at this point. **Hold back**.
E	EMPATHY	*'You have a lot on your mind.'* Or *'No wonder you're upset this morning.'*	An empathic response suggests that you have noticed the feelings. It demonstrates that you care. Empathy can be used at any point and several times; but **don't forget it** at this point. **Go slowly**
&			
T	TALK	*'Who supports you?' 'Who can you talk to?'* Make a list of the people that support them	Most of the support that a patient gets will come from family/friends and others close to them. The social support around a patient has a strong influence over their ability to cope with or manage their situation. **Find out who they've got**
H	HELP	*'How does this person or these people help?'* Each person may provide different support	It can be helpful to discuss how the people in the family/social support actually help. The support that they get from family and friends commonly involves reassurance, comfort, and problem solving. **Understand their support**
Y	YOU	*'What would help?' 'What do you think would help?'* *'What else would help?'* Make a list of the things that the patient thinks would help	Patient centredness involves asking the patient what they think would help before offering advice yourself. **Keep holding back** with your solutions Patients are likely to have more than one idea of what would help. **So ask again**
M	ME	*'Is there something you would like me to do?'*	The discussion can then turn to what you might do to help Ask the patient first. You might list what they want you to do. Repeat it back At this point you might suggest things that you think might help, **if they want you to**
E	END	Summarize their concerns (your first list), their support (your second list), what they think would help (your third list): *'Is it OK to leave it there for now?'*	A summary can contain and conclude the discussion. **Ask permission to close** the discussion for now

Reproduced with kind permission of University Hospital of South Manchester NHS Foundation Trust.

Table 24.3 The SAGE & THYME foundation level workshop

Activity	Purpose	Educational justification
Facilitated small group discussion (max. 10 learners)	Establish what learners already know about noticing and responding to patient concerns	Reflective and vicarious learning. Placing value on the pre-workshop knowledge of learners and allowing them to hear the pre-workshop knowledge of other learners
Lecture presentation by trained facilitator (max. 30 learners) Presentation of printed materials	Describe the policy and research evidence relating to helpful communication skills and emotional support. Description of the SAGE & THYME mnemonic	Theoretical learning. Placing new 'knowledge' alongside existing knowledge
Facilitated small group discussion (max. 10 learners)	Discussing the relevance of the new material: how it builds upon pre-workshop knowledge and how it could be applied in clinical practice	Reflective learning
Facilitated rehearsals (max. 30 learners) Scenarios from the learners Demonstration with trained facilitators	Engage all learners in rehearsals of helpful communication skills using SAGE & THYME	Experiential learning. Involving all learners in the choice of phrases and the sequence of the questions in the safety of the classroom
Video presentation	To show the use of SAGE & THYME in approx. 5 minutes	To reinforce the learning and demonstrate the efficiency of cue-based structured interactions with distressed patients
Facilitated small group discussion (max. 10 learners)	Draw out the learning from the workshop for each learner	Reflective learning. Vicarious learning. To reinforce and embed the learning

Reproduced with kind permission of University Hospital of South Manchester NHS Foundation Trust.

be recognized among other essential skills and procedures in cancer nursing (Dougherty and Lister 2015). It is taught within a specific three-hour workshop (the SAGE & THYME foundation level workshop, described in Table 24.3) in which learners are taught practical listening skills: the importance of creating privacy; the need to ask about emotions; the skills of reflection and summary; and then screening for further concerns. Learners are taught how to ignore the 'expert' within them which filters, prioritizes, and applies solutions while listening to the concerns. They learn how to listen to all of the concerns, even those that have no solution. The teachers of SAGE & THYME describe this as 'containing' or 'holding' rather than 'unpacking' distress (Connolly *et al.* 2010). Learners are encouraged to make written lists of the concerns (with the permission of the patient) and to use the lists to summarize the concerns (Connolly *et al.* 2010). Learners also discuss empathy and its sensitive application in practice. They are taught how to contain their own anxieties about solutions to the patient's problems, so that individual patients can think for themselves first. The sequence suggested in the SAGE & THYME workshop, therefore, holds the listener back from offering solutions until near to the end of the consultation. The purpose of this holding back is to allow the patient to draw upon their own support and their own resources and ideas about what they think would help. In these ways, SAGE & THYME attempts to be a patient-centred model for listening and responding, which uses a mnemonic to transport the research evidence from the classroom into clinical practice.

The SAGE & THYME foundation level workshop

The developers of the SAGE & THYME foundation level workshop were predominantly specialist nurses in cancer and palliative care who had been taught 'advanced level' communications skills training themselves (Connolly *et al.* 2010). Their motivation to develop a foundation level training experience for colleagues came both from policy (NICE 2004), which recommended that training at 'level 1'

was required, and from a sense of their professional responsibility to disseminate valuable learning about helpful communication skills to every health and social care worker that cancer patients would encounter (NICE 2004). A practical and pragmatic workshop was subsequently designed: practical in that it would offer more than just theory; pragmatic in that it would train large numbers of learners in a short period of time. The workshop, therefore, is three hours in duration and is suitable for up to 30 learners at a time (Connolly *et al.* 2010). In order for the workshop to be efficient, safe for learners, and effective in its goals, it requires three accredited SAGE & THYME trainers. The workshop is designed to enable people from diverse clinical backgrounds to learn together in a range of ways (discussion, theoretical learning, reflection, observation, and reflection). The learning environment is created by the three facilitators, so that learners can feel safe enough to discuss emotional support with other learners and involved enough to consider how the skills taught might apply to their individual clinical practice. Table 24.3 describes the SAGE & THYME foundation level workshop.

Three studies have been published which have looked at feedback from participants in the SAGE & THYME workshops (Connolly *et al.* 2010, 2014; Griffiths *et al.* 2015). One study reported observed changes to communication behaviours following the workshop (Connolly *et al.* 2014). All other data is self-reported: questionnaire or focus group data where workshop participants describe for themselves what they learned, changes to their motivation and any changes that they made to their interactions with patients after completing the SAGE & THYME foundation level workshop. The findings from these studies relate predominantly to hospital-based and community nurses and are summarized in Box 24.2. The SAGE & THYME foundation level workshop is a relatively recent development when compared to the well-established advanced communications training workshops and has not yet been subjected a great deal of research scrutiny. Particularly missing from

Box 24.2 The impact of SAGE & THYME workshops

Learning

- Existing communication skills had been affirmed and learners felt that they had been challenged with new skills (Griffiths *et al.* 2015).
- Gathering all of the concerns was described as a change to their practice (Griffiths *et al.* 2015).
- Elements of SAGE were mostly familiar to learners, but the elements within THYME were mostly new to them (Griffiths *et al.* 2015).
- Asking about the support surrounding the patient (Talk and Help) was a change to the practice of learners (Griffiths *et al.* 2015).
- Asking the patient what they thought would help (You) was a change to the practice of learners (Griffiths *et al.* 2015).
- Learners knew more about helpful communication behaviours after the workshop (Connolly *et al.* 2014; Griffiths *et al.* 2015) and retained this knowledge two months later (Griffiths *et al.* 2015).

Beliefs, confidence, and willingness

- Learners became more positive about the benefits of helpful communication behaviours (Connolly *et al.* 2010, 2014).
- Learners increased their belief that they personally would be able to use the helpful communication behaviours (Connolly *et al.* 2010, 2014; Griffiths *et al.* 2015).
- Learners felt more able to open and close a discussion with a patient about emotions (Connolly *et al.* 2014; Griffiths *et al.* 2015).
- Learners felt more confident and competent to talk to people about their emotional troubles (Connolly *et al.* 2010).
- Learners felt less concerned about getting too close to patients and becoming overwhelmed by the patients' emotions (Connolly *et al.* 2014).
- Learners felt that the SAGE & THYME structure would be useful in their clinical practice and described feeling highly motivated to use it (Connolly *et al.* 2010, 2014).
- Learners felt more willing to talk to people about their emotional troubles (Connolly *et al.* 2010).

Changes in behaviour

- Learners felt that their communication skills had improved (Connolly *et al.* 2014; Griffiths *et al.* 2015).
- Learners reported a marked change in their style of communication (Connolly *et al.* 2010, 2014; Griffiths *et al.* 2015).
- Learners felt that they were allowing patients to find their own solutions more after the workshop (Griffiths *et al.* 2015).
- Learners felt that they had learned how to give control to the patient (Connolly *et al.* 2014; Griffiths *et al.* 2015).
- Learners demonstrated more helpful communication behaviours in videotaped interactions after the workshop when compared to similar interactions beforehand (Connolly *et al.* 2014).
- Learners gave examples of how they had used SAGE & THYME in practice (Connolly *et al.* 2014; Griffiths *et al.* 2015).
- Learners described using the SAGE & THYME structure on several occasions with patients (Connolly *et al.* 2014; Griffiths *et al.* 2015).
- Learners felt that they had left patients feeling empowered and satisfied (Connolly *et al.* 2014; Griffiths *et al.* 2015).
- Learners felt that interactions with patients had become more structured (Connolly *et al.* 2014; Griffiths *et al.* 2015).
- Learners felt that their interactions with patients had become more focused (Connolly *et al.* 2014; Griffiths *et al.* 2015).
- Learners felt that they had been able to hold back with solving problems in order to listen fully to all of the concerns of the patient (Connolly *et al.* 2014).
- Learners felt that by holding back advice to the end of the interaction, the patients had become more empowered (Connolly *et al.* 2014; Griffiths *et al.* 2015).
- Learners felt that they were more likely to hold back with advice and information and reassurance (Connolly *et al.* 2014).

Integration into normal practice

- Learners felt that the principles taught in the workshop had been incorporated flexibly within their practice (Griffiths *et al.* 2015).
- After two months, learners described having adapted the structure of SAGE & THYME into their practice and that they had persisted with the patient-centred behaviours of listening, holding back, and helping patients to find their own solutions (Griffiths *et al.* 2015).

Further communications skills training

- Learners felt motivated to take further communication skills training (Connolly *et al.* 2014).
- Learners were highly likely to recommend the workshop to a colleague (Connolly *et al.* 2010).

the evidence base is any observed, independent evidence that learners in the workshop change their behaviour with real patients (Connolly *et al.* 2014). Neither is there any objective evidence that patient outcomes are improved directly as a result of training in this workshop. Until such research is undertaken, the developers, teachers, and commissioners of the workshop rely on the evidence reported by learners who have attended it. From this evidence it appears that learning happens; that beliefs change; confidence grows and willingness to discuss sensitive emotional concerns with patients increases. Moreover, behaviour changes and learners report using SAGE & THYME with their patients. They notice improvements for their patients and for themselves. Within two months of the workshop, learners describe incorporating the helpful listening skills, the holding back, and empowerment into their interactions with patients even if they don't use the SAGE & THYME structure quite as it was taught to them. Lastly, learners recommend the workshop to their clinical colleagues and report increased motivation to undertake further communication skills training. For these reasons, the SAGE & THYME foundation level workshop is in demand by health and social care organizations in the United Kingdom who wish to provide a short 'underpinning' or 'foundation' workshop for all of their clinical and non-clinical staff who encounter distressed patients, families, or carers.

Dissemination of the SAGE & THYME foundational level workshop

The SAGE & THYME foundation level workshop is taught in many healthcare organizations across the United Kingdom (SAGE & THYME 2015). Each organization purchases a licence and develops a training team of at least three trainers, who are then named on the licence. Trainers of the SAGE & THYME foundation level workshops are accredited though a 2.5-day 'train-the-trainers' programme (SAGE & THYME 2015). Trainers are selected for their clinical and educational strengths using a 'person specification' (Box 24.3) and are assessed for their suitability and preparedness to train against specific training competencies. In order to be accredited, trainers must demonstrate a clear understanding of the helpful communication skills being taught, as well as an understanding of the elements of the SAGE & THYME structure. Additionally, they must demonstrate competence in the three specific roles needed for the rehearsals (interactive demonstrations) used in the workshop. Once accredited, SAGE & THYME trainers work within specific licences and can run workshops for learners in their own organizations. Many such organizations establish more than three trainers in order to sustain a programme in which large numbers of staff can be equipped with the skills to support patients.

Discussion

The educational reformer John Dewey described the responsibility of teachers to craft learning opportunities that challenge learners to consider skills which are just a little more difficult than those that they already have (Dewey 2004). The SAGE & THYME foundation level workshop appears to consolidate basic listening skills and stretch learners to consider patient-centred responses. Learners seem to appreciate this challenge. Short workshops, which are tightly focused on the published evidence and which use a combination of learning styles, are a promising new approach in foundation level communications skills training (Griffiths *et al.*

Box 24.3 The background and experience of the trainers

Experience

- Background in the training of communication skills.
- Background in health or social care.
- Experience of training using experiential training/learning methods.
- Experience of running groups/workshops/seminars.
- Attended a SAGE & THYME foundation level workshop run by the developers.

Skills

- Confidence in front of a group and able to deliver a lecture to 30 learners.
- Ability to facilitate 'role play' in front of 30 learners.
- Ability to facilitate small group discussions with up to 10 learners.
- Ability to support emotionally distressed learners.
- Ability to manage a diverse group of learners.

Personal characteristics

- Motivated to become a SAGE & THYME facilitator.
- Open to new ideas.
- Have time available to become a facilitator.
- Committed to facilitating at least three or four SAGE & THYME foundation level workshops each year.
- Advocate the skills taught through the SAGE & THYME model in their practice.

Reproduced with kind permission of University Hospital of South Manchester NHS Foundation Trust.

2015). The learner can relate the new learning to prior knowledge and be safely involved in the learning process through reflection and interaction with rehearsals. Some of the key skills taught within the advanced communications skills workshops appear also to be successfully taught in three hours to larger numbers of nurses and other health workers. Learners appear to value the learning and there is some evidence that the learning positively influences their interactions with patients. The dissemination of a standardized communications skills workshop across geographically disparate healthcare organizations also appears practical. This opens the possibility of training whole workforces how to listen and respond using evidence-based and patient-centred skills, as has been described in the United States and in Holland (Stein *et al.* 2005; Ammentorp and Kofoed 2011). There is a need for further research to test how the learned skills actually change nurses' behaviours with real patients and how those behaviours affect patients. The training appears to empower the nurses; do the nurses then empower the patients?

Perhaps there are parallels between listening skills and hand-washing skills in healthcare. Careful and thorough hand-washing for the benefit of patients was once thought to be so unimportant and so easy to learn that it did not need to be taught. Equally, careful and skilful listening to patients will perhaps one day also be fully recognized to be of universal importance and deserving of skilful, evidence-based training.

References

Ammentorp J, Kofoed PE (2011). Research in communication skills training translated into practice in a large organization: a proactive use of the RE-AIM framework. *Patient Educ Couns* **82**, 482–7.

Booth K, Maguire P, Hillier V (1999). Measurement of communication skills in cancer care: myth or reality? *J Adv Nurs* **30**, 1073–9.

Butow P, Brown R, Cogar S, Tattersall M, Dunn S (2002). Oncologists' reactions to cancer patients' verbal cues. *Psychooncology* **11**, 47–58.

Choralalambous A, Papadopoulus IR, Beadsmoore A (2008). Listening to the voices of patients with cancer, their advocates and their nurses: a hermeneutic-phenomenological study of quality of nursing care. *Eur J Oncol Nurs* **12**, 436–42.

Connolly M, Perryman J, McKenna Y, et al. (2010). SAGE & THYME™: A model for training health and social care professionals in patient-focussed support. *Patient Educ Couns* **79**, 87–93.

Connolly M, Thomas JM, Orford, JA, et al. (2014). The impact of the SAGE & THYME foundation level workshop on factors influencing communication skills in health care professionals. *J Contin Educ Health Prof* **34**, 37–46.

Dewey J (2004). *Democracy and Education*. Courier Corporation, New York, US.

Dougherty L, Lister S (eds) (2015). *The Royal Marsden Manual of Clinical Procedures*, 9th edition. Wiley, Chichester, UK.

Fallowfield L, Jenkins V (1999). Effective communication skills are the key to good cancer care. *Eur J Cancer* **35**, 1592–7.

Griffiths J, Wilson C, Ewing G, Connolly M, Grande G (2015). Improving communication with palliative care cancer patients at home—a pilot study of SAGE & THYME communications skills model. *Eur J Oncol Nurs* **19**, 465–72.

Gysels M, Richardson A, Higginson I (2005). Communication training for health professionals who care for patients with cancer: a systematic review of training methods. *Support Cancer Care* **13**, 356–66.

Heaven C, Clegg J, Maguire P (2006). Transfer of communication skills training from workshop to workplace: the impact of clinical supervision. *Patient Educ Couns* **60**, 313–25.

Maguire P, Pitceathly C (2002). Key communication skills and how to acquire them. *BMJ* **325**, 697–700.

Moore PM, Rivera Mercado S, Grez Artigues M, Lawrie TA (2013). Communication skills training for healthcare professionals working with people who have cancer. *Cochrane Database Syst Rev* **28**, CD003751.

National Institute for Clinical Excellence (NICE) (2004). *Improving Supportive and Palliative Care for Adults with Cancer: The Manual*. Department of Health.

Oermann MH (1999). Consumers' descriptions of quality health care. *J Nurs Care Qual* **14**, 47–55.

SAGE & THYME (2015). Available at: www.sageandthymetraining.org.uk

Saino C, Lauri S, Erikssonn E (2001). Cancer patients' views and experiences of participation in care and decision making. *Nurs Ethics* **8**, 97–113.

Silverman J, Kurtz S, Draper J (2013). *Skills for Communicating with Patients*. Radcliffe Publishing Ltd, Oxford, UK.

Stein T, Frankel RM, Krupat E (2005). Enhancing clinician communication skills in a large healthcare organisation: a longitudinal case study. *Patient Educ Couns* **58**, 4–12.

Stiefel F, Barth J, Bensing J, et al. (2010). Communication skills training in oncology: a position paper based on a consensus meeting among European experts in 2009. *Ann Oncol* **21**, 204–7.

Wilkinson S, Perry R, Blanchard K (2008). Effectiveness of a three-day communication skills course in changing nurses' communication skills with cancer/palliative care patients: a randomised controlled trial. *Palliat Med* **22**, 365–75.

CHAPTER 25

The implementation of advanced communication skills training for senior healthcare professionals in Northern Ireland: The challenges and rewards

Anne Finn, Emma King, and Susie Wilkinson

Introduction and background

In this chapter we will describe the key challenges and rewards of the implementation and delivery of a programme of advanced communication skills training (ACST) for senior healthcare professionals working in cancer and palliative care in Northern Ireland (NI). We will also discuss the rationale for this initiative, the programme content, and the direction and priorities for sustaining this into the future. To provide some context, the chapter begins with a brief discussion on the population and provision of health services in NI and the strategic drivers influencing the need for development of a sustainable evidence-based communication programme for the region.

Northern Ireland is a region of the United Kingdom with a population of 1.8 million people. Responsibility for population health and well-being, and the provision of health and social care, is devolved to the NI Assembly from the UK Government in Westminster. Northern Ireland differs from the rest of the United Kingdom in that provision of health and social care was unified by the Northern Ireland Order (1972), giving responsibility for providing comprehensive health services to each of four geographical areas. In 2005, an independent review of these services in NI resulted in the reconfiguration of health and social care organizations, and, in particular, the creation of five health and personal social services agencies for NI. This is the model of health delivery we were working within when implementing and delivering this communication skills programme.

Anyone who faces illness or disability, loss, or bereavement needs the support of professionals who empathize with what they are going through and can display humanity (Nursing and Midwifery Council and the General Medical Council 2012). The importance of effective communication in healthcare is well documented. Surveys indicate patients with cancer place good communication with healthcare professionals high on their list of priorities (Bowling et al. 2013: Furber et al. 2013). Poor communication can have serious consequences, leading to complaints by patients and their relatives, and can also leave them feeling dissatisfied (Audit Commission 2013). They can also develop a sense of uncertainty that impairs their ability to comply with recommended treatments (Butow et al. 2002). Good communication has been shown to influence patients' emotional health, symptom resolution, function, and physiological measurements (Michie et al. 2003). It is also recognized that insufficient training in communication is a major factor contributing to stress, lack of job satisfaction, and emotional burnout in healthcare professionals (Taylor et al. 2005). Despite the knowledge that effective communication is an essential part of caring for patients with cancer, there is evidence that in practice communication continues to be problematic (NICE 2004). Rather than issues of clinical competence, many complaints reflect a perceived failure of effective communication (Neuberger 2013). Research suggests communication skills do not reliably improve with experience alone (Levin and Weiner, 2010). However, there is evidence that with appropriate teaching, these skills can be acquired and retained (Fallowfield et al. 2002: Wilkinson et al. 2008). This awareness has led to an increasing demand for communication skills training. Furthermore, the expectation is that over time all senior healthcare professionals will be able to demonstrate they have the level of competence to communicate complex information, involve patients in clinical decisions, and offer choice (DoH 2007). Thus it should be considered that communication skills need to be a core clinical skill for all who have to deal with issues relating to breaking bad news and supporting patients to make and understand decisions related to their care and treatment.

Furthermore, there is direct benefit to clinicians themselves. Effectiveness can increase, with feedback following courses indicating those who implement the learning can save consultation time. Butow *et al.* (2002) demonstrated that clinicians who respond to at least one patient cue have shorter consultation times. In the present healthcare climate, with targets and time being of the essence, this is an important factor to be considered.

The NI Framework for Cancer Prevention, Treatment, and Care (2010) and NI palliative and end-of-life care strategy (2010) also recognized the need for health and social care professionals to be skilled in communicating effectively and sensitively with people affected by cancer. Both documents stipulate that those professionals with responsibility for communicating significant news should undertake a programme of ACST. This is in line with UK-wide initiatives, which have resulted in the development of an agreed programme of training.

The importance of good communication is also reinforced by the recent report of the application of health and social care governance arrangements for ensuring the quality of care provision for NI, the Donaldson Report (2014). This report states that many patients experience disrespect for them and their families, bad communication, and poor coordination of care.

The importance of effective communication skills and an introduction to training in this area for undergraduate healthcare professionals is swiftly becoming a core component of the curriculum for many universities. For this reason, the major focus for communication skills training for our healthcare professionals in NI is in the post-graduate setting. Prior to 2009, those seeking to extend their communication skills were unable to do so in NI, as appropriate evidence-based programmes were not available locally. Accessing these programmes proved to be a costly business both financially and in the use of the healthcare professionals' time, as trips had to be made to the UK mainland to avail of the programme there. As a result, very few were able to access the training due to the high overall financial costs. Fortunately we were given the opportunity to undertake the ACST programme and the subsequent Training the Trainers course, which would allow us to share this experience and cascade the training to other senior healthcare professionals.

The evidence base

Wilkinson *et al.* (2008*a*) conducted a randomized controlled trial to evaluate the effectiveness of a three-day communication skills course in its ability to change UK nurses' communication skills. One hundred and seventy-two nurses were randomly allocated to undertake the three-day course or to control (no course). The results demonstrated that a three-day communication skills course was effective in changing nurses' behaviours up to three months post-course. In addition, the quality of the nurses' communication skills improved after attending the course, reflected by the increase in audiotaped assessment scores. The course was also shown to have a positive effect on the nurses' confidence in dealing with cancer patients.

The course has been evaluated for fourth year medical students and then repeated in their Senior House Officer (SHO) year. The results were then compared with SHO's who had not completed the three-day course; the findings confirm the efficacy and sustainability of the variant for training doctors (Mason and Ellershaw 2008).

The three-day course has also been evaluated for nurses working with patients who have heart disease, and for senior healthcare professionals caring for children and young people. Both studies demonstrate this method of training is acceptable to other clinicians and increases their confidence in communicating with patients and their carers (Wilkinson *et al.* 2008*b*).

Based on the research, and as a cohort of healthcare professions from NI had already completed this course, it was decided that the Wilkinson variant of ACST would be the programme of choice for implementation in NI.

The Wilkinson ACST model

The programme is based on Confucius' (551 BC) philosophy of: 'Tell me I will forget, show me, I may remember, involve me and I will understand.' The adult learning theories of Knowles (1978) and Rogers (1983) are also incorporated to promote a learner-centred approach, which is known to enhance effective person-centred communication and includes cognitive, behavioural, and affective components.

Core principles

The course is aimed at senior healthcare professionals working in cancer and palliative care and consists of a three-day intensive, experiential, learner-centred course, where up to 12 participants work with two facilitators on areas of communication they find personally challenging. The programme is delivered outside of the hospital setting, thus away from the workplace. Participants are bound by agreed ground rules and trained actors simulate patients in role play. The participants set the agenda for the three days by presenting complex communication scenarios they have found difficult in practice; they are then facilitated to work through their own scenario over the three-day period. As a result the facilitation process can be challenging, as with each programme the facilitators can be presented with complex participant scenarios which are completely different on each occasion. Thus it requires well-trained and experienced facilitators to ensure the programme runs smoothly and maximum learning is gained for those who participate. Facilitators delivering the programme must also deliver a minimum of three ACST programmes per year to maintain their skills.

Learning outcomes

This course enables participants to reflect and critically appraise their own and others communication skills and to demonstrate the skills required to facilitate a structured patient-centred assessment/consultation using specific strategies to handle complex communication scenarios. They should also be able to tailor complex information to meet the needs of patients and carers.

Monitoring and evaluation

At the conclusion of each programme, participants are asked to complete a four page written evaluation form; the verbal feedback they have given throughout the course is also taken into consideration. The actors are also asked to provide verbal feedback to the facilitators at the end of each day and in order to be deemed competent facilitators must complete a competency based assessment.

Development of the Northern Ireland ACST programme

The initial ACST delivery in NI began in 2009 with the original three-day course. The programme has undergone a process of evaluation and review in response to feedback from participants. One common theme arising from evaluations was the preference of participants to be able to access a two-day programme as opposed to the historical three-day version. Reasons for this were variable but included three days being too 'emotionally and physically challenging' and also 'too long', with participants citing the three-day programmes as 'becoming tedious' with query to the value of learning by the third day. In response to this feedback, the facilitators steering group agreed to trial a two-day programme throughout 2012/2013 with a maximum of six participants. Thus, the current NI ACST model is composed of a two-day course containing the learning philosophy, core components, learning outcomes, and delivery methods of the original (see Box 25.1).

A major component of the programme is the use of video-recorded learner-centred role plays based on the communication issue the participant has identified as challenging during the agenda setting process. Through the use of role play the participants are encouraged to practise their skills to address the scenarios identified as complex/difficult in a 'safe' environment. This assists them to face such difficulties in the future with more confidence.

Box 25.1 Core components of the two-day programme

- **Introductions and ground rules**

Participant-generated ground rules ensure safety and equal participation.

  Two didactic presentations delivered on day one:

- **Evidence base for training**

- **Skills required for assessment/consultations**

These presentations include the use of facilitating skills and blocking behaviours, the structuring of a patient assessment, and experiential learning methods used during the course.

- **Agenda setting**

Participants set their own agenda for the course by identifying challenging communication situations they have encountered with patients, carers, or colleagues. This process is followed to ensure the course is learner-centred and responsive to specific individual learning needs.

- **Use of trigger tapes**

Participants critique the strengths and weaknesses of the communication skills demonstrated on pre-recorded video clips known to be representative of issues identified as difficult by healthcare professionals (e.g. handling anger).

- **Discussion**

Debate and engagement is encouraged among participants around the key communication issues identified.

- **Use of role play**

Actors playing the role of patient/carer/colleague are an essential component of the programme in terms of offering **standardization** (being able to reproduce the same issue/content a number of times) and **customization** (matching the role play to learners' individual needs and level of experience). Participants are encouraged to imagine how patients in these situations may be feeling. **Patient prediction** is aimed at increasing understanding of patient perspective and encouraging the use of empathy.

Delivering the two-day programme—challenges and rewards

During the programme, the involved healthcare professionals describe, practice, and explore the issues they have highlighted as major challenges for them in communication. A number of issues and core themes are repeatedly identified by facilitators.

The reluctant participant

In NI, the concept of peer review has made ACST a mandatory requirement for certain core multidisciplinary cancer teams, and is no longer optional (National Peer Review Programme 2013). As a result, senior clinicians are frequently nominated to undertake this programme and thus are attending under duress and with a major degree of reluctance. This proves a challenge for facilitators, as the reluctant participant can easily become disengaged and can influence and disrupt the learning and participation within the group. If this is not addressed by facilitators early on, it can seriously impact on the programme with reports from facilitators of feeling uncomfortable, undermined, and distressed. In response to this challenge, NI has developed a pre-course participant contract, which requests signed agreement from participants to ensure they attend all sessions, actively participate, contribute constructively, receive valid feedback in a developmental way, and be prepared to examine and reflect on their current communication skills. In return, we as facilitators agree to provide the necessary information, teaching, and support to help them to complete the ACST course. This initiative is in its trial period and will be evaluated after an agreed time.

The time factor

Without exception on each course, the issue of 'lack of time' is raised by all of the professional groups. There is no doubt that in the present extremely pressurized clinical climate, time is a precious commodity. Often at the start of day one, medical consultants tell us they do not have the time it would take to provide the level of communication, empathy etc. they perceive the initial presentation and discussion on course content is suggesting. They continually identify a time frame officially allocated for each patient consultation as around 20 minutes. What we have found, however, raises another issue: is it the lack of time or rather the lack of appropriate use of facilitating communication skills that will allow them to engage and disengage with confidence during the consultations that is actually the problem? We have handled this in several ways (see Box 25.2).

Agenda setting

Agenda setting enables the participants to determine and dictate the content of the programme ensuring that it is learner-centred. Each participant is encouraged to explore communication issues

Box 25.2 Time factors

- Negotiating time boundaries: 'We have around 20 minutes or so to talk today would that be OK?'

- Using the time taken in trigger tapes as examples: often when watching these participants feel the time taken to perform an assessment, e.g. is longer than it actually is. Facilitators stop and start these clips at appropriate learning points; however, the overall time taken to complete a holistic assessment in the clip is a maximum of 15 minutes and often participants are astounded at this time frame.

- Monitoring time in their role play: using the camera, it is possible for the facilitator to record the time taken by a participant to complete their role play using their newly acquired communication skills and strategies. This time frame is often a pleasant surprise to them, as it is inevitably much shorter than they assume.

Box 25.3 Ideas, concerns, and expectations

Examples of phrasing when asking about patients' ideas, concerns, and expectations:

Ideas: Finds out what the patient believes and their thoughts and feelings about their condition

'What do you think might be happening?'

'You've obviously given this some thought; it would help me to know what you were thinking it might be.'

Concerns: Elicits what is a particular concern or worry to the patient at this stage of their illness

'What are you concerned that it might be?'

'Is there anything particular or specific that you were concerned about?'

Expectations: What were the patient's thoughts for the future? What were they hoping for, expecting, and what would they like to happen?

'What were you hoping we might be able to do for this?'

'How might I best help you with this?'

that are applicable to themselves and their practice, ensuring that the programme remains focused on their specific learning needs. Ownership and agreement of agenda items ensures participants do not become dissatisfied with the relevance of these issues to their work areas, and encourages active engagement with their role play scenarios. In setting the agenda, participants are invited to identify a challenging communication interaction emanating from their practice which they have found difficult in the past. These issues can be related to patients, families, or colleagues, and the content needs to be very specific involving the words spoken and emotions involved. The agenda setting is crucial to the content and development of the two days. Our challenges with this frequently arise when participants do not appear to grasp the concept of what a 'communication issue' actually is. Frequently we are faced with participants telling us the minutia involved in a scenario but failing to identify the actual core communication issue. To address these, facilitators must have the skills to identify within the minutia the specific communication issue and then employ a learner-centred approach to support the participant in identifying their actual communication scenario. Facilitator time management in this process is crucial to ensure the programme does not overrun. We endeavour to sensitively but firmly manage this situation while ensuring equity of time for all participants.

Assessment

This programme continues to highlight an apparent lack of insight and ability of some participants to undertake appropriate holistic patient assessment. Some healthcare professionals appear to consistently remain in the realms of information giving and the desire to 'fix' patients' problems; therefore often failing to identify their actual concerns. As the importance of impeccable assessment cannot be underestimated and is an integral part of medical and nursing practice, it needs to be taught in a systematic way with attention being paid not only to content, but to the structure of the interview. To this end we integrate a structured model for assessment, which from the outset is embedded into the initial role play scenarios. This concept is based on the Calgary–Cambridge guide to the medical interview, which is a recognized framework for medical assessment

(Silverman *et al.* 2005). Participants are introduced to the concept of the assessment structure, that is

- Introduction

- Information gathering

- Information giving

Most importantly participants are frontloaded with a model from the guide namely **ICE** (Ideas, Concerns, and Expectations), which allow participants to elicit the patient's key problems, establish which of these are main concerns, and enable care to be focused on the patient's individual needs. This focus assists in displaying holistic, patient-centred care, and moves away from the traditional assessment of physical symptoms only (Winterburn and Wilkinson 2010) (Box 25.3).

The frontloading is supported by the use of a video clip prior to commencement of the role play sessions. This clip demonstrates a healthcare professional undertaking a holistic assessment with a patient using ICE and the Calgary–Cambridge (2005) assessment structure. Participants are enabled and supported by the facilitators to examine and discuss the content of the clip, to identify the communication skills utilized by the nurse, and the structure and strategy used to progress through the assessment. This then equips participants with the knowledge of ICE and assessment structure, which they then can incorporate alongside other management strategies in their role play scenarios. This frontloading system has proved very successful and feedback on it has been positive.

Anger and strong emotions

This is an agenda item which inevitably reoccurs on most two-day programmes at least once, if not more often. It would appear healthcare professionals are being faced with issues such as anger and other strong emotions on a regular basis. They express a lack of confidence and say they are not equipped to deal with these situations. Participants acknowledge these feelings can be generated from a desire to protect themselves, as asking patients about their feelings can 'open a can of worms' they feel they may not be able to deal with. NICE (2004) suggest that psychological distress is a common phenomenon in people affected by cancer and is understandably a natural response to what is a very traumatic situation. They also recommend staff working in cancer services be familiar and suitably skilled in using a range of strategies to manage these situations. Hence, we facilitate participants to employ a strategy specifically for dealing with anger (Box 25.4) and then utilize ICE in combination with facilitating communication skills to hear and empathically respond to the patient's/relatives' story and jointly plan a way forward. Participants are frontloaded with a video clip showing such a situation being managed using both a structured strategy and incorporating ICE. They then plan their role play using elements from the clip contents they feel will help them manage their unique communication scenario, eliciting suggestions from their other group members to help them plan their role play. This also encourages group cohesion and a sense of unity for the members. The challenge for facilitators is to maintain at all times an enabling—rather than teaching—environment in the management of the role plays in order to maintain the experiential, learner-centred approach, which is so important in the acquisition of new skills and in changing learner's behaviour (Kurtz *et al.* 2005) (Box 25.4).

A major reward from the NI ACST initiative has been the development and production of a new and updated DVD addressing five complex communication scenarios. The choice of topics included were those consistently identified in agenda setting by participants such as those discussed above. This DVD is now in regular use by facilitators in programme delivery and has been highly evaluated by participants. Delivery of the NI ACST programme also now stretches beyond cancer service to include non-cancer specialities. In addition, healthcare professionals from a variety of specialties such as respiratory, heart failure, renal, dementia, mental health, and paediatrics have attended our programme. Overall the course has been highly evaluated by participants from all clinical areas.

Course evaluation—two days vs. three days

In 2014 an analysis was carried out to compare evaluation questionnaire feedback from 72 participants on the three-day course with the 66 participants who had completed the two-day course. The benefits of the multidisciplinary mix are seen as valuable in both cohorts and the smaller group is also preferred. The analysis report recommends the continuation of the two-day model for ACST, as no disadvantages have been identified and the programme appears to meet the needs of the participants (Rutherford and McCaughey 2014).

Conclusion and the way forward

This chapter has addressed a number of key challenges faced by facilitators delivering ACST in Northern Ireland. Using examples of actual situations from programme delivery, it has offered suggestions of how experienced facilitators have managed these issues as they arise in programme delivery. Over the last five years there has been much hard work, drive, and commitment by a core of dedicated healthcare professionals to ensure that the ACST programme is accessible to senior staff throughout NI. The demand for such training into the future is anticipated to be great when considering peer review for cancer teams and the shift of focus from cancer to include non-cancer specialities. The challenge now will be to maintain this dedication and hard work to forward plan, to ensure the programme will be self-sustaining, affordable, and accessible for years to come. Ongoing programme development has been planned for the coming year; following this time frame, ongoing progress will be reliant on the value for service users and staff which individual NI Trusts place on this quality initiative. Their continued support will be crucial to ensure its success.

References

Audit Commission (2013). *What Seems to be the Matter? Communication between Hospitals and Patients.* HMSO, London, UK.

Bowling A, Rowe G, McKee M (2013). Patients' experiences of their healthcare in relation to their expectations and satisfactions: a population survey. *J R Soc Med* **106**, 143–9.

Butow PN, Brown RF, Cogar S, Tattersall MHN, Dunne SN (2002). Oncologists' reactions to cancer patients verbal cues. *Psychooncology* **11**, 47–58.

Department of Health (2007). *Cancer Reform Strategy.* Department of Health, London, UK.

DHSSPS (2010). *Living Matters, Dying Matters: A Palliative and End of Life Care Strategy for Adults in Northern Ireland.* DHSSPS, Belfast, Northern Ireland.

DHSSPS (2010). *Service Framework for Cancer Prevention, Treatment and Care.* Available at: http://www.sor.org/system/files/article/201207/service_framework_for_cancer_prevention__treatment_and_care_-_full_document.pdf. DHSSPS, Belfast, Northern Ireland.

Donaldson L, Rutter P, Henderson M (2014). *The Right Time, The Right Place: An expert examination of the application of health and social care*

Box 25.4 Core content of teaching: Anger

- Do not say 'calm down'.
- Ignore sarcasms and put downs that would lead to more anger and argument.
- Try not to take anger personally.
- Aim to move the person from an emotional state to a more rational state.
- Acknowledge and recognize the anger by saying 'I can see you are very angry'.
- Give permission to be angry by saying 'I really want to hear what you are angry about and what you have to say'.
- If appropriate, sensitively ask 'but can you please speak more quietly so that I can hear what you have to say'.
- Establish facts, listen to the story, get as much information as possible.
- Concentrate on the person and their stress/feelings.
- Maintain eye contact.
- Recap and summarize to be clear of facts.
- Try to negotiate a solution.
- 'What can I do to help' or 'Let's work on this together'.
- Take action if appropriate.

governance arrangements for ensuring the quality of care provision for Northern Ireland. DHSSPS, Belfast, Northern Ireland.

Fallowfield L, Jenkins V, Farewell V, Saul J, Duffy A, Eves R (2002). Efficacy of a Cancer Research UK communication skills training model for oncologists: a randomized controlled trial. *Lancet* **359**, 650–6.

Furber L, Cox K, Murphy R, Steward W (2013). Investing communication in cancer consultations: what can be learnt from doctor and patient accounts of their experience? *Eur J Cancer Care* **22**, 653–62.

Health and Personal Social Services (Northern Ireland) Order (1972). Her Majesty's Stationary Office, London, UK. Available at: http://www.legislation.gov.uk/nisi/1972/1265/contents

Knowles MS (1978). *The Adult Learner: A Neglected Species*. Gulf, Houston, TX.

Kurtz S, Silverman S, Draper J (2005). *Teaching and Learning Communication Skills in Medicine*, 2nd edition. Radcliff Publishing, Oxford, UK.

Levin T, Weiner JS (2010). End-of-life communication training. Ch.19. In: Kissane D, Bultz B, Butow P, Finlay L (eds). *Handbook of Communication in Oncology and Palliative Care*. Oxford University Press, Oxford, UK.

Mason SR, Ellershaw EJ (2008). Preparing for palliative medicine; evaluation of an education programme for fourth year medical undergraduates. *Palliat Med* **22**, 687–92.

Michie S, Miles J, Weinman J (2003). Patient-centeredness in chronic illness: what is it and does it matter? *Patient Educ Counsel* **51**, 197–206.

National Institute for Clinical Excellence (2004). Supportive and palliative care for people with cancer. Available at: https://www.nice.org.uk/guidance/csgsp/evidence/supportive-and-palliative-care-the-manual-2 [Last accessed November 26, 2014].

National Peer Review Programme (2013). *Manual for Cancer Services—Lung Cancer Measures*. Version 1.1 NHS England, UK.

Neuberger J (2013). *More care less pathway: a review of the Liverpool Care Pathway*. Available at: https://www.gov.uk/government/uploads/system/uploads/attachment_data/file/212450/Liverpool_Care_Pathway.pdf (Last accessed November 26, 2014).

Nursing & Midwifery Council & General Medical Council (2012). *Joint statement on professional values*. Available at: http://www.nmc-uk.org/media/Latest-news/NMC-and-GMC-release-joint-statement-on-professional-values/ [Last accessed January 29, 2015].

Rogers CR (1983). *Freedom to Learn From the 80's*. Merrill, Columbus, OH.

Rutherford L, McCaughey C (2014). *Evaluation of the Two Day Versus the Three Day Advanced Communication Skill Training in Northern Ireland Using the Susie Wilkinson Model* (unpublished).

Silverman JD, Kurtz SM, Draper J (2005). Calgary Cambridge guide to the Medical Interview—communication process. Available at: http://www.gp-training.net/training/communication_skills/calgary/calgary.pdf [Last accessed February 3, 2015].

Taylor C, Graham J, Potts H, Richards M, Ramirez A (2005). Changes in mental health of UK hospital consultants since the mid-1990s. *Lancet* **366**, 742–4.

Wilkinson S, Linsell L, Perry R, Blanchard K (2008a). Effectiveness of a three-day communication skills course in changing nurses' communication skills with cancer/palliative care patients: A randomized controlled trial. *Palliat Med* **22**, 365–75.

Wilkinson S, Linsell L, Perry R, Blanchard K (2008b). Communication skills training course for nurses working with patients with heart disease. *Br J Cardiac Nurs* **3**, 475–81.

Winterburn S, Wilkinson S (2010). The challenges and rewards of communication skills training for oncology and palliative care nurses in the United Kingdom. Ch. 36. In: Kissane D, Bultz B, Butow P, Finlay L (eds). *Handbook of Communication in Oncology and Palliative Care*. Oxford University Press, Oxford, UK.

CHAPTER 26

Training facilitators to deliver an advanced communication course for senior healthcare professionals in cancer and palliative care

Susie Wilkinson and Anita Roberts

Communication skills

While there is general agreement on the importance of communication skills training for senior healthcare professionals (SHCPs) working in cancer and palliative care, as well as evidence that communication skills training improves communication skills (Moore et al. 2013), there is a paucity of information regarding the training, development, and support for the facilitators who deliver communication skills courses for the SHCPs in cancer and palliative care.

Several studies have evaluated training programmes for doctors: Kurtz et al. (2005) explored training general practitioners to deliver courses for GPs; Arnold et al. (2010) developed the Oncotalk programme for doctors. They identified important lessons for teaching communication skills including: the importance of trust within the group; the trainee facilitators own emotions in learning communication skills; and the importance of skills practice and positive feedback with reflection. However, to date, little has been described for training nurses and professions allied to medicine.

This chapter describes the key skills facilitators need to effectively deliver the experiential advanced communication skills training (ACST) course for SHCPs working in cancer and palliative care described in Chapter 25 (Wilkinson et al. 2008). This course, which is delivered by two facilitators, was one of three courses chosen for the national advanced communication skills programme (Connected 2012).

This chapter will focus on the content, process, and guidelines of the facilitator training course (FTC) and report on an evaluation of the effectiveness of the FTC in terms of the facilitators' levels of confidence in delivering the ACST.

The facilitator training course

The aim of the course is to:

◆ develop trainee facilitators' skills to teach and assess communication skills;

◆ enable trainee facilitators to reflect on and improve the delivery of an ACST course.

The FTC was designed to incorporate adult learning principles (Knowles 1978). Kurtz and Cooke (2010) suggest lectures alone are ineffective and do not change behaviours. Teaching should be experiential involving skills, practice, and reinforcement; learners' attitudes and emotions should be acknowledged and the learning should integrate knowledge, skills, and attitudes.

The course runs with a minimum of 6 and a maximum of 12 trainee facilitators. Each trainee facilitator must have attended the Wilkinson ACST as a learner so that they are familiar with the course they are learning to facilitate. It is important that anyone who facilitates communication skills training does so on a regular basis, to ensure that skills and competence are maintained. Therefore, trainee facilitators must also have consent from their manager, not only to attend the course, but also a commitment from their managers to release them to deliver a minimum three ACSTs per year as part of their role.

The FTC is delivered over three consecutive days in an environment away from the workplace whenever possible, to maximize involvement and commitment. As with any experiential course, a safe environment is essential, and this is created by having experienced facilitators delivering the course. It is vital to establish group ground rules and have clear regulations for running any role play. This safe environment enables trainee facilitators to make honest disclosures about any difficulties they may have experienced when teaching.

The trainee facilitators are introduced to the micro-teaching model used for the ACST course they are learning to deliver (see Fig. 26.1). This model outlines the process of teaching communication skills. As the ACST course is experiential and learner centred, participants are encouraged to identify areas that they find difficult and wish to develop. They are asked to think of examples from their practice. These issues are then explored and appropriate skills and

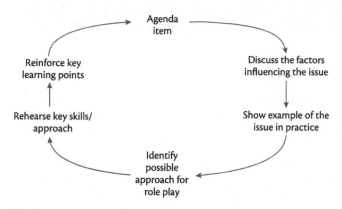

Fig. 26.1 Micro teaching model.

Reproduced with permission from Wilkinson S, *Training the Trainer Handbook*, Copyright © Susie Wilkinson 2002–14.

strategies identified. Role play is then used as a vehicle to practise these new skills.

The FTC reflects the ACST course, in that it adopts a learner-centred approach. The trainee facilitators generate their own agenda by identifying and describing a teaching scenario they have found difficult. The key issues from each scenario are identified and these are practised via role play during the course.

An example of a typical agenda for the FTC is shown in Box 26.1.

The FTC considers each element of the ACST course and the teaching methods used. This ensures that the trainee facilitators understand the underpinning rationale for each element of the ACST course and have the opportunity to practise these elements using role play to ensure that they can deliver it competently and safely.

Course introductions

The aim of this element of the course is to ensure that there is an understanding of the course participants' background and also to start the process of group cohesion.

Trainee facilitators are taught to ask the participants to state their name, role, and previous communication skills training. This enables trainee facilitators to determine the level at which they need to pitch the course. It is also helpful to explore the participants' expectations of the course, as it identifies whether their expectations are realistic, and can also highlight hidden agendas or specific considerations.

Ground rules and group safety

This section of the course aims to promote a safe environment where participants feel able to freely disclose their communication difficulties, associated feelings, and fears honestly without feeling a failure.

Trainee facilitators need to be adept in generating effective ground rules, as these provide clear boundaries should difficulties occur during the course. They are important for group cohesion and safety. Following the introductions and before any further disclosures, participants are invited to generate a set of ground rules. It is important that the term 'ground rules' is understood; clarification about what they are and why they are important may be needed. Once generated, the ground rules are written up on a flip chart and then collectively agreed by the group as rules which will be adhered to by all for the duration of the course. These rules should be displayed in the room for the duration of the course. Box 26.2 shows a typical set of ground rules.

Trainee facilitators need to make clear what the boundaries are in terms of the levels of working. For example, any discussion and exploration in the group is expected to relate to professional communication issues rather than personal issues. This prevents any participants who are experiencing emotional difficulties who have a strong desire for personal disclosure from using the ASCT group as a therapy group.

Trainee facilitators need to know how to get the group to bond as quickly as possible. The sooner participants begin to share in the

---

Box 26.1 Example of a participants' agenda for the FTC course

1. Setting the agenda—ensuring all participants needs are met.

2. Setting the role play up.

3. Managing a participant who is very reluctant to role play.

4. Managing a role play that is not going anywhere.

5. Managing a role play that is going wrong.

6. Getting participants to engage in feedback.

7. Challenging participants—'The reality is we don't have the time for this course'.

8. Dealing with a very distressed participant.

9. Dealing with the dominant (know it all) participant.

10. Dealing with a confrontational participant—'What you are saying deskills people'.

11. Dealing with an angry participant.

Reproduced with permission from Wilkinson S, *Training the Trainer Handbook*, Copyright © Susie Wilkinson 2002–14.

Box 26.2 An example of typical ground rules

♦ Participants are required to attend the whole course.

♦ Everyone should contribute throughout the course.

♦ Each participant has to undertake a role play.

♦ Participants should demonstrate respect to each other and be sensitive to enabling each participant to contribute.

♦ Feedback should be constructive, positive, non-judgemental, and specific to skills and strategies.

♦ Negative comments must be followed with constructive suggestions for alternatives.

♦ Confidentiality to be maintained. The group should negotiate what level and parameters they wish to place around the confidentiality.

♦ Participants may become distressed, and a response to this should be agreed. These should include the option of having time out and to debrief privately with a facilitator.

Reproduced with permission from Wilkinson S, *Training the Trainer Handbook*, Copyright © Susie Wilkinson 2002–14.

learning experience by contributing their ideas and responses in a constructive and helpful rather than destructive and unhelpful way, bonding will take place. As the group begins to feel safer and bonding develops, the level of disclosure will deepen from the disclosure of just the facts of the situation to facts plus feelings.

Trainee facilitators also need to be able to reinforce the bonding by being positive about disclosures from participants, by saying for example, 'That was very helpful, thank you for sharing that with us'.

It is also important to actively invite comments from quieter group members early on in the course, so they know they are expected to be involved. If participants disclose personal feelings about a communication task, for example being scared of handling a difficult question, such as 'Am I dying?', the trainee facilitator needs to reinforce their concern immediately: 'Thank you for sharing with us that you are scared about handling such a difficult question. That is very helpful and an area which we will certainly be exploring. Does anyone else find this difficult?'

This kind of response confirms and legitimizes to participants that disclosure and expression of feelings are valid and important contributions.

Deskilling of participants

An important skill for the trainee facilitators to develop is the ability to create an environment that minimizes the risk of deskilling participants and of them being harmed during their experiential learning.

Behaviours that are likely to deskill a participant include:

- when a participant makes an important disclosure which is ignored by the group or the facilitator;
- when critical feedback is given without any supportive or alternative suggestions being offered;
- criticisms from the facilitators themselves can be especially damaging.

Resistance to training

A trainee facilitator needs to be able to identify any group activity that could be damaging and be alert to the silent, domineering, hostile, angry, or withdrawn participants. When communication skills training for SHCPs in cancer and palliative care working in England became a mandatory requirement of the Cancer Services Peer Review process, some individuals reluctantly attended courses. This resulted in a resistance to training and, on occasion, hostile behaviour towards the facilitators. Signs of impending conflict can include the seating positions participants take. For example, confrontational participants may sit directly opposite a facilitator or outside the group, and may indulge in negative, sarcastic, or critical comments. Box 26.3 highlights some examples of such comments that facilitators have had to deal with.

It is usually best for issues to be addressed by engaging with such participants in a constructive, non-defensive but firm way, by acknowledging their behaviour, and inviting them to comment on how they are feeling. It is important to empathize with their situation and negotiate the way forward. This could include offering them the opportunity to leave; if they feel this is not an option as they have to attend the course, then it should be agreed that they would need to contribute and share their experiences, which could

---

Box 26.3 Examples of comments from resistant participants

- 'I know it all, done it for years.'
- 'You can't teach me anything.'
- 'I have no interest in being here.'
- 'I don't need this—it's a waste of time.'
- 'I have done thousands of consultations.'
- 'My patients are all happy.'
- 'It will make no difference.'
- 'All this touchy feely stuff!'

Reproduced with permission from Wilkinson S, *Training the Trainer Handbook*, Copyright © Susie Wilkinson 2002–14.

---

be of mutual benefit to them and the group. In this way they may be able to take something useful away from the course.

However, if negative behaviours persist, it may be necessary to invite the participants to leave the group.

Setting the course agenda

Trainee facilitators have to learn how to help groups to generate the content of the course to ensure that the course is learner centred.

To set the agenda, participants are required to identify their learning needs based on critical reflection of areas of their communication practice they have found difficult.

This ensures that participants examine an issue that is pertinent to their practice. This could be communication with a patient, relative, or colleague. Trainee facilitators need to develop the ability to encourage participants to be very specific about the communication issue and describe any specific words or phrases that were difficult to deal with. These key phrases or words need to be written on a flip chart and checked with the individual participants for accuracy. This ensures that the course remains relevant and there is also a visual reminder of their agenda items on display.

Once the agenda is set, a flexible approach is required, which needs to be revisited regularly to ensure that learning needs are being met. It is helpful to address the less complex agenda issues first, allowing the group to develop the skills to address the more complex situations as the course progresses.

Presentations

Trainee facilitators need to be conversant with the communication literature to be able to present an overview of this literature on ACST courses. This is to promote discussion and establish a common language that enables them to describe observed skills/behaviours meaningfully and effectively.

They should be able to deliver presentations that include:

- An overview of the evidence base for communication skills training;
- An outline of the micro-skills integral to all verbal and non-verbal interactions;
- The structure of a consultation;
- Strategies for handling difficult communication scenarios.

It is important to recognize that didactic teaching methods can be stimulating but may not lead to a change in behaviour or development of skills. Didactic methods enable learners to understand what it takes to communicate effectively, but do not ensure mastery and application in practice.

Managing role play with video-recording and feedback

It is vital that trainee facilitators are able to manage role play effectively. This also includes video-recording the role play and managing feedback to ensure the learning needs of participants are met.

Before embarking on a video-recorded role play, trigger tapes and discussion can be used to analyse the key factors of the communication issue under review. Trigger tapes can provide examples of practice, which can be analysed by group discussion. This can then give ideas of how the role play might be addressed and lead to the development of appropriate strategies for managing the specific situation under review.

Role play is then used as a vehicle to test, practice, and adapt suggested strategies.

The rationale for this structured approach to role play is to maximize the safety and effectiveness of the role play experience by preventing participants from repeating negative experiences such as not knowing what to say, feeling helpless, or frustrated. It allows participants to rehearse using new strategies/techniques. It also avoids the perception that participants are being 'set up to fail', as even though they have identified the issue that they role play as something they do not know how to tackle, the preparatory work ensures they have some ideas to try.

Group support helps participants to try things in a different way and move things forward if they falter or get stuck. The provision of endorsement from other participants that the strategy being used meets with their approval increases the participants' confidence. This approach ensures that the role play stays on brief, and—most importantly— that poor practice is not endorsed.

Commonly, role play and being recorded by a video camera is the dreaded part of ACST courses. Participants may also have had of previous adverse experiences of role play, so it is important that any apprehension should be addressed. 'Throw away a worry' (Box 26.4) can be a useful way of allowing participants to express concerns and worries anonymously. These worries tend to be very similar and once they have been elicited and explored, participants often feel they are not alone in their concerns, and this can enhance group bonding.

Role play regulations differ from ground rules in that they are set and not generated by a group. This is to ensure that role play sessions are conducted in a safe and effective manner. Trainee facilitators must be able to apply these regulations in a way that allows group participants to be aware of their function and helps them to feel supported. The role play regulations are outlined in Box 26.5.

Before commencing the role play

The session should begin by asking the participant to identify the specific difficulty of the scenario they are focusing on. Learning objectives for the role play need to be made clear; for example, if the participant wants feedback on how they handle an angry relative. It is important to emphasize that the role play will not be the actual scenario encountered by the participant, but will address the main difficult communication issues, the scenario needs to be developed based on the main details of the difficult situation identified, including names for patient/relative/colleague and any other relevant information. When everyone is clear what the role player wants to practise and the strategies to be used, the facilitator takes the role player and actor out of the room. This final preparation away from the group provides a safety net for the participant in

---

Box 26.4 Warm-up exercise: 'Throw away a worry'

* Participants are asked to write their concerns about role play on a piece of paper and fold the paper up.
* The facilitator then collects the papers in a 'bin'.
* Once done the facilitator asks participants to take out a concern from the bin and read it out.
* The concerns are then written on a flip chart and explored.
* The facilitator then explicitly links the concerns described to the role play regulations to demonstrate how the concerns will be addressed to maximize the safety of the role play.

Box 26.5 Role play regulations

* Confidentiality needs to be maintained by everyone in the group.
* Role players should adhere to the brief and not overcomplicate the scenario.
* Role plays will not last longer than 15–20 minutes.
* Positive feedback must be given before constructive alternatives.
* Participants role play the issue they identified in the agenda.
* Participants are not expected to perform well, as they have identified a subject that is difficult for them.
* The role playing participant should request time out if they feel stuck or unsure of which route to take.
* The facilitator can call 'time out' if the actor is not conforming to the brief or if there is a specific point that needs to be emphasized.
* The exact scenario that the participant found difficult cannot be re-enacted but the role play will be based on the communication issue they found difficult. This enables practice of a strategy that might be used in the future if the issue arose again.
* Less complex scenarios will be addressed first before moving on to the more complicated scenarios after trust/confidence in the group has been built.
* An explicit briefing will be given to the actor involved in the role play.

that it is an opportunity for the participant to disclose any sensitive information that they do not want the group to be party to.

The facilitator should check how the participant is feeling about the role play and has an idea of the strategy they wish to practise.

It is also helpful to clarify the words the participant is going to use to begin the role play. The facilitator then needs to ascertain if the actor requires any further information and remind the role player that they can call time out at any point during the role play.

The participant is invited to return to the group, while the facilitator gives the final brief to the actor outside the room. The learning objectives of the role play must be reinforced with the actor and the level of complexity/difficulty needed agreed. The facilitator should ensure that the actor is aware of the strategy or communication skill the participant is going to practise. The facilitator must reinforce actual words, phrases, or cues that the actor needs to incorporate into the role play. It is also important to ensure the actor is aware of what skills the facilitator is hoping to see during the role play, so that these can be acknowledged and rewarded during feedback. The facilitator needs to check that the actor has all the relevant clinical information, and an endpoint of the role play should be agreed.

Starting the role play

The facilitator should give the group a brief description of the scenario with the task to be undertaken before assigning observation roles; for example, of verbal and non-verbal behaviours, and of the strategy being attempted. The group should be reminded that they **must** first comment on what went well in terms of the skills used and the strategy the role player has chosen to try out, before suggestions of what could have been done differently are made.

It is helpful to check that the role players are ready to start and to give the role player an opening line, as this helps to ease them into the role play.

During the role play

If the role player calls time out it is helpful to understand the reason for stopping as this can inform the discussion. The recording of the scenario is then played back and the group asked to provide feedback on the positive aspects of the verbal and non-verbal skills and strategies and also to consider how the actor as the patient/relative/colleague may be feeling about the communication to this point. The actor should then be invited to comment on both positive and less effective moments of the interview. The trainee facilitators must learn to explore the impact of the communication by asking things such as 'how did you feel when the doctor/nurse said that?', 'which of the strategies suggested would you have preferred?'

The group should be encouraged to suggest alternative ways of dealing with difficulties encountered by the role player by saying, for example: 'We've looked at some very effective things that were done, has anyone any suggestions as to how it could have been handled differently?'

It is important to ask for specific and not general comments, for example: 'Exactly what would you have said at this point?' The group should be encouraged to suggest further strategies—'Any other suggestions about how he/she might proceed?'

Moving the role play on

The facilitator needs to ensure that the group has defined sufficient alternative strategies and only when this has been done, or if the group is stuck should the facilitator offer a strategy. The role player should be asked which strategy they would like to try and after checking that the role players are ready to continue, the facilitator should advise how the role play should continue. It is helpful again for the facilitator to provide a cue line to restart the role play.

Conclusion of role play

When the role play concludes, the role player should be allowed to comment first on the scenario played and how they are feeling. The actor followed by the group should be invited to give final comments. Then the facilitator should feedback anything not mentioned by the group, recap the key points, and link these in with any previous scenarios if appropriate.

The role player should always be asked to identify what learning they will take from having completed the role play. It is vital that trainee facilitators understand that the role player should finish the session having achieved something effectively, or the whole process will be viewed as humiliating and deskilling.

Debriefing

After each session, it is essential to check with each role player how they are feeling and to move out of the role play. If they are not able to come out of role, invite them to discuss this.

Working with actors

It is crucial that trainee facilitators are able to brief and manage the actors' participation in role play to ensure the participants' learning needs are met.

Using actors as simulated patients provides an ideal opportunity to recreate specific clinical problems and communication challenges to order. This allows consultations to be customized to a learner's level and tailored to their needs. Learners then have the opportunity to experiment and rehearse skills. Actors are able to replay parts or the whole of an interview, reacting appropriately and differently as learners try various approaches—and as such, this means that time can be used very efficiently. Actors have an important role to play in providing feedback to learners and giving insight from a lay perspective.

The use of trigger tapes

Trigger tapes can be used to provide an example of a specific communication issue. Analysis of these examples can encourage group discussion to explore the issues and help participants to generate suitable strategies which can be tested out in role play. Guidelines for using trigger tapes are outlined in Box 26.6. Trigger tapes are useful for demonstrating verbal and non-verbal skills, effective and ineffective communication and its consequences. They also allow participants practise on how to give constructive criticism in a safe environment. The replay facility is also useful as it enables key points to be highlighted.

The disadvantages of using trigger tapes are it is difficult to screen participants' reactions and they do appear sometimes to cause distress by reminding participants of an emotional situation they have encountered. This possibility should have been discussed at the beginning of the course during the ground rules session. To guard against this happening, pre-course information needs to be sent out to participants, stressing that if they have had a recent bereavement

Box 26.6 Guidelines for facilitators using trigger tapes

- Facilitators need to be familiar with the material contained within each trigger tape, noting the specific learning points to be demonstrated.

- The tape should be stopped at regular intervals to highlight learning points and encourage group discussion. Tapes should not run for longer than 5–10 minutes without pausing.

- Facilitators should encourage participants to request pauses to highlight issues.

- It is useful to assign specific tasks to participants; for example, identify specific facilitating behaviours, observe non-verbal communication, identify steps/strategies being used, etc.

- During feedback, participants should be asked to comment first on what they have seen and how they feel it is going. The group must be encouraged to give constructive feedback, firstly on what has gone well including the specific verbal and non-verbal skills, and secondly on alternative skills or strategies which could be employed.

- The group should be invited to predict how the patient/relative in the trigger tape may be feeling about the interview.

- Facilitators should only add their own comments when the views of the group have been exhausted or if poor practice is being condoned.

- When ending a trigger tape session, key points should be elicited from the group and the learning summarized using slides or flipchart.

Reproduced with permission from Wilkinson S, *Training the Trainer Handbook*, Copyright © Susie Wilkinson 2002–14.

or a recent traumatic life event they must discuss their participation in the course with the facilitator before undertaking the course.

If a participant should become distressed, one facilitator needs to stay with the group and the other should attend to the distressed person away from the group. The situation may be uncomfortable for the group and may need to be talked through with them. It follows that trainee facilitators need to be able to manage distressed participants in a supportive manner.

Another disadvantage of watching trigger tapes is that it is not an experiential activity and so may simply raise awareness of the issues rather than changing the behaviour of the participants.

Using group discussion

Discussion can be a dynamic teaching method for topics which do not require a formal lecture and are not suitable for role play, or trigger tape demonstration. Such issues may include team problems, ethical dilemmas, or spiritual issues. The advantages of using this teaching method are it uses the expertise within the group and is particularly useful when the group may be of mixed disciplines. Group members participating in the discussion will feel that their knowledge and experience is being valued by the whole group. Participants can sometimes be reluctant to join in discussion. It can be argued that it is unethical to force people to participate, but it

may be that they are simply unsure or inexperienced with the subject matter.

Evaluation of the facilitator training course

A multicentre, pre- and post-course design was used to evaluate the impact of the three-day FTC on changing participants' levels of confidence in teaching advanced communication skills. The methods and results have previously been reported (Wilkinson *et al.* 2010). A self-selected sample of healthcare professionals working in cancer or palliative care undertook the three-day FTC described above. Six courses with a maximum of 12 participants in each were held across six geographical locations across the United Kingdom. Recruitment took place between July 2006 and April 2008. Participants were eligible for recruitment if they were senior healthcare professionals working in cancer and palliative care who wanted to be actively involved in teaching communication skills, through to healthcare professionals, and those who had previously completed the ACST.

Fifty-six healthcare professionals participated. The primary outcome variable was a change in confidence in teaching scores from pre-course to post-course, as measured by the communication skills confidence questionnaire (Fallowfield *et al*. 2001). The questionnaire contained nine confidence items, each scored from 1 (not at all confident) to 10 (very confident). The results indicated there was a significant increase in total confidence scores from 6.5 pre-course to 7.9 post-course (t = 9.9, p < 0.001). Forty-eight (91%) participants had improved confidence scores, one the same, and four had worse.

The secondary outcome was the course evaluation questionnaire. Participants were asked how useful the course was overall. The majority of the participants found the course to be very useful, rating it with a score between 9 and 10. When asked if they would definitely, or perhaps recommend the course or not, to other healthcare professionals, all (n = 40) responded that they definitely would recommend it to their colleagues.

Ongoing support and assessment

On completion of the FTC, the participants (trainee facilitators) are encouraged to observe at least one ACST being facilitated by colleagues who have been assessed against a competency framework as competent to running the ACST. After such time, trainee facilitators are then encouraged to work with and be supported by an assessed facilitator on at least two ACST courses. If the assessed facilitator believes the trainee facilitator has reached an appropriate level of competency, they will be encouraged to undergo a competency assessment. All facilitators for the Wilkinson ACST are required to attend a refresher day once a year.

Conclusion

Attending an experiential communication skills course can often be a daunting and stressful experience for participants. In the hands of properly trained facilitators it can be a life changing experience. This chapter has outlined the challenges trainee facilitators face and gives ideas for handling each of these. It is hoped it will encourage more healthcare professionals to train to become facilitators for an advanced communication skills programme to further enhance patient care.

References

Arnold RM, Back AT, Baile WF, Fryer-Edwards K, Tulsky J (2010). The Oncotalk model. Ch. 54. In: Kissane D, Bultz B, Butow B, Finlay I (eds). *Handbook of Communication in Oncology and Palliative Care.* Oxford University Press, Oxford, UK.

Connected: National Communication Skills Training (2012). [*Communication skills in cancer*]. National Cancer Action Team, London, UK. Available at: http://webarchive.nationalarchives. gov.uk/20130513211237/http://www.ncat.nhs.uk/our-work/ improvement/connected-advanced-communication-skills-training [Online].

Fallowfield L, Saul J, Gilligan B (2001) Teaching senior nurses how to teach communication skills in oncology. *Cancer Nurs* **24**, 185–191.

Knowles MS (1978). The Adult Learner: A Neglected Species. Gulf, Houston, TX.

Kurtz S, Cooke L (2010). Learner-centred communication training. In: Kissane D, Bultz B, Butow P, Finlay I (eds). *Handbook of Communication in Oncology and Palliative Care.* Oxford University Press, Oxford, UK.

Kurtz S, Silverman J, Draper J, van Dalen J (2005). *Teaching and Learning Communication Skills in Medicine.* Radcliffe Publishing, London, UK.

Moore PM, Mercado SR, Atrigues MG, Lawrie TA (2013). Communications training for healthcare professionals working with people who have cancer. Cochrane Collaborative. Available at: http://onlinelibrary.wiley. com/doi/10.1002/14651858.CD003751.pub3/full [Online].

Wilkinson S, Linsell L, Blanchard K, Roberts A (2010). Effectiveness of a three-day training the trainers course in improving trainee facilitators' confidence in teaching communication skills courses to senior healthcare professionals working with cancer patients: Recent advances and research updates. Available at: www.australasiancancer.org/ journal__/download-article.php?id=450 [Online].

Wilkinson S, Linsell L, Perry R, Blanchard K (2008). Effectiveness of a three-day communication skills course in changing nurses' communication skills with cancer/palliative care patients: A randomised controlled trial. *Palliat Med* **22**, 365–75.

CHAPTER 27

Communication in the context of cancer as a chronic disease

Patsy Yates

Introduction to communication in the context of cancer as a chronic disease

Modern cancer treatments have resulted in significant improvements in survival rates. Extended survival and new treatment approaches have meant the way individuals experience their disease has changed. For many, cancer is now experienced as a chronic disease associated with ongoing or recurring physical and psychosocial sequalae. These changes require that health professionals employ communication strategies, which are responsive to the unique issues associated with living with a chronic condition. This chapter draws on frameworks developed to support individuals living with chronic conditions and considers how these frameworks can be applied to enable effective communication in this changing context of cancer care.

The cancer experience

The diagnosis and treatment of cancer has always been a complex clinical process, often associated with significant physical and psychological morbidity. But there have been important changes to the cancer treatment trajectory in recent years. Scientific advances have meant that several new treatment options are available and it is not uncommon for the active cancer treatment phase to be extended over long periods of time. Some treatments, aimed at long-term control of the disease or reducing the risk of recurrence, can be ongoing for many years after the initial diagnosis. For some, a second primary cancer can develop, or the disease can recur once or a number of times. In the latter case, individuals will face the prospect that their disease may eventually be fatal despite initially being given a positive prognosis. These individuals can sometimes be offered additional new lines of treatments that are primarily focused on control rather than cure.

No matter which trajectory an individual experiences, the physical, psychological, and social sequalae of a cancer diagnosis and cancer treatment are constantly changing and can be long term. One recent review identified that at least 50% of cancer survivors experience late treatment-related side effects, including physical, psychosocial, cognitive, and sexual abnormalities, as well as concerns regarding recurrence and/or the development of new malignancies. The review also identified that many effects are chronic in nature and that they can be severe and sometimes life-threatening. Increased unemployment rates and workplace discrimination among cancer survivors were also identified (Valdivieso *et al.* 2012).

Another systematic review of long-term symptoms post-completion of primary treatment in patients with breast, gynaecological, prostate, and colorectal cancers identified significant physical limitations, cognitive limitations, depression/anxiety, sleep problems, fatigue, pain, and sexual dysfunctions. The authors concluded that based on longitudinal and cross-sectional evidence, cancer survivors can experience these symptoms for more than 10 years following treatment (Harrington *et al.* 2010).

The psychosocial distress experienced by individuals in the years following diagnosis and treatment can be profound. One review identified fear of recurrence and disease progression existed years after initial diagnosis. The review concluded that fear of recurrence is experienced in modest intensity by most survivors, and that no significant change occurs in fear of recurrence over time. The review identified significant negative associations between fear of recurrence, quality of life, and psychosocial well-being (Koch *et al.* 2013).

Additional health concerns, such as high rates of concurrent chronic conditions, including cancer, are present in cancer survivors. The cumulative effects of such co-morbid conditions can have a substantial impact on daily functioning (Hays *et al.* 2014). In one Australian study, a total of 2,103 cases and 4,185 controls reported that for men, after adjusting for age, cancer survivors were more likely than controls to have ever had cardiovascular disease, high blood pressure, high cholesterol, and diabetes. Similarly, for women, there was an increased prevalence of high cholesterol, diabetes, and osteoporosis in cancer cases, but after adjusting for socioeconomic status; these associations were no longer significant. While no other differences in lifestyle behaviour or BMI between cases and controls were identified, the authors concluded that chronic disease management is important as part of healthcare after a diagnosis of cancer (Berry *et al.* 2014).

Models of cancer as a chronic disease

The Institute of Medicine report 'From cancer patient to cancer survivor: lost in transition' (Hewitt *et al.* 2006) advocates for a number of changes to ensure that cancer survivors are better supported in four key areas: prevention; surveillance; intervention for consequences of cancer and its treatment; and coordination between specialist and generalist providers. This changing understanding of the cancer trajectory has been associated with increasing interest in the application of chronic disease models to guide service provision.

The Chronic Care Model identifies fundamental elements of high-quality chronic disease management that focus on enabling patients, healthcare providers, and healthcare systems (Wagner 1998). A key component of chronic care models is emphasis on a person's ability to self-manage long-term effects of the disease and its treatment. For health professionals, supported self-management requires the effective use of cognitive strategies, including reframing, prioritizing, and changing beliefs (Liddy 2014). The patient is considered a co-partner in the process requiring that health professionals recognize, and are sensitive to, the position of the patient and whether the patient is willing and able to contribute (Tritter and Calnan 2002). This can be especially challenging in the context of cancer, where the illness can be experienced at certain points as chronic, but at other times requires acute intervention (Tritter and Calnan 2002).

Effective decision support is another key feature of chronic disease management. Health literacy is an important consideration in decision support. Health literacy is a construct that is described as being socially, physically, *and* contextually constructed, thus requiring an understanding of how information practices facilitate people becoming health literate, rather than a sole interest in the person's skills development (Lloyd and Bonner 2014).

Health professional communication in the context of chronic disease

Health professionals need to support individuals to deal with the day-to-day effects that cancer or cancer treatment has on their lives and to live well beyond cancer. This requires specific communication practices that focus on behaviour change, building resilience, and promoting the individual's ability to self-manage the short and longer-term effects of cancer and its treatment. In this section, the capabilities required of health professionals to enable patients to effectively manage the physical and psychological sequalae of cancer will be reviewed. Knowledge, skills, and attitude elements outlined in the publication *Capabilities for Supporting Prevention and Chronic Condition Self-Management* (Department of Health and Ageing 2009) will provide a framework for considering specific communication practices that can be used to support individuals experiencing cancer as a chronic condition.

The *Capabilities for Supporting Prevention and Chronic Condition Self-Management* resource describes 19 core capabilities identified through extensive research as necessary for healthcare professionals to successfully support patients and carers to self-manage chronic conditions. Each of these skill areas assumes an underlying knowledge and values base. See Box 27.1 for the list of capabilities.

Demonstrating such capabilities in practice requires a range of essential, as well as some more advanced communication skills. In the following section, communication practices that support individuals living with cancer as a chronic disease are explained.

Box 27.1 List of capabilities for supporting prevention and chronic condition self-management

- General patient-centred capabilities
  - Health promotion approaches
  - Assessment of health risk factors
  - Communication skills
  - Assessment of self-management capacity (understanding strengths and barriers)
  - Collaborative care planning
  - Use of peer support
  - Cultural awareness
  - Psychosocial assessment and support skills
- Behaviour change capabilities
  - Models of health behaviour change
  - Motivational interviewing
  - Collaborative problem definition
  - Goal setting and goal achievement
  - Structured problem solving and action planning
- Organizational/systems capabilities
  - Working in multidisciplinary teams/interprofessional learning and practice
  - Information, assessment, and communication management systems
  - Organizational change techniques
  - Evidence-based knowledge
  - Conducting practice-based research/quality improvement framework
  - Awareness of community resources

Reproduced with permission from Department of Health and Ageing, *Capabilities for Supporting Prevention and Chronic Condition Self-Management: A Resource for Educators of Primary Health Care Professionals*, Table 2, p. 12, Australian Government, Department of Health and Ageing, Canberra, Australia, Copyright © 2009 Commonwealth of Australia as represented by the Department of Health.

Person-centred capabilities

Person-centred care is central to modern health services because of its link with improved safety and quality of care. No consensus exists on the definition of person-centred care, although definitions typically emphasize that it exists when care is consistent with the values, needs, and desires of patients, and when healthcare providers involve patients in healthcare discussions and decisions (Mead and Bower 2000; Holmström and Röing 2010). General person-centred capabilities thus underpin all interactions with patients to enable effective therapeutic relationships to be established and maintained. Such relationships are essential to provide a context whereby the individual's strengths, needs, priorities, and concerns can be identified. Core elements of person-centred capabilities include skills in communication, collaborative care planning, and psychosocial skills enhancement.

Communication skills

Elements

◆ The ability to establish and develop mutual understanding, trust, respect, and cooperation.

◆ The ability to express oneself clearly so the other person understands.

◆ The ability to listen and interpret effectively to understand what the other person is trying to express.

◆ Includes communication between service providers.

Reproduced with permission from Department of Health and Ageing, *Capabilities for Supporting Prevention and Chronic Condition Self-Management: A Resource for Educators of Primary Health Care Professionals*, p. 13, Australian Government, Department of Health and Ageing, Canberra, Australia, Copyright © 2009 Commonwealth of Australia as represented by the Department of Health.

Table 27.1 Communication strategies associated with person-centred communication

Communication practice	Associated communication strategies
Sharing information	Active listening, asking open-ended questions, developing functional goals
Compassionate and empowering care	Being attentive, altruistic, and authentic
Careful observation	Observing and enquiring about unique patient characteristics and circumstances; acknowledging and adapting to these characteristics and circumstances

Source: data from Marissa K Constand *et al.*, 'Scoping review of patient-centered care approaches in healthcare,' *BMC Health Services Research*, Volume 14, Issue 271, DOI: 10.1186/1472-6963-14-271, Copyright © Constand *et al.*; licensee BioMed Central Ltd. 2014.

A diagnosis of cancer is associated with significant distress and results in major disruptive changes to life meaning. Effective communication requires health professionals who are able to demonstrate empathy and understand the unique meaning of the situation to each individual. Practices required to achieve these outcomes include reflective listening and open-ended questioning to assess how the person experiences the impact of cancer and its treatment, and their perception of what is needed to manage the future. A recent systematic review of communication practices in healthcare identified common features of person-centred communication, which included sharing of information (identified in 89.5% of papers reviewed); compassionate and empowering care provision (identified in 53% of papers reviewed); and sensitivity to patient needs (identified in 58% of papers reviewed) (Constand *et al.* 2014). Specific strategies associated with these three person-centred communication practices are presented in Table 27.1.

Psychosocial assessment and support skills/skills enhancement

Elements

◆ Ability to identify, build, and sustain positive aspects of psychosocial health such as resilience, strengths, and coping skills with the patient and their carers.

Reproduced with permission from Department of Health and Ageing, *Capabilities for Supporting Prevention and Chronic Condition Self-Management: A Resource for Educators of Primary Health Care Professionals*, p. 14, Australian Government, Department of Health and Ageing, Canberra, Australia, Copyright © 2009 Commonwealth of Australia as represented by the Department of Health.

The diverse and complex nature of psychosocial responses to cancer requires focused assessment to enable identification of main concerns, as well as the person's personal resources which can be used to assist with self-management. These experiences can change over time, and so require ongoing assessment. For cancer patients, it is also important to recognize that some concerns may be of a more private nature, such as impact on sexual function. Identifying such concerns is an important part of psychosocial assessment.

Good communication skills are critical to effective psychosocial assessment. These skills include practices described in the above section, and include listening, reflection, and the use of open-ended questions to encourage patients to express their main concerns. Given the complex nature of psychosocial assessment, standardized screening tools can help to facilitate communication and ensure a comprehensive, evidence-based approach. Such tools can be used at regular follow-up appointments or whenever there is a change in the person's circumstances. Consider teaching the person how to use the tools themselves to identify concerns that might prompt further action or contact with healthcare professionals. Other tools have been developed specifically for health professionals to provide a prompt to exploring challenging physical, emotional, and social concerns during interactions with patients. Some examples of such tools are presented in Table 27.2.

The selected examples in Table 27.2 are screening or practice frameworks. More comprehensive psychosocial assessment using relevant diagnostic tools may be needed when screening identifies concerns that require further understanding and action. Alongside these processes, health professionals also need to communicate in ways to promote resilience, strength, and coping skills, by identifying sources of strength, showing positive regard and acceptance, and providing encouragement.

Behaviour change capabilities

Effective management of many of the physical and psychosocial sequalae of cancer requires the person to actively engage in a range of health management behaviours. Health professionals require an understanding of various models of health behaviour change to provide a foundation to understanding human behaviour and the mechanisms involved in effecting change. To apply these models effectively in practice, health professionals need to employ specific communication skills that focus on cognitive change, motivation, and capacity building. Two capabilities will be reviewed in this section—motivational interviewing and collaborative problem identification.

Table 27.2 Screening tools and frameworks to support psychosocial assessment

Tool	Description	Used by
Distress Thermometer (National Comprehensive Cancer Center 2015)	Single item rating scale (0 = no distress to 10 = extreme distress) to identify distress from any source. If distress is four or higher, it is recommended that health professionals use a 39 item problem check list to help identify sources and types of distress in key domains including practical, family, emotional, spiritual/religious, and physical concerns	Health professional and patient versions are available
National Breast and Ovarian Cancer Centre's Psychosocial care Referral Checklist (Cancer Australia)	A referral checklist to provide a simple way for health professionals to identify patients at higher risk of psychosocial distress. The checklist includes open-ended question prompts for health professionals to facilitate discussions	Health professionals
Ex-PLISSIT (Davis and Taylor 2006)	This framework incorporates key communication processes health professionals can use to initiate discussions about the sensitive topic of sexuality, including: permission, limited information, specific suggestions, intensive therapy; explicit permission-giving at every stage (not just at the first stage). The model also emphasizes the need to review all interactions with patients and challenge your own assumptions about the patient's situation	Health professionals
Intimacy and Sexuality: A Guide for Patients with Gynaecological Cancer (Cancer Australia)	This resource has been developed to support women (and their partners) in understanding and addressing issues of intimacy and sexuality following the diagnosis and treatment of gynaecological cancer. It aims to empower women so they can ask questions that they may otherwise avoid asking due to embarrassment or other concerns	Women with gynaecological cancer (although the principles have relevance to all patients with cancer)

Source: data from National Comprehensive Cancer Center, *National Comprehensive Cancer Center Clinical Practice Guidelines: Distress Management, Version 3*, Copyright © 2015; National Breast and Ovarian Cancer Centre, *Psychosocial care referral checklist for patients with cancer*, Cancer Australia, Copyright © 2016 available from https://canceraustralia.gov.au/sites/default/files/publications/pcrg-1-psychosocial-care-referral-notes_504af02602d77.pdf; and Davis S, and Taylor B, 'From PLISSIT to Ex-PLISSIT,' in Davis S (Ed), *Rehabilitation: the use of theories and models in practice*, Churchill Livingstone, UK, Copyright © 2006.

Motivational interviewing

Elements

+ Involves encouraging the person to talk, generate self-motivational statements, deal with resistance, develop readiness to change, and negotiate a plan, developing determination and action.

+ The five principles underlying the process are expressing empathy, developing discrepancy, avoiding arguing, rolling with resistance, and supporting self-efficacy.

+ Motivational interviewing embodies cognitive change skills.

Reproduced with permission from Department of Health and Ageing, *Capabilities for Supporting Prevention and Chronic Condition Self-Management: A Resource for Educators of Primary Health Care Professionals*, p. 14, Australian Government, Department of Health and Ageing, Canberra, Australia, Copyright © 2009 Commonwealth of Australia as represented by the Department of Health.

The chronic nature of disease and treatment-related effects means individuals are often required to implement long-term lifestyle changes, such as changes in diet and exercise behaviours. For some, it can also mean long-term adherence to ongoing oral therapies. Motivational interviewing is one strategy that has been identified as especially useful to assist individuals achieve sustained behaviour change. Motivational interviewing has been defined as '*a directive, client centred counselling style for eliciting behaviour change by helping clients to explore and resolve ambivalence*' (Rollnick and Miller 1995). More specifically, it is an interpersonal style used to trigger the process of behaviour change, where the health professional's role is to direct the discussion, rather than assume the traditional role of expert giving advice to the patient. Such health professional–patient interactions thereby enable the person to accept change, and to reflect on ways to address resistance (Miller and Rollnick 2013).

For example, modifying diet to reduce or maintain weight can be important to reduce the risk of a second cancer or cancer recurrence, and to maintain optimal health. Rather than telling patients such actions are important, motivational interviewing uses strategies based on the health professional as a partner with the patient who is the expert. Communication practices therefore focus on strategies such as asking the person how they feel about changing their dietary and exercise behaviours, how they would like their health to be different, and assessing how ready they are for change. It is also important to build confidence, understanding what would help the person themselves to be confident. Understanding what action is needed to overcome any barrier to the behaviour is also required (see: Motivational Interviewing for Diet, Exercise and Weight, http://www.uconnruddcenter.org/files/Pdfs/MotivationalInterviewing.pdf).

Elements

+ Open dialogue with the patient about what they see as their main problem, what happens because of the problem, and how the problem makes them feel.

Reproduced with permission from Department of Health and Ageing, *Capabilities for Supporting Prevention and Chronic Condition Self-Management: A Resource for Educators of Primary Health Care Professionals*, p. 14, Australian Government, Department of Health and Ageing, Canberra, Australia, Copyright © 2009 Commonwealth of Australia as represented by the Department of Health.

Collaborative problem identification

The experience of cancer differs according to a range of factors that are not just disease and treatment related. This experience is influenced by factors such as culture, social circumstances, and psychological characteristics. The person's ability to adapt to their circumstances is also dependent on personal and social resources, such as health literacy and financial resources. Identifying an individual's problems and concerns therefore needs to be a collaborative process, with health professionals respecting the patient's expertise and acknowledging differences in how individuals experience and interpret their situation.

To facilitate collaborative problem solving, health professionals can guide and support the process of goal setting and action planning for patients. As with other capabilities, core communication skills, including reflective listening and open-ended questioning are critical to develop mutual understanding, trust, respect, and cooperation. This enables health professionals to enquire in a deeper way to gain a more thorough understanding of the person's current needs and to identify barriers and enabling factors to help them adjust. For example, asking the person what the most important concerns are to them is likely to be a more effective and efficient way to identify priority actions. Such questions can also help provide the clarity and motivation needed for the person to respond. Some individuals may find it difficult to express their main concerns. In these cases, taking time to explore what is important to the person can assist.

To assist with collaborative problem identification, it may also be useful to work together to devise SMART (specific, measurable, achievable, realistic and timely) goals and strategies. This can help to achieve clarity and define specific actions that are relevant and acceptable to the person's individual circumstances. Such goals can also empower the individual, by providing a guide for monitoring progress and recognizing when additional supports may be needed.

Organizational/system capabilities

Working in multidisciplinary teams/interprofessional

Elements

- Involves understanding and respecting the role and function of all members.
- Integrating care by recognizing and actively engaging service providers across systems, sectors, and agencies, not just within organizations.
- Communication skills together with the timeliness of those from and about each other to improve collaboration and the quality of care (Jessop 2007; Braithwaite and Travaglia 2005).

Reproduced with permission from Department of Health and Ageing, *Capabilities for Supporting Prevention and Chronic Condition Self-Management: A Resource for Educators of Primary Health Care Professionals*, p. 15, Australian Government, Department of Health and Ageing, Canberra, Australia, Copyright © 2009 Commonwealth of Australia as represented by the Department of Health.

learning/practice

Management of cancer as a chronic condition involves support from primary care and specialist teams across multiple care settings. The complexity of cancer patients' health needs also requires multiple disciplines to be part of the care team over time.

Communication skills are key to interacting effectively to ensure collaboration and coordination across systems, sectors, and agencies, as well as within organizations and local care teams. The National Breast Cancer Centre's *Multidisciplinary meetings for cancer care: a guide for health service providers* publication emphasizes the importance of good group dynamics and recommends teams clarify role perceptions and expectations of each other; identify your own and other professionals' competencies; explore overlapping responsibilities, and re-negotiate role assignments (National Breast Cancer Centre 2005). The National Breast Cancer Centre has found that improving communication among multidisciplinary team members may be one of the most important factors in ensuring patients feel that they are receiving care from a coordinated team. There has been a growing recognition of the importance of effective team functioning in healthcare, and an understanding of the unique set of skills that are required to optimize teamwork to

Box 27.2 Specific interprofessional communication competencies

1. Choose effective communication tools and techniques, including information systems and communication technologies, to facilitate discussions and interactions that enhance team function.

2. Organize and communicate information with patients, families, and healthcare team members in a form that is understandable, avoiding discipline-specific terminology when possible.

3. Express one's knowledge and opinions to team members involved in patient care with confidence, clarity, and respect, working to ensure common understanding of information and treatment and care decisions.

4. Listen actively, and encourage ideas and opinions of other team members.

5. Give timely, sensitive, instructive feedback to others about their performance on the team, responding respectfully as a team member to feedback from others.

6. Use respectful language appropriate for a given difficult situation, crucial conversation, or interprofessional conflict.

7. Recognize how one's own uniqueness, including experience level, expertise, culture, power, and hierarchy within the healthcare team, contributes to effective communication, conflict resolution, and positive interprofessional working relationships (University of Toronto 2008).

8. Communicate consistently the importance of teamwork in patient-centred and community-focused care.

Reproduced with permission from Inter Professional Education Collaborative Expert Panel, *Core Competencies for Interprofessional Collaborative Practice: Report of an Expert Panel*, Interprofessional Education Collaborative, Washington, DC, USA, Copyright © 2011 American Association of Colleges of Nursing, American Association of Colleges of Osteopathic Medicine, American Association of Colleges of Pharmacy, American Dental Education Association, Association of American Medical Colleges, and Association of Schools of Public Health, available from http://www.aacn.nche.edu/education-resources/ipecreport.pdf

achieve improved patient outcomes. Box 27.2 provides a list spe-

Elements

◆ Various techniques used within healthcare settings, each based on theories of organizational structure, culture, and models of change, group behaviour, and values.

Reproduced with permission from Department of Health and Ageing, *Capabilities for Supporting Prevention and Chronic Condition Self-Management: A Resource for Educators of Primary Health Care Professionals*, p. 15, Australian Government, Department of Health and Ageing, Canberra, Australia, Copyright © 2009 Commonwealth of Australia as represented by the Department of Health.

cific competencies identified as key to this capability.

Organizational change techniques

Traditional healthcare systems have not typically been designed to support long-term cancer care, with survivorship care programmes available in only a few specialist centres. Facilitating change to the way services are delivered is necessary to improve the way work is delivered to the population served. While such change is often considered to be the responsibility of managers and policy makers, individual health professionals can contribute to such improvements through good communication skills that support their important advocacy and influencing role. Such communication skills seek to persuade and educate individuals at all levels of the health system to inform service improvements. One study reported that effective team members demonstrated leadership, the ability to influence, the ability to analyse data, effective decision making, and listening. The study also reported that team members were most effective when they demonstrated respect for others, a cooperative attitude, a positive attitude, courage to disagree, and facilitated participation (Leggat 2007).

Conclusion

For many patients today, cancer is experienced as a chronic condition. This changing disease context requires that health professionals are capable of providing person-centred care, facilitating positive and sustained change in health behaviours, and promoting improvements at the organization and system level. Central to all such capabilities is effective communication practices. These communication practices require more sophisticated understandings of the patient as partner in the care process, with health professionals acting more as facilitators and supporters. Such practices represent a shift from traditional roles, but are critical if we are to achieve optimal outcomes for patients and health systems.

References

Berry N, Miller M, Woodman R, *et al.* (2014). Differences in chronic conditions and lifestyle behaviour between people with a history of cancer and matched controls. *Med J Aust* **201**, 96–100.

Cancer Australia (2012). Intimacy and Sexuality: A Guide for Patients with Gynaecological Cancer. Available at: https://canceraustralia.gov.au/publications-and-resources/cancer-australia-publications/intimacy-and-sexuality-women-gynaecological-cancer-starting-conversation [Last accessed April 20, 2016].

Cancer Australia. Psychosocial Care Referral Tool, Available at: https://canceraustralia.gov.au/sites/default/files/publications/pcrg-1-psychosocial-care-referral-notes_504af02602d77.pdf [Last accessed April 20, 2016].

Constand M, MacDermid J, Dal Bello-Haas V, Law M (2014). Scoping review of patient-centered care approaches in healthcare. *BMC Health Serv Res* **14**, 271.

Davis S, Taylor B (2006). From PLISSIT to Ex-PLISSIT. In: Davis, S (ed.). *Rehabilitation: the use of theories and models in practice*. Elsevier, Edinburgh, UK.

Department of Health and Ageing (2009). *Capabilities for Supporting Prevention and Chronic Condition Self-Management: A Resource for Educators of Primary Health Care Professionals*. Commonwealth of Australia, Canberra.

Harrington C, Hansen J, Moskowitz M, *et al.* (2010). It's not over when it's over: long-term symptoms in cancer survivors—a systematic review. *Int J Psychiatry Med* **40**, 163–81.

Hays R, Reeve B, Smith A, *et al.* (2014). Associations of cancer and other chronic medical conditions with SF-6D preference-based scores in Medicare beneficiaries. *Qual Life Res* **23**, 385–91.

Hewitt M, Greenfield S, Stovall E (2006). *From Cancer Patient to Survivor: Lost in Transition*. National Academies Press, Washington, WA.

Holmström I, Röing M (2010). The relation between patient-centeredness and patient empowerment: a discussion on concepts. *Patient Educ Couns* **79**, 167–72.

Interprofessional Education Collaborative Expert Panel (2011). Core Competencies for Interprofessional Collaborative Practice: Report of an Expert Panel. Washington, DC: Interprofessional Education Collaborative. Available at: http://www.aacn.nche.edu/education-resources/ipecreport.pdf [Last accessed April 20, 2016].

Koch L, Jansen L, Brenner H, *et al.* (2013). Fear of recurrence and disease progression in long-term (≥5 years) cancer survivors—a systematic review of quantitative studies. *Psychooncology* **22**, 1–11.

Leggat S (2007). Effective healthcare teams require effective team members: defining teamwork competencies. *BMC Health Serv Res* **7**, 17,

Liddy C, Blazkho V, Mill K (2014). Challenges of self-management when living with multiple chronic conditions: systematic review of the qualitative. *Can Fam Physician* **60**, 1123–33.

Lloyd A, Bonner A (2014). The health information practices of people living with chronic health conditions: Implications for health literacy. *J Lib Info Sci* **46**, 207–16.

Mead N, Bower P (2000). Patient-centredness: a conceptual framework and review of the empirical literature. *Soc Sci Med* **51**, 1087–110.

Miller W, Rollnick S (2013). *Motivational Interviewing: Helping People Change*, 3rd edition. Guilford Press, New York, NY.

Motivational Interviewing for Diet, Exercise and Weight. Available at: http://www.uconnruddcenter.org/files/Pdfs/MotivationalInterviewing.pdf [Accessed April 20 2016].

National Breast Cancer Centre (2005). Multidisciplinary meetings for cancer care: a guide for health service providers. National Breast Cancer Centre, Camperdown, NSW. Available at: https://canceraustralia.gov.au/sites/default/files/publications/mdm-mdc-meeting-for-cancer-care_504af02d7368d.pdf [Last accessed April 20, 2016].

National Comprehensive Cancer Center (2015). *National Comprehensive Cancer Center Clinical Practice Guidelines: Distress Management*, Version 3.

Rollnick S, Miller W (1995). What is motivational interviewing? *Behavior Cognitive Psychol* **23**, 325–34.

Tritter L, Calnan M (2002). Cancer as a chronic illness? Reconsidering categorization and exploring experience *Eur J Cancer Care* **11**, 161–5.

Valdivieso M, Kujawa A, Jones R, Baker L (2012). Cancer survivors in the United States: A review of the literature and a call to action. *Int J Med Sci* **9**, 163–73.

Wagner E (1998). Chronic disease management: What will it take to improve care for chronic illness? *Eff Clin Pract* **1**, 2–4.

CHAPTER 28

Advancing family communication skills in oncology nursing

Talia Zaider, Shira Hichenberg, and Lauren Latella

Introduction to advancing family communication skills in oncology nursing

A major imperative of supportive cancer care is to sustain the well-being of the caregiving family (Northouse 2012). This focus parallels a broader movement in medicine towards advancing family-centred care, a model of healthcare delivery which prioritizes mutually beneficial partnerships between the family and medical team (Johnson *et al.* 2008). In the oncology team, nurses are uniquely positioned to initiate and model family-centred care because of their frequent contact with families and role as a 'relational bridge' between the family and medical team (McLeod *et al.* 2010, p. 97). Yet communicating effectively with families is a complex task, requiring skill in establishing alliance with multiple stakeholders under conditions of high stress. To our knowledge, there have been no training efforts that specifically guide nurses on how to effectively collaborate with, and provide support to families in the cancer setting. In a review of the Institute of Medicine recommendations on promoting quality cancer care, Ferrell, McCabe, and Levit (2013) underscored the importance of communication skills training to empower nurses to take a leadership role in modelling effective collaboration with families.

In this chapter, we describe two formats of a new communication skills training initiative referred to as *Partnering with Families in Cancer Care* (PFCC). This training model aims to empower nurses to support and partner with caregiving families. It was developed specifically for acute care nurses, the frontline providers who interface with families and triage psychosocial care referrals during hospitalization. A brief, single-session training module targets bedside nursing staff, and focuses on managing high stress interactions with families. A second, more comprehensive (six-month) training programme targets advanced practice nurses who assist with the management of complex family situations, and whose role on the inpatient unit allows for more advanced conceptualization, assessment, and intervention with families. We will review the conceptual underpinnings of family-centred nursing care, present the content of each training format, and describe preliminary data on training efficacy among nurses who participated in each model.

The nurse–family partnership

Over the last several decades, the field of family nursing has evolved into an established body of practice and theory (Wright and Leahey 2012. Kaakinen and colleagues (2010) distinguish between engaging the family-as-*context* versus family-as-*client*. In a family-as-context approach, the predominant approach in the healthcare setting, the nurse prioritizes the patient's needs, and communicates with families in order to optimize patient care (e.g. 'Who in the family will be coming to Rosa's chemotherapy appointments?'). In a family-as-client approach, the nurse assesses the larger family's support needs (e.g. 'How has the family been adjusting to Rosa's treatment at home?'). The Calgary Family Assessment and Intervention Model, developed by Lorraine Wright and Maureen Leahey (1994) is an example of a family-as-client practice model that guides nurses in conceptualizing and intervening with families in primary care.

Family-centred nursing practices have been advanced in paediatric, palliative care, and critical care settings, where families have clearly designated roles as surrogate decision makers (e.g. Hudson, *et al.* 2005; Mehta *et al.* 2009; Tomlinson *et al.* 2011). There is growing evidence that communication practices that encourage partnership with families (e.g. family meetings, shared-decision making, family presence in hospital rounds and procedures) are associated with improved clinical outcomes, increased satisfaction with care, and decreased stress for staff (Davidson *et al.* 2007; Schaefer and Block 2009; Doolin *et al.* 2011). A nurse-led multidisciplinary task force convened by the American College of Critical Care Medicine identified both 'family coping' and 'stress related to family interactions' as two of the key areas in need of attention and improved practice (Davidson *et al.* 2007).

In the adult oncology setting, the individual patient is prioritized, with the family construed as adjunctive to his or her care. Frontline providers in acute cancer care are offered no clear guidelines about how to best engage families, particularly the subset of multistressed families whose interactions with the medical team pose difficulties. Although nurses report that working with families is one of the most rewarding aspects of their work, addressing conflictual family dynamics generates considerable stress (Traeger *et al.* 2013).

In a recent survey of 912 hospital oncology nurses, the highest rated obstacle to providing high-quality end-of-life care was 'dealing with anxious family members.' Of the top ten rated obstacles identified by oncology nurses in this study, seven pertained to families, including 'family not accepting patient's poor prognosis,' and 'nurse having to deal with angry family members' (Traeger *et al.* 2013). When relational difficulties arise within families, or between families and the medical team, the nurse's capacity to adhere to tenets of family-centred care—forging a trusting and mutually supportive partnership—is at once more crucial, and more difficult to achieve.

Barriers and facilitators of family engagement

Barriers to achieving collaboration with families have been identified at both the family level (e.g. divergent patient and caregiver needs, poor communication within the family, rejection of support) and at the institutional level (e.g. insufficient time and resources, lack of continuity of care, lack of skill, and confidence in working with families) (Hudson *et al.* 2004). Failure to create an alliance, taking sides in family conflict, and giving premature advice to families have been cited as three common missteps providers make in interactions with families (Wright and Leahey 2005). In an analysis of 'breakdowns' in ICU nursing care with families, Chesla and Stannard (1997) observed that when family-related stress mounted, there was a tendency towards increased distancing between nurses and patients or families, and nurses were then more prone to pathologizing the family.

McLeod and colleagues (2010) conducted in-depth interviews with families and oncology nurses in both inpatient and ambulatory care settings in order to elicit views on which nursing practices build collaboration and mitigate distress. Caregivers and nurses agreed on two key practices: (i) 'knowing the family,' in which nurses were able to gather information about family relationships, read non-verbal cues, and create space for families to take part in a consultation; and (ii) attending to family distress, which occurred when nurses educated families about managing the impact of cancer on the family.

Family-centred communication training

The objective of the PFCC training intervention is to strengthen the capacity of nurses to partner with caregiving families and address sources of family distress in the acute cancer care setting. Two training interventions have been developed and implemented. The first is a one-session module that was delivered to 282 oncology acute care nurses at Memorial Sloan Kettering Cancer Center (MSKCC). The second is a six-month intensive training that was administered to advanced practice nurses in acute care. Each strives to achieve the overarching goal of improving family-centred care through a set of observable skills and communication behaviours (Brown and Bylund 2008). Training content was based on the seminal work of leading theorists and practitioners in family systems care, including Wright and Leahey's *Calgary Family Assessment and Intervention Models* (Wright and Leahey 2012), William Madsen's *Collaborative Therapy with Multi-stressed Families* (Madsen 2007), and the framework promoted by our Comskil programme for teaching family-focused assessment in cancer (Zaider and Kissane 2009; Gueguen *et al.* 2009). These models emphasize the importance of adopting an appreciative and respectful stance towards families, identifying strengths and expertise within the family group, and appreciating the interdependence between patients and family members' responses to illness.

To better understand nurse's training needs, we administered a survey to 30 inpatient oncology staff at MSKCC, asking them to rate ten common family challenges on two dimensions: (i) perceived difficulty handling the challenge and (ii) training interest in the listed challenge area. Challenges rated most difficult were family conflict, poor teamwork, and discrepant views on treatment goals. Interest in training was strongly endorsed across all situations, regardless of perceived difficulty. To further tailor the didactic and experiential portions of our training, nurses were asked to anonymously submit illustrative examples of challenges they have encountered with families, by responding to the prompt, '*Describe a challenging interaction you had with a family*'. Three broad challenge areas were identified, illustrated in the next section with qualitative excerpts provided by nurse participants.

Within-family challenges

Relational problems *within the family* or *between the patient and family* can create considerable distress and complicate collaboration with the medical team. When poor family functioning is not recognized, providers become drawn into a family drama unknowingly, sometimes feeling pulled into alignment with one particular family member, or enlisted as a communication 'switchboard' for families who fail to communicate with each other directly. Examples of these challenges as described by nurses are as follows:

'… The sisters of the patient flew the parents in that night and the parents did not know the patient was dying. I was being yelled at by the sisters of the patient to not tell the elderly parents their son was dying …'

'I took care of someone whose parents were on two different ends of the spectrum. The mom wanted to keep fighting and kept thinking that the patient was coming around and making improvements even though he was terminal, and the dad was grasping the reality of the situation.'

Partnership challenges

A mismatch between the beliefs of the medical team and family about patient care is a common source of friction, sometimes requiring a kind of 'cross-cultural negotiation' (Madsen 2007, p. 24). Differences may be overt (e.g. language barriers, religious differences), but often are less salient (e.g. beliefs about who is entitled to be included in care plan discussions or who is competent to give help—physicians vs. nurses). Nurses carry their own personal beliefs (e.g. how a 'normal' family should behave), as well as professional and institutional values. In institutional cultures where restoration of health is the primary goal and failure in this regard is seen as defeat, there can be little space for nurses and families to acknowledge an impending death, or the profound impact of infirmity and loss. A common reason for distress among nurses is the discrepancy between their own beliefs and those of patients and families (Perkin *et al.* 1997). Below are examples of partnership difficulties described by nurse participants:

'A patient's husband was extremely demanding about her care, had many complaints about nursing staff's response time to his wife's calls. After spending time speaking with him, I found out that he is filled with a lot of guilt because he had discouraged his wife from visiting a doctor when she first developed symptoms and he blamed himself for her advanced disease.'

'Medical team thought patient should be end-of-life/comfort care, but the family was completely for doing everything and anything. The medical team had explained that there wasn't anything they could do more for the patient. The family was very anxious, understandably, and also hostile at times towards the staff.'

Reciprocal escalation challenges

Sequences of interaction can occur between nurses and family members, in which each party unknowingly invites further escalation. This can result in a polarizing 'us vs. them' mindset that leaves staff feeling stuck, and caregiving families feeling alienated. When a family has been labelled 'difficult,' providers may avoid encounters, prompting the family to feel criticized or kept at a distance and resulting in defensive behaviour on their part, which then confirms the nurse's view of the family. Several such negative cycles can occur, as illustrated below:

'After an unsuccessful attempt at an IV insertion, a patient's mother said, "Can we get a nurse who knows how to put in an IV?" ... I spent 30 minutes explaining the procedure to the patient and convincing her to cooperate. The patient was expressing verbal understanding, but the mother would say, "Let's just do it." After an hour of this, the team decided to cancel the patient for the day because of the inability to obtain access, and it was very upsetting for everyone involved.'

Brief training model

A brief, one-session communication skills training module was developed for bedside nurses in acute care. The module teaches strategies for responding to high stress encounters with families.

Training format

Training entails a didactic presentation (30–45 minutes) followed by a large group role play session. The didactic presentation reviewed the literature on family distress during hospitalization, general principles in collaborative care with families, and strategies for responding effectively to challenging interactions. Exemplary videos were embedded into the presentation to illustrate key skills. A trained facilitator then led a group role play in which simulated (actor) families followed pre-scripted roles. Each nurse participant was asked to practice specific strategies with the actor-family, and frequent time-outs were used to invite reflection. The role play segment enabled nurses to directly apply the new skills in a safe, supportive learning environment, with peer-led feedback to address common barriers.

Training content

The strategies reviewed during this training are described in Table 28.1. Consistent with the framework used in the larger Comskil programme (Brown and Bylund 2008), nurses are taught a set of strategies (i.e. general approaches that orient learners towards the stated goal), skills (i.e. observable, concrete behaviours performed) and process tasks (i.e. verbal or non-verbal behaviours that set the stage for effective nurse–family communication).

Strategy 1, *checking your emotional posture*, seeks to cultivate awareness of one's emotional stance prior to interacting with a family. This strategy encourages nurses to attend to their own discomfort so that they can respond skilfully to a patient or family. Nurses are encouraged to 'check their emotional temperature' (on a scale from 1 to 10) and take steps to shift their stance from reactive to curious. The 3-Minute Breathing Space is an exercise drawn from Kabat-Zinn's Mindfulness-Based Stress Reduction programme

Table 28.1 Summary of didactic content for a brief training module on responding to challenging interactions with families

Strategy	Skill	Process Task
Check your emotional posture: responsive vs. reactive	Take emotional temperature (1–10) Body scan	◆ Step out of 'fix it' mode ◆ Recognize discomfort and slow down
Be an ally to the family as a whole (within-family challenges)	Ask open questions Clarify Restate Summarize (differences)	◆ Elicit perspectives ◆ Summarize differences ◆ Highlight positive and common intentions ◆ Feedback family's dilemma
Frame choices (cross-cultural challenges)	Ask open questions Clarify Restate Summarize	◆ Be transparent with families about viewpoints of medical team and parameters of care (choices, range of possible action) ◆ Ask about hopes and intentions ◆ Acknowledge mismatch between viewpoints of family and medical team ◆ Summarize intentions of family and medical team
Provide empathic response	Acknowledge Normalize Praise family's efforts Validate Encourage expression of feelings	◆ Convey that concerns are being taken seriously ◆ Acknowledge vulnerability
Block escalation if inevitable	Review next steps Transition	◆ Disengage if escalation seems inevitable ◆ Suggest time out with plan to return ◆ Redirect volatile family members

(Pipe *et al.* 2009) that offers a technique for addressing intense anxiety. By slowing the impulse to fix the problem or react quickly, nurses are better positioned to listen openly to a family's struggle.

Strategy 2, *becoming an ally to the family*, emphasizes the importance of eliciting and acknowledging the multiple perspectives in a family group while maintaining neutrality when possible. This is accomplished by inviting each family member to articulate concerns, identifying the 'common ground' among family members, highlighting positive intentions, and aspects of the problem around which the nurse and family can unite. Identifying areas where the family may have unique expertise or strength is another way to align with the family and potentiate their natural resources.

Strategy 3, *frame choices*, describes ways to address discrepant perspectives between the family and medical team. Nurses are encouraged to be transparent with the family about available choices, and the parameters of the family's caretaking role (what can and cannot be done, what range of choices they have and what range of action is possible in the given situation). This strategy also emphasizes the importance of reviewing the nurse or medical team's positive intentions, even when their behaviour seems at variance with the family's wishes.

Strategy 4, *respond empathically*, involves acknowledging, validating and normalizing sources of anger, and/or mistakes made. Skills include normalizing the family's experiences, conveying that the family's concerns are being taken seriously, and when possible, reframing anger as worry, upset, and disappointment.

Strategy 5, *block escalation if inevitable*, recognizes those occasions when the nurse or the family become too activated and distressed to maintain constructive discussion, at which point a skilful 'time out' offer with a clear plan to return may be the best solution.

Preliminary results

Participating nurses completed surveys following their participation in the training module. Items inquired about the perceived utility and relevance of training components (e.g. skills reviewed, booklet, exemplary videos, role play experience). Nurses were also asked to rate how confident they felt responding to challenging family interactions before and after the training. Across 29 months, 282 inpatient bedside nurses (26 separate cohorts) were nominated for training by nurse leaders on their unit (acute care, paediatric, urgent care, and intensive care).

Paired *t*-tests compared nurse's confidence in responding to challenging family interactions, as retrospectively recalled before training ($M = 3.32$, $SD = 0.79$) and after completion of training ($M = 3.96$, $SD = 0.61$). Results indicated a statistically significant difference, with mean confidence ratings higher following training ($t = 14.46$, $df = 276$, $p < .001$). The majority of nurses (90%) reported confidence in transporting the skills taught into their clinical setting, and over 75% indicated that aspects of the training itself (e.g. large group role play, facilitation) were helpful in fostering development of specific skills. Whereas only 36.8% of nurses reported that they had felt confident about family care prior to the training, this increased to 78% post-training. These data demonstrate the acceptability and perceived relevance of this module, as well as its impact on nurse's self-efficacy in working with families.

Comprehensive training model

The focused training module described above addresses stressful encounters with families, and was designed for bedside nurses who are on the frontline of patient care and often bear the brunt of these acute, sometimes escalated interactions. A more comprehensive, six-month training curriculum was developed for advanced practice nurses (APN's), who assist with the conceptualization and management of a broader range of family dynamics affecting patient care. Since a significant component of their role involves education and consultation with other inpatient staff, APN's are well positioned to champion and model family-centred care practices.

Training format

The FCNC training is delivered across six months, in two phases: (i) a **Didactic phase** (six sessions), which uses direct teaching, reflection exercises, video illustrations, and actor-supported role play to teach and practice skills in engagement, assessment, intervention and referral of distressed families; and (ii) a **Consolidation phase** (six sessions), in which staff present challenges in their current caseload and discuss the application of skills learned in training. The consolidation establishes a forum for sustainable peer support around real family situations (e.g. conflict over goals of care, end-of-life decisions).

Training content

The didactic phase of training is organized around four dimensions of family-centred patient care, summarized with the acronym PACT (**P**artner, **A**ssess, **C**are, and **T**ransition to resources; see Table 28.2). Each dimension is the focus of a separate training session, which involves didactic review of skills, illustrative videos, and experiential role play with families played by actors. We review the content of each dimension below. A booklet provided to APN provides an overview of how the principles of family-centred care inform our approach to collaborating with families.

Partner

The tasks involved in building partnership with families have been referred to as 'rituals of welcome' (Bell 2011, p.4): acknowledging family members, inviting their participation in discussions, and affirming the importance of their contributions. Negotiating common goals from the outset prevents derailment and confusion about the family's role. Eliciting agenda items, summarizing and clarifying concerns from each family member ensures a diversity of perspectives, and enables the nurse to check for understanding of the presenting situation. Partnering with the family as a unit requires the capacity to legitimize and validate each member's perspective, without taking sides, or creating alliances.

Assess

A brief and focused family assessment aims to accomplish several goals: (i) to identify strengths in the family that may be useful during the patient's hospital admission and in planning his or her transition home; (ii) to identify aspects of the family's context and history, including prior experiences with illness and loss, that may be relevant to the family's adjustment to the current admission; (iii) to identify areas of psychosocial risk, support needs, or cross-cultural challenges that may require further mobilization of resources. Assessing the family includes checking their understanding of the patient's medical situation, asking about the family's strengths and concerns in adjusting to this admission, clarifying roles (e.g. who provides instrumental support, who liaises with medical providers), inquiring about developmental transitions (e.g. weddings, births), and understanding the support network available to the family.

Table 28.2 Summary of training strategies for comprehensive curriculum in Partnering with Families in Cancer Care

Strategy	Skills
Partner	◆ Acknowledge and introduce each person ◆ Invite family to join discussion ◆ Affirm importance of family's contribution ◆ Set agenda and structure interaction ◆ Elicit agenda items from the family ◆ Normalize differences in perspective ◆ Summarize chief concerns
Assess	◆ Check family's understanding of medical situation ◆ Inquire about coping responses ◆ Clarify roles in patient care ◆ Check for outside family stressors/transitions ◆ Ask about key supports ◆ Check for relevant family history
Care	◆ Normalize illness-related challenges ◆ Identify common ground/overlap ◆ Highlight positive intentions ◆ Encourage problem solving within family ◆ Label and acknowledge emotional responses ◆ Reframe ◆ Avoid defensive responses ◆ Commend family competence ◆ Restore control/empower
Transition to Resources	◆ Normalize family's dilemma ◆ Provide information about benefit of a resource ◆ Provide rationale for resources ◆ Explore potential barriers to using resources ◆ Check for consensus and understanding

Care

The care segment of training teaches brief, focused intervention strategies designed to mitigate distress. Skills include acknowledging and normalizing family members' emotional experiences, identifying and highlighting common and positive intentions, both within the family and between the family and the medical team, and facilitating collaborative problem-solving efforts. Facilitating problem solving is distinguished from giving advice, as the nurse is encouraged to elicit ideas initially from the family in order to activate their capacity for teamwork. Reframing is a skill used to promote changes in perspective and offer the family alternative ways of construing and responding to an impasse. Finally, praising family efforts and commending areas of competence reinforces internal strengths and engages them as a resource to one another. Empowering family members and assigning helping roles can restore a sense of control when situations feel chaotic.

Transition to resources

Although many distressed families are helped by brief problem solving and affirmation of strengths, a portion of family members will benefit from intensive psychosocial support. Nurses are taught strategies to help bridge the family to other resources in order to maximize uptake of referrals provided. Normalizing ambivalence mitigates discomfort or stigma attached to seeking psychosocial support. Skills include providing clear information about the resources available, providing a rationale for the referral, checking for potential barriers, as well as establishing a consensus among family members on next steps. Following these steps promotes discussion around the referral and provides an opportunity for the nurse to pre-emptively address questions or concerns.

Preliminary results

This curriculum and evaluation process was piloted with 14 APN's, enrolled in two separate cohorts. The measurement of training efficacy and impact on care was guided by Kirkpatrick's multilevel model for evaluating educational training programmes (Hutchinson 1999). More than three quarters of training participants reported that the skills they learned enabled better patient and family care, prompted them to evaluate their own skills, were reinforced through the role play, and involved a manageable time commitment. Nurses were asked to report on their perceived confidence using various family-centred care strategies reviewed in the programme (e.g. eliciting perspectives from family members, achieving consensus in the family, highlighting family strengths). The mean confidence score across all areas of family-centred care increased from pre-training ($Mean$ = 3.30, SD = 0.60) to post-didactic training ($Mean$ = 4.20, SD = 0.68) (t = 4.02, df = 10, $p < .005$). Transfer of skills to simulated and real clinical encounters was examined using a coding instrument developed specifically for this programme. An independent observer, trained to achieve 80% reliability against a gold standard rater (T. Zaider), accompanied nurses in up to three brief (5 min) family consultations in the hospital setting. The rater coded in real time the presence/absence of 22 skills in the dimensions of partner, assess, and care. Each of the skills observed was coded for 'patient' or 'family', depending on who was addressed by the nurse's communication. This real time observational coding method was conducted pre- and post-training for the eight nurses who participated in the second training cohort. Although the small sample size limited our power to detect statistically significant differences, examination of the mean number of skills observed at pre- and post-didactic training suggests promising trends. The mean frequency of skills observed across providers increased from a mean of 4.44 (SD = 1.85) at baseline to 6.63 (SD = 2.43) following the Didactic phase of training (t = 2.043, df = 5, $p < .05$). The frequency of skills directed to the family increased from a mean of 2.5 (SD = .80) to 3.5 (SD = 1.9), primarily in the category of assessment skills, whereas the frequency of skills directed towards patients increased from 1.94 (SD = 1.20) to 3.11 (SD = .95) and were more evenly distributed across engagement, assessment, and intervention.

Overall, there were fewer family assessment skills used relative to partnering and care skills. The tendency to leap from initial engagement of the family to intervention and problem solving was evident anecdotally throughout the training experience, and may limit the nurse's capacity to fully understand the family's support needs. Interpretation of these preliminary data is limited by the constraints of a real-clinic setting in which opportunities to use the skills observed varied considerably. The examination of skill transfer in standardized, simulated family consultations, and observation of skill transfer following the consolidation phase of training is currently underway, and will provide more data on the extent of skill uptake.

Conclusion

During hospitalization, the family and medical team interface more frequently, and often in a climate of greater urgency than occurs during routine outpatient visits. This temporary 'social grouping' requires the patient, family, and medical team to function together as a larger caregiving system with common concern for the ill patient (Reiss and Kaplan De-Nour 1989). Training initiatives such as the ones presented here, which are designed to strengthen the cohesiveness of this larger family-provider system will become increasingly important, as patients and their families seek a more integrated cancer care experience.

References

Bell JM (2011). Relationships: The heart of the matter in family nursing. *J Fam Nurs* **17**, 3–10.

Brown RF, Bylund CL (2008). Communication skills training: describing a new conceptual model. *Acad Med* **83**, 37–44.

Chesla CA, Stannard D (1997). Breakdown in the nursing care of families in the ICU. *Am J Crit Care* **6**, 64–71.

Davidson JE, Powers K, Hedayat KM, *et al.* (2007) Clinical practice guidelines for support of the family in the patient-centered intensive care unit: American College of Critical Care Medicine Task Force 2004-2005. *Crit Care Med* **35**, 605–22.

Doolin CT, Quinn LD, Bryant LG, Lyons AA, Kleinpell RM (2011). Family presence during cardiopulmonary resuscitation: using evidence-based knowledge to guide the advanced practice nurse in developing formal policy and practice guidelines. *J Am Acad Nurse Pract* **23**, 8–14.

Ferrell, B. McCabe MS, Levit L (2013). The Institute of Medicine report on high-quality cancer care: implications for oncology nursing. *Oncol Nurs Forum* **40**, 603–9.

Gueguen JA, Bylund CL, Brown RF, Levin TT, Kissane DW (2009). Conducting family meetings in palliative care: themes, techniques, and preliminary evaluation of a communication skills module. *Palliat Support Care* **7**, 171–9.

Hudson PL, Aranda S, Kristjanson LJ (2004). Meeting the supportive needs of family caregivers in palliative care: challenges for health professionals. *J Palliat Med* **7**, 19–25.

Hutchinson L (1999). Evaluating and researching the effectiveness of educational interventions. *BMJ* **318**(7193), 1267–9.

Johnson BH, *et al.* (2008) Partnering with patients and families to design a patient- and family-centered health care system: Recommendations and promising practices. Institute for Patient- and Family-Centered Care, Bethesda, MD. Available at: http://www.ipfcc.org/pdf/PartneringwithPatientsandFamilies.pdf [Online].

Kaakinen JR, Gedaly-Duff V, Padgett Coehlo D, Harmon Hanson SM (2010). *Family Health Care Nursing: Theory, Practice and Research*, 4th edition. F.A. Davis Company, Philadelphia, PA.

Madsen WC (2007). *Collaborative Therapy with Multi-Stressed Families*, 2nd edition. The Guilford Press, New York, NY.

McLeod DL, Tapp DM, Moules NJ, Campbell ME (2010). Knowing the family: interpretations of family nursing in oncology and palliative care. *Eur J Oncol Nurs* **14**, 93–100.

Mehta A, Cohen SR, Chan LS (2009). Palliative care: a need for a family systems approach. *Palliat Support Care* **7**, 235–43.

Northouse LL (2012). Helping patients and their family caregivers cope with cancer. *Oncol Nurs Forum* **39**, 500–6.

Perkin R, Young T, Freier MC, Allen J, Orr RD (1997). Stress and distress in pediatric nurses: Lessons from baby K. *Am J Crit Care* **6**, 225–32.

Pipe TB, Bortz JJ, Dueck A, Pendergast D, Buchda V, Summers J (2009). Nurse leader mindfulness meditation program for stress management: a randomized controlled trial. *J Nurs Adm* **39**, 130–7.

Reiss D *et al.* (1989). The family and medical team in chronic illness: A transactional and developmental perspective. *Family Syst Med*, 435–44.

Schaefer KG, Block SD (2009). Physician communication with families in the ICU: evidence-based strategies for improvement. *Curr Opin Crit Care* **15**, 569–77.

Tomlinson D, Bartels U, Hendershot E, Maloney AM, Ethier MC, Sung L (2011). Factors affecting treatment choices in paediatric palliative care: Comparing parents and health professionals. *Eur J Cancer* **47**, 2182–7.

Traeger L, Park ER, Sporn N, Repper-DeLisi J, Convery MS, Jacobo M, Pirl WF (2013). Development and evaluation of targeted psychological skills training For oncology nurses in managing stressful patient and family encounters. *Oncol Nurs Forum* **40**, E327–36.

Wright LM, Leahey M (2005). The three most common errors in family nursing: How to avoid or sidestep. *J Family Nurs* **11**, 90–101.

Wright LM, Leahey M (2012). *Nurses and Families: A Guide to Family Assessment and Intervention*. FA Davis, Philadelphia, PA.

Zaider T, Kissane D (2009). The assessment and management of family distress during palliative care. *Curr Opin Support Palliat Care* **3**, 67–71.

CHAPTER 29

Ambulatory care nurses responding to depression

Anthony De La Cruz, Richard F. Brown, and Steve Passik

Introduction to ambulatory care nurses responding to depression

A strong body of evidence demonstrates the co-existence of depression and cancer, with reported prevalence rates of depression for solid tumours ranging from 20 to 50% (Pasquini and Biondi 2007). Despite these high rates, depression often goes undetected by healthcare providers in about 50% of cases because it usually is not looked for, and often is ignored or missed (Sharp 2005; Brown *et al.* 2009). It is important for nurses to understand that depression is an illness and that its associated symptoms are not simply a normal reaction to the diagnosis of cancer (Blair 2012). Oncology nurses in the ambulatory setting are in a key position to identify and respond to a patient's emotional distress and aid in the identification of patients that are at risk for developing depression, or may already be suffering from depression. Their ability to establish a dialogue about emerging symptoms is invaluable and it is therefore crucial to be educated in both the assessment criteria and communication skills that will assist in identifying patients that are experiencing a depressive episode. In this chapter we will present a model of core communication components consisting of strategies, skills, and process tasks. This model will enable nurses to gain an understanding of the patient's experience and assist in the recognition and treatment of depression. The results of a pilot programme utilizing this model and skills will also be presented.

Nature of depression

In a comprehensive review of more than 100 studies of patients with cancer, Massie (2004) identified a wide range (0–58%) in the reported prevalence of depression spectrum syndromes. Cancer, irrespective of site, is associated with a higher rate of depression than in the general population. Despite the high incidence and devastating consequences of depression among patients with cancer, under-recognition, and inadequate treatment prevail (Bowers and Boyle 2003). Patients faced with a diagnosis of cancer experience a broad spectrum of emotions, including depressive symptoms that range from normal unhappiness, to adjustment disorder with depressed mood, to major depression.

Clinical depression is distinguished by its intensity, duration, and the extent to which an individual's functioning is compromised (Bowers and Boyle 2003). The National Institute of Mental Health, a division of the United States National Institutes of Health, describes a depressive disorder as an illness that involves the body, mood, and thoughts. It affects how a person behaves (e.g. loss of appetite, insomnia), feels about himself or herself (e.g. hopeless, worthless, guilty), and thinks (e.g. inability to concentrate; thoughts about death). These changes are pervasive and affect every aspect of the patient's being.

In diagnosing depression, mental health professionals use criteria set out in the American Psychiatric Association's Diagnostic and Statistical Manual of Mental Disorders (DSM-V). Specific criteria help distinguish between major depression, dysthymic disorder, minor depression, and adjustment disorder with depressed mood.

The perplexing symptoms a patient exhibits may leave nurses feeling ill-equipped to differentiate sadness from depression that needs treatment (Block 2000). Although the ambulatory care nurse is not expected to diagnose a depressive disorder, an understanding of the diagnostic criteria is important in recognizing a patient's symptoms. Practitioners should familiarize themselves with the latest version of the American Psychiatric Association's Diagnostic and Statistical Manual of Mental Disorders (DSM-V) for the specific criteria related to the diagnosis of a major depressive episode.

Risk factors

Patients with cancer often experience elevated levels of emotional distress as they adjust to the diagnosis, the side effects of treatments (such as chemotherapy and radiation therapy), and the burden of symptoms caused by the disease itself. The number of symptoms attributed to treatment was positively correlated with anxious mood (Thune-Boyle *et al.* 2006). In addition, stress on their family and the economic situation due to inability to work may increase their risk of developing depression. Many of the medications used to treat cancer can also trigger symptoms—corticosteroids in particular may cause the patient to be emotionally unstable, becoming tearful easily, euphoric or irritable, and can lead to a depressive episode. In addition, there are a number of metabolic abnormalities such as calcium, potassium, or sodium imbalance, and thyroid dysfunction which can lead to a depressive episode. Risk factors also include genetic factors, such as first-degree relatives with depression or prior history of depression. Cancer-related side effects such as advance staging, brain metastases, and uncontrolled pain are also factors (Snyderman and Wynn 2009).

Barriers to recognizing depression

Patients, family, and even healthcare providers can have a number of misconceptions about the recognition and treatment of depression.

One common presumption is that all people with cancer must be depressed and it is a normal consequence. This can minimize caregivers' perception, not only of the degree of suffering associated with depression but also its impact on a person's quality of life, and it frequently leads to a belief that depression is not a serious comorbid and treatable condition and may result in the undertreatment of depression (Fulcher *et al.* 2008). In addition, many patients are reluctant to bring up their sense of sadness and depression with their physician and nurse because they do not want to burden the treatment team and may fear being stigmatized (Payne 2003).

In the ambulatory setting, nurses often focus on physical aspects of treatment and the management of side effects, and avoid emotional issues, possibly because of an unfounded belief that they must 'remedy' distress (Payne 2003). Studies indicate that nurses tend to keep communication at a superficial level and avoid emotional cues. In addition, nurses may use defence mechanisms to protect themselves from the emotions of patients and families because of a lack of confidence in their ability to address these emotions. Better communication, through knowledge, support, experience, and success, may increase confidence and self-efficacy, which ultimately improves patient care (Baer and Weinstein 2012).

Cancer patients sometimes minimize their symptoms as they feel some pressure from family members, caregivers, and friends to maintain a positive outlook about their cancer and their future. There is a general perception that a positive outlook and fighting spirit may promote better outcomes. For most patients, cancer is the most difficult and frightening experience they have ever experienced. All of this hype that if you get depressed you are making your tumour grow faster invalidates people's natural and understandable reaction to a threat to their lives (Holland and Lewis 2000).

Symptoms associated with depression

Fatigue, weight loss, insomnia, and lack of appetite are somatic symptoms that are often cited as criteria used in establishing a diagnosis of depression in the physically healthy individual. But in patients with cancer, the symptoms of depression, the side effects of treatment and the symptoms of the cancer are often very difficult to distinguish. Fatigue and lack of appetite may be associated with a chemotherapy regimen or with the cancer itself. Insomnia may be the result of pain or other symptoms related to the cancer. The detection and identification of depression poses a challenge for oncology nurses due to the overlap of symptoms a patient may be experiencing.

The distinction between symptoms of normal sadness and grief, and symptoms suggesting a diagnosis of depression has important clinical implications. Feelings of sadness, shock, anger, and fear that may accompany a cancer diagnosis are normal reactive symptoms and typically resolve within two weeks. Such emotions may return at different times during the progression of the disease course, including after learning of treatment failure, relapse, or presence of metastases (Snyderman and Wynn 2009). Asking about these feelings is a way to open up a dialogue with patients who might otherwise be reluctant to discuss them.

Patients with depression may be at increased risk of suicide. Asking a patient about thoughts of, or plans for, suicide does not initiate such ideas. On the contrary, they may be relieved if they are asked directly about their thoughts and feel that you are interested in their situation (American Psychiatric Association 2013). If suicidal ideation is present, the patient should not be left alone and be referred urgently for psychiatric evaluation and the patient may even need compulsory treatment.

Strategies for responding to depression

Maguire *et al.* (1996) conducted a communication skills training workshop with 206 health professionals, predominantly nurses (65%), which involved practice in assessing patient concerns. Participants first identified the areas that were most problematic for them (e.g. breaking bad news and eliciting and discussing patients' feelings about their disease), then watched a video comparing assessment behaviours that either promote disclosure or inhibit it, and then role-played specific communication techniques. Before the workshop, each participant interviewed a simulated patient in order to elicit the patient's current problems; after training, each participant conducted a similar assessment with a different simulated patient. Maguire reported a significant increase in participants' use of facilitative behaviour (i.e. they engaged in more behaviour that elicited their patient's concerns) and a significant reduction in the use of questions that focused solely on physical issues.

In another study, 61 clinical nurse specialists took part in a three-day communication skills training workshop, after which 29 of them were randomized to receive follow-up clinical supervision for four weeks. Simulated patient assessments conducted before and after the workshop indicated that the training programme was effective in increasing nurses' ability to use key skills, respond to patient cues, and identify patient concerns. Furthermore, the nurses who received clinical supervision were better able to transfer their skills to the clinical setting (Heaven *et al.* 2006).

Wilkinson *et al.* (2008) evaluated the effectiveness of a three-day communication skills course in changing nurses' communication skills. A total of 172 nurses were randomized to the communication course or control. This randomized control trial reported that a three-day communication skills course is effective in changing nurses' behaviours up to three months post-course. In addition, the quality of the nurses' communication skills improved after attending the course, reflected by the increase in taped assessment scores. The course was also shown to have a positive effect on the nurses' confidence in dealing with cancer patients. There is evidence to suggest if nurses undertake this mode of communication skills training, patient satisfaction with nurses' communication improves and patients show a more positive general emotional state.

In another study, Wilkinson *et al.* (2002) evaluated a communication skills programme delivered to 308 oncology nurses. After the course, the nurses displayed statistically significant improvements in nine areas of assessment. The most significant improvements were in areas with high emotional content.

Key communication skills and process tasks

Well-developed communication that includes supportive and empathetic responses serves to comfort and inspire patients, and becomes a useful therapeutic intervention. (Kennedy 2005) Using an evidence-based approach, we developed six core communication strategies to assist ambulatory care nurses in recognizing and responding to a patient's depression. The six strategies were developed in collaboration with groups of ambulatory care nurses and make use of established communication techniques. Skills and process tasks have been identified for each strategy, and examples of how nurses may approach or respond to a patient are provided. The goal is to gain an understanding of the patient's experience and to assist the patient in

CHAPTER 29 AMBULATORY CARE NURSES RESPONDING TO DEPRESSION 189

Table 29.1 Strategy #1: Make a transition to a discussion about emotional issues

Process tasks: Ensure that the setting is appropriate: – seating arrangement; – be at eye level with the patient; – avoid interruptions; – have tissues on hand.		
Skill	**Description**	**Example**
Make a 'take stock' statement	Creates a pause in the dialogue to review the prior discussion and seek the patient's permission to move on	'Now, we have talked about your physical symptoms. But it seems to me that you look sad today. Would it be all right to talk about this?'
Ask open-ended questions	Questions that allow the patient to respond in any manner they choose	'So, can you tell me more about how you are feeling?'
Normalize	Respond with a comparative statement asserting that a particular emotional response is not out of the ordinary	'It is not uncommon to feel this way at a time like this'

seeking treatment. These strategies may also be incorporated into role playing scenarios or practiced independently as a way to improve communication skills. They are not meant to be used sequentially; in fact they may be repeated and occur over multiple encounters.

Strategy #1 (Table 29.1) enables the nurse to initiate a dialogue and will shift the assessment from physiological symptoms to emotional concerns. It allows the nurse to assess the patient's needs and provides an opportunity to educate the patient on issues related to depression. It involves using open-ended questions to allow the patient to respond in their own way. Even when patients give cues, healthcare professionals often fail to ask questions that would reveal symptoms of anxiety and/or depression (Butow *et al.* 2002). Nurses are in a strategic position to detect psychological distress because most nurse–patient interactions require establishing some kind of dialogue.

Strategy #2 (Table 29.2) allows nurses to assess patients' needs and also provides important information. Nurses should be direct in pursuing information when patients provide cues that indicate psychological distress. If nurses address sensitive patient concerns with self-confidence, patients may be more likely to reveal their distress (American Psychiatric Association 2003).

Strategy #3 (Table 29.3) addresses the overlap between depressive and physical symptoms which complicates the recognition and diagnosis of depression. Many of the classic symptoms of depression may be due to physical illness or depression, or both. In discussing symptoms and risk factors, the nurse will be able to identify

the patient's needs and respond. It is important to be able to pick up, acknowledge, and explore cues patients have given, particularly about experiences of key symptoms or psychological reactions (Maguire and Pitceathly 2003).

Strategy #4 (Table 29.4) allows the nurse to empathize and provide hope and reassurance. Asking questions about the impact of events—and how these events have affected aspects of the patient's life—is crucial in allowing the nurse to empathize with the patient.

Strategy # 5 (Table 29.5) allows the nurse to educate the patient about depression. Didactic training in the recognition of depression has been found to be effective in increasing nurses' awareness of symptoms (Passik *et al.* 2000). A better understanding of depression gives healthcare providers a sense of confidence in their ability to discuss the disorder with the patient. Patients may feel confused and embarrassed and reluctant to discuss emotional difficulties. It is important to try to dispel negative perceptions by explaining the causes and risk factors, as well as the many treatment options available. Providing information about treatment options and their effectiveness may ease the patient's anxiety.

Therapies for depression include a variety of pharmacological and non-pharmacological approaches. Five categories of pharmacotherapy typically used in the cancer setting are selective serotonin reuptake inhibitors (SSRIs), atypical antidepressants, tricyclic antidepressants, psychostimulants, and, rarely, monoamine oxidase inhibitors (MAOIs). Nurses should familiarize themselves

Table 29.2 Strategy #2: Discuss patient's emotional experience

Process tasks: – Discuss patient's preference for who is present for the discussion. – Ask direct questions.		
Skill	**Description**	**Example**
Encourage expression of feelings	Express to the patient that you would like to know how he or she is feeling	'It is important to me to understand how you are dealing with all of this emotionally'
Ask open-ended questions	Questions that allow the patient to respond in any manner they choose	'So, can you tell me more about how you are feeling?'

Table 29.3 Strategy #3: Discuss patient's symptoms and risk factors

Process tasks:
- Review patient's experience.
- Explore patient's previous coping mechanism and support.

Skill	Description	Example
Clarify	Ask a question to better understand what the patient is saying	'I am not sure I understand what you mean. Can you explain a little more?'
Restate	State in your own words what you think the patient is saying	'It sounds like you do not enjoy things that you used to love to do'
Check patient's medical knowledge	Ask the patient about his understanding of the medical terminology	'What do you understand depression to be?'

Table 29.4 Strategy #4: Empathize with patient's emotional distress

Process tasks:
- Provide hope and reassurance.
- Allow patient time to process feelings.

Skill	Description	Example
Acknowledge	Make a statement that indicates recognition of the patient's emotion or experience	'It sounds as if you have found all this very distressing?'
Validate	Make a statement expressing that a patient's emotional response to an event or an experience is appropriate and reasonable	'You have been through a difficult time; it is certainly understandable to feel the way you do'
Normalize	Respond with a comparative statement asserting that a particular emotional response is not out of the ordinary	'Many people feel the way you do in this type of situation'
Praise patient's efforts	Make a statement that validates a patient's attempts to cope with his emotional issues	'It sounds like you have been trying hard to keep things as normal as you can'

Table 29.5 Strategy #5: Educate the patient about depression

Process tasks:
- Provide vocabulary and avoid jargon.
- Explain sources of information.
- Allow the patient time to integrate the information.

Skill	Description	Example
Preview information	Give an overview of the main points that you are about to cover	'I would like to discuss some aspects of depression that you may not be aware of'
Summarize	Recap the main details conveyed	'So, let me summarize what we have said: there are many different approaches to treating depression'
Check patient understanding	Ask the patient about his understanding or previously conveyed information or the current situation	'We spoke about a lot of different risk factors. Can you tell me which ones you may have?'
Invite patient's questions	Make it clear to the patient that you are willing to answer questions and address concerns	'Please feel free to call me from home if you have any questions'

with these general categories and the associated side effects. SSRIs have become the first line of treatment for depression. They are effective and well-tolerated in many patients, and are not as toxic in high doses as the older tricyclic antidepressants (Winell and Roth 2004).

Psychotherapy is also frequently used in combination with pharmacological intervention. Several psychotherapeutic techniques have been successful in treating patients with cancer. Two commonly used modalities are supportive psychotherapy and cognitive-behavioural therapy (Winell and Roth 2004).

Table 29.6 Strategy #6: Discuss whether a referral would be appropriate

Process tasks:
– Explore the patient's attitude about treatment for depression.
– Maintain eye contact.

Skill	Description	Example
Express a willingness to help	Make a specific offer to help or a general statement about being available for future help with a decision	'If there is anything I can do to help you with a decision, please let me know'
Review next steps	Go over with the patient the possible next steps and make sure the patient is clear on them	'I just want to go over the next steps that we discussed to make sure we both understand the plan'
Invite patient's questions	Make it clear to the patient that you are willing to answer questions and address concerns	'What questions do you have?'
Make a partnership statement	Convey an alliance with the patient	'Let's figure out when would be the best time to continue our discussion'
Offer time to delay a decision	Reinforce the idea that the patient has time to make a decision about treatment	'There is no rush. You can decide in your own time whether you want to speak with someone or not'
Summarize	Recap the main ideas conveyed	'Let's summarize the next steps'

Strategy #6 (Table 29.6) allows time for the nurse to discuss referrals when they are appropriate. Offer the patient a variety of alternatives when discussing referrals. A psychologist, psychiatrist, or social worker can be a source of support. Depending on institutional practice, a counselling service may be available. In addition, numerous community resources may be available and accessible to the patient.

To address the communication difficulties encountered by the oncology nurse, Brown *et al.* (2009), developed and pilot tested a communication skills training workshop based on the preceding six strategies of key communication skills and process tasks. The aim of this research was to evaluate the impact of a communication skills workshop targeting specific nurse behaviours during a discussion about a patient's depression and referral for psychological support. Each workshop incorporated didactic teaching of strategies, exemplary videos modelling ideal behaviour, and a skills practice session. The skills practice session included prepared scenarios depicting patient depression and used standardized patients-trained actors taking the role of depressed patients. During the practice sessions, there was the opportunity for skills practice including instant feedback from peers, the facilitator who incorporated video feedback, and the actor. A total of 15 nurses participated in the pilot and the results indicate that in three strategies—discuss the patient's emotional experience, discuss the patient's symptoms and risk factors, and discuss appropriate referrals—ratings of successful use were statistically significantly improved before and after training. In one strategy, to empathize with emotional distress, a trend to significance was observed. These results support many other research studies reporting that communication skills training can be used successfully to alter participants' behaviour (Brown *et al.* 2009). Future research is warranted, exploring the use of this training in a larger sample of ambulatory nurses with a more diverse patient population.

Key questions to ask

Table 29.7 lists some additional questions that may be used to guide the nurse's assessment and assist in determining if a referral is needed (Roth and Holland 2003).

Table 29.7 Key questions to ask

Question	Symptoms/factors being assessed
How well are you coping with your cancer?	Well-being
How are your spirits? Do you feel down, sad, depressed? Are you crying a lot?	Mood
Are there things you still enjoy doing, or have you lost pleasure in the things you used to do?	Anhedonia; loss of interest
How does the future look to you? Are there things that you are looking forward to?	Hopelessness
Do you feel that things are out of your control?	Helplessness
Do you worry about being a burden to family or friends?	Worthlessness
Do you have pain that isn't controlled?	Pain
Do you feel exhausted or weak? Do you feel rested after sleeping? How much time do you spend in bed?	Fatigue
How are you sleeping at night? Do you have trouble falling asleep?	Sleep
How is your appetite? Have you gained or lost weight recently?	Appetite

Adapted from Roth AJ, Holland JC, 'Psychological aspects of hematological malignancies,' Table 62.3, in Wiernik PH *et al.* (Eds.), *Neoplastic Diseases of the Blood, Fourth Edition*, Cambridge University Press, Cambridge, UK, Copyright © 2003. Reprinted with permission of the Editors.

Conclusion

Establishing and maintaining a dialogue is critical in assessing and responding to a patient's depression. Understanding the illness, its symptoms, and its impact enables nurses to support and promote referrals not only for patients exhibiting signs of depression but also for those at risk. Developing key communication skills is essential to meeting the needs of our patients. Mastering these techniques will enable nurses to relinquish inhibitory behaviours and help their patients explore their feelings, no matter where on the continuum of depression they lie or how distressing they seem. Depression is treatable. Recognizing and responding to a patient's depression can greatly improve their quality of life.

References

American Psychiatric Association (2003). Practice guidelines for the assessment and treatment of patients with suicidal behaviours. *Am J Psychiatry* **160**, 1–60.

American Psychiatric Association (2013). *Diagnostic and statistical manual of mental disorders (DSM5)*. American Psychiatric Association, Washington DC, WA.

Baer L, Weinstein E (2012). Improving oncology nurses' communication skills for difficult conversation. *Clin J Oncol Nurs* **17**, E45–51.

Blair E (2012). Understanding depression: Awareness, assessment and nursing intervention. *Clin J Oncol Nurs* **16**, 463–5.

Block SD (2000). Assessing and managing depression in the terminally ill patient. ACP-ASIM End-of-Life Care Consensus Panel. American College of Physicians–American Society of Internal Medicine. *Ann Intern Med*, **132**, 209–18.

Bowers L, Boyle DA (2003). Depression in patients with advanced cancer. *Clin J Oncol Nurs* **7**, 281–8.

Brown R, Bylund C, Kline N, *et al.* (2009). Identifying and responding to depression in adult cancer patients. *Cancer Nurs* **32**, E1–7.

Butow PN, Brown RF, Cogar S, *et al.* (2002). Oncologists' reactions to cancer patients' verbal cues. *Psychooncology* **11**, 47–58.

Fulcher CD, Badger T, Gunter AK, *et al.* (2008). Putting evidence into practice: interventions for depression. *Clin J Oncology Nurs* **12**, 131–40.

Heaven C, Clegg J, Maguire P (2006). Transfer of communication skills training from workshop to workplace: the impact of clinical supervision. *Patient Educ Couns* **60**, 313–25.

Holland JC, Lewis S (2000). *The Human Side of Cancer*. Harper Collins, New York, NY.

Kennedy Sheldon L (2005). Communication in oncology care: the effectiveness of skills training workshops for healthcare providers. *Clin J Oncol Nurs* **9**, 305–12.

Maguire P, Booth K, Elliott C, *et al.* (1996). Helping health professionals involved in cancer care acquire key interviewing skills—the impact of workshops. *Eur J Cancer* **32A**, 1486–9.

Maguire P, Pitceathly C (2003). Improving the psychological care of cancer patients and their relatives. The role of specialist nurses. *J Psychosom Res* **55**, 469–74.

Massie MJ (2004). Prevalence of depression in patients with cancer. *J Natl Cancer Inst Monogr* **32**, 57–71.

Pasquini M, Biondi M (2007). Depression in cancer patients: a critical review. *Clin Pract Epidemiol Ment Health* **3**, 2.

Passik SD, Donaghy KB, Theobald DE, *et al.* (2000). Oncology staff recognition of depressive symptoms on videotaped interviews of depressed cancer patients: implications for designing a training program. *J Pain Symptom Manage* **19**, 329–38.

Payne WM (2003). A qualitative study of clinical nurses specialists' views on depression in palliative care practice. *Palliat Med* **17**, 334–8.

Roth AJ, Holland JC (2003). Psychological aspects of hematological malignancies. In: *Neoplastic Diseases of the Blood*, 4th edition. Cambridge University Press, Cambridge, UK.

Sharp K (2005). Depression: The essentials. *Clin J Oncol Nurs* **9**, 519–25.

Snyderman D, Wynn D (2009). Depression in cancer patients. *Prim Care* **36**, 703–19.

Thuné-Boyle ICV, Myers LB, Newman SP (2006). The role of illness beliefs, treatment beliefs, and perceived severity of symptoms in explaining distress in cancer patients during chemotherapy treatment. *Behav Med* **32**, 19–29.

Wilkinson SM, Gambles M, Roberts A (2002). The essence of cancer care: the impact of training on nurses' ability to communicate effectively. *J Adv Nurs* **40**, 731–8.

Wilkinson S, Perry R, Blanchard K (2008). Effectiveness of a three-day communication skills course in changing nurses' communication skills with cancer/palliative patients: a randomized controlled trial. *Palliat Med* **22**, 365–75.

Winell J, Roth AJ (2004). Depression in cancer patients. *Oncology (Williston Park)*, **18**, 1554–60; discussion 1561–2.

CHAPTER 30

Communication in the last days or hours of life

Anita Roberts

Introduction to communication in the last days or hours of life

Advances in healthcare mean that populations of developed countries are living longer and so the risk of death from chronic illness and co-morbidities increases. One impact of such changes is that people are more likely to die in institutional settings (Ellershaw and Wilkinson 2011; Bloomer *et al.* 2013). However, regardless of what setting people die in, they should receive the best care possible. This care should be based on their needs and include the family and friends as much as is possible.

Ellershaw and Lakhani (2013) describe the elements of care necessary for delivering the best care for the dying person (see Box 30.1). These elements are widely reflected in the literature describing high-quality care in the last days or hours of life (Veerbeek 2008;

Box 30.1 Ten key elements of care for the dying person (Ellershaw and Lakhani 2013)

1. Recognition that the person is dying.

2. Communication with the dying person (where possible) and always with family and loved ones.

3. Spiritual care.

4. Anticipatory prescribing for symptoms of pain, respiratory tract secretions, agitation, nausea and vomiting, dyspnoea.

5. Review of clinical interventions taking into account the dying person's wishes and best interests.

6. Review hydration needs of the dying person, including the need for commencement or cessation of artificial hydration.

7. Review nutritional needs of the dying person, including the need for commencement or cessation of parenteral nutrition.

8. Full discussion of the care plan with the dying person and relative or carer.

9. The regular reassessment of the dying person.

10. Provision of dignified and respectful care after death.

Reproduced from *The British Medical Journal*, John E Ellershaw and Mayur Lakhani, 'Best care for the dying patient', Volume 347, F4428, Copyright © 2013 British Medical Journal Publishing Group, with permission from BMJ Publishing Group Ltd.

GMC 2010; Costantini *et al.* 2011; NICE 2011; Leadership Alliance for the Care of Dying People (LACDP) 2014), and open and honest communication between dying patients, those important to them, and the staff who care for them is a critically important element in this sensitive area of care.

Death is a subject that is often feared and this can mean that it is not often discussed (Vora and Vora 2008). It is notoriously difficult and emotional for people who are dying to talk about their impending death, concerns they may have, and the emotions they are experiencing. This may also be true for their loved ones. Communication at this time can be further complicated by social taboos and interpersonal dynamics (Emanuel 2012).

Poor communication continues to be an element in complaints on end-of-life care. Healthcare professionals do not always have the open and honest conversations needed (Parliamentary and Health Service Ombudsman 2015). For three quarters of people, death is not sudden but expected, and so many benefit from end of life care (NHS England 2014). In order to provided good care in the last days or hours of life, it is essential that communication is always a proactive, two-way process with healthcare staff actively and sensitively eliciting and listening to the views and concerns of people who are dying and their family and friends, and not waiting to be asked questions (Ellershaw and Wilkinson 2011). All healthcare staff need to develop skills that enable them to communicate in a sensitive and respectful manner, which not only takes into consideration what the dying person and those important to them want, but also acknowledges what they may feel able to talk about at any particular time point (Wilkinson 2011; LACDP 2014).

This chapter discusses communication in the last days or hours of life, dealing with uncertainty, identifying the priorities of the dying person, giving information and discussing care in a sensitive and supportive manner, and communication skills training opportunities for healthcare staff.

In order to be able to engage in the complex and sensitive conversations that are part of caring for dying patients and their families, it is helpful to have a good understanding of the process of effective communication.

Effective communication

Effective communication involves non-verbal, paralinguistic, and verbal elements. Patients and relatives are more likely to engage in sensitive conversations with clinicians who are open to discussion, use facilitating skills sensitively, and who have an empathic approach.

Table 30.1 Aspects of non-verbal communication

Environment	The physical environment can invite or inhibit communication in obvious or subtle ways
Positioning	The distance participants maintain between themselves is important. Being to close can feel uncomfortable but being too distant can inhibit communication.
Touch	A powerful way of expressing emotion. Dying people may feel the need for physical contact with others but not everyone likes to be touched.
Eye Contact	This is a way of collecting information, getting feedback, and monitoring non-verbal behaviour. Eye contact can also communicate attitude and emotion. It can also be a signal for turn taking in conversation.
Facial expression	Signals attitude and emotion. Facial expressions indicate a person's true feelings by supporting or conflicting with what is being said.
Gestures	Communicate messages by emphasizing or clarifying speech. They can be used to regulate speech such as nodding to encourage the speaker to continue. Some gestures have a direct verbal equivalent (e.g. waving, nodding) and can replace verbal communication.
Posture	Can signal the strength of a person's emotion, attitude, and mood.

Non-verbal communication is an extremely complex yet integral part of overall communication and plays a vital role in discussions of an emotional nature (see Table 30.1).

Non-verbal communication provides an opportunity to reinforce or modify what is said in words. For example, people may shake their head to emphasize that they disagree with the other person, but a shrug of the shoulders and a sad expression when saying 'I'm fine' may provide an important cue that things are not really alright. This form of communication not only coveys important information about a person's emotional state, but is also an effective method of giving and receiving feedback. It also helps to regulate flow of communication, for example, by indicating that a person has finished speaking or wants to say something.

Paralanguage is the component of communication which includes rhythm, sound, pitch, volume, and intonation of what is being said.

Although the paralinguistic component is often used and interpreted unconsciously, it is a significant part of communication as it provides important cues for health professionals trying to understand people's needs. For example, it can be used as an effective way of emphasizing important information, to concur, or to contradict.

To illustrate the paralinguistic element of communication, consider the following statement:

'He said that he had been worried about his Mum for the last week.'

By adjusting the emphasis, volume, intonation, etc. of how this statement is said, it can change from a simple statement of fact to a statement that conveys you are shocked by this fact. Alternatively, it can be said in a manner that turns it into a question or in a manner that indicates it is a lie. Paralinguistic communication can also indicate emotions such as anger, shock, and distress.

Skilled verbal communication is vital if dying people are to receive high-quality care. Healthcare professionals can support dying patients and families by providing information, comfort, and empathy during this challenging time. This can be achieved by listening actively and responding in a sensitive and meaningful way. Inadequate communication can be distressing and leave a lasting impact on families. Some of the factors that can hinder communication have been identified and are outlined in Table 30.2.

Verbal skills that facilitate effective communication are outlined in Table 30.3.

Recognizing impending death

Healthcare professionals must continually assess the condition of the patient and respond accordingly to adapt care, taking the needs and wishes of the patient and family into account.

There is evidence that if clinicians recognize that a patient is expected to die within the coming days or hours, they are more likely to talk to the patient and relatives about death and the most appropriate care, including withholding futile or burdensome treatments (Houttekier et al. 2014).

If the patient is likely to die soon, this should be clearly and sensitively communicated to the patient (if conscious). The same communication must take place with those important to the patient and others involved in that patient's care. Discussion should acknowledge any uncertainty about the prognosis, and provide opportunity for any questions to be asked.

It is important that the patient and their loved ones understand why it is thought that death may be imminent but also understand that uncertainties exist at this time. It should also be made clear that if the patient's condition should change, the care and treatment will be reviewed and changed as necessary.

This is an important and complex process. In order to achieve this level of care, healthcare professionals must make time to talk with dying patients and their families.

There are many different approaches to structuring interactions with patients and families identified in the literature. One of these, the Calgary–Cambridge model (Silverman et al. 2013), provides a useful framework for healthcare professionals to structure many of the difficult, sensitive, and complex consultations that are encountered when caring for dying patients (Table 30.4). In the context of care in the last hours or days of life, a consultation could mean any planned, structured interaction with a patient or relative, for example, to assess the understanding of the situation and discuss any concerns, discussing the individualized plan of care or explaining why it is thought that the patient is likely to die.

Discussing the deteriorating condition: The patient is dying

When it is likely that the patient will die within the next few days or hours, clear communication is imperative to allow decisions to be made and actions taken in accordance with the person's needs and wishes (GMC 2010; LACDP 2014). Healthcare professionals must make time to talk regularly with not only the dying patient, but also their family. Issues and concerns must be identified, acknowledged, and responded to sensitively.

The first step in this process is to assess the understanding of patient and family. This discussion needs careful planning and

Table 30.2 Factors that can hinder communication

Inappropriate questioning	This includes the use of: ◆ leading questions which may pre-determine the response ◆ closed questions to elicit qualitative information ◆ asking a number of questions at once ◆ asking 'why' which can feel intimidating and less sensitive than asking 'how', 'what', etc.	'He looks very comfortable, doesn't he?' 'Are you feeling breathless?' rather than 'How is your breathing?' 'How are you coping? Are you comfortable?' 'Have you got any pain?' 'Why didn't you sleep?' as opposed to 'What was it that stopped you sleeping?'
Minimizing problems or concerns	This includes the use of: ◆ normalizing comments that convey lack of understanding or imply the issue is not very important ◆ stock comments used to deflect questions or issues	'Don't worry about the sound of his breathing, it's normal.' 'Everyone dies at some point' (in response to the question 'Am I going to die?')
Inappropriate reassurance	This includes both falsely reassuring patients but also trying to reassure before the full facts of the situation are clear	'We will make sure that you don't have any pain.'
Inappropriate advice or opinion	Imposing views, opinion or solutions rather than exploring the issue	'I would prefer this medication, if it was me in your position.'
Changing the focus of the conversation	This includes changing the focus away from: ◆ emotional issues to more physical issues ◆ from one person to another ◆ from one time frame to another ◆ ignoring cues	'What symptoms did you have?' (in response to 'The doctor told me I was dying. I was devastated, it was such a shock.') 'What did your husband think about about you going to the hospice?' (in response to 'The nurse suggested that it might be a good idea to go into the hospice, but I wasn't sure.') 'I think it would be better to talk to the doctor about that, rather than me.' 'How are you now?' (in response to 'It was dreadful when they told me the results, I was so upset') 'OK, so you're breathing has improved, that's good!' (in response to 'My breathing is better but I'm still feeling down.')

sufficient time. Thought must be given to the location in which such discussion will take place, with the environment being as private as possible and potential interruptions minimized. Additionally, consideration needs to be given to who needs to be involved in the discussion—the patient should be given the opportunity to have a relative with them if they so wish.

The patient and family should be encouraged to describe what they know about what is happening. It is important to establish actual understanding, rather than just what they have been told. Open questions are a helpful way to start this dialogue; some examples of such questions are given in Box 30.2.

The discussion that follows is dependent upon the patients understanding. Generally, understanding can fall into three levels:

◆ Full awareness
◆ Uncertainty
◆ No awareness

Each of these situations needs to be addressed accordingly (see Fig. 30.1).

Full awareness

If the patient or relative is fully aware of the situation, discussion can then focus on thoughts and feelings about their condition, and any specific concerns or worries they may have. An individualized plan of care can be developed, taking into account not only the patient's condition, but also their needs and preferences.

Uncertainty

Some patients or relatives may be aware that the patient's condition is deteriorating and associate this with approaching death but still be very uncertain of this. When encouraged to talk about their thoughts and feelings, they may well seek confirmation from the healthcare professional by asking questions, such as 'Am I dying?' or 'How long do you think I have got left?'

Healthcare professionals can often find such emotive questions difficult to answer because they are worried about upsetting the patient and making them feeling worse about the situation. However, such questions can be addressed in a sensitive and supportive manner (Fig. 30.1).

These questions are usually asked because the patient has been thinking about the situation, and so the first step is to encourage the patient to talk about these thoughts by using such prompts as 'Is this something you have been thinking about? What thoughts have you had about this?' If the patient seems reluctant to talk, or changes the subject this may indicate that they are not yet able to continue with the conversation as they are not ready to hear the answer at this point, and it may prudent not to force the issue but allow the patient to return to the subject when they feel ready.

However, if the patient continues to disclose thoughts relating to the deteriorating condition and the question asked, it suggests that awareness of the situation and the need for confirmation. In this case, the healthcare professional must respond honestly and confirm the patient's thoughts before going on to develop the plan of care.

Table 30.3 Skills that facilitate effective communication

Active listening	This includes: ◆ using silences ◆ acknowledgement ◆ empathy	Allows the opportunity to think about and assimilate what is being said Includes words or sounds that indicate that the person is being heard Demonstrates understanding and motivates the person to expand on what they are saying	'Right, yes, mmmh, oh' 'This situation is very worrying for you'
Picking up cues	This can be done by using: ◆ reflection ◆ open questions ◆ encouragement	Motivates the person to expand on what they are saying	'Please tell me more about how this making you feel'
Clarification	This involves: ◆ avoiding assumptions and ensuring clarity ◆ challenging discrepancies or ambiguity ◆ summarizing	Ensuring the meaning of what is being said is understood Provides feedback to the person, demonstrates that you have been listening and provides the opportunity for information to be corrected, or added to	'Could you tell me exactly what you mean when you say you feel bad' You've told me that you're ok but you've also mentioned that you're feeling a bit frightened'
Information giving	Information should: ◆ include elicitation of what is already known ◆ be tailored to the needs of the individual ◆ be given in manageable chunks ◆ be given in a clear manner that the patient can understand and deal with ◆ include checking of understanding of what has been said	Helps to identify what new information is needed and helps in understanding the level of language appropriate Drawing on the above to promote understanding and recall of information Break information into small sections to allow information to sink in. Seek permission before continuing to the next section Giving a clear indication of what it going to be discussed helps the patient to appreciate the situation and indicate issues that they are not willing/able to talk about. Avoid giving unnecessary detail and using jargon that may cause misunderstanding This aids recall and avoids misunderstanding	'It would be really helpful for me to know what you understand about what is happening' 'So, I think it would be helpful to talk about the results of the investigations, then we can discuss what we do next and also talk about any thoughts, concerns, or questions you might have. How does that sound?' 'We have discussed a lot of things today, what is your understanding now?'

No awareness

In some situations, the patient will be unaware that their deteriorating condition indicates that they may die soon and may need the healthcare professional to provide a sensitive explanation. It is important to ensure that the pace of this discussion is such that allows the patient to understand and absorb the information (see Fig. 30.1).

Table 30.4 The Calgary–Cambridge model

Structuring the conversation	Initiating the conversation	Building the relationship
	Gathering information	
Attending to flow	(Physical examination)	Involving the patient/relative
	Explanation and planning	
	Closure	Facilitating behaviours

Adapted from Jonathon Silverman, Suzanne Kurtz, and Juliet Draper, *Skills for Communicating with Patients*, *Third Edition*, Radcliffe Publishing Ltd, London, UK, Copyright © 2013 from Jonathon Silverman, Suzanne Kurtz, and Juliet Draper, with permission from CRC Press.

It is helpful to prepare the patient by explaining that something important needs to be discussed and ascertaining how much information they want. The next step is to warn the patient that tough information is going to be given. This helps to facilitate the processing of the information (Baile *et al.* 2000) and can be done by using phrases such as 'I'm afraid that I have some bad news to tell you'. Pausing after this and waiting for the patient to respond enables information to be guided by the patient's response. Information should be given in clear and simple terms and broken into small chunks. It is helpful to focus on and address the patient's responses, including non-verbal cues, explore their feelings, and elicit any concerns they may have. Frequent pauses give the opportunity for questions to be asked and also enables the healthcare professional to gauge the need for further information as patients vary in the amount of information they want.

It is not unexpected for patients or relatives become distressed after being told bad news. A strategy for handling emotional responses such as these is shown in Table 30.5. It is beneficial to acknowledge that the person is upset using phrases such as 'I can see this is upsetting for you. It's ok to be upset'. The healthcare professional should encourage the patient to talk about what they are

Box 30.2 Opening a dialogue to assess understanding

- 'What is your understanding of your illness?'
- 'What has been happening over the last few days regarding your illness?'
- 'How do you feel about what has been happening over the last few days?'
- 'What thoughts have you been having about what has been happening to you?'
- 'What sense are you making of what has been happening to you?'

finding upsetting and accept what they are told in an empathic way, for example, 'It sounds as though you are finding … particularly upsetting and I can see this is hard for you'. However, if the patient does not want to discuss what is upsetting them, this decision must be respected. It is vital that healthcare professionals can just be with the patient at this time, as well as discussing the patient's feelings in a caring and empathic manner as there may be nothing that can be changed or will make the patient feel any better. This helps to give patients hope (Koopmeiners *et al.*1997), even in the last few days or hours of life. If issues they find upsetting can be ameliorated, clearly these should be addressed.

Discussing the plan of care

The NHS Constitution (2013) gives people the right to be involved in discussions and decisions about their end-of-life care. Where appropriate, this right includes their family and carers. Many patients are likely to want the opportunity to discuss what is important to them and to be involved in deciding what care they want in the final stages of their life. Some may also want to discuss what they want to happen after they die, such as organ or tissue donation, religious observances, etc. However, not all patients are ready to think about these issues and prefer to leave decisions to a relative or the healthcare professionals. It is necessary to try to find out if there is any specific reason for this as it is important for them to understand options available to them. However, if the patient does not want to engage in such discussions, this should be respected.

The focus for care in the last few hours or days of life must be the person who is dying, and care provided must be individualized according to his or her needs and wishes. If the patient lacks capacity, decisions must be taken in their best interests in accordance with the Mental Capacity Act (2005). Best interest decisions should respect any valid advance decisions and involve anybody named by the patient as someone to be consulted, anyone engaged in caring for the patient, close relatives or friends, anyone with a lasting power of attorney, enduring power of attorney, or anyone appointed by a court for such a purpose, if at all practical and appropriate.

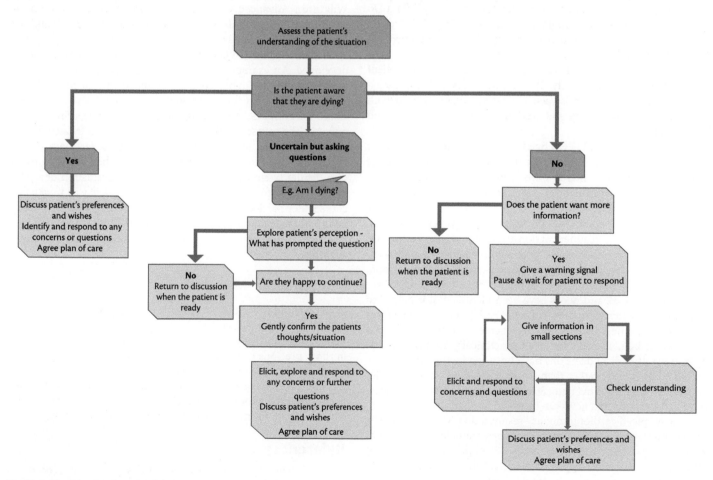

Fig. 30.1 Algorithm for discussing dying.

Table 30.5 Handling emotional responses

1. Recognize the emotion	'I can see that you are upset.'
2. Acknowledge and validate the response	'It's ok to be upset.'
3. Understand the response	'Would it be ok to talk about this? I can appreciate this is a difficult situation, is there anything specific your finding upsetting?'
4. Accept the response	'It sounds as though you are upset because …'
5. Ameliorate response (if appropriate or possible)	Is there anything that the patient would find helpful?

Families have their own needs, which should also be met as far as possible. However, it must be recognized that it is not always possible to meet the needs or wishes of all family members. This should not stop the healthcare professional keeping them involved as much as possible and listening to and acknowledging these needs, as well as explaining the decisions being made.

As the patient's condition deteriorates it may become necessary to consider treatment options such as whether artificial hydration is appropriate, whether medication needs to be discontinued or given parentally, whether a syringe driver is needed, and which interventions are appropriate.

Another important issue for consideration is the need for a Do Not Attempt Cardiopulmonary Resuscitation (DNACPR) order as this may help to ensure that the patient dies in a dignified and peaceful manner.,

All such decisions made need to be communicated to the patient (if possible) and to the family. This can be a very difficult discussion to have as the patient is very ill, relatives are often tired, both physically and emotionally, and everyone may well be anxious and frightened.

The discussion should begin by identifying the needs and wishes of the patient and family and from the perspective that all parties wish to act in the best interest of the patient. Everyone involved in this process must have the information they need, or are asking for in a way they can understand to make informed decisions about the care options. Consideration should be given to the potential benefits, burdens, and risks of treatment or non-treatment. It is very important that healthcare professionals are clear about whether they are seeking consent for specific interventions, consulting about a decision, or explaining about clinical decisions that have been made. Once preferences, wishes, and needs have been identified, it is helpful to structure this conversation by first confirming areas of agreement between all parties, then negotiating agreement about decisions that need to be made (e.g. the need for clinically assisted artificial hydration). If clinical decisions have been made, these need to be explained sensitively rather than being posed as options. Strategies such as those outlined in Figure 30.1 for responding to difficult questions and breaking bad news can be useful in such discussions

For example, if cardiopulmonary resuscitation (CPR) is felt to be futile, rather than asking 'If your Mum's heart should stop suddenly, would you like us to try to start it again?', hoping that the relative would say no, it is more appropriate to use following approach:

Describe the situation, for example, 'Unfortunately, as your Mum is so ill now, if her heart were to stop, it would be almost impossible for us to start it again'. Then pause and wait for the response if the relative is in agreement, continuing with 'and because we don't want to put her through any undue distress,we need to ensure that all the staff involved in her care are aware of the situation so that we can keep her as comfortable as possible and not put her through the trauma of trying to restart her heart'.

It is vital to check the relatives' understanding, and to elicit and address any concerns they may have. If there are any differences in opinion at any stage, these must be discussed openly and if there is a continuing difference of opinion, additional advice, including a second opinion, should be obtained. Healthcare professionals should consider getting support to facilitate communication to reach a consensus, for example from a social worker, advocacy worker, or faith community leader (LACDP 2014).

Training the workforce

Most approaches to teaching communication skills incorporates cognitive, affective, and behavioural components, and is learner-centred with the general aim of promoting greater self-awareness in the health professional.

Training is being delivered in a variety of ways, such as sessions integrated into degree or Master's studies, or short non-accredited courses and workshops using actors as simulated patients. Such courses include the Cheshire and Merseyside Communication Skills Training Programme (http://www.mcpcil.org.uk/learning-and-teaching-division/short-courses-and-study-days.aspx); the Wilkinson Advanced Communication skills training for Senior Healthcare Professionals in Cancer Care (see Chapter 26); and the SAGE & THYME course (see Chapter 24).

In addition to established training, new approaches are being developed. An example of this is a multiprofessional simulation-based care of the dying course developed by the Marie Curie Palliative Care Institute Liverpool and North West Simulation Education Network, which is supported by a virtual learning environment. The course consists of e-learning followed by a study day which focuses on four scenarios simulating the last days of life. Participants have to manage the scenarios and then this is followed by a debrief session where feedback is given. Evaluation of a pilot of this course found that participants thought it was a valuable course; they particularly liked its realism and the multidisciplinary nature of the training (Roberts *et al.* 2015). This suggests that it is an effective addition to the communication skills training currently available.

Conclusion

Each hour and day of life can be made more meaningful and worthwhile through providing the best care possible. This includes communicating effectively with dying people and those close to them in in those precious days and hours at the end of life. Conversations about dying and death are difficult, however with appropriate training and support, together with time and opportunity for reflection, healthcare professionals can develop the required skills and resilience to communicate both effectively and compassionately.

References

Baile W, Buckman R, Lenzia R, Globera G, Bealea E, Kudelkab A (2000). SPIKES—A six-step protocol for delivering bad news: application to the patient with cancer. *Oncologist* **5**, 302–11.

Bloomer MJ, Endacott R, O'Connor M, Cross W (2013). The 'dis-ease' of dying: Challenges in nursing care of the dying in the acute hospital setting. A qualitative observational study. *Palliat Med* **27**, 757–64.

Costantini M, Ottonelli S, Canavacci L, Pellegrini F, Beccaro M (2011). The effectiveness s of the Liverpool care pathway in improving end of life care for dying cancer patients in hospital. A cluster randomised trial. *BMC Health Serv Res* **11**, 13.

DH (2013). *The NHS Constitution*. DH, London, UK.

Ellershaw J, Wilkinson S (2011). *Care of the Dying: A Pathway to Excellence* (2nd edition). Oxford University Press, Oxford, UK.

Emanuel L (2012). Communication between patient and caregiver. In: Cohen J, Deliens L (eds). *A Public Health Perspective on End of Life Care*. Oxford University Press, Oxford, UK.

Houttekier D, Witkamp FE, Van Zuylen L, Van DR, Van DH (2014). Is physician awareness of impending death in hospital related to better communication and medical care? *J Palliat Med* **17**, 1238–43.

Koopmeiners L, Post-White J, Gutnecht S, *et al.* (1997) How healthcare professionals contribute to hope in patients with cancer. *Oncol Nurs Forum* **24**, 1507–13.

Leadership Alliance for the Care of Dying People (2014). *One chance to get it right Improving people's experience of care in the last few days and hours of life*. Leadership Alliance for the Care of Dying People, London, UK.

General Medical Council (2010). *Treatment and Care Towards the End of Life: Good Practice in Decision Making*. GMC, London, UK.

NHS England (2014). *Actions for End of Life Care: 2014-16* Available at: http://www.england.nhs.uk/wp-content/uploads/2014/11/actions-eolc.pdf

National Institute for Health and Clinical Excellence (2011). NICE Quality standard for end of life care for adults. NICE, London, UK.

Parliamentary and Health Service Ombudsman (2015). *Dying Without Dignity. Investigations by the Parliamentary and Health Service Ombudsman into complaints about end of life care* Parliamentary and Health Service Ombudsman, London, UK.

Roberts A, Gambles M, Hellaby M (2015). The future of palliative care: Using a novel approach to prepare the workforce. *BMJ Support Palliat Care* **5**, 107.

Silverman JD, Kurtz SM, Draper J (2013). *Skills for Communicating with Patients*, 3rd edition. Radcliffe Medical Press, Oxford, UK.

Veerbeek L (2008). *Care and Quality of Life in the Dying Phase: The contribution of the Liverpool Care Pathway for the Dying Patient*. Erasmus University Rotterdam, the Netherlands. Available at: http://hdl.handle.net/1765/13429

Vora E, Vora A (2008). A contingency framework for listening to the dying. *Int J Listen* **22**, 59–72.

Wilkinson S (2011). Communication in care of the dying. In: Ellershaw J, Wilkinson S (eds). *Care of the Dying: A Pathway to Excellence*, 2nd edition. Oxford University Press, Oxford, UK.

CHAPTER 31

E-learning as a medium for communication skills training

Hannah Waterhouse, Melanie Burton, and Julia Neal

Introduction to e-learning as a medium for communication skills training

Advanced communication skills training is inherent in the development of a health and social care workforce capable of delivering high-quality palliative care. Traditionally this training has focused on specialist healthcare professionals working in the field of oncology. However, in the Department of Health (DoH) document *The End of Life Care Strategy* (DoH 2008) it was recognized that most people died at the end of a progressive chronic illness. Included as some of the major contributors to this mortality, were cardiorespiratory disease, stroke, dementia, and neurological conditions. The follow on document from the DoH (2009) identified quality markers and measures for end-of-life care and reiterated the need for the appropriate training of both health and social care professionals in order to ensure good quality care.

Education for Health is a charity, dedicated to providing education and training to health professionals working in primary care, with the aim of improving the lives of people living with long-term conditions. In 2002 the charity first gained accreditation from the Open University for its diploma and degree level distance learning modules. Each 30 credit module is designed to be studied over a six-month period. The delivery of the modules was originally a blended learning format incorporating face-to-face contact (usually two study days per 30 credit module) with a distance learning pack. Since 2010 the module learning materials have been converted from the distance learning pack to an e-learning format and students are still able to attend the two study days if they wish. In 2012, the cardiorespiratory palliative care degree level module underwent this process. Prior to conversion of the module, the educational needs of the future healthcare workforce in relation to end-of-life care was considered. It was decided to broaden the curriculum to make it more applicable to the management of people living with and dying from a range of non-malignant conditions.

The module is aimed at any non-palliative care specialist healthcare professionals. In other words—any healthcare professional who participates in the delivery or management of healthcare provided to people with the advanced stages of common life-limiting long-term conditions (respiratory disease, heart failure, long-term neurological conditions, and dementia) who does not work as part of the specialist palliative care team. It focuses on the management of symptoms, when treatments are limited, and a proactive, palliative care approach is required, particularly at the end of life.

Communication skills are a key part of good palliative care and the module explores the effective use of advanced communication skills and consultation skills in order to facilitate holistic patient-centred care. This chapter will elaborate on the process of developing the communication and consultation skills unit into an e-learning format, looking at the advantages and disadvantages, and suggesting solutions in order to maximize the student's learning.

Communication issues in non-malignant life-limiting conditions

Unlike a diagnosis of cancer, a diagnosis of many of the life-limiting long-term conditions (chronic obstructive airways disease (COPD), chronic heart failure (CHF), multiple sclerosis (MS)) do not carry the same perception of poor prognosis with patients, their carers, and society at large (Murray *et al.* 2002; Gardiner *et al.* 2009; Golla *et al.* 2014). Often they are considered long-term conditions to be 'lived with' rather than 'died from', and there is not a realization that they have a prognosis worse than many cancers (Stewart *et al.* 2001).

However, unlike many cancers, the course of the condition is unpredictable, with periods of exacerbation followed by sudden deterioration of symptoms and quality of life, interspersed with more stable symptom control. Though it is known that the conditions (COPD, CHF, many neurological conditions) are likely to result in an early death, there tends to be uncertainty around distinguishing between an exacerbation of the condition and end-stage disease. This leads to problems in prognostication and it is cited by healthcare professionals as a barrier to initiating conversations about prognosis and end-of-life care in this patient group (Barclay *et al.* 2011; De Vleminck *et al.* 2014). It is felt that conversations about end-of-life care during an exacerbation might foster the perception of loss of hope in the person and their carers. However, there is also some evidence that even during periods of symptom stability, a significant minority of patients and carers prefer not to focus on discussions around death and dying (Momen *et al.* 2012). Patients with conditions that have an impact on cognitive function (long-term neurological conditions, dementia, hypoxic conditions) need to be managed with this potential in mind as discussions need to be timed to enable patients to have an influence on their future care even if they lose mental capacity.

The particular communication issues that arise for healthcare professionals are facilitating opportunities for discussion around prognosis with patients and carers, together with the timing of discussions around advance care planning and end-of-life care (Barclay *et al.* 2011; De Vleminck *et al.* 2014).

Technology enhanced learning for healthcare professionals

The Department of Health document, *A Framework for Technology Enhanced Learning* (DoH 2011), emphasizes the need for educators to recognize the place of technology in the provision of education and training in the healthcare sector. There has been a cultural shift in the way society works and interacts, with an increasing reliance on technology both as a means of communication and a source of knowledge. Improvement in areas such as bandwidth, storage, processing speed, and software have enabled the development of ever more responsive, flexible online learning facilities to be made available to a potentially increasing number of healthcare professionals. The NHS England *Five Year Forward View* (2014) recognizes the role technology will have in the future organization of healthcare, and learning and development should focus on supporting staff to adopt innovation, harnessing technology, and embracing change.

E-learning includes a variety of technical applications and educational approaches and can be defined as any learning taking place on a computer, usually attached to a network, either locally or via the internet (DoH 2011). It should not be used as an end in itself, but appropriately integrated into a blended approach to learning, implemented to address specific learning and clinical needs.

With the development of e-learning has come a reconsideration of the theories of learning and the recognition of the need for a new theory to fully recognize the impact and opportunities this new learning environment affords. Connectivism has been described as the 'theory for the digital age' (Siemens 2005). It looks at learning from the perspective that all learners have prior knowledge and future learning evolves from making connections with new information, people, and devices. It also recognizes that knowledge can be housed in appliances and learning can be around knowing when and how to access that information (Siemens 2005). The mix of human and non-human tools for learning is felt to be unique. Connectivism has been criticized for encouraging overreliance on continuous access to information, negating the importance of the learner to learn (Duke *et al.* 2013) or to apply critical thinking (Harper 2006) and the possibility of technological applications giving only the impression of engaging students in more active forms of learning, without necessarily being used to its full potential, has been raised (Greitzer 2002). For most however, connectivism reflects the increasingly student centred approaches being used in education (Kop and Hill 2008). 'Blended learning combines different approaches and technologies, in particular a combination of traditional (e.g. face-to-face instruction) and online teaching approaches and media' (Littlejohn and Pegler 2007). This approach was one Education for Health was keen to adopt, as student feedback indicated they valued the opportunity to attend study days and engage in interactive interprofessional learning with a clinical expert facilitating the day. However, the use of technology also offers learners flexibility with a choice of where, when, and how to engage in learning, affording busy healthcare professionals the opportunity to balance working and personal lives with a commitment to continuing professional development.

The e-learning modules developed by Education for Health provide the learner with a scaffolded approach to learning, with structured online learning materials providing the knowledge base and online activities encouraging learners to explore other resources and construct their knowledge linked to their own practice. This approach to learning is in alignment with how adults learn; that is, they are self-directed, internally motivated, problem centred, use their life experiences to contextualize new information, and need practical application of information gathered (Fidishun 2005).

Education for Health provides academically accredited courses and the approach taken to teaching and learning is based on Chickering and Gamson's (1987) Seven Principles of Good Practice in Undergraduate Education. Features of the virtual learning environment (VLE) that reflect this approach include:

- The use of a reflective diary to encourage active learning. Space is provided on each page of the e-learning resource to allow students to make notes. As well as allowing students to bookmark sections for further consideration, it encourages them to think about what they have learnt in that section, relate it to past experiences and record for future reference.

- The availability of prompt feedback in various activities including assessment tool, drag and drop, and the provision of expert answers in formative exercises.

- Time on task is maximized by providing tools such as external links to further information and evidence.

- Online messaging board that facilitates communication between the clinical lead and administrative team and the students.

- Support materials for students carrying out summative assessment and additional information in the form of an online student guide.

- The provision of a flexible environment where diverse ways of learning are respected meaning that students can learn at a time and pace in a way to suit a variety of learning styles-student centred learning, flexible, own pace, variable timescale, location independent, variable workspace, variety of learning modes and preferences are catered for.

Feedback from students has influenced the continued development of the VLE predominantly around the ease of access and navigation around the site. From the perspective of the e-learning materials, students have identified many of the features described above as advantages of the learning format and have appreciated the flexibility and interactivity of the modules (Box 31.1).

Design of consultation and communication skills unit for delivery via e-learning

When designing the unit on consultation and communication skills within the Non-malignant Palliative Care Module, consideration was given to the aims and objectives of the training (Box 31.1). Students are required to consider the importance of communicating well, develop appropriate attitudes and beliefs, and change their communication behaviours as a consequence of the unit (Fallowfield *et al.* 2003). The five learning outcomes relating to communication skills that the unit aimed to address were: understanding the importance of good communication; identifying the different facilitators and barriers to communication; identifying when these facilitators and barriers are being used/having an impact on a consultation; demonstrate ability to use facilitators and avoid/address barriers to communications; change own clinical practice to incorporate skills into consultations.

It was considered that the e-learning materials would be particularly useful in contributing to the knowledge content of the unit. The benefits of an e-learning environment enabled this information to be presented in a variety of forms that appeal to different learning styles. In addition, certain content lends itself to delivery in particular formats available within the VLE. The communication content of the e-learning unit (Box 31.2) covers a variety of topics that were felt to be key to the appropriate development of skills for the communication challenges for healthcare professionals dealing with people with life-limiting long-term conditions.

Facilitators and barriers to good communication were represented in written form, with a click and reveal format. This enabled the students firstly to assess their knowledge (suggest their own definition of each skill) then, by clicking on each icon, to build on their learning by contextualizing the skills through an audio soundtrack demonstrating the use of each skill (Fig 31.1). This page can be returned to and repeated by the student, enabling consolidation of learning.

Having enabled the students to describe and give examples of the communications skills the training is aiming to enhance, the content moves on to exploring the student's ability to recognize when these skills are being used in practice. Within a three-day advanced communication skills programme (Wilkinson 2008), this is initially done by asking students to identify the skills used in a teaching video simulation. These are expensive to produce but are an invaluable learning tool as, in contrast to 'real time scenarios' they can be revisited and rechecked by the student to facilitate deeper learning. The e-learning environment is an ideal medium for students to review simulated scenarios, and the unit not only has access to videos imbedded into the material (Wilkinson 2007), but also has external links to a variety of web-based scenarios freely available

online. Students are asked to view and review the simulated scenarios and identify how the facilitators and barriers to communication impact on the consultation being observed. Again this contextualizes their learning and deepens their understanding of the particular role of communication skills in palliative and end-of-life care.

Another feature of the VLE which is effectively used in this unit is the reflective diary facility, which enables the student to make online notes attached to each learning page. These can comprise explanatory notes and can link the student's personal experiences with the content of the units, further contextualizing the information, and facilitating deeper learning.

With the plethora of information and papers written on communication within the healthcare context, students find it useful to be guided to some initial publications to help them direct their learning. This is particularly important in assisting the student in differentiating between the different quality of the evidence available. The use of online links to publications facilitates the easy access to papers which have been chosen to enhance the students' depth of learning. These include research papers, but also pivotal government publications and NICE guidelines. Activities are included around some of the articles referred to in order to help students consider their implications on their practice (e.g. McKillop and Petrini 2011). Links can also be used to websites such as *Gold Standards Framework* and *The National Council for Palliative Care*. It is anticipated that students use these documents as a springboard for further learning and exploration of the topic.

Student activities are interspersed throughout the unit content. These address the student learning need at several levels. Some are specifically based on consolidating knowledge (e.g. reviewing videos); however, there are also activities for the student to apply in clinical practice, encouraging them to use some of the skills that they have explored within the unit (Box 31.3).

Working through the content of this unit, in the student's own time, is designed to equip them with the knowledge and recognition of the skills for communication with patients with life-limiting long-term conditions.

Face-to-face contact

Currently the timing of access to the learning materials and the start of the module means that the students are unlikely to have

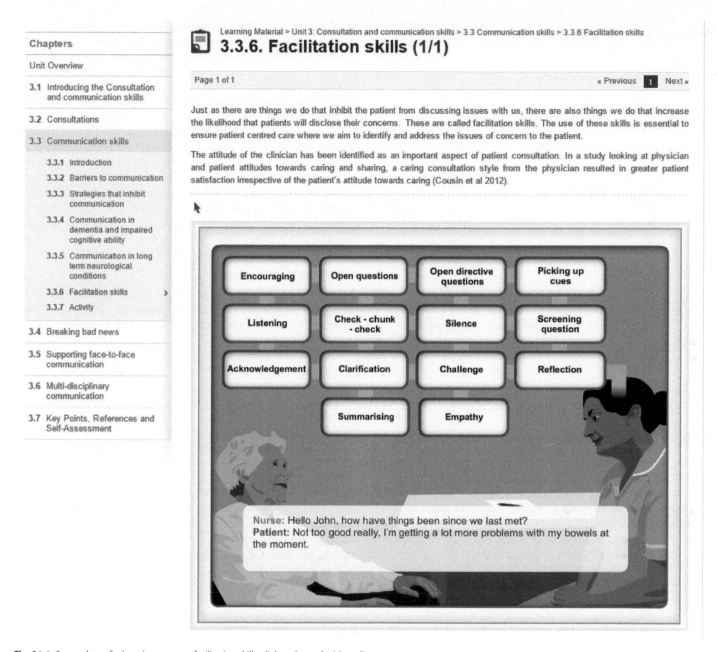

Learning Material > Unit 3: Consultation and communication skills > 3.3 Communication skills > 3.3.6 Facilitation skills

3.3.6. Facilitation skills (1/1)

Page 1 of 1   « Previous   1   Next »

Just as there are things we do that inhibit the patient from discussing issues with us, there are also things we do that increase the likelihood that patients will disclose their concerns. These are called facilitation skills. The use of these skills is essential to ensure patient centred care where we aim to identify and address the issues of concern to the patient.

The attitude of the clinician has been identified as an important aspect of patient consultation. In a study looking at physician and patient attitudes towards caring and sharing, a caring consultation style from the physician resulted in greater patient satisfaction irrespective of the patient's attitude towards caring (Cousin et al 2012).

Fig. 31.1 Screenshot of e-learning page on facilitation skills: click and reveal with audio.
Reproduced with kind permission of Education for Health.

accessed the information prior to the first study day, which is based around communication skills. The study day supports the e-learning in terms of content. It also gives the opportunity for detailed discussion of the skills being acquired and the immediate response of the trainer to student queries. Simulated scenarios are used to help the students recognize communication skills and barriers (see Box 31.4). The face-to-face contact with the trainer and other students facilitates the use of role play to enhance skill acquisition. Contact and discussion with other students is considered an important part of learning communication skills. This contact is currently restricted to the face-to-face sessions, but other methods of incorporating student interaction within the VLE will be discussed in the section on future development of the unit.

Student support

It is recognized that students require support for a variety of different aspects of their course. A VLE guide has been produced to facilitate the students' initiation into the e-learning environment. Frequently asked questions are addressed and a step-by-step guide on how to get started has been developed. A session on using the VLE has also been included in the first study day to ensure all students get the most out of the available learning materials. A team of administrators is also provided who can help guide the student through technical issues around the VLE, as well as administrative issues around the running of the course.

As a blended/primarily distance learning course, there is a limit to the face-to-face contact the student has with both their peers

---

Box 31.3 Consultation and communication skills unit content

1. Introduction
2. Consultations
3. Communication skills
   i. Introduction
   ii. Barriers to communication
   iii. Strategies that inhibit communication
   iv. Communication in dementia and impairment cognitive ability
   v. Communication in long-term neurological conditions
   vi. Facilitation skills
   vii. Activity (video review)
   viii. Breaking bad news: link to article for review
   ix. Activity: contact other member of MDT and set action plan to on how to work more closely together
4. Breaking bad news
5. Support for face-to-face consultations
6. Multidisciplinary team communication
7. Key points and references

Reproduced with kind permission of Education for Health.

---

and the trainer. However, Education for Health has put in place strategies to improve the student experience and reduce the sense of isolation and lack of motivation that can occur when students undertake a distance learning course (Abrami and Bures 1996). The module has a designated clinical lead and the contact details are given to the students at the start of the course and during the study days. The clinical lead can also be contacted through the online environment, as well as via more conventional methods (email and telephone). The support provided is usually in relation to the

---

Box 31.4 Student activity

Choose two patients with long-term life-limiting conditions and explore their perspective on adherence to health advice or treatment. Here are some topics to consider that may help you shape your research:

1. Do you know what they believe about their health?
2. How do they perceive their illness?
3. What threats do they believe that the illness poses to their health?
4. What do they believe about the necessity for treatment?
5. How effective do they perceive the treatment to be?
6. What are their concerns about treatment?

Reproduced with kind permission of Education for Health.

---

development and writing of the summative assignments, but may also be around study skills and the course materials.

There is currently no structured peer-to-peer support, but students within cohorts are often employed by the same healthcare provider and are geographically close to each other. Informal links are fostered in the study days and students often keep in contact with each other via email.

As adult learners working within a healthcare environment, they are also guided to seek out suitable clinical experience to support their learning of advanced communication and consultation skills. This includes recommendations to work with or shadow local clinicians with the appropriate skills and experience. However, in order to be as inclusive as possible, and recognizing that this support is not always available to students, this is neither a structured mentorship nor a compulsory aspect of the course.

Assessment of students

The key aim of the unit on consultation and communication skills training is to improve the skills of the students so that they can be more effective in their clinical practice, and so facilitate better patient outcomes.

In the Cochrane review that investigated the effectiveness of communication skills courses in training healthcare professionals working with people with cancer, the outcome measures were around the students demonstrating that they had used the skills they had learnt from the course and measures of how that impacted on patient satisfaction and anxiety (Moore *et al.* 2013). When designing the summative assignment for the unit, various methods were considered to incorporate the assessment of the students' communication skills, together with ensuring that the assessment was at the appropriate academic level. There is no formal mentorship of the student within their clinical practice, which excludes the use of a form of work based clinical assessment of skills. It was considered whether the assessment could be based around the critical review of a simulated scenario that could be viewed online by the students. However, this would only demonstrate that the student could recognize the skills being used and would not assess whether they had taken the further step to use the skills in practice.

Consequently, a reflective assignment has been developed which asks the student to analyse their personal experience of a patient consultation with someone who has a life-limiting long-term condition. In the assignment they are asked to be specific about the skills they used, and use quotes from the consultation to demonstrate those skills. They are also asked to explore the evidence base around the techniques used and look for alternative communication solutions if the consultation was not effective. This goes some way to establishing the assessment of the students' use of the skills they have developed from studying the unit.

Future developments

A downside of distance learning can be a sense of isolation, which can be perpetuated within the online environment (Wilkinson *et al.* 2004). The importance of human contact cannot be overestimated and the blended approach has proved to be of benefit in providing the opportunity for learners to meet face-to-face to share their learning and practice experience. A future development will be to provide additional opportunities for students to come together; mindful of the difficulties healthcare professionals face in finding time to attend face-to-face days, online communication tools will be used to connect and motivate students (Westbrook 2012). These communication tools will be embedded in the VLE alongside the online learning materials.

Asynchronous online discussion forums afford text-based communication and collaboration, which students can contribute to at any time that suits them rather than needing to be available at an allocated time (synchronous). The asynchronous characteristic of the activity has the added benefit of providing students and tutors with the time and space for reflection before contributing.

The forums can be used to support some of the same types of activity that occur at the face-to-face study days. Online formative activities designed to encourage reflection on practice can be re-designed to encourage students to share these reflections with one another in the forum and to provide peer feedback on others' reflections. However, it is also recognized that the use of forums requires careful introduction. Consideration should be given to the skills required of the tutor to facilitate the online discussion, as well as the support and time required for students to familiarize themselves with this online environment before they are comfortable contributing (Westbrook 2012).

Another development will be to provide students with scheduled synchronous online tutorials. Using a webinar or virtual classroom tool, this will provide students with an opportunity to come together online at the same time. This will enable some of the formative activities to be re-designed to encourage group work. One example would be the streaming of one of the simulated scenario videos, followed by a structured feedback session facilitated by the tutor to encourage critical reflection on the video.

Both of these developments will enhance the student experience by moving beyond the online learner-content interaction and providing the opportunity for increased learner-learner and learner-tutor interaction, the value of which is increasingly being recognized.

Conclusions

Communication skills training is an important part of the education of healthcare professionals who care for people with long-term life-limiting conditions. Training has traditionally been provided by three-day interactive workshops. However, this method of training has disadvantages associated with the release of staff to attend courses and the labour intensive nature of the workshops.

Much of the learning that is required to develop the necessary communication skills lends itself to being delivered in an e-learning format. This facilitates the ability to address students' differing learning styles, as well as allowing flexibility of how, when, and where to engage in learning. Despite this, the importance of face-to-face contact is also recognized. Therefore, a blended approach to learning via a mixture of study days and e-learning is probably the most effective method to adopt. With the continued development of technology, peer-to-peer contact and peer-to-tutor contact will increasingly be feasible within the e-learning environment, which will further enhance the learning experience.

References

Abrami PC, Bures EM (1996). Computer-supported collaborative learning and distance education. *Am J Dist Educ* **10**, 37–42.

Barclay S, Momen N, Case-Upton S, Kuhn I, Smith E (2011). End-of-life care conversations with heart failure patients: a systematic literature review and narrative synthesis. *Br J Gen Pract* **61**, 49–62.

Chickering AW, Gamson ZF (1987). Seven principles for good practice in undergraduate education. *The American Association of Higher Education Bulletin*. Available at: http://www.aahea.org/articles/sevenprinciples1987.htm [Accessed February 17, 2015].

Department of Health (2008). End of Life Care Strategy: promoting high quality care for all adults at the end of life. DoH, London, UK.

Department of Health (2009). The End of Life Care Strategy: quality markers and measures for end of life care. DoH, London, UK.

Department of Health (2011). A Framework for Technology Enhanced Learning. Available at: https://www.dh.gov.uk/publications [Accessed February 15, 2015].

De Vleminck A, Pardon K, Beernaert K, *et al.* (2014). Barriers to advance care planning in cancer, heart failure and dementia patients: A focus group study on general practitioners' views and experiences. *PLoS One* **9**, e845905.

Duke B, Harper G, Johnston M (2013). Connectivism as a digital age learning theory. *The International HETL Review Special Issue*, pp. 4–13.

Fallowfield L, Jenkins V, Farewell V, Solis-Trapala I (2003). Enduring impact of communication skills training: results of a 12-month follow up. *Br J Cancer* **89**, 1445–9.

Fidishun D (Circa 2005). Andragogy and technology: integrating adult learning theory as we teach with technology. Available at: www.lindenwood.edu/education/andragogy/andragogy/2011/Fidishun_2005.pdf [Online].

Gardiner C, Gott M, Small N, *et al.* (2009) Living with advanced chronic obstructive pulmonary disease: patients concerns regarding death and dying. *Palliat Med* **23**, 369–97.

Gold Standards Framework. Available at: www.goldstandardsframework.org.uk [Last accessed February 15, 2015].

Golla H, Galushko M, Pfaff H, *et al.* (2014). Multiple sclerosis and palliative care- perceptions of severely affected multiple sclerosis patients and the health professionals: a qualitative study. *BMC Palliat Care* **13**, doi: 10.1186/1472-684X-13-11.

Greitzer F (2002). *A cognitive approach to student centred e-learning: proceedings of Human Factors and Ergonomics Society*, 46th annual meeting, pp. 2064–8.

Harper J (2006). Transformation in higher education: the inevitable union of alchemy and technology. *Higher Education Policy* **19**, 135–51.

Kop R, Hill A (2008). Connectivism: Learning theory of the future or vestige of the past? *Int Rev Res Open Dist Learn* **9**, 1–13.

Littlejohn A, Pegler C (2007). *Preparing for Blended e-Learning*. Routledge, Abingdon and New York.

McKillop J, Petrini C (2011). Communicating with people with dementia. *Ann Ist Super Sanità* **47**, 333–6.

Momen N, Hadfield P, Kuhn I, Smith E, Barclay S (2012). Discussing an uncertain future: end-of-life care conversations in chronic obstructive pulmonary disease. A systematic review of the literature and narrative synthesis. *Thorax* **67**, 777–80.

Moore PM, Mercado SR, Atrigues MG, Lawrie TA (2013). Communications training for healthcare professionals working with people who have cancer. *Cochrane Collaborative*. Available at: http://onlinelibrary.wiley.com/doi/10.1002/14651858.CD003751.pub3/full [Online].

Murray S, Boyd K, Kendall M (2002). Dying of lung cancer or cardiac failure: prospective qualitative interview study of patients and their carers in the community. *BMJ* **325**, 929–32.

NHS England (2014). Five Year Forward View. Available at: http://www.england.nhs.uk/wp-content/uploads/2014/10/5yfv-web.pdf [Last accessed: February 21, 2015].

Siemens G (2005). Connectivism: A learning theory for a digital age. *Int J Instructional Technol Dist Learn* **21**. Available at: http://itdl.org/Journal/Jan_05/article01.htm [Last accessed: February 16, 2015].

Stewart S, MacIntyre K, Hole DJ, Capewell S, McMurray JVJ (2001). More malignant than cnacer? Five year survival following first admission for heart failure. *Eur J Heart Fail* **3**, 315–22.

The National Council for Palliative Care. Available at: www.ncpc.org.uk [Online].

Westbrook C (2012). Online collaborative learning in health care education. *Eur J Open Dist E-learn* [online]. Available at: http://www.eurodl.org/index.php?article=475 [Last accessed February 19, 2015].

Wilkinson A, Forbes A, Bloomfield J, Fincham Gee C (2004). An exploration of four web-based open and flexible learning modules in post-registration nurse education. *Int J Nurs Studies* **4**, 411–24.

Wilkinson S (2007). Communication skills in heart disease; Training for health care professionals (DVD) British Heart Foundation.

Wilkinson S, Perry R, Blanchard K, *et al.* (2008). Effectiveness of a three-day communication skills course in changing nurses' communication skills with cancer/palliative care patients: a randomised controlled trial. *Palliat Med* **22**, 365–75.

SECTION D

A specialty curriculum for oncology

Section editor: Phyllis N. Butow

CHAPTER 32

Enrolment in clinical trials

Richard F. Brown and Terrance Albrecht

Introduction to clinical trials

Despite recent advances, the five-year survival rates for many cancers remain low, and there is a continued need for research to improve cancer outcomes. Clinical trials are research studies designed to improve cancer prevention, diagnosis, treatment, and survivorship. This research base necessarily involves enrolling cancer patients and others (e.g. family members for genetic linkage studies, healthy community volunteers to serve as matched controls) into clinical trials. Clinical trials demonstrate the efficacy of new therapies and are the mechanism through which research is translated into standards of care. The effectiveness of this translational process is greatly dependent on the number and representativeness of participants enrolled in trials, yet less than 5% of all adult cancer patients enter clinical trials. Despite a nearly 20-year effort by the National Institutes of Health (NIH) to enhance clinical trial accrual, these rates are not improving and even lower participation rates are reported in minority populations, including African Americans (AA).

The goal of this chapter is to outline issues involved in recruitment to clinical trials, to describe the ethical principles underlying informed consent and provide suggested strategies to aid communication between healthcare providers and patients about clinical trials.

Types of cancer clinical trials

According to the US National Cancer Institute, cancer clinical trials are generally categorized into one of the following phases of research: **Phase I trials** are initial studies with humans that usually enrol limited numbers of people. Their main purpose is to evaluate dosage safety and the frequency and method by which new drugs should be administered (e.g. either orally, or by injection into the bloodstream or muscle). **Phase II trials** are designed to further evaluate drug and dosage safety and to begin assessing the impact of drugs in treating specific types of cancer. **Phase III trials** test new drugs, new drug combinations, or new surgical procedures by comparing them against current standards of care. A participant will usually be randomly assigned to the standard (control) group or the new treatment group. Phase III trials often require, by design, large numbers of enrolees and data may be collected at multiple clinical sites across the United States and abroad.

Accrual to clinical trials

Patients are typically offered the opportunity to enrol in a clinical trial as a treatment option by their oncologists. The base rate of accrual at a cancer centre depends on the number of trials available to eligible patients at a given point in time. As noted above, low accrual rates have been reported in the literature and can be attributed to many factors, including the communication process that occurs when oncologists talk to patients (and families or companions, if present) about joining clinical trials (Fallowfield *et al*. 1997; Albrecht *et al*. 2003; Brown *et al*. 2007). Albrecht and colleagues suggest from their data at two cancer centres that low rates may be partially due to the extent to which physicians do and do not explicitly offer trials to their patients, and, in turn, are partially due to the extent to which patients understand that they have, or have not, been offered enrolment in a trial.

The challenge to physicians lies in the multiple and sometimes conflicting communication goals they face in communicating with patients and their families/companions in the outpatient clinic setting. Physicians must establish relational trust in the encounter, provide high quality care, ensure that patients are sufficiently informed to authentically provide 'informed consent' or 'informed refusal' in making treatment choices and when enrolling in clinical trials (accrual rates are actually performance measures for physicians at some institutions). Through this process, physicians are mandated to honour ethical and scientific principles of neutrality and full disclosure to protect their patients. This is a tall order; the full range of ethical concerns associated with clinical trials are described below.

Ethical concerns

Beneficence and the move from paternalism

These two concepts of beneficence and paternalism became linked in the Corpus Hippocraticum, with the doctors of ancient Greece undertaking to:

> 'come for the benefit of the sick, remaining free of all intentional injustice and of all mischief', while at the same time withholding the patient's diagnosis and prognosis and diverting the patient's attention away from the illness and treatment. (Hippocrates 1986) The notion of beneficent paternalism persisted in the medical tradition through to the 18th century when philosopher/physicians attempted to regulate professional conduct by formulating and publishing codes of conduct aimed at establishing medicine in an ethical framework (Lord 1995).

Beneficence remains a fundamental ethical principle guiding medical practice; however, the traditional paternalistic role of the doctor has become increasingly unacceptable in the light of changes in patient attitudes towards medical practice in the late twentieth century. Individuals no longer presume that the doctor knows best and many prefer an approach that involves greater patient involvement in decision-making and respect for individual autonomy. An examination of trends in physician behaviour over four decades suggests that physicians have shifted away from paternalistic styles, characterized by withholding information from patients about their prognosis, diagnosis, and treatment options in the belief that such information would be beyond patients' comprehension and cause them excessive fear, anxiety, and loss of hope, thus worsening patient outcomes (Novack *et al.* 1979). Contemporary medical practitioners acknowledge the importance of providing accurate information to patients. Various reasons have been offered to account for this shift, including an increased fear of litigation among physicians, legal requirements, the publication of guidelines for the disclosure of diagnoses, and an improvement in therapies for cancer patients through technological advancement. Importantly, the law has been vital in promoting the concept of informed consent to standard and experimental treatments.

Active participation in the consultation requires negotiation between the physician and the patient, which is discouraged by the traditional paternalistic model. Patients are now seeking information to enable them to make decisions about treatment options, to understand prognostic issues, and to be clear about treatment side effects.

Autonomy

Autonomy in general refers to the individual's right to self-determination. According to Faden and Beauchamp (Hippocrates 1986), an individual acts autonomously if three conditions are satisfied. That is, the individual acts (a) *intentionally*, (in accordance with a plan or one's inner knowledge), (b) *with understanding*, and (c) *free from controlling influences*.

The extreme view of patient autonomy suggests that patients make their own decisions about treatment, while the doctor adopts a passive role. A more reasonable view argues in favour of the physician who inquires about the patient's preferences and values, thus developing an understanding of the patient as a person before a treatment decision is reached, which maximizes the patient's treatment goals.

In the experimental context, particularly the case of the randomized clinical trial, Kodish *et al.* argue that patient autonomy can only be ensured if the patient is 'free to choose any therapy which they might have received by participating in the RCT and is equally free to choose the randomization alternative' (Kodish *et al.* 1990). Moreover, Kodish *et al.* emphasize the right of a patient to make the choice to refuse any treatment, even when a treatment is proven, as an essential component of autonomous decision-making (Kodish *et al.* 1990).

Equipoise

Individual equipoise

Equipoise is defined as the point at which a rational and well-informed person has no preference between two (or more) available treatment options (Lilford and Jackson 1995). Thus, a physician who is convinced that one treatment option offers a better possibility of benefit for his/her patients than another, cannot ethically recommend random allocation as a means of making a treatment choice. The potential benefit to the patient must be the paramount consideration in the treatment decision. On the other hand, if the

physician is uncertain about the difference in potential benefit between two (or more) treatments offered in a clinical trial, it is ethically acceptable to defer control of the treatment decision to the randomization process.

However, the practical application of equipoise as a means of justifying the selection of randomization as an ethical means of making treatment decisions remains controversial. Equipoise has also been named the 'uncertainty principle', reflecting the prominence of the physician's inability to choose (based on lack of evidence) between comparative treatment benefits. Critics of equipoise question the degree of uncertainty physicians apply to the process of choosing between known and experimental treatments, and recent articles have added qualifiers such as 'reasonably', 'substantially', and 'genuinely' to uncertainty to try and further describe the physician's belief about the treatment options. However, this raises the question of who decides what counts as reasonable or substantial uncertainty. This seems largely left to the conscience of the physician.

Collective equipoise

Clearly, from the physician's perspective, reaching individual equipoise, weighing uncertainty, is a difficult process. However, another level of complexity is added by the introduction of the concept of collective equipoise. According to Chard *et al.* (Chard and Lilford 1998) collective equipoise relates to the uncertainty of a profession as a whole about a particular treatment modality. While individual equipoise may not be achieved (i.e. there is a preference for a particular treatment), this is balanced by others in the profession holding the opposing view (a preference for the alternate treatment). Thus, overall the profession is in collective or clinical equipoise. Clinical equipoise recognizes that it is the community of physicians that establishes best practice standards, and not the individual physician.

Supporters of the primacy of collective equipoise have suggested that in a case where clinical equipoise exists, a randomized controlled trial (RCT) is an ethical imperative to avoid retaining ineffective modes of treatment. In this situation, collective equipoise should override the physician's individual equipoise; thus even if the physician has a preference for a particular treatment (of those being compared), s/he would be expected to recruit patients to the trial (Freedman 1987). Conversely, while clinical equipoise appears to offer a neat solution for the physician committed to research but conflicted by degrees of clinical uncertainty, there are a number of compelling arguments suggesting that equipoise is inherently unethical as a justification for randomized trials. Enkin (Enkin 2000) and others point out that if moral authority is granted to the medical community as a whole, the individual responsibility of physicians is devalued and the needs of the patient for guidance are overlooked (Hellman 1979). While the medical community may be certain about the effectiveness of a treatment at one time, this certainty can change, and the preferences of individuals do count. In addition, clinical equipoise may pose a threat to the transparency of the doctor–patient relationship. If the physician is participating in a trial justified by collective equipoise and does not disclose a particular treatment preference, then a basic ethical tenet has been violated. Again, this poses a dilemma for the physician who must balance his/her clinical opinion, enthusiasm for research, the weight of clinical uncertainty, and the best interests of the patient in order to make an ethical treatment recommendation.

Justice

The ethical principle of justice refers, in the current context, to the application of rules of fairness and equality to the clinical trial process. This can be realized as: (a) fairness in the distribution of the harm and benefit of trial treatments; and (b) equitable criteria for the inclusion of potential trial participants.

In the first instance, it is argued that injustices occur when individuals are advantaged through medical research at the expense of others. Marquis (Marquis 1983) clarifies this point in noting that few would condone a society in which people are sacrificed for their functioning organs in order to benefit the needs of the society in general. However, ethical conflicts can arise and ethical principles surrounding individual versus social benefit need to be recognized and balanced. Trial patients (particularly those participating in Phase I studies) are commonly treated with promising new treatments that are not guaranteed to provide any personal benefit but which may benefit others in the future. The crucial difference between Marquis' example and the plight of trial patients is that trial patients are routinely informed of the uncertainty of treatment benefit prior to trial entry. Thus, gaining informed consent guards against such an ethical problem. However, as the quality of information provision about trials is variable and as patients can misunderstand this information, it is possible to question the validity of the safeguard of informed consent.

Low representation of minority patients in clinical trials results in inequity in access to the latest technologies and cancer treatments, compromises the generalizability and external validity of trial results, and may fail to identify important positive or negative treatment effects among underrepresented populations. Inequitable access to state-of-the-art cancer care contributes to health disparities in cancer mortality and survival.

Informed consent

Informed consent can be defined as an autonomous action taken by a patient giving permission for doctor to undertake a medical plan. Informed consent became part of US law in 1914. However, while this legal instruction instituted patient authorization as part of the treatment process, it did not define the nature of the information that should be provided to the patient about their illness or possible treatments.

Gert et al. (Gert et al. 1997) provide a considered view of the bioethics of the consent process (both for clinical trials and standard treatments). They differentiate between the moral rules governing this situation that are more or less compulsory and governable by law (including provision of adequate information, lack of coercion, and assessment of patients' competence to make a choice) and moral ideals, to which doctors aspire but cannot necessarily fulfil in all instances; for example, providing information about alternative treatments in a way which does not overemphasize the attractiveness of one, or belittle another. The consent process involves the doctor presenting information to the patient about their illness and the options for treatment, and making an appraisal about the patient's response to the information, including the degree to which the patient understands the information provided (Gert et al. 1997). The rationale underlying the doctrine of informed consent is to protect patient autonomy and to ensure that patients have an active role in making barriers to recruitment.

Physician barriers

Gaining informed consent to clinical trials is problematic for doctors. Many doctors experience problems initiating clinical trial discussions and find the dual roles of caring physician and experimenter difficult to resolve (Fallowfield 1995). Prospective studies have reported that 70–80% of non-accrual is attributable to the doctor. Doctors' reasons for not accruing patients to trials include concerns over (a) damaging the doctor–patient relationship; (b) acknowledging the uncertainty of treatment benefits; and (c) practical issues such as rigid protocol designs, patient inconvenience, and extra work for physician. These results suggest that efforts to improve doctors' participation in clinical trials need to address communication difficulties experienced by doctors when recruiting patients to trials. Communication difficulties with patients are evident in three key areas: (i) oncologists omit critical information or the information is poorly presented leading to patient misunderstanding and poor recall of information; (ii) oncologists underestimate their patients' information needs and overestimate the amount of information they give; and (iii) in spite of evidence-based calls to routinely involve patients in decision-making, patients are often not involved and their decision-making preferences are not being met. These difficulties are compounded with minority patients, as physicians use less supportive and positive talk, and for example, are less patient-focused with African American patients than white patients. Moreover, AA patients have been shown to be less active communicators than white patients (Street et al. 2005). Such racial disparities in physician–patient communication could lead to less exchange of information and less patient involvement, in turn leading to less informed decisions (Gordon et al. 2006) and lower trust in physicians.

Patient barriers

Many eligible patients who are invited to participate in a trial, decline (though estimates widely vary from 23–50%). Reasons for trial refusal by eligible patients include concerns regarding experimentation, and uncertainty and loss of control over treatment decisions. Many patients and the general community do not understand the role of randomization in avoiding bias in treatment selection (Ellis et al. 1999). Other barriers have been identified such as race, gender, and lack of knowledge of the requirements of trial participation, and the possibility of receiving a placebo. Studies suggest that racial differences in patient barriers to clinical trial participation are due in part to non-clinical factors related to: (a) a paucity of culturally relevant information that is evident in minority patients' lack of trial knowledge and understanding of important trial procedures such as dose escalation and randomization; (b) higher mistrust of the research enterprise and the medical system among AA patients, which is reflected in concerns regarding experimentation and loss of control over treatment decisions; (c) factors related to the patient–physician relationship; and (d) family pressures. Patients who actively participate in their healthcare by asking questions and involving themselves in making treatment decisions have improved outcomes such as lower anxiety and increased perceived control over their disease as compared to patients who are passive. Cancer patients vary in their ability to be active communicators. Previous studies have found that physicians are more informative, accommodative, and supportive with more actively communicating patients and that, with appropriate support, the participatory level of patients can be increased.

Improving the recruitment process of patients to clinical trials

Physician communication

Patients' decisions about enrolling in trials are affected by *what* physicians tell them about the clinical trial and *how* physicians tell them the information. Content messages are what physicians tell patients about the trial. These include legally proscribed aspects of the study protocol (essentially the information on the consent document), and the potential adverse effects (side effects) that the patient is likely to experience from the drug therapies. Albrecht and colleagues have added three additional types of content messages that they have found important for patient understanding of clinical trials. These include messages of reassurance and support, specifically regarding the patient's experience of each potential side effect, reassurance and support regarding the patient's decision to enrol in the clinical trial (whether s/he decides for or against enrolment) and discussion regarding the benefits and drawbacks of clinical trial participation.

Finally, perhaps the most important content message from the physician is to recommend to a patient that s/he enrol in a trial. Such recommendations do influence patients' decisions (Eggly *et al.* 2008). In observing clinical offers, Eggly and colleagues have shown that most physicians do recommend the trials that they are offering to their patients. Indeed, in contrast to the equipoise principle, many do so in a more directive, not general manner, such as saying, 'I recommend this trial for you', as opposed to saying 'I recommend this trial'.

The patient's perspective: Improving the decision process

From the patient's perspective, the decision of whether to enrol in a clinical trial is complicated by the reasons used to arrive at the conclusion and the affective and cognitive aspects of the decision as it is made and afterwards. Reasons for the decision made vary widely and include personal factors (perceived quality of life, length of survival), family members, and significant others' opinions, perceptions of the potential side effects, and perceptions of the financial costs involved in enrolling in the trial. Physician communication behaviours also factor in to patients' judgements, especially how well they seemed to listen and answer questions, how the patient perceived the way the physician interacted with his/her family or companions, and how well explanations were given and the level of empathic support provided.

Cognitive and affective aspects of the decision involve the degree to which the patient is confident in the decision s/he is making, the extent of agreement shared with the physician and family/companions regarding the nature of the decision, and the level of positive relational effect perceived with the physician, and the family/companion as they face the decision and the treatment process together (Albrecht *et al.* 2008).

Communication about clinical trials

The development of communication skills training has been suggested as a promising way forward to aid clinicians in the difficult task of clinical trial recruitment. Brown *et al.* in a series of articles have developed and pilot tested an informed consent communication skills workshop. The results of this programme of research revealed four areas where communication training could aid physician–patient communication (Brown *et al.* 2004*b*, c; Brown *et al.* 2007). These included: (a) shared decision-making strategies; (b) the sequence of moves in the consultation; (c) the type and clarity of the information provided; and (d) disclosure of controversial information and coercion. These themes reflect the clinical judgement and theoretical perspectives of linguists, psycho-oncologists, ethicists, and oncologists involved in the analysis.

Shared decision-making strategies

Participation in treatment decision-making, at the patient's preferred level of involvement, was identified as an essential component of seeking informed consent to the clinical trial. Fourteen strategies contributing to a collaborative decision-making framework were identified. They are summarized in Box 32.1.

Importantly, language that portrays the patient as an active agent in the process of deciding about and enacting their own healthcare encourages the sense of an autonomous self among patients. Grades of agency occur; the most active participant is portrayed as the doer, decider. The least active participant is portrayed as the person or object 'done to' (the one who is treated, told, or organized).

Sequence of moves in the consultation

The analysis led to an understanding of the importance of sequence in the interaction. Thus, the consultation data were categorized into a series of phases and an ideal sequence of these phases was identified. This model was developed to promote patient understanding of information, to ensure equal weight was given to the discussion

---

Box 32.1 Strategies for doctors to encourage collaborative decision-making

- Introduce joint decision-making process.
- Use language which realizes and reflects patient autonomy.
- Check preferred decision-making style (involved or not).
- Check information preferences of patient.
- Invite questions and comments.
- Check medical knowledge of patient.
- Check patient understanding.
- Explicitly offer choice of treatment.
- Acknowledge uncertainty of treatment benefits.
- Declare professional recommendation.
- Provide opportunity for amplification of patient voice.
- Provide time and opportunity to discuss patient concerns in detail.
- Offer decision delay.
- Offer ongoing decision support/answers to future questions.

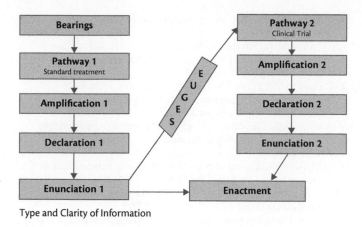

Type and Clarity of Information

Fig. 32.1 The recommended sequence of moves (Brown *et al.* 2004*a*).
Reprinted from *Social Science and Medicine*, Volume 58, Issue 2, R.F Brown *et al*, 'Developing ethical strategies to assist oncologists in seeking informed consent to cancer clinical trials', pp. 379–390, Copyright © 2004 Elsevier Science Ltd, permission from Elsevier, http://www.sciencedirect.com/science/journal/02779536

of standard and experimental treatments, and to avoid potential coercion (see Fig. 32.1).

Within Pathways 1 and 2, a number of facts need to be communicated in order for the patients to give ethical informed consent. However, merely including these facts will not necessarily ensure understanding. The fullness and clarity of the explanation needs also to be considered.

Disclosure and coercion

Issues that could be covered include: (a) that in many instances the participating doctors may be investigators on the trial and thus have a potential conflict or duality of interest; (b) the accessibility of trial treatments after the trial has ceased; (c) the availability of other potentially suitable trials.

Words used by doctors, who may be quite unaware of their ramifications, may encourage or perhaps coerce patients into participating in clinical trials. These are outlined next.

Doctor preferences

If the doctor does not explicitly state their views on clinical trial participation, while acknowledging patient choice, patients may feel unspoken pressure to participate. Preferences may be covertly suggested in many ways; for example, by spending more time talking about the trial treatment versus standard treatment.

Terms

Doctors commonly use the term 'you are eligible for this trial'. This phrase, however, can imply that the patient is 'lucky' to have been selected, or should be hopeful that their disease status allows them to participate in the trial. We suggest using the phrase 'the trial is suitable for you'.

Appealing to altruism

A common motivation for patients to enter clinical trials is a sense of making a contribution to medical knowledge which will benefit others, or altruism. Finding the balance between recognizing and appreciating patient altruism and using it in a coercive fashion can be difficult. Once again, the terms used can make a difference. Thus the use of terms such as '*You* can benefit future generations'

is perhaps more coercive than 'This will help us find the answer to this question'.

Framing

Coercion may also occur when the potential value of a clinical trial treatment is presented with a positive frame versus negative framing for the standard treatment (or vice versa). Research suggests that some patients prefer positively framed information ('you have a 70% chance of cure') as this encourages a positive outlook, while others prefer negatively framed information ('you have a 30% chance of the cancer coming back') as this emphasizes the importance of additional treatment.

Evaluation data and modification to programme for MSKCC

A modified version of this physician-focused communication skills training programme, based on the COMSKIL model (Brown and Bylund 2008) was implemented and evaluated as part of a larger programme of communication skills training at Memorial Sloan Kettering Cancer Center. At the completion of the communication skills training module, participants were asked to complete an evaluation. They were asked to rate aspects of their own sense of confidence and self-efficacy in dealing with the communication challenge targeted by the module. Participants were presented with a list of question and asked to indicated their response on a Likert scale from 1–5 with anchors at 1—'Strongly disagree' to 5—'Strongly agree'.

We compared scores on the self-evaluation data pre- and post-training using paired sample *t* tests. Participants' confidence in making shared treatment decisions, including discussing of a clinical trial, increased significantly pre- and post-training. Three other post-training questions about self-efficacy and confidence all received average scores above four, indicating that the participants strongly agreed that they would use newly acquired skills, provide better care after training, and had been prompted to critically evaluate their own communication skills (Table 32.1).

Table 32.1 Course evaluation data: Mean rating for shared treatment decision-making module

Course evaluation items	Mean (sd)
	N = 101
Before this workshop I felt confident making shared treatment decisions	3.17 (.86)
Now that I have attended the workshop I feel confident to make shared treatment decisions	4.04 (.66) (*p* < .05)
I feel confident that I will use all the skills that I learned today	4.41 (.55)
The skills I learned today will allow me to provided better patient care	4.33 (.62)
The workshop prompted me to critically evaluate my own communication skills	4.39 (.62)

Adapted from Brown RF *et al.*, Developing patient—centered communication skills training for oncologists: Describing the content and efficacy of training, *Communication Education Special Edition*, Volume 59, Issue 3, pp. 236–249, Copyright © 2010, with permission of the authors.

Summary and conclusions

Seeking informed consent to cancer clinical trials presents a significant communication challenge for oncologists and patients. Improving this communication may lead to increased accrual to clinical trials. Strategies aimed to aid this communication focus on four areas designed to ensure a transparent dialogue, underpinned by ethical informed consent and free from coercion.

The authors continue to pursue research agendas that explore gaps in communication about clinical trials and factors that affect decision-making about clinical trials. In addition, the authors are evaluating the utility of interventions that aid both physicians and patients in communicating about trials.

References

Albrecht TL, Eggly SS, Gleason ME, *et al.* (2008). Influence of clinical communication on patients' decision making on participation in clinical trials. *J Clin Oncol* **26**, 2666–73.

Albrecht TL, Penner LA, Ruckdeschel JC, *et al.* (2003). Understanding patient decisions about clinical trials and the associated communication processes; a preliminary report. *J Cancer Educ* **18**, 210–14.

Brown RF, Butow PN, Boyle F, Tattersall MH (2007). Seeking informed consent to cancer clinical trials: evaluating the efficacy of communication skills training. *Psychooncology* **16**, 507–16.

Brown RF, Butow PN, Butt DG, Moore AR, Tattersall MH (2004*a*). Developing ethical strategies to assist oncologist in seeking informed consent to cancer clinical trials. *Soc Sci Med* **58**, 379–90.

Brown RF, Butow PN, Butt DG, Moore AR, Tattersall MH (2004*b*). Developing ethical strategies to assist oncologists in seeking informed consent to cancer clinical trials. *Soc Sci Med* **58**, 379–90.

Brown RF, Butow PN, Ellis P, Boyle F, Tattersall MH (2004*c*). Seeking informed consent to cancer clinical trials: describing current practice. *Soc Sci Med* **58**, 2445–57.

Brown RF, Bylund CL (2008). Communication skills training: describing a new conceptual model. *Acad Med* **83**, 37–44.

Chard JA, Lilford RJ (1998). The use of equipoise in clinical trials. *Soc Sci Med* **47**, 891–8.

Eggly S, Albrecht TL, Harper FW, Foster T, Franks MM, Ruckdeschel JC (2008). Oncologists' recommendations of clinical trial participation to patients. *Patient Educ Couns* **70**, 143–8.

Ellis P, Dowsett SM, Butow PN, Tattersall MH (1999). Attitudes to randomised clinical trials among outpatients attending a medical oncology clinic. *Health Expect* **2**, 33–43.

Enkin MW (2000). Clinical equipoise and not the uncertainty principle is the moral underpinning of the randomised controlled trial. *BMJ* **321**, 756–8.

Fallowfield L (1995). Can we improve the professional personal fulfilment of doctors in cancer medicine. *Br J Cancer* **71**, 1132–3.

Fallowfield L, Ratcliffe D, Souhami R (1997). Clinicians' attitudes to clinical trials of cancer therapy. *Eur J Cancer* **33**, 2221–9.

Freedman B (1987). Equipoise and the ethics of clinical research. *N Eng J Med* **317**, 141–5.

Gert B, Culver CM, Clouser KD (1997). *Bioethics: A Return to Fundamentals.* Oxford University Press, New York, NY.

Gordon HS, Street RL Jr, Sharf BF, Souchek J (2006). Racial differences in doctors' information-giving and patients' participation. *Cancer* **107**, 1313–20.

Hellman S (1979). Editorial: randomised clinical trials and the doctor—patient relationship. An ethical dilemma. *Cancer Clin Trials* **2**, 189–93.

Hippocrates (1986). *A History and Theory of Informed Consent*, Oxford University Press, New York, NY.

Kodish M, Lantos JD, Siegler M (1990). Ethics of randomised clinical trials. *Cancer* **65**, 2400–5.

Lilford RJ, Jackson J (1995). Equipoise and the ethics of randomisation. *J R Soc Med* **88**, 552–9.

Lord RS (1995). Informed consent in Australia. *Aust N Z J Surg* **65**, 224–8.

Marquis D (1983). Leaving therapy to chance. *Hastings Cent Rep* **13**, 40–7.

Novack DH, Plumer R, Smith RL, Ochitill H, Morrow GR, Bennett JM (1979). Changes in physician attitudes towards telling the cancer patient. *J Am Med Assoc* **241**, 897–900.

Street RL, Gordon HS, Ward MM, Krupat E, Kravitz RL (2005). Patient participation in medical consultations: why some patients are more involved than others. *Med Care* **43**, 960–9.

CHAPTER 33

Working as a multidisciplinary team

Jane Turner

What is a multidisciplinary team?

A multidisciplinary team has been defined as: 'A collection of individuals who are interdependent in their tasks, who share responsibility for outcomes, who see themselves and are seen by others as an intact social entity embedded in one or more larger social systems' (Cohen and Bailey 1997).

The importance of multidisciplinary teams

As cancer treatment becomes increasingly complex, it is obvious that no one individual can maintain knowledge and skills across all domains of care. This means that a collaborative approach is required to ensure that expertise is available to assist in decision-making and planning of treatment, which is evidence-based and focused on the needs of the individual patient, taking into account their social and family context. Team composition should be broad in focus, extending beyond the obvious medical and nursing members. For example, interventions by speech pathologists and dieticians can reduce the risk of problems such as aspiration for patients treated for head and neck cancer. Similarly, patients with lymphoedema or difficulties with mobility require assessment and treatment by physiotherapists, or occupational therapists. As survivorship emerges as an important area of clinical focus, rehabilitation specialists and exercise physiologists may also be team members.

Benefits of a multidisciplinary approach

An increasing body of evidence is demonstrating the benefits of care delivered by multidisciplinary teams including: decreased unplanned admissions to hospital; improved access to healthcare; enhanced continuity of care; and improved clinical outcomes (Mickan 2005). Other advantages include:

Survival

A recent review by Hong *et al.* (2010) reported results from 12 studies demonstrating a significant association between multidisciplinary care and survival.

Support and information for patients

The National Breast Cancer Centre specialist nurse project team (2003) evaluated the impact of providing specialist breast care nurses for women with breast cancer. The report revealed that women valued the support provided by the nurses. Women who received care from breast care nurses were also more likely to receive hospital fact sheets, which may in turn reduce distress and anxiety.

Evidence-based treatment

Optimal evidence-based treatment is more likely to be implemented in a multidisciplinary context in which knowledge is shared. A survey of over 2,000 cancer health professionals in the United Kingdom found that over 90% of respondents believed that multidisciplinary care was associated with improved clinical decision-making and evidence-based treatment, leading to improved quality of treatment (Taylor and Ramirez 2009).

Clinical trials

The National Breast Cancer Centre's specialist nurse project (2003) reported that women with breast cancer are more likely to participate in clinical trials when a breast care nurse was part of the team. It has also been noted that patients attending a multidisciplinary clinic for treatment of lung cancer have higher rates of recruitment into trials than those not treated by multidisciplinary teams (Magee *et al.* 2001).

Cost effectiveness

Inclusion of members with psychosocial expertise into a multidisciplinary team has cost implications. A meta-analysis found that 90% of studies reported a decrease in medical service utilization following a psychological intervention (Chiles *et al.* 1999).

Impact on health professionals

Oncologists face inherently difficult tasks ranging from breaking bad news, discussing transition from curative to palliative goals of treatment, to end-of-life decision-making. Being able to draw on the expertise and support of team members trained in communication skills and psychosocial care is likely to be of considerable assistance for health professionals facing such challenging clinical problems, leading to reduced distress for patients and increased professional satisfaction.

Characteristics of well-functioning teams

According to Mickan and Rodger (2005), the key features of effective teams are:

♦ Clear purpose—relevant to patients and linked to the organization;

- Goals—need for members to agree and be able to clearly describe these in measurable terms;
- Good leadership—leaders need to set and maintain structure, manage conflict, coordinate tasks, and provide feedback;
- Regular patterns of communication, clear well-written records;
- Cohesion—sense of camaraderie and involvement generated by working together over time;
- Mutual respect—open to talents and beliefs of each person in addition to their professional contribution.

Evidence about communication in teams

Evaluation of team communication is complex because communication is not confined to face-to-face meetings. Informal 'corridor discussions' are frequent and may not be recorded, despite the fact that the discussion has led to action (Rowlands and Callen 2013).

Interprofessional communication

A recent survey of psychologists working in cancer settings revealed that more than 40% used verbal communication or emails to give feedback to the referrer about initial assessment (Thewes *et al.* 2014). While provision of feedback verbally and by email has the benefit of being quick, there is the drawback that relevant details are confined to an individual and may not be shared with the rest of the team. Of more concern is the fact that 22% of psychologists who participated in this survey did not routinely provide feedback to the referrer. This may be because of concerns about confidentiality and disclosure of sensitive information, for example about past trauma or substance abuse. However, in the absence of feedback or advice the rates of referral may decline, meaning that patients with psychosocial concerns do not receive the treatment they require.

The development of electronic records systems ideally means that all members of a treatment team can access information and update clinical notes in 'real time'. As with any technology there are risks of systems failures, 'downtime' for technical upgrades, and problems with data exchange between services which employ different software and security measures.

Clarity of role

Position descriptions are often written to satisfy institutional requirements and over time practitioners commonly develop new skills and expertise which may variously expand on or deviate considerably from their original role description. Some changes may be subtle. Others may be more major—such as moving to confine clinical practice to a particular tumour stream or disease stage. There is a risk that these changes are not explicitly conveyed to all members of the multidisciplinary team. Lack of awareness of the role and activities of other team members can lead to duplication of effort and inefficient use of resources. It also poses the risk that patients who are already anxious will perceive inconsistencies or differences in emphasis in information that is provided.

Misperceptions and lack of clarity of role can also influence referral patterns. For example, palliative care may be perceived as providing end-of-life care only (Rowlands and Callen 2013) that potentially denies patients referral for symptom control, which may have a considerable impact on quality of life.

Impact of poor communication

Poor communication within multidisciplinary teams can impact on patients and their families, as well as staff members.

Adverse patient outcomes

A surgical review of 444 malpractice claims from four liability insurers in the United States evaluated 258 errors which led to patient injury. A single communication breakdown was cited in 72% of cases, in 23% of cases there were two communication breakdowns, and in 5% there were three or more (Greenberg *et al.* 2007).

The National Confidential Enquiry into Patient Outcome and Death (2008) reported on the care of patients who had died within 30 days of receiving systemic anti-cancer therapy. The report cited multiple instances of communication failures including: failure to clarify which clinician was ordering investigations; poor documentation of risks and benefits of treatment including curative or palliative aims of treatment; poor documentation of toxicity related to previous cycles of treatment; limited communication and access to clinical records across clinical services; use of electronic records which could not be accessed by all members of the treatment team, and poor communication with community services, including general practitioners.

Impact on family and carers

In the absence of a well-functioning team, patients and family members bear the burden of repeatedly informing different health practitioners about changes in treatment plans and medication. This can lead to misunderstandings and errors, erode patient confidence, and engender anxiety about the quality of care.

Staff stress

This is a significant issue. For example, more than one-third of nurses in an Australian survey reported dissatisfaction with the degree to which they felt they were part of a team (Barrett and Yates 2002). In the case of patients with advanced cancer, oncology nurses report that they find it especially stressful if the physician does not communicate with them about a patient's poor prognosis or clarify the goals of treatment, as this limits their ability to support the patient (Turner *et al.* 2007).

What underpins communication difficulties?

The culture

There is increasing pressure and cost associated with gaining entry into medical school and completing training. The process of necessity rewards those who are highly disciplined and focused, and possibly inward-looking. While being autonomous and self-reliant are advantages in the competitive world of medical education, these characteristics do not necessarily lend themselves to being open and collaborative within a multidisciplinary team. Existing hierarchies in health mean that senior medical practitioners may dominate discussion, making it difficult for less experienced team members to make comments in team meetings (Rowlands and Callen 2013). Interns are also likely to feel apprehensive about raising concerns because they perceive that they could be unfavourably evaluated by consultants. However, education may not be solely to blame for stereotyped attitudes about status and roles. Formal assessment of healthcare students reveals that even on entry into their education they have defined attitudes towards different health professional groups; for example, perceiving some as more caring than others (Lindqvist *et al.* 2005).

Training

Differences in emphasis and style of training can lead to difficulties in having one's concerns about patients understood by another professional group. Terminology can also cause confusion. For example, a newly graduated psychologist who is told by a distressed patient that their pathology report is 'positive' may interpret this as being a favourable result, and fail to appreciate that in fact it is an adverse result.

The organization

While it is accepted that hospitals will often be large centres comprised of specialist departments, the ways in which these can be accessed and the preferred method of communication is often poorly described or not articulated at all. If an intern is concerned that a patient might be depressed but feels uncertain about how to access the social worker or other psychosocial professional, there is real potential for the patient's needs to remain unmet. The ethos of the organization can also be affected by budgetary restraints. Focus on the 'bottom line' rather than quality care inevitably affects the ability of a team to function.

Concerns about time

Improvements in survival have occurred because of prevention and early detection, as well as advances in treatment. However, many of these treatments are complex to deliver and potentially toxic with the risk of error. Hence development of protocols for treatment and quality control are essential; however, adherence to protocols and completion of necessary documentation can be time-consuming. When staff feel under pressure, making allowances for 'extra' commitments, such as attendance at a team meeting, may seem very difficult or 'not worth it'.

Stigma and misperceptions

An inclusive approach to multidisciplinary treatment is not always embraced. The status of some members of the team is reflected in pejorative terms used in the past, and even now psychiatry and psychology can attract critical comments disguised as humour. If psychosocial care is considered by health professionals to be based on 'soft science' rather than research-derived evidence, this will inevitably affect communication within the team and potentially reduce referrals of patients who are anxious or depressed.

Geographic isolation

Initial assessment and development of a management plan for many cancers such as lung cancer typically occurs at a tertiary referral centre, with later treatment being delivered in a location close to the patient's home, family, and supports. However, this necessitates the development of a referral network by the local health professional, who may encounter logistic difficulties in obtaining information from different health services.

Personality style and personal issues relating to team members

Team members inevitably will have different personality styles, some being more amenable to discussion than others. Members of a poorly functioning team may unconsciously scapegoat a team member who is different by virtue of training and experience, sex, or race. This can lead to escalating tension, the development of factions, and further deterioration in team function. Of particular concern is evidence that professionals working in oncology report high levels of stress. The individual who feels burdened by their role may not only withdraw from the patient, but may be a less assertive and communicative member of the multidisciplinary team.

General problems with meetings

Direct application of business models for meetings is not necessarily appropriate to healthcare settings; nevertheless, some themes are generic. These include the need to have an agenda, a time frame for the meeting, a defined method of arriving at decisions and implementing these, and facilities adequate in size with access to appropriate technology (Taylor and Ramirez 2009). Failure to address these practical issues can create an atmosphere of frustration, leading to devaluation of the role of the multidisciplinary team.

Improving communication in multidisciplinary teams

Interventions to improve communication are likely to require a multifaceted approach. It is naïve to assume that historical boundaries and hierarchical structures will magically dissipate on formation of a multidisciplinary team, and these issues are likely to require specific attention (Fleissig *et al.* 2006). It is also critical to recognize that a team is not a static entity. Membership is typically fluid, and increasingly complex cancer treatments will mean an expanding diversity of team members—all of whom have interconnected roles, relationships, and interaction with the clinical environment (Varpio *et al.* 2008).

The following recommendations are based on the best-available evidence, and grounded in clinical experience in an oncology setting:

Communication skills training

Amos *et al.* (2005) have demonstrated that participation in workshops involving role plays designed to enhance awareness of the roles of other members of the team leads to self-reports of increased listening. This study also reported a trend of decreased staff turnover.

Hall *et al.* (2007) designed an intervention in a palliative care unit to promote enhanced clinical roles of nurses, combined with a more explicit pattern of communication with the physician. The intervention was associated with greater nurse confidence, and physicians also reported high satisfaction. During the pilot study, a number of key themes emerged, including the need to address potential blurring or overlap of roles, and strategies to resolve conflict. The study further highlighted the importance of team cohesion and the value of professional confidence and leadership.

Staff orientation and role clarification

Although most institutions have mission statements about the importance of care of patients, few acknowledge the status of staff and their interrelationships. A directory of staff expertise to supplement existing service directories can provide accurate information about skills, referral processes, and roles. All team members need to be aware of the roles and abilities of other team members and have a clearly defined process to facilitate contact, especially in urgent cases. Being unable to contact emergency supports or critical information can lead to adverse outcomes including mortality (National Confidential Enquiry into Patient Outcome and Death 2008).

Use of structured proforma

Structured communication tools show promise in improving clarity of interprofessional communication by telephone. One such tool is ISBAR:

Identify—the caller should identify themselves by name, state their professional position, location, and role, as well as clearly state the patient's name, age, sex, and location

Situation—give the reason for contacting the person including the degree of urgency

Background—describe the clinical context, current problem, test results, current management including medications

Assessment—statement of what the caller thinks is happening clinically (e.g. 'The patient is pale and hypotensive. I think that he may be bleeding following the liver biopsy')

Request—what the person being called is asked to do (e.g. 'I am not able to manage this situation and need urgent assistance. Can you come to help?')

> Reproduced from *Quality and Safety in Health Care*, Marshall S, Harrison J, and Flanagan B, 'The teaching of a structured tool improves the clarity and content of interprofessional clinical communication', Volume 18, Issue 2, pp. 137–140, Copyright © 2009 BMJ Publishing Group Ltd and The Health Foundation, with permission from BMJ Publishing Group Ltd.

Medical students trained in this technique demonstrated superior skills to those not trained; however, assessment was in close proximity to training and it is not clear that improvements would be sustained over time (Marshall *et al.* 2009).

Similarly, a structured template may be helpful in written communication, for example to guide allied health professionals and psychologists to provide information to referring practitioners (Thewes *et al.* 2014).

Use of technology

Case conferencing by videolink is acceptable to team members, and has the potential to overcome geographic impediments to effective team communication (Taylor and Ramirez 2009).

Simulated patients are commonly used in medical education, and there is potential to expand and modify these technologies, to give students in different institutions the opportunity to assume different professional roles and communicate with colleagues about a simulated patient. Sijstermans *et al.* (2007) have reported results of a study using simulation in which the technology helped students learn to define the domains of different specialties and improve their interprofessional communication.

Review of focus

Discussion of problems and resolution of difficult clinical issues is important, but reflection on successes is likely to promote team pride and optimism. Unfortunately, in most teams there is an emphasis on identification of problems, rather than reflection on what has worked, and the factors which have contributed to a good outcome.

Interprofessional education

There is emerging evidence that interprofessional education enhances awareness of colleagues' scope of practice and improves confidence in communication (Solomon and Salfi 2011) as well as the provision of mutual support (Brock *et al.* 2013). Given the evidence about preconceptions of students about those from other disciplines it is important to consider embedding interprofessional education rather than providing opportunistic or ad-hoc training. However, barriers exist at many levels, including funding, lack of demonstration of long-term benefit, and the complexities of incorporation into existing curricula. Lawlis *et al.* (2014) provide a comprehensive overview of enablers and barriers to interprofessional education, noting that while an individual academic may be resistant because of territory or 'turf wars' it is equally possible that a local champion can be a powerful advocate.

Inclusive approach

As knowledge expands and treatments become more complex it is clear that no individual can be expected to have universal competencies. Hence it may be appropriate to reflect more broadly about composition of teams. A pilot study of inclusion of a pharmacist in a community-based palliative care team demonstrated that when team members acquired improved medication-related knowledge and skills, medication management was improved and medication-related errors reduced (Hussainy *et al.* 2011).

Clerical staff do not treat patients, but they represent the 'frontline' and their comments and attitudes can influence clinical interactions. Patients who have been warned by the receptionist that 'the doctor is very busy' may be reluctant to discuss their concerns because they do not want to 'waste the doctor's time' with potential for adverse clinical impact. Inviting the opinions of clerical and administrative staff could lead to practical improvements to patient flow through re-design of reception areas and intake processes.

Recognition of the emotional dimensions

There is a body of research on stress and burnout, and while these terms are popularly used, there is often little acknowledgement of the emotional demands of working in oncology. Exposure to the suffering and grief of patients can be distressing and rekindle grief about personal experiences of loss (Turner *et al.* 2007). Validation of the grief and sadness inherent in the care of patients with cancer is an important step, as is giving staff the chance to reflect on their personal context.

Realistic approach

Accept that personality differences will occur and have clear professional boundaries.

Practical exercises

1. You have been asked to design a brochure for patients being treated in your cancer service. Your task is to explain the purpose

of the multidisciplinary team, including a list of members and their roles.

2. Construct a template to assist an intern to provide a discharge summary for a patient who has required inpatient treatment for neutropenia related to an infected catheter line. Include all members of the team who should receive a copy of the summary, and any expectations in terms of wound care, prescription of antibiotics, and follow-up.

3. Imagine that you are a junior nurse on night duty in an inpatient oncology unit. One of your patients is an elderly man admitted for management of poor oral intake during radiotherapy for head and neck cancer. The patient has become agitated and distressed: you are not sure if this is because of pain, or if he is developing delirium. Describe in detail what you would say when you make a phone call to the intern on duty.

4. Imagine that you are a patient who has recently undergone surgical treatment for cancer. Your task is to write to the hospital administration congratulating them on the excellent nursing care provided in their institution, giving specific examples.

5. You are assuming the role of radiation therapist giving a lecture to nurses about radiotherapy treatment of patients with head and neck cancer. Provide details to the nurses about the information you would want them to provide if they wanted you to review a patient with severe desquamation.

6. Write a paragraph to be included in a patient information brochure describing the importance of psychosocial care for patients with cancer and their families. Include a description of the training of social workers, psychologists, and psychiatrists.

Clinical exercises

1. Danny is a 23-year-old single man undergoing treatment for a germ cell tumour. He says that anxiety has been a long-standing problem and he doesn't think he can go through with the treatment as he feels too anxious.

   (a) Describe to Danny how a social worker or psychologist could assist him.

   (b) How would you respond if a team member expressed frustration about Danny saying he 'just needs to get on with it'?

2. Ruby is a 38-year-old woman who has three young children. She has advanced breast cancer which has progressed despite extensive chemotherapy. She has been admitted to hospital for assessment following a seizure and investigations have received a solitary cerebral metastasis. Her oncologist has made a referral for neurosurgical review. Ruby says that she is pleased about this, as she is confident that the cancer can be removed and things will be fine.

   (a) Imagine that you are one of the nurses caring for Ruby. You are concerned that she does not understand her prognosis, particularly in view of her disclosure that her children do not know about her cancer diagnosis. How could you discuss your concerns with her oncologist?

   (b) Imagine that you are the oncologist who has been treating Ruby since her original diagnosis of breast cancer four years ago. Describe to your intern how it feels to have a patient develop progressive disease despite your best efforts.

References

Amos MA, Hu J, Herrick CA (2005). The impact of team building on communication and job satisfaction of nursing staff. *J Nurses Staff Dev* **21**, 10–16.

Barrett L, Yates P (2002). Oncology-haematology nurses: a study of job satisfaction, burnout, and intention to leave the specialty. *Aust Health Rev* **25**, 109–21.

Brock D, Abu-Rish E, Chiu DC-R, *et al.* (2013). Interprofessional education in team communication: working together to improve patient safety. *BMJ Qual Saf* **22**, 414–23.

Chiles JA, Lambert MJ, Hatch AL (1999). The impact of psychological interventions on medical cost offset: a meta-analytic review. *Clin Psychol Sci Pr* **6**, 204–20.

Cohen SG, Bailey DE (1997). What makes teams work: group effectiveness research from the shop floor to the executive suite. *J Manage* **23**, 239–90.

Fleissig A, Jenkins V, Catt S, Fallowfield L (2006). Multidisciplinary teams in cancer care: are they effective in the UK? *Lancet Oncol* **7**, 935–43.

Greenberg CC, Regenbogen SE, Studdert DM, *et al.* (2007). Patterns of communication breakdowns resulting in injury to surgical patients. *J Am Coll Surg* **204**, 533–40.

Hall P, Weaver L, Gravelle D, Thibaulth H (2007). Developing collaborative person-centred practice: A pilot project on a palliative care unit. *J Interprof Care* **21**, 69–81.

Hong NJ, Wright FC, Gagliardi AR, Paszat LF (2010). Examining the potential relationship between multidisciplinary cancer care and patient survival: An international literature review. *J Surg Oncol* **102**, 125–34.

Hussainy SY, Box M, Scholes S (2011). Piloting the role of a pharmacist in a community palliative care multidisciplinary team: an Australian experience. *BMC Palliat Care* **10**, 16.

Lawlis TR, Anson J, Greenfield D (2014). Barriers and enablers that influence sustainable interprofessional education: a literature review. *J Interprof Care* **28**, 305–10.

Lindqvist S, Duncan A, Shepstone L, Watts F, Pearce S (2005). Development of the 'Attitudes to Health Professionals Questionnaire' (AHPQ): A measure to assess interprofessional attitudes. *J Interprof Care* **19**, 269–79.

Magee LR, Laroche CM, Gilligan D (2001). Clinical trials in lung cancer: evidence that a programmed investigation unit and a multidisciplinary clinic may improve recruitment. *Clin Oncol* **13**, 310–11.

Marshall S, Harrison J, Flanagan (2009). The teaching of a structured tool improves the clarity and content of interprofessional clinical communication. *Qual Saf Health Care* **18**, 137–40.

Mickan SM (2005). Evaluating the effectiveness of health care teams. *Aust Health Rev* **29**, 211–17.

Mickan SM, Rodger SA (2005). Effective health care teams: A model of six characteristics developed from shared perceptions. *J Interprof Care* **19**, 358–70.

National Breast Cancer Centre's Specialist Breast Nurse Project Team (2003). An evidence-based specialist breast nurse role in practice: a multicentre implementation study. *Eur J Cancer Care* **12**, 91–7.

National Confidential Enquiry into Patient Outcome and Death (2008). For better or worse? Available at: http://www.ncepod.org.uk/2008report3/Downloads/SACT_report.pdf (Last accessed January 18, 2015).

Rowlands S, Callen J (2013). A qualitative analysis of communication between members of a hospital-based multidisciplinary lung cancer team. *Eur J Cancer Care* **22**, 20–31.

Sijstermans R, Jaspers MW, Bloemendaal PM, Schoonderwaldt EM (2007). Training inter-physician communication using the Dynamic Patient Simulator®. *Int J Med Inform* **76**, 336–43.

Solomon P, Salfi J (2011). Evaluation of an interprofessional education communication skills initiative. *Educ Health (Abingdon)* **24**, 1–10.

Taylor C, Ramirez AJ (2009). Multidisciplinary team members' views about MDT working: Results from a survey commissioned by the National Cancer Action Team. National Cancer Action Team, London, UK.

Thewes B, Butow P, Davis E, Turner J, Mason C (2014). Psychologists' views of inter-disciplinary psychosocial communication within the cancer care team. *Support Care Cancer* **22**, 3193–200.

Turner J, Clavarino A, Yates P, Hargraves M, Connors V, Hausmann S (2007). Oncology nurses' perceptions of their supportive care for parents with advanced cancer: challenges and educational needs. *Psychooncology* **16**, 149–57.

Varpio L, Hall P, Lingard L, Schryer CF (2008). Interprofessional communication and medical error: a reframing of research questions and approaches. *Acad Med* **83**(10 Suppl), S76–81.

CHAPTER 34

Communicating genetic risk

Clara Gaff, Louise Keogh, and Elizabeth Lobb

Introduction to communicating genetic risk

As cancer is common, many people have a personal and/or family history of cancer. The discovery of cancer predisposing genetic mutations has heightened community awareness of the link between family history, genetic constitution, and personal risk. The component of an individual's cancer risk that is due to their genetic make-up can be described as their 'genetic risk'. Knowledge of genetic risk can assist both individuals with cancer and unaffected individuals to make decisions about healthcare and inform relatives who may share that genetic risk. Accordingly, patients seek advice about their risk and its implications and management from general practitioners (primary healthcare physician) or cancer specialists (Nippert et al. 2014).

Risk communication has been described as 'the open, two-way exchange of information and opinion about risk, leading to better understanding and better (clinical) decisions' (Ahl et al. 1993); that is, risk communication is more than the act of telling the patient a risk figure, it also encompasses the personal meaning that is made of that information. In summarizing 20 years of research and process in risk perception and communication, Fischhoff (1995) suggests that risk communication requires summarizing the relevant science, analysing recipients' decisions, assessing their current beliefs, drafting messages, evaluating their impact, and repeating the process, as needed. Accomplishing these tasks, he concludes, can significantly reduce the chances of producing messages that go against good practice in communication.

In this chapter, we discuss the interlinked processes of risk assessment, risk perception, and risk communication in the context of genetic risk of cancer. While this is only one component of an individual's risk of cancer—other factors including lifestyle, medical history, and environmental exposures—the principles of risk communication are applicable to each of these individual risk factors.

Risk assessment

The first task of the health professional is to determine the patient's genetic risk. Generally speaking, this assessment is based on either the patient's family history of cancer or, less commonly, relatedness to a family member known to carry a cancer predisposing mutation.

Family history

Numerous tools are available to calculate the likelihood an individual has a cancer predisposing mutation based on family history (Riley et al. 2012). The results of risk calculation tools can vary depending on the underlying assumptions and figures applied.

Nonetheless, individuals can be broadly but usefully classified into three genetic risk categories for a specific cancer: average risk, moderate risk, and high risk.

- Individuals at average risk either do not have a family history of cancer or the cancers in the family are 'spontaneous'; that is, the cancer can be attributed to cumulative chance events and environmental factors. Their lifetime risk of developing a cancer is the same as the population risk of that cancer.

- Individuals at moderate risk have some relatives affected with the same type of malignancy, usually diagnosed at a similar age to the age of onset in the general population. The causes of these 'familial cancers' are not usually apparent but are likely to be due to multiple interacting factors, clusters of spontaneous cancer, or the presence of (multiple) gene mutations, each with a weak effect.

- Individuals at high genetic risk are suspected or known to have an inherited cancer syndrome. This can be indicated by a family history of closely related affected family members, often with an earlier age of onset than the general population. These family histories are caused by mutations in genes regulating DNA repair, cell growth, and cell division. Usually, these are inherited in a dominant fashion, with an affected parent having a 50% chance of passing the mutation on to each child. The lifetime risk of an individual who carries the mutation is usually greater than the population risk, but less than 100%. The degree of risk will depend on the inherited cancer syndrome and the specific cancer. For instance, people with a mutation causing Lynch Syndrome—an inherited colorectal cancer syndrome—have on average a cumulative lifetime risk of developing colorectal cancer of 50–80% and women have a 25–60% risk of uterine cancer (Kohlmann and Gruber 2004).

Genetic testing

Genetic testing can ascertain if a person has a mutation(s) known to increase the risk of cancer. Ideally, genetic testing to identify a causative mutation is offered first to an affected member of a high-risk family. If such a mutation is found, then predictive testing can be offered to other at-risk family members to determine if they have inherited the cancer-causing mutation or a normal copy of the gene. The absence of a mutation only definitively reduces risk to that of the population if there is a known mutation in the family.

Risk perception

As responses to information are influenced by pre-existing perceptions, and risk perception is known to be a factor in health-related behaviour, it is important to have an understanding of how individuals construct and use their belief about the likelihood of personal harm ('perceived risk') (Weinstein and Klein 1995). Perceived risk may be expressed qualitatively ('It is inevitable that I will get cancer') or quantitatively ('My chance of getting cancer is 60%') and how individuals come to understand their own personal risk is influenced by a number of factors.

> Risk perception has to be understood as a communication process along a chain from the sender to receiver, with different stations in between that may amplify or attenuate risks. Such stations can be social (e.g. news media), individual (e.g. attention filter), or institutional (e.g. political and social actions) (Bodemer and Gaissmaier 2015, p. 11).

For patients at high risk of cancer, some of the factors known to influence perceived risk for cancer include: the extent of family history; beliefs about preventability and severity of cancer; ability to process numerical information and demographic factors (Tilburt et al. 2011). Thus, two women with the same objective risk of developing breast cancer but different experiences of breast cancer in their family, beliefs and abilities are likely to respond differently to risk information (Keogh et al. 2011). Similarly, if we consider two women who see themselves having a one-in-three risk on breast cancer, one may think they will definitely get cancer, and another may think they will definitely not get cancer. It seems reasonable to assume that this is true of hereditary cancer more broadly. A summary of the influences on risk perception is reproduced in Table 34.1

A number of theoretical models have been proposed to describe how representations of illness are developed, how risk information is processed, and how these influence decisions and behaviour (Tilburt et al. 2011).

Of particular relevance is the Heuristic-Systematic Model (Chen and Chaiken 1999), which proposes that risk information can be processed cognitively and/or affectively when a decision is being made. Systematic processing involves careful examination and analysis of the content of the information provided, such as cancer risks and the management options discussed in a cancer genetics consultation. Consequently, it requires considerable cognitive effort. Heuristic processing is more intuitive, using rules-of-thumb or 'shortcuts' to make sense of information. The use of heuristics has been demonstrated in cancer genetics (Kenen et al. 2003). The belief that physical or temperamental similarity with an affected individual confers higher risk for cancer is an example of a 'representativeness' heuristic: information about similarity and stereotypes is used to make a judgement, in this case about personal risk. Heuristic processing requires relatively little effort and is more likely to occur when, inter alia, the information has low personal relevance, there is time pressure, the individual is experiencing an affective response to risk such as worry, and when there is ambiguity in the information (Etchegary and Perrier 2007). Informed decision-making is assumed to be the result of systematic processing and it has been argued that the provision of genetic risk information should be given in conditions that promote systematic processing; for example, with sufficient, unambiguous information and without time constraints (Etchegary and Perrier 2007).

Table 34.1 Factors that influence risk perception and understanding

Factor	Description
Individual factors	
Cognitive/emotional traits	Personality traits such as optimism versus pessimism, risk-taking attitudes, and preferences for numerical format of risk figures
Numeracy	The ability to understand numerical values and probability (the numerical equivalent of literacy)
Consequences	The range of consequences related to the risk information; consequences can be positive, negative, life altering, neutral, etc.
Uncertainty and the need to reduce uncertainty	The uncertainty associated with risk figures and the emotional need to reduce this uncertainty
Experiential factors	
A priori beliefs	Initial beliefs about risk level
Availability	Prior experiences (i.e. real-life experiences that are cognitively 'available' to the client when the risk is presented)
Representativeness	Inferences from a small sample (e.g. a family) to a larger group (e.g. a specific population)
Other factors	
Anchoring	Bias introduced by the first concept or risk figure introduced
Binarization	The tendency to simplify risk information and reorient it towards the possible outcomes rather than the likelihood of those outcomes (i.e. viewing numerical risk in two categories—50/50, present/absent, will/will not happen—regardless of the probability presented)
Complexity	The generally complex nature of risk figures, particularly multiple related risk figures presented together, or in sequence

Adapted with permission from the *Annual Review of Genomics and Human Genetics*, Volume 14, Denise M. Lautenbach et al., 'Communicating Genetic Risk Information for Common Disorders,' pp. 491–513, Copyright © 2013 Annual Reviews, http://www.annualreviews.org. Source: data from Uhlmann, WR. et al. (Eds.) *A Guide to Genetic Counseling, Second Edition*, p. 624, Wiley-Blackwell, Hoboken, NJ, USA, Copyright © 2009; and Weil, J., Psychosocial Genetic Counseling, p. 41, *Oxford Monograph of Medical Genetics*, Oxford University Press, New York, USA, Copyright © 2000 by Oxford University Press, Inc.

Presenting risk to patients

Conveying genetic risk to patients must cover a great conceptual distance—from probabilities based on mathematics derived from populations, to the communication of individual risk, and then to the interpretation and meaning made of personal risk by individuals. Accurate risk comprehension among patients in genetic counselling programmes may be critical to their decision-making about whether to have a genetic test and, among those who test positive, to their decision-making about risk management (Sivell et al. 2008). We also know that individuals are likely to have different needs of risk counselling depending on their medical and demographic background (Roshanai et al. 2012).

Perhaps unsurprisingly, the literature on communication of risk in familial cancer focuses on numerical probability (Sivell et al. 2008), as numerical risks appear to present precise information regarding the probability that a health problem will occur and convey authority. When clinicians present numerical probability information, they rely on the premise that patients will respond to a given probability in a consistent manner. That is, a 10% risk should be interpreted as a 10% risk, regardless of whether it is presented as a percentage, an odds ratio, or whether it is presented as numerically or pictorially.

Despite the appearance of precision inherent in numerical presentation, in fact studies of different populations and subgroups show that individuals presented with the same numerical figure have divergent ways of interpreting what the figures mean (Hallowell et al. 1997). People also make errors when asked to transform percentages into proportions and vice versa, and they confuse information about the frequency of an event with its rate of occurrence. Thus, it would appear that numerical probability statistics cannot be relied on to ensure patients have adequate understanding of genetic risk.

An alternative expression of risk is verbal probability (e.g. there is a high risk). This is often used by doctors to express uncertainty, or when there is a lack of information from empirical research or conflicting results from published studies (Timmermans 1994). Budescu argues that most laypeople understand words better than numbers and typically handle uncertainty by means of verbal expressions; for example, 'I think that …', 'chances are …', 'it is unlikely that' (Budescu et al. 1988). He argues that words are perceived as more flexible and less precise in meaning. Studies in genetic counselling settings have shown that, when provided with numerical estimates, patients appear to spontaneously transform their probability information into discrete categories, for example high or low risk (Bottorff et al. 1998), supporting a notion that words are easier and more comfortable to process than numbers.

The provision of risk information may be simplified by asking the patient for his/her preferences relating to the format of the risk information (words, numbers, or both) and the type of risk information sought (e.g. lifetime risk, 10-year risk). Publications have typically failed to support this premise, however. For example, Lobb et al. (2003) found that there was no association between the way genetic risk was communicated in familial cancer consultations and women's accuracy of risk recall or satisfaction with the consultation. Women who were given risk information, both as words and numbers, or in their preferred format, were not more accurate or satisfied than those who were not. These findings suggest that risk is a difficult concept to grasp, and that it may be important spending time in the consultation exploring a patient's understanding of risk in different contexts and formats.

Strategies for practitioners

Health professionals face the challenging task of conveying complex risk information to patients with different pre-existing experiences, beliefs, and perceptions. At the very least, a patient at high risk will be expected to integrate information about the likelihood there is a genetic susceptibility in the family, the risk of inheriting or transmitting the predisposing mutation, and the risk of then developing the disease (Lobb et al. 2003). They are then expected to make medical and behavioural decisions on the basis of this understanding.

A 'contextually based approach' is recommended by cancer genetic risk assessment and counselling guidelines (Riley et al. 2012), and appears to be applied in practice (Lobb et al. 2005). A first step is to enquire about the patient's specific concerns and expectations, for example for facts, practical support or emotional support (Roshanai et al. 2012). In Table 34.2 we provide some strategies with exemplars for communicating about genetic risk. These aim to support the development of a relationship which supports two-way communication; the identification of the influences on the patient's personal beliefs about their risk, as well as convey factual information.

Risk communication can be supported by use of tools, such as decision aids. The Ottawa Hospital Research Institute provides a repository of decision aids (https://decisionaid.ohri.ca). Some are designed for use in the consultation, while others are designed as adjuncts to the clinical interaction. Some decision aids are proven to produce higher knowledge scores, lower decisional conflict, and more active patient participation in decision-making (O'Connor et al. 1999).

Genetic risk information has the potential to affect the individual's beliefs about the cause of a disease and consequently its controllability. It is not a great leap to recognize that it could thereby affect emotional adjustment and motivation to engage in behaviour that might reduce risks. For example, provision of DNA-based genetic risk information about hereditary heart disease resulted in an increased belief in the genetic causation of heart disease, leading to a reduced expectation that behavioural change (e.g. diet) would be effective in reducing risk, and an increased expectation that biological means (e.g. medication) would be effective (Marteau and Weinman 2006).

Emotional disturbances, such as misplaced anxiety, that may prevent at-risk individuals seeking appropriate care, can become apparent during this process. Addressing these may facilitate the systematic processing of information and decision-making (Etchegary and Perrier 2007).

Patient communication of risk to relatives

In most areas of medicine, the risks discussed are relevant only to the patient in the consultation. However, inherited risk is shared within families, and the genetic risk status of one family member has implications for others. Consultations about genetic risk,

Table 34.2 Key strategies for communicating about genetic risk

Goal	Exemplar
Clarifying patient's expectations and setting the agenda	'Before I start, perhaps you could tell me what you would like to find out today?'
Goal setting	'I can talk about the chances of you developing cancer and, although we cannot completely prevent breast cancer, I can talk about the options for reducing your risk. Would that be helpful?'
Explaining the process	'A while back, you sent me information about the cancers in your family. I'll go through that now and check that I have the facts straight, then talk to you about the likelihood that cancer might be inherited in your family and what your chance of developing cancer is. Then we can talk about what you might be able to do about that risk.'
Identifying patient's beliefs and perceptions	'Before I start talking about our interpretation of what is happening in your family, could you tell me what you believe has caused the cancers in your family?'
Checks patient's genetic knowledge	'There is a lot about "genes" in the news nowadays and everyone has some idea of what this means. Could you tell me what you imagine when I talk about a gene.'
Check information preference	'Is that something you want to know?'
Check concerns	'Is that something that concerns you?'
Checks understanding	'I've given you a lot of information today and I know you want to talk to your family about this. What do you think you might say to them?'
Invite questions	'Please ask me any questions … interrupt me … if I use any words that don't make sense tell me "I just didn't understand that" and we'll go back.'
Validate the patient	'You seemed to have picked that up really well, is that fairly clear?'
Begin to personalize the information	'So, on the basis of three people in your family having developed … cancer, closely related to one another, and with these two people at the younger end … we'd certainly be very suspicious that there's an inherited predisposition to … cancer.'
Ask patient's opinion	'Is that something that you've considered/thought all along?'
Explain medical terminology	'Now if we find an alteration, the technical term is a mutation, in one of those two genes BRCA1 or BRCA2.'
Use a diagram	
Check preference for risk information?	'Did you want the numbers on that?'
Re-frame	'So to put that another way …'
Discussing family history to minimize distress	Explain the process, take note of special dates, e.g. date of diagnosis or death of other family member, explore emotional concerns, identify patient beliefs and perceptions, and validate the patient's experiences

therefore, consider the relevance of the information to relatives of the patient. For example, if a known cancer predisposing mutation is identified, then at-risk relatives can be tested for this mutation. The patient will be advised of this in the consultation and asked to inform those now eligible for testing. However, while it is rare that the patient will refuse to inform relatives, few inform all at-risk relatives about the availability of genetic testing (Gaff *et al.* 2007).

A number of strategies may be needed to assist patients to communicate with family members. Time may be required for the patient to adjust to their own risk before they are prepared to pass information on to family members. The patient considering disclosure to relatives may consider the perceived vulnerability of the recipient, as well as the time and manner of the disclosure (Gaff *et al.* 2007). Other family members may assist. Koehly *et al.* (2009) found in hereditary breast ovarian cancer families, that 'disseminators' of genetic information are more likely to be female, in the older or same generation, have a cancer history, and provide emotional and tangible support. The consultation itself could also be important: a multifaceted intervention which included coaching in communication skills significantly increased the number of women who communicated about genetic risk to relatives (Bodurtha *et al.* 2014).

Verbal dissemination of risk information within families can be supplemented with other complementary means of communication.

Box 34.1 Case study: A young woman at potentially high risk of hereditary bowel cancer

Jane Brown is 32 years old and has been married to Peter for 10 years. They have a daughter, Mia (5 years), and Jane works part-time as a sales assistant in a department store. Jane and Peter met while still at school and Peter has a management position in a bank. His work is quite stressful and takes him away from home on a regular basis.

Jane moved to the city when she married, but her mother Glenda and a sister still live in the country. Jane is the youngest of three children. She has a 38-year-old sister, Jean, and a brother, Michael who is 35. Jane's father David, was diagnosed with advanced bowel cancer at 38, and died 2 years later leaving Glenda to raise the three children.

Jane was 10 years old at the time of her father's illness and has strong memories of trips to the hospital at the time of her father's treatment. Her mother was weepy and tired. The father's diagnosis and death are not discussed in the family and Glenda has subsequently re-married.

Jane has one paternal aunt (Monica) who has recently been diagnosed with bowel cancer at 52, another paternal aunt (Joanne) was affected by endometrial cancer at 48 and has subsequently passed away. One maternal cousin of Jane (Bob) was also diagnosed with bowel cancer in his fourties, has completed treatment and remains well.

Since her cousin's diagnosis, Jane has become increasingly anxious about her own risk of bowel cancer. She has attended for colonoscopy and has had polyps removed. She is attending the familial cancer clinic to discuss her own risk of developing bowel cancer.

For example, a combination of verbal and written communication with family members resulted in more relatives contacting genetic services about their risk than either form of communication alone (Suthers *et al.* 2006).

Conclusion

As described, in the past there has been a focus on the impact of interventions such as decision aids, audiotaped consultations, written summaries, and genetic counselling consultations, on shifting inaccurate baseline risk perceptions (Edwards *et al.* 2008). However, a more meaningful outcome may relate to one of the key activities of genetic counselling, facilitating adjustment. In this context, adjustment to living with increased risk of cancer may be achieved by exploring the personal meaning of that risk and its implications. Current models of risk communication suggest that this will have a positive effect on social and medical decision-making. The case study in Box 34.1 provides an opportunity to try out some of these strategies.

References

Ahl A, Acree J, Gipson P, McDowell R, *et al.* (1993). Standardization of nomenclature for animal health risk analysis. *Revue scientifique et technique (International Office of Epizootics)* **12**, 1045–53.

Bodemer N, Gaissmaier W (2015). Risk perception. In: Cho H, Reimer T, Mccomas KA (eds). *The SAGE Handbook of Risk Communication.* Sage Publications, Thousand Oaks, CA.

Bodurtha J, McClish D, Gyure M, *et al.* (2014). The KinFact intervention : a randomized controlled trial to increase family communication about cancer history. *J Women's Health (Larchmt)* **23**, 806–16.

Bottorff JL, Ratner PA, Johnson JL, *et al.* (1998). Communicating cancer risk information: the challenges of uncertainty. *Patient Educ Couns* **33**, 67–81.

Budescu DV, Weinberg S, Wallsten TS (1988). Decisions based on numerically and verbally expressed uncertainties. *J Exp Psychol Hum Percept Perform* **14**, 281.

Chen S, Chaiken S (1999). The Heuristic-Systematic Model in its broader context. In: Chaiken S, Trope Y (eds). *Dual-process Theories in Social Psychology.* Guilford Press, New York, NY.

Edwards A, Gray J, Clarke A, *et al.* (2008). Interventions to improve risk communication in clinical genetics: systematic review. *Patient Educ Couns* **71**, 4–25.

Etchegary H, Perrier C (2007). Information processing in the context of genetic risk: implications for genetic-risk communication. *J Genet Couns* **16**, 419–32.

Fischhoff B (1995). Risk perception and communication unplugged: twenty years of Process1. *Risk Analysis* **15**, 137–45.

Gaff CL, Clarke AJ, Atkinson P, *et al.* (2007). Process and outcome in communication of genetic information within families: a systematic review. *Eur J Hum Genet* **15**, 999–1011.

Hallowell N, Green J, Statham H, Murton F, *et al.* (1997). Recall of numerical risk estimates and counsellees' perceptions of the importance of risk information following genetic counselling for breast and ovarian cancer. *Psychol Health Med* **2**, 149–59.

Kenen R, Ardern-Jones A, Eeles, R (2003). Family stories and the use of heuristics: women from suspected hereditary breast and ovarian cancer (HBOC) families. *Sociol Health Illn* **25**, 838–65.

Keogh LA, McClaren BJ, Apicella C, Hopper JL (2011). How do women at increased, but unexplained, familial risk of breast cancer perceive and manage their risk? A qualitative interview study. *Hered Cancer Clin Pract* **9**, 1–11.

Koehly LM, Peters JA, Kenen R, *et al.* (2009). Characteristics of health information gatherers, disseminators, and blockers within families at risk of hereditary cancer: implications for family health communication interventions. *Am J Pub Health* **99**, 2203.

Kohlmann W, Gruber SB (2004). Lynch syndrome. In: Pagon RA, Adam MP, Ardinger HH, *et al.* (eds.) *GeneReviews.* University of Washington, Seattle, WA.

Lobb E, Butow P, Meiser B, *et al.* (2003). Women's preferences and consultants' communication of risk in consultations about familial breast cancer: impact on patient outcomes. *J Med Genet* **40**, e56.

Lobb EA, Butow P, Barratt A, Meiser B, Tucker K (2005). Differences in individual approaches: communication in the familial breast cancer consultation and the effect on patient outcomes. *J Genet Couns* **14**, 43–53.

Marteau TM, Weinman J (2006). Self-regulation and the behavioural response to DNA risk information: a theoretical analysis and framework for future research. *Soc Sci Med* **62**, 1360–8.

Nippert I, Julian-Reynier C, Harris H, *et al.* (2014). Cancer risk communication, predictive testing and management in France, Germany, the Netherlands and the UK: general practitioners' and breast surgeons' current practice and preferred practice responsibilities. *J Community Genet* **5**, 69–79.

O'Connor AM, Rostom A, Fiset V, *et al.* (1999). Decision aids for patients facing health treatment or screening decisions: systematic review. *BMJ* **319**, 731–4.

Riley BD, Culver JO, Skrzynia C, *et al.* (2012) Essential elements of genetic cancer risk assessment, counseling, and testing: updated recommendations of the National Society of Genetic Counselors. *J Genet Counsel* **21**, 151–61.

Roshanai AH, Lampic C, Ingvoldstad C, *et al.* (2012). What information do cancer genetic counselees prioritize? *J Genet Counsel* **21**, 510–26.

Sivell S, Elwyn G, Gaff CL, *et al.* (2008). How risk is perceived, constructed and interpreted by clients in clinical genetics, and the effects on decision making: systematic review. *J Genet Couns* **17**, 30–63.

Suthers GK, Armstrong J, McCormack J, Trott D (2006). Letting the family know: balancing ethics and effectiveness when notifying relatives about genetic testing for a familial disorder. *J Med Genet* **43**, 665–70.

Tilburt JC, James KM, Sinicrope PS, *et al.* (2011). Factors influencing cancer risk perception in high risk populations: a systematic review. *Hered Cancer Clin Pract* **19**, 2.

Timmermans D (1994). The roles of experience and domain of expertise in using numerical and verbal probability terms in medical decisions. *Med Decis Making* **14**, 146–56.

Weinstein ND, Klein WM (1995). Resistance of personal risk perceptions to debiasing interventions. *Health Psychol* **14**, 132.

CHAPTER 35

Supporting patients considering reconstructive surgery

Diana Harcourt and Alex Clarke

Introduction to supporting patients considering reconstructive surgery

The diagnosis and treatment of cancer can have a significant, negative impact on patients' psychosocial well-being, body image, sexuality, and sense of self. 'Reconstructive surgery' refers to procedures carried out to improve function and restore a 'normal' appearance for patients whose appearance is considered to be 'different' for any reason, including the effects of diseases such as cancer and its treatment. Reconstruction is commonly assumed to offer improved body image and quality of life.

This chapter uses the example of breast reconstruction to consider ways in which patients faced with complex decisions about reconstructive surgery might be helped to make the choice that is best for them, as an individual. It begins by outlining common breast reconstruction options, including choices around the type and timing of surgery, and then considers women's motivation for surgery, satisfaction with outcomes, and interventions to help to them make their decision.

Breast care teams (including breast surgeons, plastic surgeons, and specialist nurses) play a crucial role in helping women decide whether or not to undergo reconstruction and managing their expectations of the outcome of surgery. Some patients report it being difficult to discuss body image and appearance concerns in a clinic setting where health professionals' priority is on treating the cancer. Creating an ethos in which appearance-related issues can be discussed as routinely as physical and medical issues (such as pain and treatment side effects), and feeling confident in conversations about these issues, should be an aim of any health professional. We therefore hope that the content of this chapter will support clinicians working with cancer patients who are candidates for reconstructive surgery, as well as those interested in research in this field.

Breast reconstruction

The term 'breast reconstruction' describes a range of surgical procedures that intend to recreate a breast shape for women who have lost a breast as a result of a mastectomy, either following diagnosis of cancer, or after confirmation of an increased risk of developing the disease. It is sometimes described as 'quality of life surgery', since it does not treat the cancer itself, nor does it affect the detection of future tumours or impact on recurrence or survival in any way.

In the United Kingdom, guidelines for the provision of care for women diagnosed with breast cancer stipulate that the possibility of breast reconstruction should be discussed with all those for whom mastectomy is an option. However, research in the United States suggests that clinicians do not discuss it with all their patients and that they are less likely to offer it to women from lower income households, even when health insurance is taken into account (Chen *et al.* 2009). Although some women choose not to recreate a breast shape by any means, the majority use an external prosthesis, but some find them to be an uncomfortable reminder of the treatment they have had and worry that the prosthesis will move or become dislodged, and therefore be noticeable to others. A patient audit in England (National Mastectomy and Breast Reconstruction Audit 2011) reported that more than 15,000 women underwent mastectomy each year and, of those, more than 5,000 chose to undergo breast reconstruction.

Timing of breast reconstruction

Breast reconstruction typically involves numerous separate procedures, a post-surgical inpatient stay, and several months' recovery. It can take place in the same operation as the mastectomy (known as immediate reconstruction) or as a separate procedure weeks, months, or years later (delayed reconstruction). Decisions about the timing of breast reconstruction are individual, and will be informed by a number of factors including the stage of breast cancer, a woman's medical history, her psychological and social situation, the potential need for post-operative radiotherapy (which can impact on scarring, aesthetic outcome, and increase the likelihood of capsular contracture) and, most importantly, her own goals and expectations.

Some women find immediate reconstruction appealing as it offers the possibility to avoid living without a breast for any period of time, and thereby reduce the distress associated with feeling 'different' or 'disfigured' after a mastectomy. It can also reduce the number of surgical procedures, anaesthetics, and hospital stays compared to delayed reconstruction, although recovery is longer after immediate reconstruction than after mastectomy alone. However, others choose to delay breast reconstruction because they feel overwhelmed by the number of decisions they are required to make around the time of diagnosis and initial mastectomy. Some women feel they need to focus on their cancer before they are psychologically and physically ready to proceed with restoring their breast. Delayed breast reconstruction allows women more time to make their decision, the opportunity to experience mastectomy with and without a prosthesis before deciding for or against further surgery, and has the potential to restore a more positive body image for those who dislike their post-mastectomy appearance.

Types of reconstruction

The options for how breast reconstruction is carried out are numerous and potentially complicated, using either implants or autologous procedures that move tissue from another part of the woman's own body (the most commonly used techniques involve the lower abdomen or back). In some instances, a combination of different surgical techniques is used. A reconstructed breast will not precisely match the patient's natural breast, and she may therefore face further choices about whether to reduce or lift the opposite (contralateral) breast in order to improve shape, establish symmetry, and match the reconstructed breast.

All surgical procedures have risks, and discussions about the possible complications arising from reconstruction must be taken into consideration when discussing the options available to any potential patient. Breast implants (usually filled with saline or silicone) eventually wear out and are likely to need to be replaced in the future. There is also a possibility of capsular contracture, whereby the body forms a layer of scar tissue around the implant which may, occasionally, be so hard and strong that it causes pain and distorts the shape of the reconstructed breast, with the resulting need for further surgery to relieve these symptoms and, possibly, the need to remove the implant entirely. Recent developments in implant surgery include the use of mesh inserts to support the implants, which can result in a more natural shape and feel than using an implant alone.

Breasts reconstructed by using the woman's own body tissue (autologous procedures) are usually soft, have a more natural shape than those created by an implant, and age much like a natural breast. However, they do not look or feel exactly the same as a natural breast and patients can expect potentially significant scars at the donor site—for example, a long scar across the abdomen or a horizontal scar (usually hidden along the bra line) on the back, depending on the type of procedure carried out. Furthermore, the initial operation for an autologous reconstruction is longer and more complicated than implant surgery, and there is greater potential for complications and 'failure', both on the site of the reconstructed breast and at the donor site. For a small percentage of patients undergoing free flap techniques, microsurgery fails to re-establish circulation to the transplanted tissue, resulting in complete flap loss.

The psychological impact of complications after breast reconstruction has received very little attention from researchers to date, although Gopie et al. (2013) have reported higher levels of anxiety and depressive symptoms among women who self-reported any kind of surgical complication post-reconstruction. Interestingly, more patients reported complications compared with their surgeon's reports.

The most appropriate method of reconstruction depends on several factors, including the size and shape of the patient's breasts, the amount of body tissue that the woman has at potential donor sites, and whether or not she has had, or will receive, radiation therapy. If more than one method is suitable, the patient is faced with the choice, which can involve processing complex information about the advantages and disadvantages of each option.

Nipple reconstruction

Depending on the type of mastectomy carried out, a woman is likely to lose her nipple when her breast is removed. There are several options available to restore this aspect of the breast including temporary, prosthetic stick-on nipples, or surgical techniques that use the skin and fat of the reconstructed breast together with a skin graft from the upper thigh to recreate the areola, followed by a 'tattoo' procedure to match the colour of the woman's natural nipple and areola. However, regardless of procedure, a reconstructed nipple will not have any sensation. Research (e.g. Harcourt et al. 2011) has highlighted the importance of providing information about these additional choices (including photographs of possible outcomes and information about likely sensation) when the possibility of breast reconstruction is first raised.

Scarring

All patients will have some permanent scarring after a mastectomy and breast reconstruction, but it can be difficult to predict the personal impact this will have. Scars on the stomach, back, thigh, and buttocks can often be easily covered in clothing; however, some women feel very conscious of the area of the body that was used as the donor site. Women who have undergone TRAM or DIEP flap procedures (which move tissue from the abdomen) have reported feeling dissatisfied with and unprepared for the scarring across their abdomen (Abu-Nab and Grunfeld 2007). Although scarring is unavoidable, women are likely to be better prepared for the outcome if they have realistic expectations about the likely location and appearance of scars.

In summary, any type and timing of breast reconstruction requires the patient to be completely committed to what is an ongoing and often drawn-out process, typically involving several procedures over a period of months or years. It is a choice requiring careful consideration; if a woman is already feeling overwhelmed about her diagnosis, the pending surgery, and other anxieties, then decision-making can be very difficult.

Women's reasons for seeking reconstructive breast surgery

There are many reasons for electing for or against breast reconstruction and it is important not to assume that reconstruction is the preserve of younger women—some older women would not contemplate mastectomy without reconstruction, while some younger women do not feel the need to undergo the additional surgery that it entails. Motivations for surgery include wanting to avoid using an external prosthesis, to restore a sense of balance and body integrity, and to not feel restricted when choosing clothing. Many women describe wanting to restore 'normality' after mastectomy, but the phrase 'normal' can mean many different things. Women may want to look normal (i.e. normal appearance), to fulfil everyday activities (i.e. normal behaviour), establish a new sense of what they consider to be normal (i.e. reconstructing normality) and to no longer consider themselves to be ill (i.e. normal health) (Denford et al. 2011). Clarifying each patient's perceptions of what they would consider to be a 'normal' outcome is one way of exploring their expectations of surgery (the importance of clarifying patient expectations and goals is discussed later in this chapter).

Some women elect for reconstruction because they are concerned that a mastectomy alone will impact negatively on their feelings of attractiveness and experiences of sexual intimacy. However, reconstructive surgery does not necessarily allay these concerns and some women report feeling sexually and physically unattractive several years after reconstruction. Even couples who had a strong intimate relationship before surgery are likely to have to renegotiate this aspect of their relationship, at least in the short term. Male partners have reported concerns that touching the reconstructed breast might be painful for their partner and worries that they might reopen surgical wounds. Although this reluctance is driven by concern for their partner, a woman who is conscious of her altered appearance and is looking for reassurance that she is still attractive to her partner might easily misinterpret this lack of contact. This has the potential to create difficulties within the relationship that open communication between both parties could alleviate. It has been suggested (Rowland and Metcalfe 2014) that interventions that effectively support men could enable them to be better placed to support their partners, thereby benefitting women who are making decisions about surgery, and potentially improving communication between them.

Satisfaction with outcomes

While some research has shown that breast reconstruction offers benefits in terms of improved body image and quality of life for many mastectomy patients (Al-Ghazal *et al.* 2000), other studies have found it is not a universal remedy for all the challenges and distress associated with losing a breast (Harcourt and Rumsey 2004). Although women often report being satisfied with their decision to undergo reconstruction, a reconstructed breast can never be an exact replacement for the natural breast and they can still experience difficulties adjusting to their new appearance and incorporating their reconstructed breast(s) into their body image. Adjusting to the changes that take place during any type of reconstruction process (not only reconstructive breast surgery) is an ongoing, often challenging process, and patients may need specialist support to help them before, during, and after surgery (Fingeret *et al.* 2014). A recently developed screening tool for cancer patients undergoing reconstructive surgery has potential to help health professionals identify those who are dissatisfied with outcomes and who may benefit from additional support around body image concerns (Fingeret *et al.* 2014).

In recent years, the Breast-Q (Pusic *et al.* 2009) has become the most widely used measure of patient satisfaction with surgical outcomes and quality of life after breast reconstruction. Using the Breast-Q, the National Mastectomy and Breast Reconstruction Audit in England (2011) reported that, 18 months after surgery, one-third of immediate reconstruction and 22% of delayed reconstruction patients could not describe the outcome as 'excellent' or 'very good'. Forty per cent of immediate reconstruction patients were unsatisfied with how their breast looked compared to before they had surgery (although it is important to acknowledge that participants were asked to report, retrospectively, on how satisfied they were with the appearance of their breasts before surgery—there was no pre-surgical baseline measure. Similarly, it is arguable that the appropriate comparison is not the pre-operative breast but the breast post-mastectomy).

Elsewhere, research has reported regret about the decision to undergo reconstruction among 47% (Sheehan *et al.* 2007) of participants. This figure supports research that has discussed dissatisfaction with breast reconstruction in terms of scarring (particularly at the donor site), pain, and asymmetry of the two breasts (Harcourt and Rumsey 2004), rather than surgical complications or need for revisions (Benditte-Klepetko *et al.* 2014). Sheehan *et al.* (2007)

related satisfaction to women's expectations of surgical outcome or process, supporting the view that dissatisfaction is associated with unrealistic, and therefore unmet, expectations.

A patient's own, subjective perception of the outcome of reconstruction is typically a better predictor of levels of distress and satisfaction, and might not agree with that of her significant others or her surgeon. While a surgeon might be keen to perform further procedures, such as scar revisions, the patient might be satisfied with the outcome of surgery and not want to undergo any further operations. Similarly, patients might be unhappy with the results of surgery that their surgeon is very pleased with. Such disparity could reflect differing pre-operative expectations about the likely outcome of surgery. If a surgeon has not ascertained what the patient hopes to achieve from reconstruction, then they are unlikely to have a good understanding of their expectations and wishes. In such circumstances, it is not surprising that they may not have concurring views on the success of a procedure—further supporting the importance of clearly understanding women's pre-surgical expectations about post-surgical outcomes.

Facilitating shared decision-making

Making the decision for or against breast reconstruction can be difficult and daunting for patients, largely because of the need to consider new and complex information, and possibly because of the influence, consciously or unconsciously, of other people including the patient's partner. If immediate reconstruction is an option, then initial decisions must be made around the time of diagnosis and when the possibility of mastectomy has just been raised, a time during which information overload is not uncommon and it can be particularly difficult to understand and process complex information. Understandably, women's ability to consider the details of breast reconstruction at this stage may be hampered by their concerns about their cancer diagnosis and treatment options. They might perceive themselves to have relatively little time to make their decision because they are keen for the cancer-treating surgery to take place as soon as possible and fear that delaying their decision could have implications for their health (Harcourt and Rumsey 2004). A major challenge for healthcare staff is how to give potential breast reconstruction patients sufficient information, time, and support to make their decision within the confines of a busy hospital service.

Information provision

While some women feel able to make a decision very quickly and might then seek information that will support the choice they have made, others need to obtain and assimilate a complex mass of information before they are able to decide. A small but important group find it very difficult to make a choice, irrespective of the amount of information they are given (Harcourt and Rumsey 2004).

Ensuring patients have easy access to reliable, up-to-date information that addresses both the possible physical and psychosocial consequences of surgery is essential in order to enable them to start considering their options, personal values, and preferences, and may also reduce the likelihood and extent of regret about their decision at a later stage.

Information should be available in a variety of formats (including trusted websites, patient handouts, educational sessions, photos, interactive computer programs and audio tapes) to meet women's varying information needs. All information should have the source clearly identified together with the date. Inaccurate or outdated information can be misleading and contribute to unrealistic expectations. Rather than relying on images in surgical textbooks (which can be hard for patients to relate to), surgeons should provide a library of photographs of their own patients (from whom consent for the use of the image has been obtained). Images of women of diverse ethnicity, age, physique, and at various stages in their post-surgical recovery can help women to consider their own priorities and aspirations. Although images of less successful aesthetic outcomes may be upsetting for some women, it is important to have a range of photos available and to discuss the possible likelihood and outcome of both less and more successful procedures.

Meeting other patients who have already had breast reconstruction can help decision-making and provide an opportunity to discuss the situation with someone who is not a clinical expert but has personal experience to share. However, this does have to be carefully managed in order that potential patients are not overly swayed by those who are particularly enthusiastic about their own surgical results. Some aspects of the outcome of surgery are particularly difficult to describe to those contemplating reconstruction. For example, what is considered to be 'mild tingling' to one woman could be 'persistent pain' to another. The use of language to convey these experiences accurately is a very difficult task for healthcare professionals who have not experienced the surgery themselves. When meeting other patients in person is not possible, websites that share patient experiences (e.g. www.healthtalkonline.org) can be helpful. Such resources can provide a personal point of view and may also help to remind the patient that they are not alone in their experience. Accounts from former patients can be very powerful and useful resources, but women might also be overwhelmed by graphic accounts and the amount of information available.

Clarifying patients' expectations and goals

One of the reasons why decision-making about breast reconstruction may be particularly difficult is that it is 'preference sensitive' (Lee *et al.* 2010) because the 'right choice' depends on each woman's personal preferences, including not wanting reconstruction. Therefore, clarifying each patient's motivations, preferences, and values is imperative, central to shared decision-making (Makoul and Clayman 2006) and a key aspect of patient-centred care. Being aware of each individual patient's pre-surgical expectations for reconstruction is paramount for health professionals who are supporting them through the decision-making and surgical processes; two women who have undergone apparently successful surgery with good wound healing (from an objective perspective, such as that of the surgical team) may have very different perceptions of their reconstructive result, depending on their pre-operative expectations.

Qualitative research (Snell *et al.* 2010) has explored women's expectations of implant-based reconstruction in terms of appearance, physical impact, and procedure and recovery, describing those that were not met as unclear, unrealistic, and unfulfilled. Our experience suggests that women who are dissatisfied with the outcome of reconstruction because their expectations were not met are likely to seek further, corrective surgery (with implications for resources and patient distress), and may maintain avoidance behaviours (e.g. intimacy, choice of clothing) that surgery was intended

to reduce. It is therefore feasible to surmise that if women have realistic expectations, then patient dissatisfaction, well-being, and requests for additional surgery could improve.

However, although health professionals need to ask women about their priorities and concerns (Lee *et al.* 2010), promote realistic expectations (Pusic *et al.* 2012; Snell *et al.* 2010), and support them making high-quality decisions by empowering them in shared decision-making, there is a dearth of interventions to help them elicit patients' values, expectations, and preferences. Instead, support typically focuses on information provision. However, increasing the amount of information available does not address erroneous expectations since it reinforces patients as passive recipients (Sherman *et al.* 2014) rather than actively engaged in setting clear, patient-centred goals (an approach associated with positive experiences and outcomes; Dept of Health 2010). Shared decision-making (defined as a collaborative process that allows patients and their providers to make healthcare decisions together, taking into account the best scientific evidence available, as well as the patient's values and preferences) has been heralded as a means of improving patient reported outcomes and satisfaction with cancer care, particularly concerning preference sensitive decisions. However, implementing shared decision-making processes is difficult and slow (Sivell *et al.* 2012).

Decision aids can help all patients faced with treatment decisions, particularly those who find decision-making very difficult, by decreasing decisional conflict and increasing satisfaction with the decision-making process. Some decision aids for mastectomy patients are available (see Caldon *et al.* 2010; Lam *et al.* 2013) but they are not breast reconstruction-specific or focused around a face-to-face discussion centred on patients' individual needs and the practicalities and possibilities of surgery, nor do they explicitly help health professionals and patients with the challenge of implementing shared decision-making in this difficult and emotive situation. For example, clinicians report concerns that the online decision aid BRESDEX.com cannot be tailored to patients' individual needs, and could replace nurses' roles and induce patient anxiety if not provided under clinical supervision (Caldon *et al.* 2010). The Breast Reconstruction Option Grid (www.optiongrid.org) is a brief tool to help patients compare the answers to questions that patients frequently ask clinicians about mastectomy, immediate and delayed reconstruction, typically used as the basis of a conversation within the surgical consultation. While the content of the option grid is evidence-based, the tool is purely a comparison of surgical outcomes by procedure type so includes no individual factors which have to be generated separately in order to produce a patient-centred decision.

In response to patients' increasing use of the internet when seeking information about reconstruction, Heller *et al.* (2008) developed an interactive education aid that included animated graphics, patient testimonials and pre-and-post-surgical photographs as a means of increasing women's knowledge about surgery in order to promote informed decision-making. Findings from a randomized controlled trial demonstrated greater knowledge of facts about reconstruction, lower levels of anxiety, and greater satisfaction post-operatively among those patients who received the interactive education aid rather than standard information. One of the benefits of interactive aids like this is that they can be used away from the clinical setting, at a time and place that suits the patient, and can be shared with family and friends who may be supporting her through the decision-making period. However, while this resource increased women's knowledge about reconstruction, it was an educational tool rather than a decision aid aimed at facilitating shared decision-making.

BRECONDA is a breast reconstruction-specific computer-based interactive decision aid (Sherman *et al.* 2014) that addresses both cognitions and effects associated with making a choice about surgery. It includes information about various options, an exercise to encourage women to clarify their own values, and information and support for partners. Interventions such as this and the education aid developed by Heller *et al.* (2008) could potentially be used by patients alongside other, more individual goal-directed interventions that facilitate shared decision-making within the clinic setting.

Recently, attention has shifted to decision coaching to facilitate patients' preparation for shared decision-making about preference sensitive decisions (Stacey *et al.* 2012). PEGASUS (Patients' Expectations and Goals: Assisting Shared Understanding of Surgery) is a new intervention that uses this approach to facilitate shared decision-making by helping patients and health professionals clarify each woman's motivations for reconstructive surgery by eliciting her own expectations of what she wants reconstruction to achieve, facilitate setting patient-centred goals, and aid discussion of both physical and psychosocial expectations, goals and outcomes with their surgical team (Harcourt *et al.* 2015). Unlike a purely paper-based intervention (e.g. Lam *et al.* 2013), PEGASUS involves a meeting with a decision coach (such as a specialist nurse or psychologist trained in its use) during which the patient elicits her individual breast reconstruction goals and what would indicate a successful outcome, and then rates the importance of each goal. She takes the completed PEGASUS sheet into the surgical consultation, where it is used to set shared goals and promote concordance between the patient and surgeon, so they approach surgery as a shared endeavour (in keeping with Stevenson *et al.* 2004). Feedback on the PEGASUS intervention from both patients and health professionals has been very positive, and highlighted the benefits that this approach offers in terms of helping patients be clear about their own goals and helping surgeons understand what the patient hopes surgery will achieve.

Interventions like PEGASUS that encourage patients to prepare for and actively engage in consultations effectively improve satisfaction and health outcomes (Gattellari *et al.* 2001). The PEGASUS intervention facilitates the disclosure and discussion of expectations, enabling the surgeon to decide the extent to which they are realistic and, if necessary, take appropriate steps to address unrealistic expectations (e.g. by explaining the likely outcomes further, showing more photographs, exploring the options for meeting other patients). Snell *et al.* (2010) urge clinicians to explore patients' pre-surgical expectations in order to increase post-surgical satisfaction, but this rarely happens, possibly because staff have not felt confident or supported in doing so. PEGASUS is a tool that can help health professionals in this respect.

Conclusion

The decision to undergo breast reconstruction can be difficult for women who are already dealing with a cancer diagnosis. Increasingly, the importance of health professionals understanding the psychosocial impact of mastectomy, being able to discuss body image, sexuality and intimacy, and being aware of each patient's individual expectations and goals is being recognized. New ways of supporting both patients who are faced with this choice and clinicians who are looking to provide the best evidence-based care are helping to understand patient expectations and facilitate shared decision-making within the surgical patient pathway, with the aim of improving patients' satisfaction with the outcome of reconstruction.

While this chapter has focused on breast reconstruction, we hope it is also of benefit to health professionals working with other groups of patients who are confronted by the option of different reconstructive surgical procedures. We encourage those with an interest in this area to consider other groups of reconstruction patients, such as those treated for head and neck cancer, when looking at ways of supporting them through these appearance-altering treatment decisions, and as an area for future research.

Case example

Margaret is a 57-year-old woman who identified a lump in her breast and has undergone a mastectomy within a short time of diagnosis. Although offered an immediate reconstruction of her breast, she has been very clear that she wishes to complete the treatment for her cancer and to consider her reconstructive options at a later date. She is referred for consideration of delayed reconstruction six months after her original surgery.

After being provided with written information about the different reconstructive options, Margaret meets with a psychologist using the PEGASUS approach to shared decision-making. At this appointment, the psychologist structures a conversation aimed at helping Margaret identify the priorities and outcomes that she hopes surgery will achieve for her. These include not only the physical changes in appearance, such as achieving symmetry of breast size, but the psychosocial goals that are associated with these outcomes. Margaret is clear that she would like to symmetrize her breasts with the psychosocial goals of avoiding the use of a prosthesis, wearing clothes that feel familiar and feeling confident in intimate situations. A second goal for Margaret is to maintain as much function in her arm with the goal of continuing to play regular tennis. Margaret also has a purely psychosocial goal in that she hopes to complete the reconstruction process as a means of modelling an effective coping response for breast cancer to her daughters, who are likely to be at risk for the condition.

A paper record form is used throughout the session and as each goal for physical change is elicited, it is recorded together with its related psychosocial outcome(s). Copies of this record are given to Margaret and added to her patient record. When she comes to meet her surgeon, he has the record form in front of him and he structures his own surgical consultation about the procedure in terms of Margaret's priorities and goals.

Margaret spontaneously comments that this session has been very helpful in assisting her to think through her reasons for seeking surgery and what she expects to change. Her surgeon reports that this approach helps him to be very clear about exactly what she is trying to get out of surgery and to think about it from her perspective, as well as a technical procedure.

References

Abu-Nab Z, Grunfeld EA (2007). Satisfaction with outcome and attitudes towards scarring among women undergoing breast reconstructive surgery. *Patient Educ Counsel* **66**, 243.

Al-Ghazal SK, Sully L, Fallowfield L, *et al.* (2000). The psychological impact of immediate rather than delayed breast reconstruction. *Eur J Surg Oncol* **26**, 17–19.

Benditte-Klepetko HC, Lutgendorff F, Kastenbauer T, Deutinger M, van der Horst CMAM (2014). Analysis of patient satisfaction and donor-site morbidity after different types of breast reconstruction. *Scand J Surg* **103**, 249–55.

Caldon LJM, Collins KA, Reed MW, *et al.* (2010). Clinicians' concerns about decision support interventions for patients facing breast cancer surgery options: understanding challenge of implementing shared decision making. *Health Expect* **14**, 133.

Chen JY, Malin J, Ganz PA, *et al.* (2009). Variation in physician-patient discussion of breast reconstruction. *J Gen Intern Med* **24**, 99–104.

Denford S, Harcourt D, Rubin L, Pusic A (2011). Understanding normality: a qualitative analysis of breast cancer patients' concepts of normality after mastectomy and reconstructive surgery. *Psychooncology* **20**, 553.

Department of Health (2010). *Equality and Excellence: Liberating the NHS.* Dept of Health, London, UK.

Fingeret MC, Nipomnick S, Guindani M, Baumann D, Hanasono M, Crosby M (2014). Body image screening for cancer patients undergoing reconstructive surgery. *Psychooncology* **23**, 898.

Gattellari M, Butow PN, Tattersall MHN (2001). Sharing decisions in cancer care. *Soc Sci Med* **52**, 1865–78.

Gopie JP, Timman R, Hilhorst MT, Hofer SOP, Mureau MAM, Tibben A (2013). The short-term psychological impact of complications after breast reconstruction. *Psychooncology* **22**, 290–8.

Harcourt D, Griffiths C, Baker E, Hansen E, White P, Clarke A (2015). The acceptability of pegasus: an intervention to facilitate patient-centred consultations and shared decision-making with women contemplating breast reconstruction. psychology, health and medicine. Available at: http://www.tandfonline.com/doi/full/10.1080/13548506.2015.1051059 [Online].

Harcourt D, Rumsey N (2004). Mastectomy patients' decision-making for or against immediate breast reconstruction. *Psychooncology* **13**, 106–15.

Harcourt D, Russell C, Hughes J, White P, Nduka C, Smith R (2011). Patient satisfaction in relation to nipple reconstruction: the importance of information provision. *J Plast Reconstr Aesthet Surg* **64**, 494.

Heller L, Parker PA, Youssef A, Miller ML (2008). Interactive digital education aid in breast reconstruction. *Plast Reconstr Surg* **122**, 717.

Lam WWT, Chan M, Or A, Kwong A, Suen D, Fielding R (2013). Reducing treatment decision conflict difficulties in breast cancer surgery: a randomized controlled trial. *J Clin Oncol* **31**, 2879–85.

Lee CN, Hultman CS, Sepucha K (2010). Do patients and providers agree about the most important facts and goals for breast reconstruction decisions?. *Ann Plast Surg* **64**, 563–6.

Makoul G, Clayman ML (2006). An integrative model of shared decision making in medical encounters. *Patient Educ Couns* **60**, 301–12.

National Mastectomy and Breast Reconstruction Audit (2011). 4th *Annual Report*. NHS Information Centre, Leeds, UK.

Pusic AL, Klassen AF, Scott AM, Klok JA, Cordeiro PG, Cano SJ (2009). Development of a new patient reported outcome measure for breast surgery: The BREAST-Q. *Plast Reconstr Surg* **124**, 345–53.

Pusic A, Klassen, AF, Snell L, *et al.* (2012). Measuring and managing patient expectations for breast reconstruction: impact on quality of life and patient satisfaction. *Expert Rev Pharmacoecon Outcomes Res* **12**, 149–58.

Rowland E, Metcalfe A (2014). A systematic review of men's experiences of their partner's mastectomy: coping with altered bodies. *Psychooncology* **23**, 963–74.

Sheehan J, Sherman KA, Lam T, Boyages J (2007). Association of information satisfaction, psychological distress and monitoring coping style with post-decision regret following breast reconstruction. *Psychooncology* **16**, 342–51.

Sherman KA, Harcourt DM, Lam TC, Shaw L-K, Boyages J (2014). BRECONDA: Development and acceptability of an interactive decisional support tool for women considering breast reconstruction. *Psychooncology* **23**, 835–8.

Sivell S, Edwards A, Manstead ASR, *et al.* (2012). Increasing readiness to decide and strengthening behavioral intentions: evaluating the impact of a web-based patient decision aid for breast cancer treatment options (BresDex: https://www.bresdex.com). *Patient Educ Counsel* **88**, 209–17.

Snell L, McCarthy C, Klassen A, *et al.* (2010). Clarifying the expectations of patients undergoing implant breast reconstruction: a qualitative study. *Plast Reconstr Surg* **126**, 1825–30.

Stacey D, Kryworuchko J, Bennett C, Murray MA, Mullan S, Legare F (2012). Decision coaching to prepare patients for making health decisions: a systematic review of decision coaching in trials of patient decision aids. *Med Decis Making* **32**, E22–33.

Stevenson FA, Cox K, Britten N, Dundar Y (2004). A systematic review of the research on communication between patients and health care professionals about medicines: the consequences for concordance. *Health Expect* **7**, 235–45.

CHAPTER 36

Discussing unproven therapies

Penelope Schofield and Michael Jefford

Introduction to discussing unproven therapies

The use of unproven therapies or complementary and alternative medicine (CAM) continues to evoke strong debate and diverse views within the medical community. Many doctors are concerned about the lack of scientifically credible research to support the claims of CAM proponents (ASCO 1997). However, a large and growing number of cancer patients use CAM (Eisenberg *et al.* 1998; Schofield *et al.* 2003; Flannery *et al.* 2006; Ge *et al.* 2013). Evidence indicates that clinicians neglect to appropriately discuss issues surrounding CAM use with their patients (Adler and Fosket 1999; Tasaki *et al.* 2002; Schofield *et al.* 2003; Juraskova *et al.* 2010). Improving CAM-related communication between clinicians and cancer patients has been widely advocated by researchers, medical practitioners, CAM practitioners, and patients (Eisenberg *et al.* 1998; Tasaki *et al.* 2000; Schofield *et al.* 2003; Juraskova *et al.* 2010; Ho *et al.* 2012; Koenig *et al.* 2012; Hunter *et al.* 2014; Lee *et al.* 2014).

CAM comprises a very heterogeneous group of practices, health systems, and products; used with different motivations and anticipated benefits, and ranging from promoting physical and psychological well-being to curing cancer. Hence, communication strategies will be influenced by each unique situation. While this complexity is challenging, assisting clinicians to initiate and engage patients in discussions about CAM is an essential contribution to improving health-related communication. Implications for improving the ways in which doctors discuss CAM use with their patients are wide-reaching, impacting directly upon the medical and psychological well-being of patients. This chapter presents a definition of CAM, the rationale supporting the need to improve communication about CAM, and evidence-informed guidelines about how to discuss CAM in a conventional oncology setting. The practical application of these guidelines is then described through the development and implementation of a communication skills workshop for health professionals.

Defining complementary and alternative medicines

Defining what constitutes CAM has been the subject of much debate. The US National Center for Complementary and Integrative Health (NCCIH) defines CAM as 'the array of health care approaches with a history of use or origins outside of mainstream medicine' (NCCIH 2015). What constitutes CAM changes continually as new CAMs are introduced and therapies with scientifically demonstrated safety and efficacy are integrated into conventional care (NCCIH 2015).

There are a number of different, but overlapping, terms that fall under the CAM umbrella:

◆ Complementary treatments are used together with conventional medicine. There may or may not be evidence of safety or effectiveness. The anticipated outcomes may be aimed at improving quality of life, reduced side effects, and/or survival benefits.

◆ Alternative medicine is used in place of conventional medicine. Often, the anticipated outcome is a benefit in survival. Unproven therapies usually refer to treatments that have not been rigorously tested for safety or efficacy.

◆ Integrative or integrated medicine combines CAM for which there is some high-quality evidence of safety and effectiveness with treatments from conventional medicine.

The need for improving communication about CAM

Many cancer clinicians struggle with discussions around CAM, which is perhaps not surprising given the complexity inherent in the area. Some cancer patients invest considerable amounts of time, money, and energy pursuing CAM with uncertain benefit, and which may even be harmful (MacLennan *et al.* 1996; Lowenthall 2005; Markovic *et al.* 2006). People with cancer rely on their doctors for information and guidance regarding treatment decisions (Degner and Sloan 1992). Physicians' knowledge of commonly used CAM has been found to be low in studies from the United States (Lee *et al.* 2014), Australia (Newell and Sanson-Fosher 2000), Canada (Bourgeault 1996), Israel (Giveon *et al.* 2003), and Italy (Crocetti *et al.* 1996). A US study found few physicians felt comfortable discussing CAM with patients, and the majority (84%) thought they needed to learn more about CAM to adequately address patient concerns (Corbin Winslow and Shapiro 2002). Another recent US study found that lack of knowledge and medical education about herbs/supplements and potential adverse reactions was a barrier to initiating discussions and answering patient questions about these CAMs (Lee *et al.* 2014).

Patients and clinicians do not routinely discuss CAM use (Begbie *et al.* 1996; Oldendick *et al.* 2000; Giveon *et al.* 2004; MacLennon *et al.* 2006; Hunter *et al.* 2014; Lee *et al.* 2014; Chang and Chang 2015). By analysing the audiotapes of 314 initial oncology consultations, Schofield and colleagues (Schofield *et al.* 2003) found CAM use was referred to in just 29% of consultations, with patients and kin initiating the bulk of these discussions. Moreover, approximately a third of patient-raised CAM references were ignored or glossed over by the doctor (Schofield *et al.* 2003). Another audio tape study by Juraskova and colleagues (Juraskova *et al.* 2010) found that CAM was discussed in 24% of initial oncology consultations, with patients initiating 73% of these conversations. Similar to previous work, 20% of the patient-initiated CAM comments were ignored by the treating oncologist. Clinicians may simply not know how to respond to questions about CAM, supporting the need for clear and accepted guidelines in this area. Compared to patients with cancer, oncologists are less likely to believe that CAM use may improve immunity, quality of life, cure disease, or prolong life (Richardson *et al.* 2004). These discrepant views are likely to contribute to the communication gap.

Guidelines for discussing complementary and alternative medicines in conventional oncology settings

The aim of these guidelines was to articulate a set of evidence-based recommendations to enable clinicians to have respectful, well-informed, and balanced discussion with patients about CAM. A systematic review of the relevant literature was conducted to develop the recommendations (Schofield *et al.* 2009). The recommendations for effectively discussing CAM in an oncology consultation are presented in Table 36.1.

Understand

Elicit the patient's understanding of their situation before asking about CAM use. This will provide the clinician with insights about the patient's perceptions of their situation, which will assist the clinician in responding to the issue of CAM use. Effective communication between health professional and patient assists coping, aids decision-making, and is the most effective protection against harmful CAM use. *Ask open questions with a psychological/existential focus to determine their concerns and goals.* Understanding an individual's concerns and hopes for the future assists understanding of the reasons underpinning interest in CAM.

Respect

Respect cultural and linguistic diversity and different belief systems. Attitudes towards conventional Western medicine and CAM may be influenced by a person's belief systems and their cultural background. Some people may believe that external forces, such as spirits, caused cancer. Others may blame themselves for getting cancer because of lifestyle factors, such as exercise, diet, stress, or even their thought patterns. It is a popular belief that changing lifestyle or thought patterns, particularly being positive, can influence survival. Patients are not necessarily looking for clinicians' belief in or endorsement of a particular CAM, but value characteristics such as open-mindedness, respect, and active listening.

Ask

Ask questions about CAM use often and at critical points in the illness trajectory. By asking about CAM, clinicians indicate that this is an acceptable topic of conversation. It is recommended that enquiries about CAM be part of routine initial history-taking, and again raised at critical times in the illness trajectory, such as the commencement of a new treatment regimen or after the diagnosis of recurrence. It is also important to consider CAM as a possible explanation for unusual side effects or test results.

Adopt an inquisitive, open-minded approach. Being judgemental or dismissive is likely to inhibit disclosure. Similarly, terms such as 'complementary', 'alternative', or 'unproven' can be considered value-laden, and may be interpreted differently by different patients, or may sound dismissive.

Explore

Explore details of CAM use and actively listen. Clinicians should ask direct, probing questions about their patients' CAM use, as well as follow-up questions to elicit motivations for pursuing, and expectations of, CAM use. It is critical that motivations and expectations are understood. Active listening facilitates accurate understanding to provide advice that supports patient choice and minimizes risk.

Provide balanced, evidence-based advice in relation to the CAM. It may be useful to describe the Western medical approach to acquiring and implementing research findings. Discussion may be needed to help some patients understand this process and outline how conventional therapies are evaluated, to allow a discussion about scientific evidence and unproven treatments.

Help respond to advice from family and friends. Patients may be recommended to pursue CAM by friends and family members, who may also offer anecdotal evidence of benefit. Patients may therefore need assistance from their health professional on how to respond to advice from family and friends.

Respond

Respond to the person's emotional state and express empathy. Given that the motives for using CAM often arise from the hope of a cure when either a cure is not possible, or in the setting of illness-related physical or emotional distress, it is important to explore the person's emotional state, and respond appropriately. Empathic comments are also helpful by illustrating interest and understanding of the person's situation.

Support the desire for hope and control. It appears that many people use CAM in an effort to gain hope and control. Research has found that patients with advanced disease who raised CAM with their oncologist linked CAM use with the desire to explore all possibilities of a cure, increase their survival time, or improve their quality of life. Offering to answer questions about CAM and being willing to personally talk to CAM practitioners, may support hope in this context.

Discuss

Discuss relevant concerns about the CAM while respecting the person's belief systems. It is important to indicate clearly throughout discussions that the patient will not be abandoned, even if the patient's beliefs regarding CAM differ from the clinician's own. If there are reasonable concerns that the CAM practitioner may be behaving unethically, it is important to explore this issue with the patient and suggest seeking more information about the practitioner.

Concerns may include:

Safety and efficacy. It may be advisable for the clinician to conduct an objective assessment of available evidence related to efficacy and safety. Then, discuss possible adverse effects (pharmacological or due to possible contaminants) and whether CAM may worsen the patient's condition, or interact with standard therapy.

Table 36.1 Recommended steps for effectively discussing CAM

Recommended step	Working with the patient	Example of question to ask
Understand	Elicit the patient's understanding of their situation and clarify their information preferences, before asking about CAM use	What is your understanding of things at this point? What have you been told about the test results?
	Ask open questions with a psychological/existential focus to determine their concerns and goals	What concerns you most about your illness? What are your hopes for the future?
Respect	Respect cultural and linguistic diversity and different belief systems	What do you believe might have caused your illness?
Ask	Ask questions about CAM use often and at crucial points in the illness trajectory	Are you currently doing or considering doing anything else for this condition/the side effects you're experiencing/your overall health or well-being?
	Adopt an inquisitive, open-minded approach, as appearing judgemental or dismissive will reduce disclosure	It's really important for me to know what other things you are doing to address your illness so I can help you in the best way possible
Explore	Explore details of CAM use and actively listen	Can you tell me more about <this CAM> please? What does it involve? How often do you use it? What are you hoping for from <this CAM>? Do you know if there has been any research done on the effects of <this CAM>?
	Provide balanced evidence-based advice in relation to the CAM	In Western medicine, a therapy is considered effective if a large group of patients who receive the therapy show an improvement compared with those who did not receive the therapy. It sounds like the effectiveness of <this CAM> is based on individual cases
	Help respond to advice from family and friends	Others want the best for you, let's talk about these suggestions What do you think of these suggestions?
Respond	Respond to the person's emotional state, and express empathy	This is a pretty tough time; I can understand you want to do everything possible
	Support the desire for hope and control	It's natural that you feel the need to explore all possible options to help you survive this disease; I fully support you in that
Discuss	Discuss relevant concerns about the CAM while respecting the patient's belief systems Concerns may include ◆ unknown effect and unknown quality; ◆ high financial or time cost; ◆ potential for psychological harm	Might the time involved prevent you from doing other things you would like to do? Is this cost going to cause financial hardship for you or your family? How do you think you might feel if you followed this advice but did not achieve the outcome you had hoped for?
	Discuss a trial period, what might be a reasonable timeframe to assess benefit/efficacy	How long would you expect it to take to see a benefit from <this CAM>?
Advise	Encourage use of CAM that may be beneficial and, if appropriate consider making a referral to a CAM practitioner	I'd encourage you to use <this CAM>; the evidence suggests it could really help you
	Accept use of CAM for which there is no evidence of physical harm or benefit. Support the patient's decision, even if it conflicts with your private view	We don't know much about <this CAM>. It doesn't seem to be harmful and it may even be helpful. I respect that's what you wish to do
	Discourage use of CAM where there is good evidence it will be unsafe or harmful	I respect and support your right to make this decision. However, as we have discussed I firmly believe that you have a better chance of a good outcome if you follow this treatment plan
	Balance advice with an acknowledgement of the patient's right for self-determination and autonomy	While there is little evidence for us to know if <this CAM> will be helpful, of course, the decision is yours, and I will support your right to choose
Summarize	Summarize main points of discussion, check their understanding, and for final questions. Provide evidence-based information sources	We have covered a lot today. Just so that I can check I've explained things properly, can you summarize what we have discussed? If you like I am happy to have a discussion with your <CAM provider>
Document	Document discussion in medical records	
Monitor	Follow-up discussion about CAM at the following consultation	

Financial, time, and psychological costs. Encourage patients to consider how much time, money, and hope they are willing to invest in the CAM. Even with CAM for which there is no evidence of physical harm, there may be potential psychological risks. Beliefs linking a positive thinking or fighting spirit and survival represent this type of risk. A patient who holds this belief and whose cancer advances, may feel at least partially responsible for their poor outcome (Giveon 2004). In the event of a patient forgoing conventional treatment, it is critical to discuss with patients the potential opportunity cost.

Discuss a trial period. For some CAM, close follow-up may be warranted, particularly if the CAM risks being potentially harmful. When CAM use commences, use of a symptom diary may help determine whether the therapy is beneficial or harmful, or has no effect for the individual patient.

Advise

It is reasonable to encourage or discourage the use of a particular CAM based on the relative risk or benefit that is likely to ensue.

Encourage. A number of therapies classed as CAM have been shown to be safe and efficacious and might reasonably be recommended. It may be appropriate to make a referral to a qualified CAM practitioner.

Accept use of CAM for which there is no good evidence of physical harm or benefit. Support the patient's decision, even if it conflicts with your private view.

Discourage. It is reasonable for clinicians to discourage treatment by unlicensed professionals, the injection of substances not approved by regulatory bodies, and any CAM that might delay or potentially impair conventional treatments with proven efficacy. If the patient is rejecting potentially curative treatment in favour of an unproven CAM, a short document—written and signed by the treating health professional and outlining the recommended conventional treatment options—could be offered. However, the health professional should avoid any implication of abandoning the patient.

Balance advice with an acknowledgement of the patient's right for self-determination and autonomy. A model of shared decision-making about CAM between physician and patient is recommended, with the physician providing information about the possible risks and benefits and the patient providing information about their values. Patients should be able to participate in decision-making according to their own preference for involvement.

Summarize

Summarize main points of discussion and check understanding. A summary is a useful way to ensure there are no misperceptions, and signals the end of the consultation. Refer patients to credible resources to get up-to-date, evidenced-based CAM information. Advice should be reiterated and, if there is reasonable evidence of potential for harm, reiterate concerns for the patient's safety.

Document

Document the discussion. A summary of the consultation should be documented in the patient's medical record. In addition, members of the person's broader treatment team should be informed about the discussion, especially if the CAM use is potentially harmful.

Monitor

Follow-up discussion about CAM at the next consultation. It is critical that any discussions about CAM, particularly use of potentially harmful CAM, is followed up in subsequent consultations.

How to structure learning

Intensive workshops combining facilitated discussions drawing on evidence-based communication research and clinical experience, and the use of role play with simulated patients and structured feedback, have been demonstrated to achieve the greatest learning gains. A recent randomized controlled trial tested a brief nursing education intervention intended to increase communication regarding CAM. The intervention comprised a 20-minute video and use of a laminated card to prompt discussions about CAM and resources. The low intensity and lack of role play in the intervention were identified as possible reasons that the intervention was successful in changing nurses' perceptions of their behaviour, but not actual behaviour as reported by their patients (Parker *et al.* 2013).

This section describes the intensive communication training module that we developed to teach effective communication about CAM in a conventional oncology setting. Modelling of behaviour and role play are central components of the training.

The Cancer Council Victoria (an Australian state-based cancer charity) through its Victorian Cancer Clinicians Communications Program (VCCCP) developed a workshop 'Effectively discussing complementary and alternative medicine with cancer patients, their families and friends' in collaboration with the National Breast and Ovarian Cancer Centre (now Cancer Australia) and the Peter MacCallum Cancer Centre. This training programme adds to a suite of communication skills training modules.

Format of the workshop

The format of the CAM workshop follows the standard VCCCP format. VCCCP implements evidence-based, small group, interactive workshops that promote active learning through role play. Workshops comprise a maximum of 10 participants, two trained health professional co-facilitators and a trained actor, playing the role of a patient. Participants are encouraged to consider the difficulties and challenges they encounter in clinical situations, share these issues in discussion, and work on them during the role play. A relaxed and secure environment is encouraged to allow participants to experiment with techniques and approaches they may not normally use. There are two facilitators: a psychosocial expert who is familiar with facilitation of small groups and relevant communication skills, and a clinical specialist who can discuss relevant clinical information.

In general, workshops run for four-and-a-half hours and commence with a short presentation on relevant research evidence, followed by a DVD modelling ideal communication, then a group discussion of the verbal and non-verbal skills displayed in the DVD. Evidence-based communication guidelines on the topic are then presented and compared to the group observations. The simulated 'patient' is then introduced to the group (an 'open chair' discussion between 'patient' and participants). A brief medical history of the 'patient' is provided and then each participant asks one question of the 'patient' to obtain a social history. Each learner then participates in a series of role plays with the simulated patient over 10 to 20 minutes. The role play is individually tailored to the participant's learning goals. Role plays can be stopped at any time by the participant who is encouraged to seek assistance from the group. Otherwise, role plays are stopped after three to four minutes by the facilitators, who then lead a constructive group discussion and seek suggestions for alternative strategies to be tried by the learner.

Actor training and setting up the scenario

VCCCP have a pool of professional actors who have undertaken both simulated patient training as well as module specific training. The actors are provided with a detailed case scenario including the illness narrative, detailed personal history, and characterization. For the CAM module, the actors were provided with information about the use of CAM in the cancer population and participated in an interactive discussion with a behavioural science researcher (PS), medical oncologist (MJ), and a cancer survivor who had used CAM during her treatment. This assists the actor to understand the feelings and emotions of a patient and motivations around CAM usage. To create the scenarios in the CAM workshop, we managed the complexity inherent in a CAM discussion by using three strategies. First, each of the participants were surveyed prior to the workshop to determine under what circumstances they have CAM discussions, what were common challenges or difficulties, and what were their learning goals for the workshop. We also enquired about learning objectives at the beginning of the workshop. Second, we limited the range of patient and CAM variation. We specified a particular time in the patient's illness trajectory (advanced, incurable cancer, having chemotherapy with palliative intent), and limited

possible CAM use to four—a highly restrictive diet; Reiki, microwave therapy, and use of high-dose vitamin C. These were chosen as they allowed us to quite quickly create scenarios that incorporated a great range of challenges in communication around CAM. Third, the facilitators and actor met prior to the workshop to tailor and practice the pre-arranged scenarios to meet the learner's needs and ensure that all scenarios felt realistic.

Developing a DVD and workshop manuals

Based upon the above guidelines and other communication recommendations, workshop manuals for both facilitators and participants were developed that support implementation of this workshop and to act as an ongoing resource for participants. The facilitator's manual provides all of the necessary tools and materials (including PowerPoint slides) for facilitators to run an interactive workshop effectively and includes a suggested workshop outline that can be adjusted to reflect their personal style or participant needs. A DVD was also created to complement the workshop. Two scenes were devised and scripts were drafted drawing on the recommended guidelines articulated in 'Guidelines for discussing complementary and alternative medicines in conventional oncology settings' section this chapter. The first scene focuses on a patient taking multivitamins and herbal preparations while having neoadjuvant (pre-operative) chemoradiation for curable rectal cancer. The second scene involves the same patient four years later. The patient now has advanced incurable disease and is contemplating a range of CAM therapies while also considering palliative chemotherapy. Table 36.2 displays the dialogue for the second scene and links the doctor's responses to the recommended guidelines.

Table 36.2 A discussion between a medical oncologist and a patient about complementary and alternative medicine: Script for a DVD scene

Character	Dialogue	Recommendation addressed
BARRY	So let me get this straight, the most you can guarantee with the chemo is 24 months, assuming all goes well.	
MEDONC	Twenty-four is an average. Around 50% of people will live longer than that; some for many years. I have one patient who was in a very similar situation to you still coming in to see me three years down the track.	Supporting hope
BARRY	OK, and the other 50%?	
MEDONC	Yes, could be less as well. It's not a lot, I know.	Empathy
BARRY	No. I need to do everything I can. There are some other things I'm considering as well. There's an interstate clinic that offers a range of treatments. I want to hit it from every angle.	
MEDONC	I can understand that. Can I ask, what sorts of things are they offering?	Ask about CAM
BARRY	I haven't brought the papers in … ozone treatment I think, Hoxsey diet, some sort of hyperthermia or something—as you people say, a real cocktail. Have you heard of them?	
MEDONC	I've heard of some of them. What are you hoping these treatments will offer you?	Explore expected outcome
BARRY	More time, 24 months isn't much. On their website they say some people have lived for years and years. Look, they're not being irresponsible and promising cure, but there are lots of satisfied customers, and I wouldn't mind being one of them. I thought that maybe I should do this before the chemo. What do you think?	
MEDONC	Well I'm not an expert on these treatments but your question is a really important one and I can understand you'd want to look into every option possible. It would be good to talk a little about what they are offering, and how they work. What do you know about the treatments, for example, what do they involve?	Open, inquisitive approach, and exploring details

(continued)

Table 36.2 (continued)

Character	Dialogue	Recommendation addressed
BARRY	It'd involve me going up there for three or four months—I'd stay with my son. I think it's pretty intensive, daily treatment, so I don't think I'd be able to have chemo at the same time—so I'm wondering about maybe chemo before or after?	
MEDONC	It sounds to me that if you started this you wouldn't be able to start chemo for three to four months?	Active listening
BARRY	That's right.	
MEDONC	I'd be really reluctant for you go interstate for three or four months and delay having the chemotherapy, which has good evidence behind it. If these other treatments don't work, your health may in fact deteriorate over the next three or four months, and your body might not be able to tolerate the chemotherapy if that happens. The chemotherapy is based on many international studies that involve thousands of people. That means we can be confident in knowing that the chemo is the best available treatment we can offer.	Discuss concerns and provide evidence-based advice
MEDONC	What do you know about these other treatments? Have they been studied in the same way, or are they basing outcomes on individual cases?	Explore evidence underpinning CAM
BARRY	To be honest I don't know … My son's been badgering me. He really thinks I should try this first.	
MEDONC	I'm sure he wants the best for you. However my concern is that we don't know much about the chances of these treatments working for you.	Discuss concerns
BARRY	Hmm. Maybe I should look into it more closely.	
MEDONC	Could you bring any information in to our next appointment? We could look at it together. I'm also wondering how much this treatment is going to cost.	Explore cost of CAM
BARRY	I don't know, I'm not particularly concerned about the money, but I'm not going to throw it at nothing—I could be spending my time in the Bahamas!	
MEDONC	That raises issues about how you want to be spending your time. I think this is something else that needs to be weighed up.	Discuss concerns
BARRY	Yeah, there's a lot for me to think about, and I don't want to miss out on the chemo but I really like the sound of these other treatments.	
MEDONC	When you bring in the information at the next appointment, do you want to see if your wife and son can come along and anyone else that you would like?	Revisit and monitor
BARRY	I know that Barbara would probably like that. I'll see.	
MEDONC	OK great. Of course the decision is ultimately yours and I understand that you need to explore all options, but I'd like to be sure that you understand I do have some serious concerns about the evidence behind these treatments, their side effects, and that it may delay the chemotherapy. We need to look at this closely to make sure you're making the right decision. Ultimately I'll support you whatever you decide.	Balanced advice acknowledging patients right for self-determination
BARRY	Thanks, sure.	
MEDONC	There are a number of good websites and written resources you might be interested in. Can I give you some written information to take away?	Provide evidence-based information sources
BARRY	Yes, thanks. *medical oncologist hands the literature*	
MEDONC	Barry we've covered a lot today. Do you have any other questions or is there anything else you'd like to discuss?	Check for final questions
BARRY	No. I don't think so. I just want to get the best outcome. What you've said makes sense but I guess I need to think about it.	

Reproduced with kind permission from Penelope Schofield.

Barry was a 65-year-old married man when he first experienced symptoms of bleeding from the bowel, four years ago. His general practitioner organized a colonoscopy, which showed that Barry had a rectal cancer. Barry was advised to have neoadjuvant (pre-operative) chemoradiation followed by surgery. He completed this treatment and a further four months of post-operative adjuvant chemotherapy. He was well for the subsequent three and a half years, but has recently been diagnosed with advanced, incurable disease. He has been told that the average (median) survival for people in this circumstance is about 20 months. He is thinking about pursuing alternative treatments, but also wishes to try conventional chemotherapy, that he has been told has a very good chance of improving his survival, though cannot cure his disease.

Acknowledgements

Justine Diggens, Sue Hegarty, Catherine Charleson, Rita Marigliani, and Caroline Nehill contributed to the previous version of this chapter. Hilary Schofield assisted in the references. Professor Ron Epstein, University of Rochester, provided invaluable comments on earlier drafts of the recommendations. Pam MacLean Communication Centre assisted in the development of the script.

References

Adler SR, Fosket JR (1999). Disclosing complementary and alternative medicine use in the medical encounter: a qualitative study in women with breast cancer. *J Fam Pract* **48**, 453–8.

ASCO (1997). The physician and unorthodox cancer therapies. *J Clin Oncol* **15**, 401–6.

Begbie SD, Kerestes ZL, Bell DR (1996). Patterns of alternative medicine use by cancer patients. *Med J Aust* **165**, 545–8.

Bourgeault IL (1996). Physicians' attitudes toward patients' use of alternative cancer therapies. *CMAJ* **155**, 1679–85.

Chang HY, Chang HL (2015). A review of nurses' knowledge, attitudes, and ability to communicate the risks and benefits of complementary and alternative medicine. *J Clin Nurs* **24**, 1466–7.

Corbin Winslow L, Shapiro H (2002). Physicians want education about complementary and alternative medicine to enhance communication with their patients. *Arch Intern Med* **162**, 1176–81.

Crocetti E, Crotti N, Montella M, Musso M (1996). Complementary medicine and oncologists' attitudes: a survey in Italy. *Tumori* **82**, 539–42.

Degner L, Sloan JA (1992). Decision making during serious illness: what role do patients really want to play? *J Clin Epidemiol* **45**, 941–50.

Eisenberg DM, Davis RB, Ettner SL, *et al.* (1998). Trends in alternative medicine use in the United States, 1990–1997: results of a follow-up national survey. *JAMA* **280**, 1569–75.

Flannery M, Love M, Pearce K, Luan J, Elder W (2006). Communication about complementary and alternative medicine: Perspectives of primary care clinicians. *Altern Ther Health Med* **12**, 56–62.

Ge J, Fishman J, Vapiwala N, *et al.* (2013). Patient-physician communication about complementary and alternative medicine in a radiation oncology setting. *Int J Radiat Oncol Biol Phys* **85**, 1–6.

Giveon SM, Liberman N, Klang S, Kahan E (2003). A survey of primary care physicians' perceptions of their patients' use of complementary medicine. *Complement Ther Med* **11**, 254–60.

Giveon SM, Liberman N, Klang S, Kahan E (2004). Are people who use "natural drugs" aware of their potentially harmful side effects and reporting to family physician? *Patient Educ Couns* **53**, 5–11.

Ho EY, D'Agostino TA, Yadegar V, Burke A, Bylund CL (2012). Teaching patients how to talk with biomedical providers about their complementary and alternative medicine use. *Patient Educ Couns* **89**, 405–10.

Hunter D, Oates R, Gawthrop J, Bishop M, Gill S (2014). Complementary and alternative medicine use and disclosure amongst Australian radiotherapy patients. *Support Care Cancer* **22**, 1571–8.

Juraskova I, Hegedus L, Butow P, Smith A, Schofield P (2010). Discussing complementary therapy use with early-stage breast cancer patients: exploring the communication gap. *Integr Cancer Ther* **9**, 168–76.

Koenig CJ, Ho EY, Yadegar V, Tarn DM (2012). Negotiating complementary and alternative medicine use in primary care visits with older patients. *Patient Educ Couns* **89**, 368–73.

Lee RT, Barbo A, Lopez G, *et al.* (2014). National survey of US oncologists' knowledge, attitudes, and practice patterns regarding herb and supplement use by patients with cancer. *J Clin Oncol* **32**, 4095–101.

Lowenthal R (2005). Public illness: How the community recommended complementary and alternative medicine for a prominent politician with cancer. *Med J Aust* **183**, 576–9.

MacLennan AH, Myers SP, Taylor AW (2006). The continuing use of complementary and alternative medicine in South Australia: costs and beliefs in 2004. *Med J Aust* **184**, 27–31.

MacLennan AH, Wilson DH, Taylor AW (1996). Prevalence and cost of alternative medicine in Australia. *Lancet* **347**, 569–73.

Markovic M, Manderson L, Wray N, Quinn M (2006). Complementary medicine use by Australian women with gynaecological cancer. *Psychooncology* **15**, 209–20.

NCCIH (2015). Time to talk: Ask your patients about their use of complementary and alternative medicine. Available at: https://nccih.nih.gov/timetotalk

Newell S, Sanson-Fisher RW (2000). Australian oncologists' self-reported knowledge and attitudes about non-traditional therapies used by cancer patients. *Med J Aust* **172**, 110–13.

Oldendick R, Coker AL, Wieland D, *et al.* (2000). Population-based survey of complementary and alternative medicine usage, patient satisfaction, and physician involvement. South Carolina Complementary Medicine Program Baseline Research Team. *South Med J* **93**, 375–81.

Parker PA, Urbauer D, Fisch MJ, *et al.* (2013). A multisite, community oncology-based randomized trial of a brief educational intervention to increase communication regarding complementary and alternative medicine. *Cancer* **119**, 3514–22.

Richardson MA, Masse LC, Nanny K, Sanders C (2004). Discrepant views of oncologists and cancer patients on complementary/alternative medicine. *Support Care Cancer* **12**, 797–804.

Schofield P, Diggens, J, Charleson, C, Marigliani, R, Jefford M (2009). Effectively discussing complementary and alternative medicine in a conventional oncology setting. *Patient Educ Couns* **79**, 143–51.

Schofield PE, Juraskova I, Butow PN (2003). How oncologists discuss complementary therapy use with their patients: an audio-tape audit. *Support Care Cancer* **11**, 348–55.

Tasaki K, Maskarinec G, Shumay DM, Tatsumura Y, Kakai H (2002). Communication between physicians and cancer patients about complementary and alternative medicine: exploring patients' perspectives'. *Psychooncology* **11**, 212–20.

CHAPTER 37

Promoting treatment adherence

Kelly B. Haskard-Zolnierek, Tricia A. Miller, and M. Robin DiMatteo

Introduction to treatment adherence

Patient adherence (also referred to as compliance or concordance) represents the extent to which a patient follows through with the medical recommendations of the healthcare provider. The recommended regimen may involve medications, screenings, appointment attendance, dietary change, and/or other lifestyle changes. Persistence refers to following a course of treatment for the entire period of time it is prescribed. In cancer treatment, adherence may, for example, be required in the context of adjuvant hormone or targeted therapy, chemotherapy, or radiation appointment attendance, follow-up screening attendance, and/or dietary or exercise change. Although adherence has important documented effects on cancer outcomes, many factors influence whether or not patients adhere. This chapter describes the following:

◆ the value of adherence, as well as the reasons why adherence may be challenging for patients;

◆ the significance of providers' recognition of their patients' non-adherence, and their open communication and partnership to help their patients achieve adherence; and

◆ the process of communication that facilitates adherence.

We also explain specific strategies within healthcare provider–patient communication that can promote adherence.

Rates of adherence

Meta-analytic research finds that across medical conditions and regimens, the average rate of patient adherence is approximately 75%; thus, a quarter of all patients, on average, do not follow through with their treatment recommendations (DiMatteo 2004b). Across studies of different types of cancer, medication adherence to oral chemotherapy can be as high as 80% (van Dulmen et al. 2007). Rates of non-adherence to endocrine treatment for breast cancer have been found to range from 20 to 40%, depending on the setting (focusing on adherence and persistence over four or more years of treatment (Chlebowski and Geller 2006)). Findings on adjuvant chemotherapy for lung cancer patients demonstrate that only about 50% of patients follow through with all recommended cycles of chemotherapy (Alam et al. 2005). Studies of adjuvant chemotherapy treatment for colon cancer show approximately 78% adherence (Dobie et al. 2006).

Outcomes of non-adherence

Non-adherence may have negative effects on patients' health outcomes. The literature identifies major consequences of non-adherence to patients' health status and clinical outcomes, including poor symptom control, and/or disease recurrence. Non-adherence with treatment has also been associated with shortened survival time (DiMatteo et al. 2012). Patient non-adherence may also involve financial consequences, through unused prescriptions or unnecessary hospitalizations, and may reduce the trust between physicians and their patients.

In addition, outcomes are affected when patients neglect to regularly attend scheduled appointments, such as for chemotherapy or radiation treatments. Research on colon cancer has shown increased risk of mortality when patients fail to complete treatment (Dobie et al. 2006). Certain levels of adherence may be necessary for achievement of better outcomes, such as in early stage breast cancer care, where patients who are more than 80% adherent to their adjuvant aromatase inhibitor medication regimen have significantly better outcomes than those with lower rates of adherence (Partridge et al. 2008).

Barriers to adherence in cancer

Successful patient adherence to the complex treatment regimens associated with cancer may be influenced by numerous factors. Many aspects of the patient's life that predict his or her adherence behaviours have been discussed extensively in the theoretical and empirical adherence literature. Some barriers to adherence can indicate intentional non-adherence, whereas others may be unintentional. Intentional non-adherence in the context of cancer, for example, could result from a patient's non-persistence with adjuvant medication treatment, due to serious side effects in order to prevent recurrence and increase chances for survival. A patient might also purposely miss follow-up appointments, or take incomplete doses of a medication because they feel asymptomatic or do not believe in the purpose of the treatment. Unintentional non-adherence, on the other hand, involves misunderstanding the details of the regimen (e.g. timing or dosing), or forgetting to follow through because of personal reasons or interferences with one's lifestyle.

Patient factors

A simple model of predictors of adherence

A complete explanatory model of adherence to treatment does not exist, and many predictors have been offered in the research literature. A useful model involving three broad categories of factors provides a framework for understanding patient non-adherence. This model is known as the Information-Motivation-Strategy model of adherence (DiMatteo *et al.* 2012). This model describes, respectively, the cognitive, motivational, and resource-related factors that influence adherence

Information

A crucial factor in determining patients' adherence is their understanding of the treatment. In the process of cancer care, patients must usually process extensive information about their disease and accompanying treatments, including following a medication-taking schedule, managing side effects, the necessity of regular screenings, and how to follow a health-promoting diet and exercise regimen. Many patients have trouble remembering what they have been told by their physicians, and depressed or anxious states may particularly increase the chance of forgetting.

Motivation

Patients also must be motivated to adhere. Patients' beliefs, attitudes, and perceptions all factor into improving motivation. Patients with greater self-efficacy about their ability to discuss treatment options with their healthcare providers are more adherent (Demissie *et al.* 2001). Other research indicates that discontinuation of tamoxifen is associated with patient beliefs that the costs of treatment outweigh the benefits (Lash *et al.* 2006). Patients who seek support and information, actively solve problems, and express concerns regarding their illness and treatment directives may be more motivated to adhere, compared to patients who avoid the challenges of treatment management.

Strategy

Possessing adequate resources (e.g. monetary, time, and access to medical care) can be critical to adherence. Patients might miss appointments because of work or family commitments, for example. Social support plays a role; patients who have less tangible and emotional support and have less cohesive families are at greater risk of non-adherence (DiMatteo 2004*a*). Adherence may be promoted by strong social networks, which may somehow affect physiological processes. Research has indicated that greater social support is associated with better adherence to chemotherapy treatment for colon cancer (Dobie *et al.* 2006).

Mental health

Adherence, and each of the patient-related predictors listed above, can also be affected by 'distressed psychological states', such as depression, anxiety, or stress, which can accompany serious illnesses such as cancer. Other emotional reactions such as guilt, fear, anxiety, stress, pain, lowered quality of life, and fatigue can also predict non-adherence. Emotional distress can decrease adherence to methods for cancer detection. For example, colon cancer screening and mammography utilization occur significantly less often in distressed older adults than in their non-distressed counterparts (Thorpe *et al.* 2006). Psychological distress can also influence lifestyle factors such as diet, exercise, and sleep.

Severity of disease

Although separate from the three-factor model of adherence predictors listed above, severity of disease may also influence adherence. A meta-analysis reported that in more serious diseases, including cancer, patients who reported poorer health were significantly less likely to adhere to treatment (DiMatteo *et al.* 2007). According to objective measures of disease severity (e.g. blood pressure), in less serious diseases (e.g. hypertension), patients in poorer health were more likely to be adherent. However, in more serious diseases such as cancer, patients who were objectively more seriously ill (such as those with later stages of the disease, or who had a serious abnormality) were less likely to be adherent to their regimens (DiMatteo *et al.* 2007). These findings suggest that the difficulties faced by the most severely ill cancer patients may interfere with their adherence for a myriad of reasons, including their doubts about the efficacy of treatment, or their struggles with the demands of the disease.

Interaction-level or regimen factors

Treatment side effects

Non-adherence may occur when the regimen is particularly complex or when side effects are severe. For cancer patients, managing oral chemotherapy side effects can be particularly challenging; problems with side effects can contribute to discontinuation of the treatment regimen before it is completed and can lead to problems with patient autonomy (Regnier Denois *et al.* 2011). In breast cancer, for example, adjuvant therapy can be accompanied by side effects such as hot flashes and joint pain (Cella and Fallowfield 2007). For the treatment of many cancers, patients must regularly attend radiation therapy appointments, which can be physically and mentally exhausting and attended by negative side effects. Patients in partnership with their doctors may make a decision to not begin, postpone, or to discontinue treatment prematurely because of the negative effects on quality of life.

Communication and interactional dynamics

Effective physician–patient communication can improve adherence and health outcomes (Zolnierek and DiMatteo 2009) (see Box 37.1 for essential physician healthcare provider adherence-related communication skills). Some research, for instance, has shown that more physician support and more shared decision-making increase adherence (Kahn *et al.* 2007). Furthermore, patients have an increased likelihood of adherence to breast and cervical cancer screening recommendations when their healthcare providers promote it (Castellano *et al.* 2001). Research on cancer screening in a sample of low-income women found that one predictor of following screening recommendations was a longer, more positive relationship with a healthcare provider (O'Malley *et al.* 2002). A survey of oncology healthcare providers indicated that more than 85% believed effective communication improved patient adherence (Roberts *et al.* 2005). Unfortunately, trusting, collaborative communication does not always transpire. A study of oncologist–patient communication about adjuvant hormonal therapy for breast cancer revealed that many issues related to medication-taking, challenges with adherence, and struggles in regimen persistence were not ever discussed by physicians with their patients (Davidson *et al.* 2007). Reducing the interaction-level barriers to patient adherence requires recognizing the importance of a trusting physician–patient relationship to ensure the efficient transfer of medical information. Improving the interaction involves building provider–patient partnerships, concentrating on the patient's quality of life, and addressing the specific barriers that patients may face.

Box 37.1 Essential physician/healthcare provider adherence-related communication techniques and examples

1. Work with patients to understand their treatments and how to follow them.

   - Use the 'teach-back method' to clarify the patient's understanding of the details of the regimen (Cartwright *et al.* 2014) For example: 'Can you repeat back to me how you will take this medication so we can be sure that I have explained it clearly?'

   - Invite the patient to ask questions. For example: 'I hope you will ask me any questions you have about the treatment process during our visit.'

   - Provide patients with written information. For example: 'You may find it helpful to use this checklist, and as we talk you can check off any relevant issues (side effects, strategies to deal with them, etc.) that may concern you. Then before you leave today, we will provide you with some written materials related to those items.'

2. Motivate patients to believe in the treatment, and want to adhere to it.

   - Explain the relationship between adherence and outcomes. For example: 'The evidence from the studies that have been conducted shows that when patients take this medication for five years, the chances of recurrence are reduced.'

   - Discuss the risks and benefits of treatment as well as alternative treatment options. For example: 'As with any treatment, there may be some side effects, but the long-term benefits may outweigh those.' 'It seems you're concerned this might not be the best treatment for you. Why don't we discuss your concerns, as well as alternative options?'

   - Encourage problem-focused and proactive coping. For example: 'Many patients have difficulty remembering to take their medication at the same time every day. Let's list some things that may help you to remember so that we can plan for the possibility of forgetting to take your medication before it happens.'

   - Promote positive expectations about the outcomes of treatment. For example: 'I am hoping for a very good outcome, and I feel confident that your following the treatment exactly as recommended will very much improve your health.'

3. Recognize barriers to adherence and help patients follow treatment. Focus on the following:

   - The patient's views about the challenges of the regimen. For example: 'I know that it will be a change to fit the radiation appointments into your schedule each week but I believe it is very important for your health. Perhaps you can think of this as a significant way that you are taking care of yourself.'

   - The patient's support network and building social support. For example: 'How has your husband responded to your diagnosis?' 'Have you considered joining a support group so that you can talk with other women who are having similar experiences?'

   - The patient's mental health. For example: 'Tell me about how your moods have been. Sometimes when patients are feeling down or depressed, they have difficulty taking their medication as prescribed for a number of different reasons. Let's discuss some of the ways you might handle that.'

   - Available resources. For example: 'Do you have a way to get to and from the pharmacy to pick up your chemotherapy medications?'

   - Helpful reminder methods. For example: 'It can be quite helpful to put your medication next to the coffee pot or tea kettle. Then you remember to take it every morning when you have your cup of coffee or tea.'

Effective communication as a route to promotion of adherence

Overview

Effective communication in the medical visit involves both verbal and non-verbal communication, including voice tone, eye contact, facial expressions, use of touch, gestures, and body orientation or 'synchrony'. Effective communication focuses on affective elements of care, as well as the tasks of the medical visit, such as information transfer. Particularly in the context of treatment of a serious illness such as cancer, communication is more critical, as it involves delivering bad news, making major decisions about treatment, discussing participation in clinical trials, navigating communication with family members, and developing physician–patient rapport. Communication about adherence itself can be challenging, but is particularly important because of the implications for patient outcomes. Healthcare professionals may not know their patients are non-adherent, or may be unaware of barriers to adherence in

their patient's life. Thus, provider–patient communication requires openness about expectations of treatment, support in handling the challenges of adherence, and assistance with effective strategies to improve adherence. Discussions focused on reducing barriers to adherence should not involve blaming the patient but should instead foster opportunities and encouragement for the open exchange of information and building a partnership to improve patients' adherence, health outcomes, and quality of life.

One of the most important steps to achieving adherence involves the development of rapport, in a trusting partnership. Open communication and establishing goals and desired outcomes are essential to promoting adherence. From the first visit, a collaborative relationship between provider and patient must be developed and then strengthened over future visits, throughout the course of illness and treatment. Showing empathy involves understanding the patient's perspective of living with illness, as well as clearly expressing that understanding to the patient. This empathic behaviour and understanding should also extend towards the difficulties of disease management and medication-taking. Healthcare providers should also actively seek to understand coping with the challenges of adherence from the patient's perspective.

It is important that oncology healthcare providers and their patients communicate effectively and discuss openly their perceptions of the intended treatment plan. One study found that physicians and cancer patients reported differences in whether or not there was even discussion of how treatment would affect the patient's quality of life (Meropol et al. 2003). However, in this same study, patients self-reported that this was one of the most important topics that they wanted to discuss with their physicians. Providers' failure to discuss the negative effects of medication-taking on patients' quality of life can significantly decrease adherence to treatment (Meropol et al. 2003).

Exchange of information

Patients differ in the amount of information they want to receive, and physicians also fluctuate in how much information they actually give. Information is a form of social support that can give cancer patients knowledge about their disease, and thus increases in knowledge could potentially increase adherence behaviours. Communication that is initiated by physicians, where there is discussion of patients' specific disease and treatment, both can establish and promote patients' beliefs and confidence that they have treatment options, and may also improve their satisfaction with the provided care. When providing information to increase patient adherence, physicians should avoid using excessive medical jargon and instead provide important information in written form, and actively confirm complete comprehension of information, to be sure that their patients understand.

Partnership, involvement, and shared decision-making

Although patients may vary in their interest in being involved in decision-making, many patients do value and want to be involved in the process of their medical decision-making. If patients are not encouraged to be active participants in their medical care, their rates of adherence may suffer, as shown in one study of adherence to tamoxifen (Kahn et al. 2007). Achieving concordance in the management of medication regimens in cancer involves understanding what is important to patients, acknowledging the importance of quality of life, keeping track of symptoms, and communicating with all members of the healthcare team (Chewning and Wiederholt 2003). Shared decision-making occurs when both physicians and their patients work together in partnership towards a treatment plan that is most conducive to the patient's lifestyle.

Communication about patient's emotional state and resources

Patients' mental health can be a barrier to adherence. Understanding and memory, motivation and attitudes, and social support and resources can all be negatively affected by poor mental health. Patient mental health can influence adherence. Thus, it is important for physicians and healthcare providers to be aware of, and ask about, symptoms and behaviours that may indicate a patient is battling depression or anxiety (see Box 37.2).

It is also important to discuss resources, including the financial aspects of treatment, and the availability of instrumental and emotional support from loved ones. Both types of resources, social

---

Box 37.2 Clinical case

Jane Smith is a 35-year-old woman with early stage oestrogen receptor-positive breast cancer. She is a single parent to two daughters, Lily (who is five) and Lauren (who is eight). Jane owns a small web design business, which she runs from her own home office. Jane had a lumpectomy and radiation therapy; her oncologist is now recommending adjuvant hormonal therapy to prevent recurrence of her cancer. Jane is hesitant to begin adjuvant hormonal therapy because of what she has heard about the side effects associated with the recommended medication and the commitment to a five-year medication treatment plan. Jane worries about how the medication side effects will negatively interfere with her life; particularly, in the care of her daughters given that they are so young and need her attention. Jane also worries that the medication side effects will inhibit her from working and running her business. Jane often doubts that the benefits of this new recommended treatment would outweigh the drawbacks. Additionally, since her diagnosis, Jane has been struggling with depression and feels that she doesn't have anyone to turn to for practical or emotional support.

In efforts to make Jane feel more comfortable, her oncologist sits down with her to discuss the efficacy of the medication and its relationship to the outcomes of her cancer. The oncologist discusses the likelihood of various potential side effects and some strategies to cope with them and reduce their severity if they do occur. Together they also go over ways to fit the medication schedule into her busy lifestyle and about memory aids (e.g. medication journal or smartphone applications) to help remind her when a dose should be taken. Jane's oncologist also recognizes her psychological state and recommends that she seek professional counselling, suggesting that it might be helpful to have someone to talk with given everything she has been through.

---

and economic, can make a difference in a patient's willingness and capacity for following through with recommended treatments.

Communication and the healthcare team

All members of the patient's healthcare team have a potential role to play in communicating about adherence. Most empirical research on this topic has focused on physicians, although nurses, pharmacists, and other healthcare team members also have important opportunities to answer patients' questions, give information, and counsel patients about adherence. Nurses, for example, are often primarily involved in patients' follow-up communication after surgery.

Strategies to improve memory and simplify medication-taking

Problems understanding and remembering medication regimens can negatively affect adherence; thus, memory aids (e.g. reminders, cues, lists, calendars, pillboxes, timers, smartphone applications, etc.) can play a crucial part in helping patients to remember to take their medications properly. Healthcare providers can recommend such tools to their patients and can also be involved in providing appointment reminders, for example, via email, text message, or phone call. In practice, of course, it can be challenging to assist large numbers of patients with the support and reminders that are needed to help them adhere; new technologies can make this more feasible. For example, one innovative study involved the development of a computer database tracking system for cervical and colon cancer screening (Bock and Kwan 2007). The database kept track of lab results, produced letters to patients informing them of their results, and sent appointment reminders; this system resulted in significant increases in screening.

Interventions to improve communication about adherence

Effective communication may not be easy, but it is a trainable skill; intervention studies show that training in communication skills can make a difference. Skills such as information giving and active listening can be enhanced, and the positive effects of training can persist over time (Fallowfield *et al.* 2003). A meta-analysis examining 21 studies of patient adherence as an outcome of physician communication skills training interventions reported a positive significant effect on adherence across all studies (Zolnierek and DiMatteo 2009).

Conclusion

Improving provider–patient communication and reducing patient barriers are significant steps towards improving cancer patient adherence. Research on specific communicative behaviours in oncology and their relationship to adherence is somewhat lacking. There is a need for more specific research focused on describing the communication behaviours that are most beneficial to adherence. Follow-up research should then assess the design of interventions to improve those behaviours. In practice, healthcare providers can help patients improve adherence by communicating openly, sharing in decision-making about treatment, and being aware of the challenges associated with adherence. Developing a trusting therapeutic relationship focused on fitting a treatment regimen into a patient's life is a key to promoting adherence in cancer patients.

References

Alam N, Shepherd FA, Winton T, *et al.* (2005). Compliance with post-operative adjuvant chemotherapy in non-small cell lung cancer. An analysis of National Cancer Institute of Canada and intergroup trial JBR.10 and a review of the literature. *Lung Cancer* **47**, 385–94.

Bock GW, Kwan BM (2007). Encouragement of patient self-management and adherence through use of a computerized tracking system for cervical and colon cancer screening. *J Am Board Fam Med* **20**, 316–19.

Cartwright LA, Dumenci L, Siminoff LA, Matsuyama RK (2014). Cancer patients' understanding of prognostic information. *J Cancer Educ* **29**, 311–17.

Castellano PZ, Wenger NK, Graves WL (2001). Adherence to screening guidelines for breast and cervical cancer in postmenopausal women with coronary heart disease: an ancillary study of volunteers for hers. *J Womens Health Gend Based Med* **10**, 451–61.

Cella D, Fallowfield LJ (2007). Recognition and management of treatment-related side effects for breast cancer patients receiving adjuvant endocrine therapy. *Breast Cancer Res Treat* **107**, 167–80.

Chewning B, Wiederholt JB (2003). Concordance in cancer medication management. *Patient Educ Couns* **50**, 75–8.

Chlebowski RT, Geller ML (2006). Adherence to endocrine therapy for breast cancer. *Oncology* **71**, 1–9.

Davidson B, Vogel V, Wickerham L (2007). Oncologist-patient discussion of adjuvant hormonal therapy in breast cancer: results of a linguistic study focusing on adherence and persistence to therapy. *J Support Oncol* **5**, 139–43.

Demissie S, Silliman RA, Lash TL (2001). Adjuvant tamoxifen: predictors of use, side effects, and discontinuation in older women. *J Clin Oncol* **19**, 322–8.

DiMatteo MR (2004a). Social support and patient adherence to medical treatment: a meta-analysis. *Health Psychol* **23**, 207–18.

DiMatteo MR (2004b). Variations in patients' adherence to medical recommendations: a quantitative review of 50 years of research. *Med Care* **42**, 200–9.

DiMatteo MR, Haskard KB, Williams SL (2007). Health beliefs, disease severity, and patient adherence: a meta-analysis. *Med Care* **45**, 521–8.

DiMatteo MR, Haskard-Zolnierek KB, Martin LR (2012). Improving patient adherence: A three-factor model to guide practice. *Health Psychol Rev* **6**, 74–91.

Dobie SA, Baldwin LM, Dominitz JA, Matthews B, Billingsley K, Barlow W (2006). Completion of therapy by Medicare patients with stage III colon cancer. *J Natl Cancer Inst* **98**, 610–19.

Fallowfield L, Jenkins V, Farewell V, Solis-Trapala I (2003). Enduring impact of communication skills training: results of a 12-month follow-up. *Br J Cancer* **89**, 1445–9.

Kahn KL, Schneider EC, Malin JL, Adams JL, Epstein AM (2007). Patient-centered experiences in breast cancer: predicting long-term adherence to tamoxifen use. *Med Care* **45**, 431–9.

Lash TL, Fox MP, Westrup JL, Fink AK, Silliman RA (2006). Adherence to tamoxifen over the five-year course. *Breast Cancer Res Treat* **99**, 215–20.

Meropol NJ, Weinfurt KP, Burnett CB, *et al.* (2003). Perceptions of patients and physicians regarding phase I cancer clinical trials: implications for physician-patient communication. *J Clin Oncol* **21**, 2589–96.

O'Malley AS, Forrest CB, Mandelblatt J (2002). Adherence of low-income women to cancer screening recommendations. *J Gen Intern Med* **17**, 144–54.

Partridge AH, LaFountain A, Mayer E, Taylor BS, Winer E, Asnis-Alibozek A (2008). Adherence to initial adjuvant anastrozole therapy among women with early-stage breast cancer. *J Clin Oncol* **26**, 556–62.

Regnier Denois V, Poirson J, Nourissat A, Jacquin JP, Guastalla JP, Chauvin F (2011). Adherence with oral chemotherapy: results from a qualitative study of the behaviour and representations of patients and oncologists. *Eur J Cancer Care (Engl)* **20**, 520–7.

Roberts C, Benjamin H, Chen L, *et al.* (2005). Assessing communication between oncology professionals and their patients. *J Cancer Educ* **20**, 113–18.

Thorpe JM, Kalinowski CT, Patterson ME, Sleath BL (2006). Psychological distress as a barrier to preventive care in community-dwelling elderly in the United States. *Med Care* **44**, 187–91.

Van Dulmen S, Sluijs E, Van Dijk L, De Ridder D, Heerdink R, Bensing J (2007). Patient adherence to medical treatment: a review of reviews. *BMC Health Serv Res* **7**, 55.

Zolnierek KB, DiMatteo MR (2009). Physician communication and patient adherence to treatment: a meta-analysis. *Med Care* **47**, 826–34.

CHAPTER 38

Communication strategies and skills for optimum pain control

Melanie Lovell and Frances Boyle

Introduction to communication strategies

Pain is a significant cause of suffering for people living with cancer. The onset of pain can trigger a host of fears of death, disability, disfigurement, dependence, and distress. The role of the healthcare professional (HCP) is to offer competent pain management with compassion and commitment to excellence, central to which is communication with the patient (Lovell *et al.* 2014).

Pain is not an event in isolation. It occurs in a personal and physical environment influenced by the social, cultural, spiritual, and biological inheritance of the patient. (Lickiss 2003) The experience of pain therefore has unique impact on and meaning for each individual. At the time of assessment, factors such as associated fatigue, depression, and anxiety may result in the pain becoming overwhelming (Twycross 1994). Assessing the pain involves not only measuring the level and determining its nature, so as to diagnose the aetiology and mechanism of pain, but also exploring the 'deeper level of pain experience'. Failure to do so can result in poor pain control and a lost opportunity for transformation of the experience and healing of the individual (Kearney 1992).

Pain prevalence and impact

Pain is a problem on a large scale for patients with cancer, despite evidence that pain can be effectively treated. A meta-analysis of prevalence studies showed the prevalence of pain rates in patients at all stages of disease was 53% (CI 43–63%) and of those, one third graded their pain as moderate or severe (Van Den Beuken-van Everdingen *et al.* 2007). Patients with pain may have more than one pain. Some groups have been shown to be at higher risk of poor pain control. These include paediatric patients, the elderly, cognitively impaired patients, those with a past history of substance abuse, and patients from culturally and linguistically diverse backgrounds.

Patients with unrelieved severe pain have reduced function and quality of life and increased levels of anxiety and depression. Pain also has a significant impact on caregivers. Despite these research findings, and the fact that most pain in cancer responds to analgesics and adjuvant therapies, there is evidence from many studies that cancer pain is frequently undertreated (Deandrea *et al.* 2008), and there are many barriers which may contribute to suboptimal pain management.

Barriers to optimal pain control

The American Pain Society (APS) identified contributing barriers due to lack of patient, professional, and public knowledge, lack of institutional commitment, regulatory concerns, and limited access to or reimbursement for interdisciplinary care. The APS further recommends addressing these barriers to improve pain management through physician leadership and a multilevel approach addressing healthcare providers, institutions, and patients and their families. Crucial prongs in the approach include quality improvement activities, evidence-based pain management practice, and patient involvement in decision making (Gordon *et al.* 2005).

Patient-related barriers can be broadly classified as those associated with myths regarding morphine and other opioids and those associated with communicating about the pain experience (Potter *et al.* 2003). Patients and their caregivers may be afraid of injections, becoming addicted to morphine, becoming tolerant to its effects, or that morphine may put them at risk of unpleasant side effects, or even death. These fears are long-standing, cross-cultural, and pervasive and relate to confusion concerning the therapeutic use of morphine versus the deleterious effects of morphine as a drug of abuse (Hanks *et al.* 2001). Despite clinical evidence that these fears are unfounded, these barriers persist and are common (Luckett *et al.* 2013).

Interventions to reduce barriers directed at patients

There is evidence from randomized controlled trials that educating patients about pain and its management can reduce these barriers and, in some studies, reduce pain levels. The interventions which have been found to be most effective are those which enable patients to self-manage their pain and included pain diaries, personalized pain management plans, and patient goal setting (Marie *et al.* 2013).

Interventions to improve pain control directed at healthcare professionals (HCPs) and institutions

Interventions to improve clinicians' knowledge and attitudes and change behaviour are notoriously challenging and few have been shown to be effective. Audit and feedback can be effective, especially when the feedback is provided in written format and verbally by a respected senior colleague on multiple occasions, and accompanied by strategies for improvement in performance (Ivers *et al.* 2012). Q stream education has also been found to be effective. This is case-based education delivered online with an email being sent every few days (Shaw *et al.* 2011).

Numerical Rating Scale

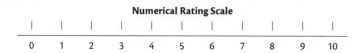

Fig. 38.1 Numeric rating scale.

Categorical (Descriptive) Scale

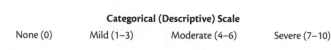

Fig. 38.2 Categorical (descriptive) scale.

Meta-analysis of studies of involvement of specialist palliative care teams has shown improved pain control and patient satisfaction (Higginson *et al.* 2003).

Measuring and describing pain

Pain is a subjective experience (Ferrell *et al.* 1993) and its management is dependent on patient reporting of pain experience. A numeric rating scale is a valid, reliable tool for accurately measuring the intensity of an individual's pain (Jensen *et al.* 1986) (see Figs 38.1 and 38.2).

A proportion of patients will find this difficult to use and they may be able to use categorical scales (none, mild, moderate, or severe). Patients who are unable to communicate verbally, such as paediatric patients or those with dementia must be assessed by the HCP using a scale such as the faces scale (Wong and Baker 1988). Screening for pain enhances communication by improving detection of pain, more discussion on quality of life and increased referral (Etkind *et al.* 2015).

Patients should be advised on how to use a pain diary to record pain scores triggers and relieving factors, and response to analgesia. There are a number of validated pain diaries available online.

Descriptors that are reliable for neuropathic pain are a matter of ongoing research. In one study, those which most significantly correlate with neuropathic pain include pain evoked by stroking the skin, bedclothes against the skin or heat, sensations of pins and needles, pricking, jumping-bursting, and stabbing-shooting (Bennett 2001). Nociceptive pain may be described as aching, cramping, stabbing, throbbing, gnawing, pressure, or sharp.

The goal of each clinical encounter and guidelines to complete it

The goal of the clinical encounter is diagnosis of aetiology and mechanism of pain and optimal management of the pain in the context of the whole patient. This includes the goal of empowering the patient (Abernathy *et al.* 2006). The patient is thereby able to more effectively communicate about and manage pain. There are a number of key messages which need to be understood by both HCP and patient to enable this:

◆ The majority of cancer pain can be safely, quickly, and effectively relieved.

◆ Pain can be measured effectively using rating scales.

◆ Pain can be monitored effectively using a daily pain diary.

◆ It is important to screen patients for pain at each visit.

◆ Patients should be encouraged to report pain.

◆ Common myths about pain and pain control should be explored and discussed.

◆ Addiction and tolerance are rarely a problem when opioids are used for cancer pain management.

◆ Patients should be instructed on how to communicate effectively about their pain.

◆ It is important to treat the pain early and get the best control possible.

◆ Side effects of opioids can be managed.

◆ Patients should be provided with written instructions about pain relief.

Key communication skills

Firstly establish rapport with patient and family

Screening for pain

'It is very important to know if you are experiencing pain so we can manage it early.' 'Can you tell me how severe your pain is now using a scale of 0–10 where 10 is the most severe pain you can imagine and 0 is no pain?' 'Can you please rate your pain on a scale of none, mild, moderate, or severe?'

'What was your pain score when it was at its worst in the last 24 hours?'

1. Identifying presence of pain(s) and likely aetiology and underlying mechanism

Site: 'Can you point with one finger to where the pain is worst?' 'Do you have other pains?' 'Where is each one worst?'

Temporal factors: 'How long ago did you first get the pain?' 'When did it get worse?' 'Is it constant or does it come and go?' 'How often do you get the pain?' 'How long does each episode last?'

Exacerbating and relieving factors: 'Does there appear to be a trigger causing the pain?' 'What makes the pain worse?' 'What makes the pain better?'

Response to treatment: 'What are you doing or taking for the pain?' 'On our rating scale, what number does that change the pain from/to?' 'How long does it take to work and how long does it work for?'

To determine if pain is neuropathic: 'Can you describe the pain?' 'Is the pain worse when the skin is stroked, touched by the bedclothes, or touched by something warm?' (Bennett 2001)

Breakthrough pain—'Do you ever get a flare of the pain?' Above questions should also be applied to any breakthrough pain.

2. Documenting the pain in a daily diary

Please rate your pain on a scale 0, 0 being no pain, and 10 being the worst pain imaginable. Please note your **average** pain for the preceding 24 hours at the same time each evening, say 7:00 pm, and also if you have breakthrough pain (a flare of your pain) (see Table 38.1).

3. Negotiating a pain management plan

Patients and health professionals should negotiate a pain management plan including written instructions about how to use the medication including for breakthrough pain, how to prevent and manage side effects, and when and how to call the healthcare professional. An example is available at http://wiki.cancer.org.au/australia/Guidelines:Cancer_pain_management/Patient_awareness_%26_self-management (Australian Adult Cancer Pain

Table 38.1 Documenting the pain in a daily diary

Day	Time	Pain level	Pain relief—dose	Pain level 1 hour later	Comments
Thursday					
Friday					
Saturday					
Sunday					
Monday					
Tuesday					
Wednesday					

Management Guideline Working Party 2013). Patients may also be shown how to communicate effectively with clinicians. In a randomized controlled trial, the following script was shown to be an effective tool for this purpose (Miaskowski *et al.* 2004). An example is shown in (Box 38.1).

4. Determining the impact of pain

'What effect does the pain have on your ability to sleep/walk/work/your mood and your relationships?'

5. Determining the meaning of pain

'What do you think the pain means?' 'What do you think is the cause of the pain?' 'What do you expect will happen now with respect to the pain?' 'Is there anything you are worried about related to the pain?'

6. Identifying beliefs which may act as barriers to pain control

Beliefs regarding pain and pain communication which are potential barriers to pain relief include: fear of progressive disease; fear of distracting the doctor from curing or treating the cancer; stoicism; fatalism; fear of death or disability. 'Some people feel they want to be brave and put up with pain—does that describe you?' 'Do you feel pain is an expected part of living with cancer?'

It is important to reassure patients: 'Managing pain is a crucial part of your overall cancer treatment.'

7. Identifying patient-related barriers to opioid use

Addiction: 'Some people believe that they will get addicted to this type of medication—are you afraid that might happen to you?' The key message is: 'Addiction is not a problem when morphine is used appropriately for cancer pain management.'

Tolerance: 'Some people are afraid that they might get used to the medication and they will need more and more for it to work, or that there will not be anything strong enough if the pain gets worse.'

Box 38.1 Negotiating a pain management plan

'Hello, I'm calling to talk with you about the pain I have … Over the past week, my pain has been___on a 0–10 rating scale and up to __. The pain has been so severe that I have not been able to sleep or ___ . I've been taking ____ for pain. I've also been taking ___ additional doses of medicine every day. Even with this my pain is not controlled. Can we change the pain medicine please?'

It can be explained as follows: 'If the pain gets worse, the dose can be increased as needed and if the pain gets better, for example in response to anti-cancer treatment, the dose can be decreased.'

Side effects: 'Are you concerned about potential side effects of the medication?'
'Morphine does cause some side effects which can be managed.'

Fear that morphine will hasten death: 'Some people think that starting morphine is the beginning of the end—morphine is the best strong pain reliever we have and many people are on it for months or years.'

Fear of masking the pain: 'Are you concerned that treating the pain will mask what is going on in your body?'

8. Identifying cultural issues affecting pain communication

'Are there beliefs in your culture about pain?' This needs to be explored with sensitivity and without preconceptions. This is discussed in greater depth in Chapter 41.

9. Spiritual issues affecting communication

'How do you see your pain with respect to your faith?'; 'Do you have any spiritual practices to help you manage pain?'

10. Dealing with difficult pain communication situations

History of substance abuse: This is a special situation and previous substance abusers are at risk of poor pain control (Kirsh and Passik 2006). Kirsh and Passik suggest a number of strategies: involve the multidisciplinary team; take a full non-judgemental history explaining that it is important for the clinician to know previous drug use to prevent withdrawal and prescribe adequate analgesia; set realistic goals recognizing that abstinence and compliance may not be realistic, providing social, emotional support, and setting limits; evaluate and treat comorbid psychiatric disorders; consider the therapeutic implications of tolerance reassessing regularly and involving significant others; use written agreements, be clear that no extra medication or prescription will be supplied for missed appointments or unaccounted for missing home drug supplies; try to identify family members who will be a source of strength or support—or conversely may attempt to buy or sell the patient's medications. The aim is a therapeutic alliance with the patient, supporters or family members, and clinicians.

Paediatric patients. The key to assessing pain in children is observing behaviour (Miaskowski *et al.* 2005) There is one tool developed specifically for hospitalized children aged 2–6 years with cancer pain called the Douleur E'chelle Gustave-Roussy (DEGR(R))instrument (Gauvin-Piquard *et al.* 1999). It evaluates chronic pain behaviours, such as appearing depressed or withdrawn.

Older persons: Pain is a common problem in the elderly and assessment can be difficult as older patients may be more reluctant to report pain. Sensory or cognitive impairment may make communication difficult (AGS Panel on Persistent Pain in Older Persons 2002).

Cognitively impaired: Communication with this group is discussed in Chapter 52. Behaviour in this group may indicate that pain is present. Changed behaviour should also trigger an assessment for pain (AGS Panel on Persistent Pain in Older Persons 2002).

It is also helpful to get a history from carers to determine behaviour in response to movement such as turning. Using a tool such as the Abbey Pain Scale can enhance assessment of pain in patients with cognitive impairment.

11. Medication adherence in further discussed in Chapter 37

Module summary

- Establish rapport and explain importance of good, rapid pain control
- Screen for pain using a pain rating scale
- Be aware of groups at higher risk of pain: the very old or young; cognitively impaired; those with a history of substance abuse; minority groups; low socioeconomic status
- Identify site, character, timing, and exacerbating and relieving factors to determine mechanism and aetiology
- Determine impact of pain
- Ask about barriers to communicating pain or using analgesia especially addiction, tolerance, side effects, and address the barriers
- Ask about beliefs about the pain—cause, expectations, cultural aspects, spiritual aspects
- Ask about meaning of the pain
- Show patient how to use a pain diary
- Teach patients how to communicate effectively about pain
- Develop a pain management plan with the patient and caregiver

Exemplary clinical scenarios across the range of common cancers to guide role plays

Breast cancer and bone metastases

Elizabeth is a 40-year-old woman who had early breast cancer four years ago, treated with surgery, chemotherapy, radiotherapy, and tamoxifen (daily tablet, ongoing). This week she lifted her five-year-old son and felt severe pain in her mid-thoracic spine. She has been resting, and taking simple analgesia, but it's not been controlled. The pain is in the middle of her back, constant and aggravated by movement, and radiates around the right side of her ribs, with a burning quality and paraesthesia. Differential diagnosis includes crush fracture, benign (e.g. low bone density from hormonal therapy) or malignant, or less likely, a disc prolapse. When seen she is splinting her movement, trying to downplay the severity for fear or an ominous diagnosis, and very anxious.

- Key examination: local tenderness, rule out spinal cord compression (sensation, reflexes, plantar responses).
- Key investigations: X-ray, MRI, or CT.
- Key communication issues: measuring pain, breaking bad news of possible relapse, ensuring acute analgesia with short acting opioid while investigating urgently.
- For the actor: trying to suppress both anxiety and movement cause a rigid thorax and shallow breathing. No hair loss.

Bowel cancer and presacral mass

Alan is a 65-year-old man who had rectal cancer three years ago, which was treated with radiotherapy, chemotherapy, and surgery. One year ago he relapsed locally in the pelvis, with pain in the sacral area, radiating to both thighs. He has had further chemotherapy with some initial improvement, but is now suffering from increasing pain which limits activity at home. His partner rings to say that he is not sleeping but will not take his medication (long-acting oral opioid) due to poor efficacy and constipation, but has not been 'telling the truth' at his visits. He is also 'very grumpy and irritable' with her.

- Key communication issues: eliciting fears about pain and analgesia, communicating about interference with sleep and ADL, eliciting symptoms of depression, negotiating alternative approaches to analgesia with lower side effects (e.g. adding co-analgesics, fentanyl patch, spinal pump).
- For the actor: move slowly to the chair, as if legs unsteady. Avoid eye contact, short answers, and little spontaneous speech. Hard to convince that there are better ways, and not at all convinced that he is depressed (not that kind of guy). He would not have hair loss.

Bone marrow transplant patient with mucositis pain

Graham is a 19-year-old in hospital for a bone marrow transplant. Chemotherapy was given last week and marrow reinfused three days ago. His mouth and throat are becoming very painful, his anxiety is increasing, and he is almost hysterical with pain '20 out of 10'.

- Key communication issues: separating anxiety from pain, explaining cause (mucositis from chemo), establishing confidence with IV analgesia with patient control, negotiating a pain scale.
- For the actor: lots of movement and anxiety, but muffled speech as if mouth is sore. Need to conceal hair.

Possibility of substance abuse

Steve is a 30-year-old male with metastatic melanoma, in hospital to have radiotherapy to a mass of lymph nodes in the groin. His pain in the leg and back is described as 'severe', but at times he is seen up walking outside to smoke and laughing with friends, and staff are concerned that his pain is not 'real'. He has been an injecting heroin addict in the past, although claims to have been clean for several years.

- Key communication issues: cross checking reports of pain with other interference measures (e.g. sleep). Assessing tolerance for opioids when he is given short acting break through doses (i.e. checking pain response). Using co-analgesics to spare opioids. Opening an honest conversation.

◆ For the actor: casual dress and a slightly evasive manner covering up real concern that he is not being taken seriously. No hair loss. Walks with a limp.

In summary, effective communication in the consultation is essential for optimal pain assessment and management.

References

Abernathy A, Currow D, Hunt R, *et al.* (2006). A pragmatic 2 × 2 × 2 factorial cluster randomized controlled trial of educational outreach visiting and case conferencing in palliative care—methodology of the Palliative Care Trial [ISRCTN 81117481] *Contemp Clin Trials* **27**, 83–100.

AGS panel on persistent pain in older persons (2002). The management of persistent pain in older persons. *J Am Geriatr Soc* **50**, 205–24.

Australian Adult Cancer Pain Management Guideline Working Party (2013). Cancer pain management in adults. Sydney, Australia.

Bennett M (2001). The LANSS Pain Scale: the Leeds assessment of neuropathic symptoms and signs. *Pain* **92**, 147–57.

Deandrea S, Montanari M, Moja L, Apolone G (2008). Prevalence of undertreatment in cancer pain. A review of published literature. *Ann Oncol* **19**, 1985–91.

Etkind SN, Daveson BA, KWOK W, *et al.* (2015). Capture, transfer, and feedback of patient-centered outcomes data in palliative care populations: Does it make a difference? A systematic review. *J Pain Symptom Manage* **49**, 611–24.

Ferrell B, Rhiner M, Ferrell B (1993). Development and implementation of a pain education program. *Cancer* **72**, (11 Suppl) 3426–32.

Gauvin-Piquard A, Rodary C, Rezvani A, Serbouti S (1999). The development of the DEGR(R): A scale to assess pain in young children with cancer. *Eur J Pain* **3**, 165–76.

Gordon D, Dahl J, Miaskowski C, *et al.* (2005). American Pain Society recommendations for improving the quality of acute and cancer pain management: American Pain Society Quality of Care Task Force. *Arch Intern Med* **165**, 1574–80.

Hanks G, De Conno F, Cherny N, *et al.* (2001). Morphine and alternative opioids in cancer pain: the EAPC recommendations. *Br J Cancer* **84**, 587–93.

Higginson I, Finlay I, Goodwin D, *et al.* (2003). Is there evidence that palliative care teams alter end-of-life experiences of patients and their caregivers? *J Pain Symptom Manage* **25**, 150–68.

Ivers N, Jamtvedt G, Flottorp S, *et al.* (2012). Audit and feedback: effects on professional practice and healthcare outcomes. *Cochrane Database Syst Rev* **13**, CD000259.

Jensen M, Karoly P, Braver S (1986). The measurement of clinical pain intensity. *Pain* **27**, 117–26.

Kearney M (1992). Palliative medicine- just another specialty? *Palliat Med* **6**, 39–46.

Kirsh K, Passik S (2006). Palliative care of the terminally ill drug addict. *Cancer Invest* **24**, 425–31.

Lickiss NJ (2003). Approaching death in Multicultural Australia. *Med J Aust* **179**, S14–16.

Lovell MR, Luckett T, Boyle FM, Phillips J, Agar M, Davidson PM (2014). Patient education, coaching, and self-management for cancer pain. *J Clin Oncol* **32**, 1712–20.

Luckett T, Davidson PM, Green A, Boyle F, Stubbs J, Lovell M (2013). Assessment and management of adult cancer pain: a systematic review and synthesis of recent qualitative studies aimed at developing insights for managing barriers and optimizing facilitators within a comprehensive framework of patient care. *J Pain Symptom Manage* **46**, 229–53.

Marie N, Luckett T, Davidson PM, Lovell M, Lal S (2013). Optimal patient education for cancer pain: a systematic review and theory-based meta-analysis. *Support Care Cancer* **21**, 3529–37.

Miaskowski C, Cleary J, Burney R, *et al.* (2005). *Guidelines for the Management of Cancer Pain in Adults and Children.* American Pain Society, Glenview, IL.

Miaskowski C, Dodd M, West C, *et al.* (2004). Randomized clinical trial of the effectiveness of a self-care intervention to improve cancer pain management. *J Clin Oncol* **22**, 1713–20.

Potter V, Wiseman C, Dunn S, Boyle F (2003). Patient barriers to optimal cancer pain control. *Psychooncology* **12**, 153–60.

Shaw T, Long A, Chopra S, Kerfoot BP (2011). Impact on clinical behavior of face-to-face continuing medical education blended with online spaced education: a randomized controlled trial. *J Contin Educ Health Prof* **31**, 103–8.

Twycross R (1994). *Pain Relief in Advanced Cancer,* London, Churchill Livingstone.

Van Den Beuken-van everdingen MH, De Rijke JM, Kessels AG, Schouten HC, Van Kleef M, Patijn J (2007). Prevalence of pain in patients with cancer: a systematic review of the past 40 years. *Ann Oncol* **18**, 1437–49.

Wong D, Baker C (1988). Pain in children: comparison of assessment scales. *Pediatric Nurs* **14**, 9–17.

CHAPTER 39

Discussing adverse outcomes with patients

Andy S.L. Tan and Thomas H. Gallagher

Introduction to discussing adverse outcomes with patients

Few communication challenges are as difficult for healthcare providers as talking with patients about adverse events, especially when the adverse event was due to a medical error. Ethicists and professional organizations have long endorsed open communication with patients about adverse events and errors in their care. Over the past decade, however, there has been a substantial increase in attention being paid to transparent communication with patients. Many countries, including Australia, the United Kingdom, and Canada have undertaken major disclosure initiatives. The Joint Commission, the body responsible for the accreditation of most US healthcare facilities, requires that patients be informed of all outcomes in their care, including 'unanticipated outcomes'.

However, there is increasing evidence of a significant gap between expectations for open communication with patients and actual clinical practice. Studies in a variety of countries suggest that fewer than one-third of adverse events due to errors are disclosed to patients. Other research suggests that when these conversations do take place, they often fall short of meeting patient expectations. Healthcare workers endorse the general concept of disclosure, but struggle with how to turn this principle into practice, especially when it comes to choosing their words when talking with patients about adverse events. Significant fear persists among both healthcare workers and institutions that more open disclosure of adverse events and errors could increase the likelihood of a medical malpractice suit being filed.

Communication dilemmas associated with disclosure of adverse events and errors to patients exist at multiple levels, ranging from the individual patient–provider encounter, to issues of national health policy. In this chapter, we will explore the special aspects of disclosure in the oncology context; international developments in disclosure; patients' and providers' attitudes and their experiences with disclosure; impact of disclosure on outcomes including litigation; disclosure in an interprofessional context; how healthcare institutions are responding to calls for greater transparency; health policy challenges associated with disclosure; and key communication strategies for disclosing errors to patients. The chapter concludes by considering a disclosure case study, and discussing next steps for disclosure in oncology.

Adverse events and errors in the oncology context

It is important to distinguish between *adverse events, unanticipated outcome*, and *medical errors*. An *adverse event* is defined as any harm that is caused by medical management and that results in measurable disability. Adverse events are relatively common, and the vast majority of them are not caused by medical errors. (Similarly, an *unanticipated outcome* is defined as any unexpected result from any aspect of diagnosis or treatment that may or may not be associated with an error—a broad definition that it is not particularly useful.) The most commonly used definition of a *medical error* is from the US Institute of Medicine: 'The failure of a planned action to be completed as intended or the use of a wrong plan to achieve an aim' (Institute of Medicine (US) Committee on Quality of Health Care in America 2000). As strictly defined here, medical errors are, in fact, quite common. The vast majority of errors are not associated with an adverse event, either by chance or timely intervention, are known as *near misses*.

There is a general expectation that healthcare workers will communicate openly with patients about all adverse events, whether due to medical error or not. However, talking with patients about adverse events not due to error is more straightforward than talking with patients about adverse events due to error. Therefore, the remainder of this chapter will focus on the challenges associated with disclosing adverse events that were due to medical errors, also known as *harmful medical errors*, to patients.

While disclosing harmful medical errors to patients can be difficult in any clinical context, the oncology environment poses special challenges. Oncology care is fraught with uncertainty, and it can be difficult to know whether a medical error occurred and, if so, whether the error was associated with harm. This is further complicated by the toxic nature of most oncology therapies, where adverse events are commonplace. The psychological burdens associated with cancer make oncology patients especially vulnerable, but the consequences of medical errors in oncology can also be severe for the provider, with emotional distress among oncologists being common. In addition, medicolegal issues associated with oncology can pose difficult challenges. Delayed diagnosis of cancer, and breast cancer in particular, is one of the most frequent precipitants of medical malpractice lawsuits in the United States.

Despite these challenges, the oncology community is ideally positioned to take a leadership role within the medical profession in enhancing the disclosure of adverse events and errors to patients. The oncology community has led in developing a knowledge base and set of practical skills for a related communication dilemma, namely the delivery of bad news to patients. There is good reason to believe that 10 years from now, healthcare workers will approach the disclosure of harmful medical errors to oncology patients very differently than they do at present.

International developments in disclosure

Important developments related to disclosure have been taking place across the world. In 2001 The Joint Commission, the United States organization that accredits hospitals and healthcare organizations, required that hospitals and healthcare organizations disclose all outcomes of care to patients including 'unanticipated outcomes', leading many hospitals and healthcare institutions to develop formal disclosure policies. By 2005, nearly 70% of healthcare organizations in the US had established disclosure policies.

The Australian Council for Safety and Quality in Healthcare's *Open Disclosure Standard*, a national standard for open communication in public and private hospitals following an adverse event in healthcare, aims to ensure open, honest, and timely communication with patients to meet the needs of the affected patient and improve patient safety. Healthcare personnel, patients, and family members at 21 pilot sites indicated strong support for open disclosure among all stakeholders, although participants were uncertain about the implementation and effects of open disclosure (Iedema *et al.* 2008). Among 119 Australian patients and family members who experienced a severe medical incident and received disclosure about the incident, most felt that the disclosure did not meet their needs and expectations—they perceived a lack of preparation for the disclosure, shared dialogue about the error, follow-up support, appropriate closure, and information about improvements to patient safety (Iedema *et al.* 2011a). While most participants were aware of health service risks and incidents, and had insights about ways to minimize risks of incidents, they experienced challenges when attempting to voice their concerns with clinicians (Iedema *et al.* 2012).

In the United Kingdom, the National Patient Safety Agency of the National Health Service launched the 'Being Open' program in 2003 (updated in 2009). As in Australia, extensive educational material for healthcare organizations, providers, and patients have been developed and pilot projects are underway to determine the impact of this new policy. To our knowledge, however, outcomes data from either Australia's *Open Disclosure* or the UK's *Being Open* projects have not been published.

The Canadian Patient Safety Institute first issued its 'Canadian Disclosure Guidelines' in 2008 and updated the guidelines in 2011. These guidelines focus on the disclosure of adverse events, and emphasize that healthcare providers and organizations have an obligation to communicate to a patient about any harm that has occurred in their care. The Canadian guidelines articulate a thoughtful approach to disclosure and encourage an expression of regret following adverse events. However, the Canadian guidelines, as with the disclosure programs in Australia and the United Kingdom, highlight an important area of persistent ambiguity that complicates the disclosure process. The Canadian guidelines

emphasize the importance of 'avoiding the use of "error" in the context of disclosure'. They note that while healthcare provider error may appear to be the most obvious contributing factor to an adverse event, there are often system breakdowns and other latent conditions that are more important contributors. On the other hand, the guidelines call for patients to be informed about 'the facts' of the event, and 'actions taken as a result of internal analysis that have resulted in system improvements'. The guidelines do note that 'if applicable, and when all the facts are established, a further expression of regret that may include an apology with acknowledgement or responsibility for what has happened as appropriate' can be included in the disclosure. It can be difficult for providers and organizations to know how best to comply with the dual requirements for open and transparent communication about adverse events that were clearly due to error, while not admitting fault or using 'error' language.

Patients' and physicians' attitudes and experiences regarding disclosure

Several studies have shed considerable light on patients' preferences for disclosure (Mazor *et al.* 2012, 2013). Patients uniformly desire the disclosure of all harmful errors in their care, even when the harm was relatively minor. Patients also desire a consistent set of information about harmful errors, including an explicit statement that an error occurred, an explanation of what the error was and its implications for their health, why the error occurred, and how recurrences will be prevented. These last two pieces of information (why the error occurred and how recurrences will be prevented) are highly valued by patients, as they show that a lesson has been learned from the event and that recurrences are less likely. Patients also value an apology as recognition of the emotional impact of the error on them personally.

Cancer patients who reported encountering a preventable and harmful problem (i.e. with their medical care and/or a communication breakdown) frequently experienced physical and emotional harm, disruption of life, damaged relationships with their clinician, and financial expense (Mazor *et al.* 2012). In only about one-third of cases, patients had a discussion about the event with the responsible clinician; the majority of patients did not voice their concerns about the adverse event. In a minority of cases where a conversation occurred, the responsible clinician had initiated discussions about the adverse events or assumed responsibility for the event. More often, the patient or a family member initiated the discussion, or no one took responsibility.

Recent research has also shed new light on how healthcare workers approach disclosure. Several large survey studies of physicians suggest that they strongly endorse the general concept of disclosure, but struggle with how to turn this principle into practice. One study compared the disclosure attitudes of physicians in the United States and in Canada, countries with significantly different malpractice climates (Gallagher *et al.* 2006b). The US and Canadian physicians' disclosure attitudes and experience were much more similar than different, suggesting that the external malpractice environment may not be as powerful a determinant of physicians' disclosure attitudes as once thought. However, despite this general support for disclosure, many physicians struggled with what words to say to patients following harmful errors (Gallagher *et al.* 2006a). The study also showed that healthcare workers may disclose less information about errors that would be unapparent to the patient, and that medical and surgical physicians approached disclosure differently. Another study of how surgeons would approach disclosure also showed that many surgeons failed to use recommended skills (Chan *et al.* 2005). For example, only 8% of surgeons mentioned anything to the hypothetical patients involved in this study about prevention of error recurrences.

Communication breakdowns in cancer care, which occur frequently, further complicate clinicians' ability to approach disclosures in the oncology context (Prouty *et al.* 2014). For instance, clinicians perceive that patient factors (lack of understanding, unrealistic expectations, emotional distress, and withholding information, and unwillingness to voice concerns about their care) were important contributors of communication breakdowns. In addition, provider factors (e.g. providers delivering inaccurate or conflicting information, inability to balance hope with reality about prognosis, and poor information exchange among providers) and healthcare system issues (e.g. insufficient time with patients, unclear treatment protocols and responsibilities) contributed to communication breakdowns in cancer care.

Impact of disclosure on outcomes

Anecdotal reports are beginning to clarify the impact disclosure has on reducing litigation and liability costs while improving patient safety (Kachalia *et al.* 2010; Boothman *et al.* 2012). Patients who sue often cite both the perception that the truth was hidden from them, as well as deficient communication skills as important reasons for why they filed a lawsuit. Full disclosure may reduce patients' intention to sue and promote faster settlements and lower awards (Mazor *et al.* 2006; Helmchen *et al.* 2010). The relationship between disclosure and litigation, however, continues to be a complex and contentious issue. The vast majority of patients injured by medical care never sue, which may in part reflect their lack of awareness that a medical error caused their injury. If this is true, open disclosure could stimulate rather than mitigate lawsuits. Even in those studies that have shown a generally positive relationship between open disclosure and intent to sue, this relationship is often diminished for the most serious errors. Such uncertainty about the impact of disclosure on litigation is likely to persist for the foreseeable future.

Despite this uncertainty, several US institutions have developed communication-and-resolution programs (CRPs) for open disclosure of adverse events and errors, and reported favourable impacts on their litigation experiences (Mello *et al.* 2014). The two distinct models implemented among these early adopters of CRPs are the early settlement and limited reimbursement models (Mello *et al.* 2014). The first of these programs, at the Lexington, Kentucky Veterans Hospital, which encouraged full disclosure of harmful errors and facilitation of compensation in selected circumstances, did not appear to have a deleterious impact on volume or pay-outs of the institution's malpractice claims. More recently, the University of Michigan reported that their CRP utilizing the early settlement model had a dramatic positive impact on their number of malpractice claims, time to resolution, and pay-outs (Kachalia *et al.* 2010; Boothman *et al.* 2012). The best-known CRP in the private sector has been developed by COPIC Insurance Company, which has implemented a limited reimbursement program since 2000 called the 3Rs program—Recognize, Respond, and Resolve. Their

'3Rs' program encourages open disclosure following unanticipated outcomes and provides compensation for patients' lost time and other out-of-pocket expenses up to $30,000. The 3Rs program has important exclusion criteria, including patient death, attorney involvement, written demand for payment, gross negligence, or complaint to the medical board. Since the program's inception in 2000 through December 31, 2009, COPIC has handled over 8,000 cases through the 3Rs program, and a total of 1,829 patients have received an average payment of $4,977 (Lembitz 2010). Of the 3Rs cases, 60 patients subsequently filed a claim or suit and only 11 of these claims or suits have resulted in indemnity payments through the tort system (Lembitz 2010). While the generalizability of these case reports is uncertain, they do provide some support for the concept that at least a subset of adverse events and errors can be effectively handled through such programs. Key success factors among early adopters of CRPs included the presence of a strong institutional champion for the program, marketing the program to clinicians, and clarifying expectations that transformative change requires time (Mello *et al.* 2014).

Interprofessional issues in error disclosure

Up to this point, disclosure has primarily been conceptualized as a conversation between an individual patient and his or her physician. However, the patient safety movement has done much to highlight the role that system breakdowns play in most medical errors. In the field of oncology, delivery of healthcare by teams of providers is the norm, including physicians as well as nurses, therapists, technicians, dieticians, and psychologists. When harmful errors happen to patients in the setting of interprofessional care, multiple team members may discuss the event with one another, and may or may not discuss the event with the patient. However, no clear standards currently exist for how interprofessional healthcare teams should discuss errors among themselves and with patients, although the benefits and challenges of achieving transparency among clinicians about errors have recently received greater attention among patient safety experts (Conway *et al.* 2011; Gallagher *et al.* 2013; Roundtable on Transparency 2015).

Studies among nurses suggest that they were less likely than physicians to disclose errors to patients, particularly regarding cognitive versus medication errors (Hobgood *et al.* 2004), possibly because nurses believe that disclosing a cognitive error to a patient would be equivalent to denouncing their physician colleagues. Other reasons include their reluctance to admit human frailty, lack of knowledge about how to disclose errors skillfully, as well as the lack of institutional support for healthcare workers who have made a serious error. Overall, nurses supported the importance of disclosure overall but questioned disclosure to anxious patients and litigious families, as well as disclosure of minor errors (Shannon *et al.* 2009). They emphasized the team dimensions of disclosure, and described many episodes of poor communication among team members about what patients had been or would be told, which resulted in nurses responding to patients' and families' questions with deception or avoidance. Nurses wanted to be involved in the error disclosure process, in part to avoid being blamed for errors, yet reported lacking adequate knowledge and experience to skilfully discuss errors. These nurses also highlighted the critical role that their nurse managers played in operationalizing institution disclosure policies on the patient care floors.

Considerable work has yet to be done about the optimal inter-professional approach to disclosure. Team disclosure conversations naturally involve a planning phase, where the team members discuss the event, and plan whether and how to disclose the event to the patient. Once this team discussion and planning process is complete, the team discloses to the patient and/or the family. Given the inherent power differentials present on such teams, strong communication and conflict resolution skills are required to discuss the event and its disclosure in a mutually supportive and blame-free way. There is also considerable work yet to be done regarding the roles different team members play in the disclosure process. Often the physician will lead the disclosure process, and may or may not want additional members of the healthcare team present for the disclosure. While nurses have expressed an interest in participating in disclosures, it is unclear how to structure team disclosures in ways such that they support, rather than overwhelm the patient. Furthermore, the role of the physician in disclosing events that were strictly nursing errors to the patients has yet to be determined. The oncology community, with its considerable experience in inter-professional healthcare delivery, is ideally positioned to explore interprofessional best practices in the disclosure of harmful errors to patients.

Another important interprofessional issue in disclosure of errors involves situations when clinicians are confronted with an apparent error of another colleague. There is presently little guidance on how clinicians should handle the disclosure of such medical errors with the responsible colleague, the institution, and patients. An expert working group convened in 2013 to develop recommendations for clinicians and institutions on communicating with patients about colleagues' harmful errors (Gallagher et al. 2013). Three key principles guided the working group's recommendations. First, patients' and families' needs should come first before clinicians' concerns of damaging collegial relationships. Second, clinicians should commit to explore and not ignore potential errors. They are obligated to obtain the facts about potential errors starting with a conversation with the involved colleague, determine how to communicate with the patient, and involve the institution for assistance where needed. Third, institutions should lead in establishing due process and a culture to support disclosure of colleagues' errors. Institutions are responsible for ensuring high-quality disclosure conversations take place with patients, supporting conversations between clinicians in exploring potential errors (e.g. through just-in-time disclosure coaching programs), utilizing existing formal and informal mechanisms to address questions about potential errors (e.g. morbidity and mortality rounds or 'kerbside consults' with a risk manager), and strengthening 'just cultures' in the institution to encourage and even reward clinicians to report adverse events.

Institutional factors promoting disclosure

Transparency is increasingly being conceptualized as a property of a system, and not just of individual healthcare providers. For instance, institutional policies and procedures related to disclosure can either facilitate or inhibit error disclosure to patients. Yet, few institutional disclosure policies provide specific guidance in how disclosure of harmful errors to patients should be carried out. Furthermore, in many institutions healthcare workers receive mixed messages about disclosure: formal institutional policies encourage disclosure, even as institutional risk managers advise and promote caution.

Institutions looking to expand their policies and procedures around disclosure can draw on the 2010 US National Quality Forum (NQF) Safe Practice on disclosure and recent expert panel reports and recommendations on transparency for patient safety (Conway et al. 2011; NQF 2010; Roundtable on Transparency 2015). The common elements across these policies and reports include a commitment to open disclosure of all serious unanticipated outcomes to patients, providing guidance on ways to promote transparency and open disclosure, and offering practical approaches for organizations and health professionals to prevent and manage serious medical adverse events when they occur. Most importantly, the Safe Practice articulates the key components of an institutional disclosure support system, which includes training in disclosure for healthcare workers, emotional support for patients and healthcare workers following unanticipated outcomes, and the availability of disclosure coaching around the clock to assist healthcare workers with disclosure tasks.

Legislative approaches to promoting disclosure and apology

Recognition of current inadequacies in the disclosure and apology process has led many countries to take legislative action. Healthcare workers' and institutions' fear of litigation is a frequently cited barrier to disclosure and apology (Iedema et al. 2011b). Thus, one common legislative strategy to promote disclosure and apology has been to adopt laws protecting some aspects of the disclosure and apology process from being considered admissions of liability. In the United States, states have used two approaches to promote disclosure and apology. As of 2010, 34 US states and the District of Columbia have enacted 'apology laws' that protect portions of these conversations from being used as evidence of liability. Nine US states have adopted 'disclosure laws' which typically mandate that serious unanticipated outcomes be disclosed. Apology laws have also been adopted in other countries including Australia, Canada, and the United Kingdom.

The variety of US apology laws reflects the range of apology laws that have been enacted elsewhere in the world. While these laws represent important endorsements of transparency, analysis of the US apology laws highlights their significant limitations (Mastroianni et al. 2010). Notably, statements acknowledging the injury but not causation or explanation ('I'm sorry this happened') will be protected, while portions of a statement explaining or acknowledging fault or responsibility ('I'm sorry I hurt you' or 'I'm sorry I made a mistake when I administered the wrong medication') could be used in litigation. Four US states with apology laws protect the entire disclosure statement, allowing a provider to express remorse and admit fault to the patient without concern that the information disclosed could be used in court as evidence of fault. Even in these few US states that protect admissions of fault, the act of communicating this information might still stimulate a lawsuit. Given these limitations, many physicians, healthcare institutions, and risk managers are likely to remain concerned about the legal risks associated with disclosure and apology.

Communication strategies

Communication training has an important role to play in improving the disclosure process. Most physicians report that they have not had formal training in disclosure, and lack confidence in their disclosure communication skills. Physicians frequently cite these communication skills deficits as important barriers to having these conversations with patients (Chan *et al.* 2005). Fortunately, physicians' experience in related communication dilemmas, such as breaking bad news to patients, can be a helpful starting point when considering how to approach disclosure of harmful medical errors. But there are important differences between disclosure of harmful errors and breaking bad news; for example, when the physician may be partly responsible for the event having taken place. Therefore, physicians should not assume that their bad news delivery skills transfer directly to the disclosure of adverse events.

Disclosure conversations have two key components: information sharing and emotion handling. Both must be attended to if a disclosure conversation is to be successful. If healthcare workers focus only on what information to disclose to the patient without carefully considering the patient's emotions, the patient may feel well informed about the event but perceive the healthcare worker as aloof and cold. If a healthcare worker focuses primarily on responding to the patient's emotions, the patient may feel well-supported, but confused about exactly what happened. Other sections of this book cover the topic of empathic communication in detail. Therefore, the remainder of this chapter will focus on the information sharing dimensions of disclosure.

There are several core principles healthcare workers should keep in mind when approaching disclosure. First, disclosures will typically take place over more than one conversation. Disclosure conversations can be uncomfortable enough that some healthcare workers might wish to have the conversation once and be done with it. Yet breaking a disclosure into several conversations has a number of advantages. First, information about the event's cause and plans for preventing recurrences often take time to develop. Waiting to tell the patient about a harmful error until a full analysis has been completed would result in a delay that many patients would consider excessive. Therefore, an initial conversation should be held with the patient as soon as the event is discovered. This conversation can then be followed up with subsequent conversations as additional information about the event becomes apparent. Breaking disclosure conversations into multiple discussions also allows patients time to digest the information and ask questions, as well as providing the opportunity to attend to any breaches in the patient/provider relationship the error may have caused.

Error disclosure can be thought of as involving four key steps.

Step one: Get help

The emotional distress that accompanies harmful medical errors can distort healthcare workers' judgement about what happened, as well as judgement about whether and how to disclose the event to the patient. Therefore, it is essential that healthcare workers avail themselves of institutional resources to assist them in the disclosure process. Patient safety analysts and quality officers are key resources who can assist in conducting a thorough analysis to determine whether the event in question was an error and to help formulate plans for prevention. Other important sources of help include risk managers, medical directors, department chairs, or other supervisors. Careful consultation with these institutional disclosure support resources can help ensure patients receive accurate information about the event. Those providing such support to frontline clinicians should be cognizant of the emotional impact these events have on providers and be prepared to offer support services as needed.

Step two: Plan the initial disclosure conversation

Consultation with the disclosure support resources should allow for careful discussion of whether the event should be disclosed and if so, what should be said. Breakdowns in the disclosure process often occur because of lack of such planning. It is especially important to anticipate patients' likely questions about the event and consider thoughtful responses. When the harmful error involved a healthcare team, the entire team should be involved in the disclosure planning, with careful consideration given to the roles of each team member in the disclosure process, and how to respond to questions the patient is likely to ask about the event.

Step three: Hold the initial conversation

Box 39.1 details initial disclosure skills developed for a program to train doctors in disclosing unanticipated outcomes to patients (Gallagher TH, personal communication, March 2015). The initial conversation should be held within the first 24 hours after the event is discovered. Relatively little may be known about the event at this point, and so it is important not to speculate about whether the event was an error, what caused the error, or who was responsible. Often these initial conversations consist of letting the patient know that an adverse event has taken place, what the event was, and its implications for the patient's health, clinical steps that have been taken to mitigate the event, and that the event will be thoroughly investigated and the results shared with the patient. An expression of regret is appropriate during the initial conversation for all adverse events. The initial conversation concludes with the opportunity for the patient to ask questions.

Step four: Follow-up conversation

The follow-up conversation provides the opportunity for healthcare workers to share with patients new information about the event, whether it was due to an error, and if so, how recurrences of the event will be prevented. If a formal event analysis reveals that the adverse event was due to a medical error, a formal apology should be provided. The follow-up conversation also provides an additional opportunity for patients to ask questions, and healthcare workers should ensure that patients know how to contact them if they have future questions. This is also often the proper time to introduce discussions of compensation, as appropriate. Such discussions are typically conducted by the institutional risk manager or other administrator, and clinicians should generally avoid addressing compensation issues with patients unless explicitly authorized to do so by the institution.

Some organizations emphasize the importance of taking responsibility as part of the disclosure process. While patients appreciate an explicit statement of acceptance of responsibility, there are numerous unanswered questions about how best to incorporate accepting responsibility into disclosure discussions. Attending physicians may feel uncomfortable accepting responsibility when leading disclosure of events in which they only played a small role. In some organizations, senior administrators make statements of responsibility on behalf of the institution to the patient. It is unclear what specific obligations flow from a healthcare worker or institution accepting responsibility for an error. Individual clinicians, for example, may feel powerless to affect a change in the systemic factors that led to the event. Additional research is needed to explore

Box 39.1 Key initial disclosure skills

1. **Get ready:**
   - Review the event, with team members as applicable, so that you are familiar with relevant information
   - Anticipate the patient's emotional response and plan how you will respond empathically
   - Consider whether a surrogate or family member should be present
   - Anticipate likely questions from the patient
   - Consider rehearsing the discussion with a disclosure coach, if available
   - Consider including one or more team members in the discussion with the patient
   - Recognize that this is likely to be one in a series of discussions with the patient about the event
   - Consider your own feelings and seek support as needed

2. **Set the stage:**
   - Turn off/sign out beepers and phones, if possible
   - Find a suitable, private room
   - Sit down
   - Describe the purpose of the conversation

3. **Listen and empathize throughout:**
   - Assess the patient's understanding of what happened
   - Identify the patient's key concerns
   - Actively listen to the patient
   - Acknowledge and validate the patient's feelings

   (Use these same skills with the family, if present)

4. **Explain the facts:**

   What happened?
   - Identify the adverse event early in the disclosure
   - Explain what happened in a way that is easy to understand
   - Explain what is known about why the adverse event occurred; do not speculate
   - Tell the patient whether the adverse event was preventable

   What are the consequences?
   - Tell the patient how the event will be treated or managed
   - Tell the patient how the event may impact his/her long-term healthcare and what will be done to care for the patient now

5. **Apologize:**
   - Say you are sorry for the adverse event in a sincere manner early in the conversation

6. **Responsibility:**
   - Explain your role in the event
   - Avoid blaming others or 'the system'

- If the event was preventable (due to error):
  - Consider using the word 'error' or 'mistake', after consultation with a disclosure coach or risk manager
  - Tell the patient what should have happened
  - Tell the patient what will be done differently to make recurrences less likely, or that a plan to prevent recurrences will be developed

7. **Close the discussion:**
   - Discuss next steps and plan for a follow-up conversation
   - Ask the patient if s/he has any final questions and provide responses
   - Designate a contact person the patient and family can reach with questions or concerns

Always remember to:

- **Show empathy**
  - ALLOW the patient to express his/her emotions
  - ACKNOWLEDGE the patient's emotions
  - VALIDATE the patient's emotions by saying that their response is understandable

- **Be honest**
  - EXPLAIN the facts about the adverse event without the patient having to do a lot of probing
  - GIVE direct answers to the patient's questions
  - If you do not know the answer to the patient's questions, state this directly, and explain your plan to learn more.

- **Utilize effective communication strategies**
  - SHOW sincere interest in the patient's questions and concerns
  - USE good non-verbal expression (e.g. eye contact)
  - AVOID medical jargon
  - CHECK for the patient's understanding of the information throughout the conversation
  - BE yourself!

Reproduced from Thomas H. Gallagher, *Training Doctors to Disclose Unanticipated Outcomes to Patients: Randomized Trial* (Gallagher, T-PI). Developed by AHRQ grant #1RO1HS016506.

how to best meet patients' needs for acceptance of responsibility around harmful errors in ways that are comfortable for both healthcare workers and institutions.

Other organizations are focusing primarily on the apology dimensions of the disclosure process. These organizations seek to follow the lead of scholars who advocate that an 'authentic' apology is one that 'acknowledges the legitimacy of the violated rule, to admit fault for its violation, and three, expresses genuine remorse and regret for the harm caused by the violation' (Taft 2005). An authentic apology 'invites forgiveness, which is the door to reconciliation'. This view of apology contrasts sharply with an 'expression of regret', in which the healthcare worker tells the patient, 'I'm sorry this happened to you', but does not admit fault or seek forgiveness. While substantial theoretical considerations support some dimensions of this push towards 'authentic apologies', there is only limited empirical evidence about how patients perceive specific apology strategies. Patients may be most interested in whether an apology seems sincere to them, rather than about what specific words were used in the apology itself. How best to integrate apology into the disclosure process is another important area of future research.

Role play scenario

As with any other communication dilemma, practising error disclosure is critical if healthcare workers are to improve their skills in this area. An error disclosure case is provided below.

Frank Jones is a 63-year-old patient diagnosed with metastatic non-small cell lung cancer who was admitted to the intensive care unit with seizures. Head CT shows a large mass, presumably another metastasis. In the ICU, he is treated with a loading dose of dilantin, 300 mg three times daily, then switched to dilantin 300 mg once daily when his dilantin levels are therapeutic. He is being transferred to the floor, and the physician writing transfer orders mistakenly writes for the patient to receive dilantin 300 mg three times daily rather than the once daily dose the patient was currently receiving. This medication error is not noticed by the floor nurses nor by the pharmacist. Two days later, the patient experiences dilantin toxicity and becomes confused, disoriented, and falls on their way to the bathroom striking his head on the sink. A dilantin level at the time of the fall was very elevated at 30. A head CT after the fall shows a new but small subdural haematoma. How should the attending physician, the floor nurse, and the medical social worker approach the disclosure about this medication error to the patient?

Conclusion

The gap between expectations that harmful errors be disclosed to patients and current clinical practice should prompt healthcare workers, institutions, professional organizations, and policy makers to adopt new approaches to communicating with patients following these events. The oncology community's expertise in sharing bad news with patients makes it an ideal group to take a leadership role in developing enhanced standards for disclosure conversations as well as to undertake research on the impact of different disclosure strategies on important patient outcomes such as trust and satisfaction in the cancer care setting.

References

Boothman RC, Imhoff SJ, Campbell DA (2012). Nurturing a culture of patient safety and achieving lower malpractice risk through disclosure: lessons learned and future directions. *Front Health Serv Manage* **28**, 13–28.

Chan DK, Gallagher TH, Reznick R, Levinson W (2005). How surgeons disclose medical errors to patients: A study using standardized patients. *Surgery* **138**, 851–8.

Conway J, Federico F, Stewart K, Campbell M (2011). *Respectful Management of Serious Clinical Adverse Events (Second Edition)*, IHI Innovation Series white paper, Institute for Healthcare Improvement, Cambridge, MA. Available

at: http://www.ihi.org/resources/Pages/IHIWhitePapers/RespectfulManagementSeriousClinicalAEsWhitePaper.aspx [Last accessed March 19, 2015].

Gallagher TH, Garbutt JM, Waterman AD (2006a). Choosing your words carefully: how physicians would disclose harmful medical errors to patients. *Arch Int Med* **166**, 1585–93.

Gallagher TH, Mello MM, Levinson W, et al. (2013). Talking with patients about other clinicians' errors. *New Eng J Med* **369**, 1752–57.

Gallagher, TH, Waterman, AD, Garbutt, JM, et al. (2006b). US and Canadian physicians' attitudes and experiences regarding disclosing errors to patients. *Arch Int Med* **166**, 1605–11.

Helmchen LA, Richards MR, McDonald TB (2010). How does routine disclosure of medical error affect patients' propensity to sue and their assessment of provider quality? Evidence from survey data. *Med Care* **48**, 955–61.

Hobgood C, Xie J, Weiner B, Hooker J (2004). Error identification, disclosure, and reporting: Practice patterns of three emergency medicine provider types. *Acad Emerg Med* **11**, 196–9.

Iedema R, Allen S, Britton K, Gallagher TH (2012). What do patients and relatives know about problems and failures in care?. *BMJ Qual Saf* **21**, 198–205.

Iedema R, Allen S, Britton K, et al. (2011a). Patients' and family members' views on how clinicians enact and how they should enact incident disclosure: the "100 patient stories" qualitative study. *BMJ* **343**, d4423.

Iedema R, Allen S, Sorensen R, Gallagher TH (2011b). What prevents incident disclosure, and what can be done to promote it? *Jt Comm J Qual Patient Saf* **37**, 409–17.

Iedema RAM, Mallock, NA, Sorensen, RJ, et al. (2008). The National Open Disclosure Pilot: evaluation of a policy implementation initiative. *Med J Aust* **188**, no. 7. Available at: https://www.mja.com.au/journal/2008/188/7/national-open-disclosure-pilot-evaluation-policy-implementation-initiative [Last accessed March 19, 2015].

Institute of Medicine (US) Committee on Quality of Health Care in America (2000). *To Err is Human: Building a Safer Health System*. Kohn LT, Corrigan JM, Donaldson MS (eds). National Academies Press (US), Washington (DC Available at: http://www.ncbi.nlm.nih.gov/books/NBK225182/) [Last accessed March 19, 2015].

Kachalia A, Kaufman SR, Boothman R, et al. (2010). Liability claims and costs before and after implementation of a medical error disclosure program. *Ann Intern Med* **153**, 213–21.

Lembitz A (2010). *Litigation alternative: COPIC's 3Rs program*. Available at: http://www.aaos.org/news/aaosnow/sep10/managing7.asp [Last accessed March 19, 2015].

Mastroianni AC, Mello MM, Sommer S, Hardy M, Gallagher TH (2010). The flaws in state "apology" and "disclosure" laws dilute their intended impact on malpractice suits. *Health Affairs* **29**, 1611–19.

Mazor KM, Greene SM, Roblin D, et al. (2013). More than words: Patients' views on apology and disclosure when things go wrong in cancer care. *Patient Educ Couns* **90**, 341–6.

Mazor KM, Reed GW, Yood RA, Fischer MA, Baril J, Gurwitz JH (2006). Disclosure of medical errors: what factors influence how patients respond?. *J Gen Int Med* **21**, 704–10.

Mazor KM, Roblin DW, Greene SM, et al. (2012). Toward patient-centered cancer care: Patient perceptions of problematic events, impact, and response. *J Clin Oncol* **30**, 1784–90.

Mello MM, Boothman RC, McDonald T, et al. (2014). Communication-and-resolution programs: The challenges and lessons learned from six early adopters', *Health Affairs* **33**, 20–9.

National Quality Forum (NQF) (2010). *Safe Practices for Better Healthcare— 2010 Update: A Consensus Report*. NQF, Washington DC, WA Available at: http://www.qualityforum.org/Publications/2010/04/Safe_Practices_

for_Better_Healthcare_%E2%80%93_2010_Update.aspx [Last accessed March 19, 2015].

Prouty CD, Mazor KM, Greene SM, *et al.* (2014). Providers' perceptions of communication breakdowns in cancer care. *J Gen Intern Med* **29**, 1122–30.

Roundtable on Transparency (2015). *Shining a Light: Safer Health Care Through Transparency*, National Patient Safety Foundation's Lucian Leape Institute, Boston, MA. Available at: http://c.ymcdn.com/sites/

www.npsf.org/resource/resmgr/LLI/Shining-a-Light_Transparency.pdf [Last accessed March 26, 2015].

Shannon SE, Foglia MB, Hardy M, Gallagher TH (2009). Disclosing errors to patients: Perspectives of registered nurses. *Jt Commission J Qual Patient Saf* **35**, 5–12.

Taft L (2005). On bended knee (with fingers crossed). *DePaul Law Review* **55**, 601.

CHAPTER 40

A health equity care model for improving communication and patient-centred care: A focus on oncology care and diversity

Kimlin Tam Ashing, Noé Rubén Chávez,
and Marshalee George

Introduction to a health equity care model

Worldwide human migration is climbing rapidly. Across countries there is increasing migration from developing nations to developed nations, as well as internal migration within countries across different regions (Segal *et al.* 2010). Thus, our societies are increasingly multiethnic, multicultural, and multilingual. Differences are often seen as increasing intergroup tensions and conflicts, but this diversity can also be seen as inherently engendering increased knowledge and opportunities that enrich quality of life for all. Therefore, human services systems within countries and communities must respond to this diversity to serve all residents, and healthcare systems are among the most challenged. Hence, those we serve to prevent illnesses, maintain health, cure diseases, heal, manage symptoms and comfort, are more and more likely to look and speak differently from us (the healthcare provider). There are not only language differences, but our patients and consumers have different sets of experiences, culture, beliefs, values, and practices that influence health status, health behaviour, provider–patient interactions, and potentially health outcomes as well. Societal diversity also reflects a complexity of different factors, including socioeconomic, educational, sociopolitical, and contextual, that also contribute to provider–patient interactions and health outcomes. Therefore, addressing diversity in healthcare settings has direct implications for improving health and addressing health inequities (Weech-Maldonado *et al.* 2012). The oncology setting presents probably the greatest opportunities and challenges in caring for diverse, in particular cultural and linguistic minorities, patients, and their families.

Cancer is probably one of the most complex and profound diseases. In an optimal care setting, cancer requires multiple levels of diagnostic procedures and therapeutic interventions from various oncology specialists. Clinical oncology has benefitted from tremendous advancements in screening, diagnostic, and therapeutic care, such that some cancers are preventable and curable, with even more cancers now viewed as highly treatable and considered chronic

illnesses. Still, cancer treatments are costly and lengthy with potential debilitating side effects, including risk for cancers, toxicities, bodily dysfunction, compromised quality of life, and pain. Cancer conjures up fear, grief, loss, hopelessness, anger and even shame (IOM Report 2008). Providing quality cancer treatment and care demands attending to the reality of the complexity of cancer care, as well as appreciating the fact that cancer care is increasingly occurring in a context of increasing patient diversity.

Adequately addressing population diversity in healthcare, particularly in the oncology setting, is most intricate and delicate. Hence, we are challenged to rethink dominant paradigms of diversity or multicultural care, ways of practising medicine, and providing healthcare in cross-cultural settings. Thus, we are inspired to expand our approaches to optimize how we relate to and communicate with patients and families from non-dominant cultures and diverse backgrounds.

In addressing diversity in healthcare various terms such as 'cultural competence', 'multi-cultural education', 'culturally appropriate', or 'culturally sensitive' are part of the lexicon. The concept of 'culture' is central to any model or effort at implementing clinical practice that reflects competency or sensitivity to diversity. Therefore, understanding what is meant by 'culture' is essential to understanding any paradigm or model aiming to address human diversity in healthcare settings. The current chapter will briefly examine the concept of culture, discuss communication within cancer care, and provide a brief overview of the prevailing paradigm to addressing human diversity in healthcare, and present some of the challenges of this work. Finally, we will discuss an enhanced approach for providing quality healthcare to diverse patients with a focus on addressing patient–provider communication in cancer care.

Conceptualizing culture

Culture has many definitions. Just within anthropology, arguably the field where culture was originally conceptualized, there exist various definitions (Thackrah and Thompson 2013). Definitions highlight a system of shared meanings or guidelines that contextualize historical and current social norms and practices, and provide the lens through which to view the world (Kagawa-Singer 2012). Also, stressed as essential units of 'culture' are norms, beliefs, values, identity, language, and practices that vary across different groups (Thackrah and Thompson 2013). Based on a socioecological framework, these elements are manifested or expressed differently based on the level of analysis—individual, familial, community, or societal (Hughes *et al.* 1993). In addition to being multidimensional and multilevel, culture is also a dynamic and fluid process, constantly evolving and changing over time and across different contexts (Kleinman and Benson 2006).

Culture is broad and intertwined with economic, political, religious, psychological, and biological conditions (Kleinman and Benson 2006). It is important to note that although culture is sometimes used interchangeably with 'ethnicity' or 'race', it is not the same but is a distinct construct. Ethnicity and race are also broad constructs. Ethnicity is typically used to refer to groups with a common culture, language, or nationality (Phinney 1996). Ethnicity, like culture is multidimensional, consisting of at least three dimensions along which individuals and samples vary: cultural norms and values; strength, salience and meaning of ethnic identity; and experiences and attitudes associated with minority status (Phinney 1996). Race is commonly used to classify persons by phenotypic characteristics, such as skin colour, facial features, and hair type. However, race is scientifically rejected as a valid biological construct (McCann-Mortimer *et al.* 2004). There is consensus, however, that race is a useful social construct that is historically shaped and a sociopolitically driven process anchored to power, status and oppressive structures (Cornell and Hartmann 1998).

In the United States for example, broad categorical groups based on ethnicity and/or race are heterogeneous in many respects. Within the ethnic category of Latino/Hispanic, or racial category of Asian/Pacific Islander and African American, there exists great heterogeneity in nationality, cultural traditions, language, socioeconomic status, beliefs, and practices. Although it can be argued that there is an 'essence' or general norms associated with these broad groupings, the diversity within these groups is so great that any generalization is problematic and perpetuates stereotypes (Ashing-Giwa 2005). Healthcare providers need to provide care that both acknowledges and respects the cultural experiences of patients, as well as their individuality.

The process and context of immigration also adds another layer of complexity. Immigrants or refugees are acculturating to their new society and local community; and are thus experiencing a process of cultural change, preservation, resistance, and integration, leading to new identities and ways of life, or even to a reinforcing of native cultural values and practices (Phinney 2006). Immigrant enclaves or communities provide resources and support for preservation of the native culture. However, generational issues are prominent, and there are differences with the children of immigrant parents developing fluency in the language and culture of the receiving society. This process and context of acculturation creates diversity not only within communities, but within families (Birman 2006). This diversity creates a challenge (e.g. intergenerational conflict, gender role issues) and opportunity (e.g. community liaison/advocate, resource) in healthcare, and especially when involving the family in patient care.

Furthermore, culture is inherently complex, as culture is characterized by both stable (e.g. shared history, geography) and dynamic processes (e.g. education, socioeconomic) and context. Culture directly influences our worldview and helps us make sense or meaning of life (Kagawa-Singer 2012). For example, it provides the ways to make sense of difficult and challenging experiences, and helps us cognitively and emotionally survive—or even thrive—through these experiences, such as through a cancer diagnosis, treatment, and post-treatment (Kagawa-Singer 2012; Surbone 2012). We engage in this deeply emotional process of meaning-making, not in isolation, but in the context of family and community relationships. This reality increases the significance of including the family and community in healthcare decision-making.

Communication in oncology care

Communication, similar to culture, is itself a complex process influenced by various factors. In the context of healthcare, the differences in knowledge, perspectives, resources, and goals between patients and providers create a challenge for communicating and understanding each other. Additional differences in lived experience between patients and providers are noteworthy. These differences particularly in cultural values, norms, and practices, add another layer of complexity. In oncology care, the challenges are great, especially given the nature of the types of treatment, care plans, team of providers, and the psychosocial difficulties affecting both patients and family as they cope and survive through a cancer diagnosis, treatment, survivorship, or end-of-life issues.

For example, a qualitative study examining the perspective of patients and their families regarding communication with their oncologist, underscored the importance of patient-centred care (Mazor *et al.* 2013). Patients and family members wanted a clinician who was sensitive and caring. Pateint and family members specifically expressed that they wanted a provider who carefully and empathetically listened and responded to their questions and concerns, and who provided information they needed in a timely, clear and understandable matter. (Mazor *et al.* 2013).

Another qualitative study exploring the perspective of cancer patients in regards to what they valued most in patient–provider communication, also discussed the centrality of patients believing and feeling that their oncologist cared about and respected them as 'individual persons' (Skea *et al.* 2014). They emphasized how communication in this context of patient-centred care is not just about the 'transfer of information' related to cancer care, but also about the relational aspect, where patients feel they are treated with dignity and respect, and are afforded autonomy in their care (Skea *et al.* 2014).

The actual practice of patient-centred care is the ideal but in reality it is challengening to achieve 100% of the time with every patient. There exist various barriers that need to be overcome in order to provide the type of care that satisfies the relational, emotional or psychosocial needs of patients. A study by Fagerlind and colleagues (2013) examined the perspective of oncologists to understand their barriers to successfully engaging in quality patient-centered, psychosocial communication. Most oncologists acknowledged the importance of addressing the psychosocial needs of their patients. Still, they also describedthe barriers that get in the way of achieving patient-centered, psychosocial communication , including insufficient consultation time, lack of patient centered measures and metricsconcerning patient focused assessments and outcomes of their psychosocial health; and lack of support from administrators due to staffing and payment issues, and guidelines regarding how to handle issues concerning patient's psychosocial health (Fagerlind, *et al.* 2013, p. 3817). Meeting the psychosocial needs of cancer patients and their caregivers are indeed challenging.

In order to more fully understand the various psychosocial needs of patients and how best to address them, we also need to understand their sociocultural context and experiences. Understanding their sociocultural context and experiences requires an explicit examination of the 'cultural competency' of the oncology care team including surgeons,oncologists, psychooncologists, social workers, spiritual care and other providers.

Cultural competence: The prevailing paradigm of healthcare with diverse populations

In the past few years there has been a surge of 'culturally competent' trainings, curriculum, and best practices, which have been designed in order to develop the ability, skills, and knowledge of healthcare providers to provide the most sensitive, 'culturally tailored', and effective healthcare services to immigrants, ethnic minorities, and other underserved and underrepresented communities (Kripalani *et al.* 2006). The 'cultural competency' initiatives that have become the objective of healthcare systems and medical school education are well-intentioned efforts at improving health outcomes and reducing health disparities for ethnic minority and underserved communities. However, these well-intentioned efforts often fall short of addressing the complexity of multiculturalism in environments of disparities (Dean 2001; Kleinman and Benson 2006).

Cultural competence, like the concept of culture, has different definitions, resulting from different perspectives, as well as the unit or level of analysis applied. Broadly speaking, cultural competence within a healthcare system involves a set of attitudes, practices, and policies that promote and support effective cross-cultural or cross-linguistic interactions and communication (Betancourt *et al.* 2003). When thinking at the level of patient–provider interactions, cultural competence entails a set of knowledge, attitudes, values, skills, and behaviour enacted by providers to more effectively engage with patients in ways that reflect a certain level of understanding, sensitivity, and respect for cultural or linguistic differences (Betancourt *et al.* 2003).

Some goals for implementing cultural competent care, in addition to achieving clear and effective communication include providing quality healthcare, minimizing medical errors, enhancing positive health outcomes, as well as promoting health equity (Betancourt *et al.* 2003). A systematic review of 34 studies found some evidence that cultural competent training improved knowledge, attitudes, and skills of health professionals, along with having a positive effect on patient satisfaction (Beach *et al.* 2005). One study, examining a large database of 66 hospitals in the state of California (United States) found that hospitals with greater cultural competency (assessed with the Cultural Competency Assessment Tool of Hospitals, CCATH) had patients who reported greater satisfaction with communication with their doctors and nurses, gave hospitals a higher rating for quality, and were more likely to recommend the hospital to others (Weech-Maldonado *et al.* 2012). Although there is some evidence that cultural competent care can be effective, in healthcare settings there is little known on the impact on health disparities, patient outcomes, as well as conceptual and practical challenges.

Conceptual and practical challenges in cultural competent care

Cultural competent care faces conceptual challenges related to the definition of 'culture' as discussed above, as well as practical challenges with implementation of 'competent' clinical practices that are responsive and optimally embraces *diversity*. Cultural competent care for practical reasons may simplify 'culture' and focus on communication and practices that unintentionally homogenize and perpetuate stereotypes of groups, especially those based on ethnicity, religion, or nationality (Kleinman and Benson 2006). As previously stated, the diversity within different groups, communities, and families both challenges and creates opportunities to better communicate across cultural and language differences. One challenge stems from the lack of healthcare providers—including physicians, oncologists, nurse practitioners, psychologists, and social workers—who share ethnic, cultural, or linguisitc realities with their patients. This reality, especially in the United States, or other Western nations with large numbers of immigrants further highlights the need for not only more competent medical interpreters (Brisset *et al.* 2013) but also for a more diverse healthcare workforce with second language capacity (Fernández and Pérez-Stable 2015).

Another challenge lies in the assumption that health providers should possess specific knowledge and skills of a particular 'cultural group' in order to effectively communicate and provide care to patients of that group (Sue 2006). It is unrealistic to think that providers will be able to learn about every group or community, or even learn multiple languages. Even when providers possess a good understanding of a particular ethnic group or community, because of cultural diversity , it is difficult to assume the general attitudes, values, or health practices of that group. Providers should aim to view patients as unique individuals without ignoring their lived experiences. Patients' lived experiences are shaped by the intersection of their culture, religion, gender, sexual orientation, socioeconomic status, acculturative experience, and other sociocontextual factors. In addition to the challenges created by cultural diversity, there are opportunities to engage the perspective of family and community to gain understanding into patients' lived experiences. Information obtained from support system interviews do not only provide deeper understanding into cultural aspects of the patient, but it highlights their personality traits, temperament, desires, strengths and weaknesses. When the provider views the patient as an individual, and observes their interaction with internal (family) and external (society) environments, the patient–provider relationship can be fruitful, thus yielding improved health outcomes for the patient.

Conceptually, some go as far as critiquing whether or not it is possible to develop 'skills' in cultural competency (Dean 2001; Kleinman and Benson 2006). They argue that culture is not something that can be reduced to a set of skills or detailed instructions on how to treat patients from various ethnic backgrounds (Kleinman and Benson 2006). It is difficult to be culturally competent when culture is continually changing (Dean 2001). Furthermore, given the complexity of the broad context in which culture is defined, what seems to be a prevailing aspect of concern for culture is the socioeconomic status and poverty level of the patient, which are contributors to health disparities (Betancourt *et al.* 2003). The reality is that many ethnic minority, indigenous, immigrant, and refugee populations are overrepresented among the lower socioeconomic status groups in most nations. Ethnic minority status may be an unfortunate proxy for low socioeconomic status (Ashing-Giwa 2005).

Therefore, in the process of seeking to be culturally competent, healthcare providers need to also develop an understanding for the socioeconomic experience andbroader social issues encountered by their patients. For example, medical education curriculums have been developed within the United States to increase knowledge and a critical awareness of social justice and racism that are relevant to understanding the impact of social determinants on health (Kumagai and Lypson 2009). Also, researchers have argued that there is a lack of a connection between cultural competency and health outcomes or reduction in health disparities, because the focus of cultural competency efforts has been narrow and does not adequately address social determinants of health, such as institutional racism or poverty (Drevdahl *et al.* 2008; Marmot *et al.* 2012; Alcaraz *et al.* 2016; Chávez 2015).

For example, a review by Beach *et al.* found little evidence that cultural competency improves patient adherence to therapy, health outcomes, or equity of services across ethnic/racial minorities, while Truong *et al.* (2014) concluded that research on cultural competency is broad and complex and will yield a relatively weak evidence base. Similar to Beach *et al.*, Truong *et al.* also concluded that, in general, there was moderate evidence of improvement in provider outcomes, as well as healthcare access and utilization outcomes, with weaker evidence of improvements in patient outcomes. Some of the reasons for poor empirical evidence of the effectiveness of cultural competence included issues with the quality of research, such as improving the conceptual clarity of cultural competence, measure validation, and methodological rigour, as well as identifying what and how specific cultural competent practices are related to particular health outcomes (Truong *et al.* 2014). This latter issue relates to the practical challenge of understanding how to achieve cultural competence in practice. There is a need for an enhanced approach that further examines what elements are essential for providing effective healthcare in contexts of diversity.

Towards a humanistic approach

First, since it is more than just an individual characteristic, culture is not just something that is brought to the clinic by the patient, but an interlinked complexity that also structures the societal and healthcare environment. This complexity is an interconnection of larger historical, sociopolitical, economic, and cultural worldviews. There is, for example, inadequate attention paid to how the 'culture' of the society and the healthcare system or biomedicine influences how providers unconsciously or consciously behave towards their patients (IOM Report 2002; Fox 2005; Kleinman and Benson 2006). There is also little attention given to how the sociocultural background of the provider influences how they interact with patients cross-culturally (Fox 2005). Although there has been a momentum towards developing more cultural consonant healthcare, there is relatively little attention to the socioecological milieu.

Secondly, the prevailing biomedicine and healthcare systems are rooted primarily in a Western worldview. This particular worldview is characterized as viewing the 'self' as primarily 'independent' as opposed to 'interdependent'. The interdependent view of self is predominant across many parts of the world including Eastern, Pacific Islander, and African cultures (Triandis 1995). Policies, norms, and everyday practices within the healthcare system tend to focus on

individual level problems, decontextualize these problems, reduce problems to genetic or biological mechanisms, and aim to reduce or eliminate pathology without also focusing on strengths of patients and promotion of well-being (Baer *et al.* 2003). This predominant thinking structures healthcare and affects how individual providers relate to and communicate with their patients. A more holistic view of patients that takes a more comprehensive look at how the complexity of culture and social structures impacts patient–provider relationships is needed.

In order to develop greater capacity for communicating sensitively and effectively across diversity, there first needs to be a willingness of healthcare providers to reflect deeply about their own identity and biases rooted in their sociocultural background and socialization in the culture of biomedicine and healthcare systems. There needs to also be a sustained engagement with not only patients within healthcare settings, but also outside these settings, as well as engagement with families and communities. This is critical for developing an in-depth and comprehensive appreciation, not abstract or stereotypical knowledge, of patients from diverse backgrounds. This deep sense of self and contextual awareness, a type of mindfulness, is part of a process that can enhance cultural competency efforts. Examining other emotional and moral qualities, in addition to cognitive skills, can provide insights for furthering these efforts.

Cultural humility

The concept of 'cultural humility' was developed by Tervalon and Murray-Garcia (1998) as a way to address what they saw as limitations with the concept of cultural competence. Cultural humility is defined as 'a lifelong commitment to self-evaluation and self-critique, to redressing the power imbalances in the patient-physician dynamic, and to developing mutually beneficial and nonpaternalistic clinical and advocacy partnerships with communities on behalf of individuals and defined populations' (Tervalon and Murray-Garcia 1998, p. 117). Work by Chang *et al.* (2012) with health promotion in the Chinese immigrant community in the United States, along with guiding wisdom from Chinese philosophy, promoted a similar cultural humility framework, QIAN (humbleness): importance of self-Questioning and critique; bi-directional cultural Immersion; mutually Active listening; and the flexibility of Negotiation. Central elements of cultural humility in this framework involve first starting with an open self-awareness; engaging in mutual learning with patients; developing mutually respectful partnerships with patients, families, and communities; and lifelong engagement in this process (Chang *et al.* 2012). These qualities and actions resonate nicely with the experiential wisdom shared by Surbone (2012), based on her extensive work with multicultural populations in oncology settings.

Surbone highlights how illness in general, and the cancer experience in particular are interpreted and understood in different ways by patients and providers, given the inherent differences in positions, perspectives, goals, and sociocultural contexts. These differences can challenge the patient–provider communication. It is the responsibility of the healthcare provider to engage with patients and families in ways that provide a more holistic understanding of cancer and treatment, and how it is experienced and understood by patients and their families (Surbone 2012). She states that virtues such as humility and respect are fundamental for better communication with all cancer patients, especially with those who are 'more vulnerable by the physical, psychological, and existential pain of cancer' (Surbone 2012, p. 35). An inclusion of these types of values/virtues in a cultural competency framework is fundamental.

Health equity care: Advancing the cultural competency framework

Based on previous work on cultural competency and cultural humility, as well as our experiences as health and cancer survivorship researchers conducting community-engaged research, we propose an enhanced framework to address diversity in the patient–provider encounter. We term this new framework—health equity care. Health equity care is pertinent in all healthcare interactions, but it is particularly relevant in multicultural contexts when the patient is not a member of the provider's ethnic group and the patient is a member of a minority and/or marginalized population. Health equity care is fundamental to improving effective and quality care in oncology and other health areas, including better communication between patients and healthcare providers. The three pillars of health equity care are: (i) cultural competency—the cognitive aspect of the relationship addressing the necessary skills and competencies such as language and learned techniques of how to work with the patient; (ii) cultural humility—the moral aspect inclusive of qualities such as lifelong self-evaluation with the aim towards justice and respect for the patient; and (iii) cultural empathy—encompasses the emotional aspect engendered by deep admiration, appreciation, and understanding of the whole patient and all that s/he brings to the clinical interaction.

It is our belief that even when working among the complexities of culture and the social context, culturally effective care is highly achievable. There can definitely be ambiguity or uncertainty tied to understanding how culture and social context influences patient–provider communication. However, uncertainty itself is commonly recognized as an inherent aspect in communication between cancer patients and oncologists (Surbone 2012). Thus, it is important to recognize culture and social context as another source of uncertainty and be sensitive to and honest regarding how one feels about this uncertainty. This aspect in oncology care is difficult for everyone involved. It is difficult for the provider, who because of her/his authority may be perceived as having all the answers, but may not. It is difficult for the patient and family, who want to know for certain that 'everything will be okay', or overcome the fear during remission of a cancer recurrence. Whatever the specific concern or anxiety, the general feeling of uncertainty is an experience shared among patients, their families, and the oncology team. As such, this process can be viewed as potentially building solidarity while breaking down the barrier of 'otherness', which may be even more salient when there are cultural and linguistic differences.

The experience among the oncology team, patients, and families can be deeply emotional and at times, such as during palliative and end-of-life care, can be soul wrenching. Thus, it is both a cognitive and emotional process. Communicating effectively in this context requires not only a foundation in systematic science, but artful humanism. It requires both skills and virtues. Cultural competency is necessary but not sufficient. Cultural empathy and cultural humility can ease the communication in situations where systematic skill is not enough. These virtues may facilitate an authentic relationship between patients, families, and the oncology team, including medical interpreters, as well as improve communication and understanding. Table 40.1 presents the core domains of each of

Table 40.1 Three pillars, core domains, and learning process of health equity care

Pillars	Core domain	Methods for teaching	Continuous learning
Cultural competency	Cognitive	Didactic and experiential	Reflection on the implementation of skills in patient–provider interactions
Cultural humility	Moral	Experiential and reflective/mindfulness	Engagement in advocacy efforts
Cultural empathy	Emotional	Experiential and reflective/mindfulness	Immersion in culture and community outside of clinic

the pillars of health equity care, along with the best approaches for teaching or stimulating their development in healthcare providers.

General guidelines for engendering and providing health equity care

There is no one course or set curriculum that can impart and nurture the three pillars of health equity care. Just as the purpose is not to develop specific skills and knowledge unique to every culture and language—that is impossible—the purpose is to offer suggestions for lifelong learning and experiences towards achieving health equity care. In fact, we view cultivating health equity care as a multidimensional process as well as a framework. We briefly want to offer some general guidelines for learning this type of care and spark further discussion of what is essential for providing care that is sensitive to diversity and promotes equity. We discuss five guidelines for nurturing and sustaining the three pillars of health equity care:

1. Didactic methods can increase knowledge and skills of cultural competency. However, experiential methods are more effective and are the most suitable for nurturing cultural humility and cultural empathy.

2. Cultural competency and especially cultural humility and cultural empathy require deep, ongoing reflection and mindfulness in order to cultivate and genuinely integrate the values and practices of cultural humility and empathy.

3. Enhanced learning of health equity care necessitates stepping outside the traditional healthcare setting and immersing oneself in diverse cultures, as well as engaging with families and communities in their real life contexts.

4. Achieving positive health outcomes and equity based on the health equity care approaches extends beyond the realm of traditional Western medicine, and expands healthcare into integrating whole person care that provides or offers referrals for social services, behavioural, psychological, spiritual, and financial care. Thus, to grow in cultural humility, we must consider the moral and social justice component of health equity care. Thus, at some level, providers must also engage in advocacy work for the benefit of the underserved or marginalized group.

5. Health equity care is a lifelong process requiring patience, optimism, and an ongoing commitment towards nurturing cultural

empathy with the self as the instrument of healing: and therefore, the healer provides the environment where human dignity, acceptance, warmth, and wellness thrives.

Conclusion

Healthcare providers in oncology and other health areas are increasingly challenged to provide quality and effective treatment and care that are responsive and appreciative of cultural and linguistic diversity. The multifaceted and dynamic interplay of culture and context shaping the patient–provider encounter, especially in more sensitive situations of oncology care, calls for a more comprehensive framework to facilitate healthcare communication. Providing humanistic care to the whole patient, which honours their cultural and other lived experiences, requires skills and values. The prevailing approach is the cultural competency model. There is evidence that cultural competent training can improve cultural knowledge and culturally informed interventions, as well as patient satisfaction (Beach *et al.* 2005; Truong *et al.* 2014). However, the cultural competency approach has proven to be necessary but not sufficient. It is important to be educated on and understand cultural practices and beliefs, yet we must be cautious not to overgeneralize and stereotype. One size does not fit all, even in patients from the same ethnic group. Each patient should be treated as a person with the right to the best care available, and with dignity. Therefore, to further advance health communication and quality care, we presented a health equity care model that embraces three pillars—*cultural competency, cultural humility,* and *cultural empathy.*

Case study

Jenny Jones a 42-year-old African American female, worked as a civil engineer and felt a left breast mass after accidentally falling face down while on the job on July 10.

Interval history

Mrs Jones has no known family history of breast or ovarian cancer and never had a screening mammogram. Her mother was a native of Jamaica and she has one uncle (aged 68 years) who is a five-year survivor of prostate cancer. Her father was born in Los Angeles, California, and she has two living paternal uncles—one with a history of prostate cancer, and the other with colon cancer (both diagnosed after age 60).

Her maternal grandmother lived with them (the Joneses), and turned the kitchen into a sanctuary for Jamaican herbs, some used for medicine and others in 'flavourful' dishes such as 'Ackee & Salt Fish', 'Jerk Chicken', 'Rice and peas', 'Callaloo', 'Escoviche Fish'; and she also had her daily cup of the 'famous Blue Mountain Coffee'. She visited Jamaica every year during the summer as a child; and she continues to participate in local Jamaican or Caribbean events.

Mrs Jones has been married to Tom Jones for 17 years and they have two children: one daughter (7 years old) and one son (14 years old). Their daughter takes ballet lessons and their son is on the high school football team. Mr Jones is a computer programmer for the Federal government and works long hours at times. Mrs Jones is premenopausal, healthy with no history of hypertension, diabetes, or any breast changes. She never smoked cigarettes and consumes very little alcohol. She has a six-year history of oral contraceptive use, which her primary care provider discontinued on July 8.

Follow-up for left breast mass

Mrs Jones went to her primary care provider Dr Jonathan Charles on July 14 to evaluate the left breast mass and she was then referred for further breast imaging. On July 16 she had a 3D TOMO bilateral diagnostic mammogram and left breast ultrasound and speculated mass measuring 4.0 cm in diameter at 9 o'clock position 3 cm lateral to the left nipple was found, and was consistent to the location of the left breast mass that Mrs Jones felt. She then had a left axillary ultrasound that was negative for suspicious lymph nodes and a left breast ultrasound guided core biopsy was performed by Dr Smith.

Biopsy results

Dr Smith contacted Mrs Jones on July17 at 3:45pm and told her over the telephone: 'Mrs Jenny Jones, your pathology results from your left breast biopsy shows that you have breast cancer. I have sent a message to your primary care provider Dr Charles and he will discuss treatment options with you on Monday.'

Mrs Jones became worried and anxious. She was thinking that she may die or become very ill and be unable to work and support her family. Even though she is an African American, her culture is influenced strongly from her Jamaican parent and relatives. Therefore, she decided to keep her news of breast cancer private, confiding only in 'God'. Dr Charles did not call her on July 20, so she called him to discuss treatment. Dr Charles scheduled her to see Dr Han, a surgical oncologist, on July 31. At that visit, Dr Han said: 'Mrs Jones since the left breast mass is 4 cm, and you are African American, many women like you die from breast cancer. I recommend that you have a bilateral mastectomy (both breasts removed) so you do not have to worry about cancer coming back.' Mrs Jones left that consult appointment feeling hopeless, as Dr Han did not provide any treatment options, nor did he inquire about her needs. He also did not provide her with any resources or advise of her right to a second opinion. Dr Han, and many of her physicians, so far, seem to be responding to her from a disease perspective and not from a person perspective. Their approach and manner do not embody cultural competence and empathy.

Mrs Jones contemplated on the lifestyle that she currently had with her family and her work; she was active with her family, civic society, and had a dynamic role on the local netball team. She then decided not to get treatment right away since she had no symptoms. She will rely on prayer and use natural herbs that her grandmother used when she was younger to reduce joint swelling or inflammation in the body and to strengthen her immune system.

Case analysis via the three pillars of health equity care

How could the three pillars—cultural competency, cultural humility, and cultural empathy facilitate health equity care?

Cultural competency requires the provider to have the necessary skills to understand relational concepts, language, norms, and communication strategies to meet patients' needs within their sociocultural context. Cultural humility requires the providers to be aware of 'self' and their 'ideal self' where they are able to set aside their personal biases, in order to beneficently and justly give patients the care they deserve with dignity, respect, and equity. Cultural empathy is being non-judgemental and the provider putting themselves in the patient's place and seeing the world through their eyes. This process provides a deep understanding and appreciation of the patient's diversity and the fabric patients bring to the clinical encounter and the cancer care team.

Scenario 1

Let's go back to when Mrs Jones received her biopsy results. If cultural competency, cultural humility and cultural empathy were practiced in her provider–patient interaction, the radiologist would have given the biopsy results to Mrs Jones differently. Even though the radiologist Dr Smith may have given breast biopsy results over the phone to patients without negative feedback, it does not negate that there may be patients who would prefer their biopsy results be delivered in a different way. The only way to find out patients' preference for the delivery results is through assessment, which could be done at the time of the biopsy, where Dr Smith could have asked 'How would you like me to give you the results of the biopsy, over the phone, in the mail, or would you like to come in to discuss the results?' Active listening is an essential skill within the assessment phase where the provider uses verbal and non-verbal cues to understand patients' preference. Cultural competency calls for flexibility and the willingness of providers to remove self and place their attention on meeting the health needs of the patient and in this case, the provider may have to add a time on the image schedule to meet and discuss the biopsy results with the patient.

Scenario 2

Dr Charles, as a primary care provider to Mrs Jones, should have built a patient–provider trusting relationship so that he could have recommended that she included her spouse or at least a support person at the surgical oncology consult with Dr Han. At that discussion Mrs Jones may have revealed to Dr Charles her inherent health beliefs and behaviours that may be unique to her, and these beliefs and practices may play a role in her perception of her breast cancer and treatment. As the referring physician to Dr Han, Dr Charles should pass on any information about Mrs Jones that he thinks is pertinent to her being receptive of her diagnosis and treatment options. In contrast, if Dr Han did not get that additional information from Dr Charles in addition to Mrs Jones's medical history, he should assess her social, cultural, and spiritual history to help him determine the best approach for discussing her diagnosis and treatment options. Dr Han was also bias in giving Mrs Jones one treatment option; he should have removed his biased opinion and provide her with all recommended treatment options that are part of National Comprehensive Cancer Network (NCCN) treatment guidelines for breast cancer. Such guidelines include neoadjuvant chemotherapy, lumpectomy with radiation, mastectomy with or without breast reconstruction, targeted therapy, and endocrine therapy. He should also encourage Ms Jones to share her needs. Mrs Jones may have chosen to have a lumpectomy with radiation if she was given a choice, because of wanting to conserve her breast or even explored mastectomy with reconstruction (to preserve body image). In addition, if Dr Han understood Mrs Jones's spiritual/religious and cultural traditional beliefs and coping mechanisms, he could have integrated those beliefs and practices within the framework of his breast cancer treatment discussions, thus increasing Mrs Jones engagement, acceptance, and adherence to treatment.

These scenarios discussed in this case study exemplify how the provider can be culturally competent, humble, and empathetic to their patients; which are essential attributes to delivering equitable, patient-responsive healthcare across various cultural and ethnic groups.

References

Alcaraz K, Sly J, Ashing K, Fleisher L, et al. (2016). The ConNECT Framework: A Model for Advancing Behavioral Medicine Science and Practice to Foster Health Equity. *J Behav Med* [in press].

Ashing-Giwa KT (2005). The contextual model of HRQoL: A paradigm for expanding the HRQoL framework. *Qual Life Res* **14**, 297–307.

Baer HA, Singer M, Susser I (2003). *Medical Anthropology and the World System*, 2nd edition. Praeger Publishers, Westport, CT.

Beach MC, Price EG, Gary TL, et al. (2005). Cultural competency: A systematic review of health care provider educational interventions. *Med Care* **43**, 356–73.

Betancourt JR, Green AR, Carrillo JE, Ananeh-Firempong 2nd O (2003). Defining cultural competence: a practical framework for addressing racial/ethnic disparities in health and health care. *Public Health Reports* **118**, 293–302.

Birman D (2006). Measurement of the "acculturation gap" in immigrant families and implications for parent-child relationships. In: Bornstein MH, Cote LR (eds). *Acculturation and Parent-Child Relationships: Measurement and Development*, pp. 113–34. Lawrence Erlbaum Associates Publishers, Mahwah, NJ.

Brisset C, Leanza Y, Laforest K (2013). Working with interpreters in health care: A systematic review and meta-ethnography of qualitative studies. *Patient Educ Couns* **91**, 131–40.

Chang E, Simon M, Dong X (2012). Integrating cultural humility into health care professional education and training. *Adv Health Sci Educ* **17**, 269–78.

Chávez NR (2015). The challenge and benefit of the inclusion of race in medical school education. *J Racial and Ethn Health Disparities* **3**, 183–6.

Cornell S, Hartmann D (1998). Mapping the terrain: Definitions. In: *Ethnicity and Race: Making Identities in a Changing World*, pp. 15–38. Pine Forge Press, Thousand Oaks, CA.

Dean RG (2001). The myth of cross-cultural competence. *Families In Society: The Journal of Contemporary Human Services* **82**, 623–30.

Drevdahl DJ, Canales MK, Dorcy KS (2008). Of goldfish tanks and moonlight tricks: Can cultural competency ameliorate health disparities? *ANS Adv Nurs Sci* **31**, 13–27.

Fagerlind H, Kettis A, Glimelius B, Ring, L (2013). Barriers against psychosocial communication: Oncologists' perceptions. *J Clin Oncol* **31**, 3815–24.

Fernández A, Pérez-Stable EJ (2015). ¿Doctor, habla Español? Increasing the supply and quality of language-concordant physicians for Spanish speaking patients. *J Gen Intern Med* **30**, 1394–6.

Fox RC (2005). Cultural competence and the culture of medicine. *N Engl J Med* **353**, 1316–19.

Hughes D, Seidman E, Williams N (1993). Cultural phenomena and the research enterprise: Toward a culturally anchored methodology. *Am J Community Psychol* **21**, 687–703.

Institute of Medicine, National Research Council of The National Academies (2002). Unequal treatment: Confronting racial and ethnic disparities in health care. The National Academies Press, Washington, WA.

Institute of Medicine, National Research Council of The National Academies (2008). Cancer care for the whole patient: Meeting psychosocial health needs. The National Academies Press, Washington, WA.

Kagawa-Singer M (2012). Teaching cultural competent communication with diverse ethnic patients and families. In: Surbone A, Zwitter M, Rajer M, Stiefel R (eds). *New Challenges in Communication with Cancer Patients*. Springer, New York, NY.

Kleinman A, Benson P (2006). Anthropology in the clinic: The problem of cultural competency and how to fix it. *PloS Med* **3**, 1673–6.

Kripalani S, Bussey-Jones J, Katz MG, Genao I (2006). A prescription for cultural competence in medical education. *J Gen Intern Med* **21**, 1116–20.

Kumagai AK, Lypson ML (2009). Beyond cultural competence: Critical consciousness, social justice, and multicultural education. *Acad Med* **84**, 782–7.

Marmot M, Allen J, Bell R, Bloomer E, Goldblatt P (2012). WHO European review of social determinants of health and the health divide. *Lancet* **380**, 1011–29.

Mazor KM, Beard RL, Alexander GL, *et al.* (2013). Patients' and family members' views on patient-centered communication during cancer care. *Psychooncology* **22**, 1–14.

McCann-Mortimer P, Augoustinos M, LeCouteur A (2004). Race and the human genome project: constructions of scientific legitimacy. *Discourse & Society* **15**, 409–32.

Phinney JS (1996). When we talk about American ethnic groups, what do we mean? *Am Psychol* **51**, 918–27.

Phinney JS (2006). Acculturation is not an independent variable: Approaches to studying acculturation as a complex process. In: Bornstein M, Cote L (eds). *Acculturation and Parent-Child Relationships: Measurement and Development.* pp. 79–95. Lawrence Erlbaum Associate Publishers, Mahwah, NJ.

Segal UA, Elliott D, Mayadas NS (eds) (2010). *Immigration Worldwide: Policies, Practices, and Trends.* pp. 47–63. Oxford University Press, Oxford, UK.

Skea ZC, MacLennan SJ, Entwistle VA, N'Dow J (2014). Communicating good care: A Qualitative study of what people with urological cancer value in interactions with health care providers. *Eur J Oncol Nurs* **18**, 35–40.

Surbone A (2012). From truth telling to truth in the making: A paradigm shift in communication with cancer patients. In: *New Challenges in Communication with Cancer Patients.* Surbone A, Zwitter M, Rajer M, Stiefel R (eds). Springer; New York, NY.

Sue S (2006). Cultural competency: From philosophy to research and practice. *J Commun Psychol* **34**, 237–45.

Tervalon M, Murray-Garcia J (1998). Cultural humility versus cultural competence: A critical distinction in defining physician training outcomes in multicultural education. *J Health Care Poor Underserved* **9**, 117–25.

Thackrah RD, Thompson SC (2013). Refining the concept of cultural competence: Building on decades of progress. *MJA* **199**, 35–8.

Triandis HC (1995). *Individualism and Collectivism.* Westview Press, Boulder, CO.

Truong M, Paradies Y, Priest N (2014). Interventions to improve cultural competency in healthcare: A systematic review of reviews. *BMC Health Serv Res* **14**, 1–17.

Weech-Maldonado R, Elliot MN, Pradhan R, Schiller C, Hall A, Hays RD (2012). Can hospital cultural competency reduce disparities in patient experiences with care? *Med Care* **50**, 48–55.

CHAPTER 41

Challenges in communicating with ethnically diverse populations: The role of health literacy

Bejoy C. Thomas and Rebecca L. Malhi

Introduction to challenges in communicating with ethnically diverse populations

Every day, people make large and small decisions that affect their health: should I get an influenza shot or not? When should I take my sick child to the doctor? How much coffee per day is safe to drink? At what age should I start to have a mammogram? Or, when the instructions on a pill bottle read 'Take one tablet twice a day', does this mean that I take one tablet every 12 hours or is it a ½ tablet each time? Whether an individual will make good health-related decisions or not is highly dependent on his or her ability to access and understand the information required to make these choices. Despite a substantial amount of health-related information that is available in healthcare facilities and through the media, evidence indicates that most adults have some degree of difficulty using the information to manage their health. The growing focus on **health literacy** worldwide is an acknowledgement that this is a critical issue for society to address. Moreover, health literacy is an often overlooked problem in cancer communication. Healthcare providers, especially those in oncology, must consider the patient's health literacy in all aspects of communication.

What is health literacy?

The concept of health literacy has evolved over many years. While early definitions of health literacy focused primarily on literacy skills, such as the ability to read health-related materials, current conceptualizations extrapolate beyond literacy alone to recognize the complexity of skills that are required to make informed decisions in the health system. One definition is: 'The ability to access, comprehend, evaluate, and communicate information as a way to promote, maintain, and improve health in a variety of settings across the life-course' (Public Health Agency of Canada 2014). This definition only hints at the level of skills required for an individual to be considered 'health literate'. In addition to possessing fundamental literacy (e.g. reading and writing skills, knowledge of

basic mathematics, speech and comprehension skills), people are expected to have some knowledge of anatomy, healthy behaviours, and the workings of the healthcare system (Nielsen-Bohlman et al. 2004; US Department of Health and Human Services 2010). Other skills include critical thinking and the ability to ask questions of health professionals and understand the answers provided. Also, individuals must continually learn new health information (e.g. such as health threats like the Ebola virus or understanding treatment options for a new cancer diagnosis), evaluate contradictory information from multiple sources, and unlearn outdated information (Kickbusch et al. 2005).

Lacking some or many of these skills will present obvious challenges for patients interacting with healthcare providers. In fact, until recent years, health literacy (or the lack of it) has usually been viewed as the individual's responsibility. However, analyses of health literacy problems have also implicated health professionals and health systems in failing to provide information in a manner appropriate to their audiences. The US Institute of Medicine emphasizes this dual responsibility: 'Health literacy emerges when the expectations, preferences, and skills of individuals seeking health information and services meet the expectations, preferences, and skills of those providing information and services' (Nielsen-Bohlman et al. 2004).

Scope of the problem

Limited health literacy is a common and concerning issue all over the world. For example, a European health literacy survey revealed that 47% of the respondents had inadequate to problematic health literacy skills (World Health Organization 2013). An estimated 60% of adult Canadians scored below the minimum literacy level needed to actively participate in society (Canadian Council on Learning 2008). The US Department of Education found similarly dismal results, with only 12% of the respondents demonstrating proficient health literacy (Kutner et al. 2006). Importantly, ethnically diverse populations are particularly vulnerable to having limited health literacy levels (Canadian Public Health Association

2006; Rootman *et al.* 2008). Low/inadequate health literacy affects all levels of society and is associated with significant negative health outcomes, including:

◆ poor self-reported health status (Canadian Council on Learning 2008);

◆ less likelihood of participating in cancer screening programmes (Davis *et al.* 2001; Lindau *et al.* 2002);

◆ greater difficulty in managing chronic health conditions like diabetes, asthma, etc. (Berkman *et al.* 2004);

◆ increased health risks because of difficulty interpreting prescription labels and managing medication usage (Wolf *et al.* 2006);

◆ greater incidence of preventable hospital visits and admissions (Nielsen-Bohlman *et al.* 2004; Berkman *et al.* 2004);

◆ increased risk of mortality, particularly among older adults (Baker *et al.* 2007; Sudore *et al.* 2006).

In addition to severe impact on health status, people with limited health literacy skills may incur higher medical costs than patients with better health literacy. Indirect costs to individuals may include development of chronic comorbidities, lost wages, and poorer quality of life (US Department of Health and Human Services 2010). At national levels, the additional expense of limited health literacy is estimated at 3–5% of the total healthcare cost per year (Eichler *et al.* 2009). In Canada, that could translate to an extra eight billion dollars per year spent on healthcare as a result of low health literacy.

An illustrative case example

Mrs Priscilla Adeyemi (pseudonym) is a 74-year-old woman who was born in Nigeria and immigrated to Canada 18 years ago. Mrs Adeyemi is a widow and lives in an apartment close to her daughter's house in Toronto. She has a Master's degree in Education and worked as a mathematics teacher in Lagos, Nigeria until her retirement. Mrs Adeyemi had no health concerns until August 2013, when her doctor noticed a small lump in her breast during a routine examination. Biopsy results confirmed that Mrs Adeyemi had breast cancer. She met her oncologist, Dr Patrick Watson (pseudonym), for the first time in his office at the cancer centre.

Dr Watson has over 30 years of experience specializing in breast cancer. He has a very heavy clinical workload, so he is not able to spend as much time with his patients as he would like. Over the years, he has had many immigrant patients and if needed, he has used a phone interpretation service for people with limited English proficiency. However, when he met Mrs Adeyemi, he was pleased to find that she was well-educated and spoke English with relative fluency.

During the appointment, Dr Watson discussed treatment options with Mrs Adeyemi and as she was noticeably upset by the diagnosis, reassured her that the survival rate was very high. He asked her several times whether she had any questions, but each time, Mrs Adeyemi smiled and shook her head. Dr Watson told her that his staff would provide her with more information to take home and read. He stressed that if there was anything that was not clear, she should phone his office and get clarification. Mrs Adeyemi left the office with a booklet and several pamphlets describing the treatment options and available services and resources. Dr Watson was satisfied with the consultation and confident that Mrs Adeyemi had all the information necessary to make a good decision regarding her health. Unfortunately, he was wrong.

Mrs Adeyemi was hopelessly confused during the consultation but was too ashamed to admit that she didn't understand what Dr Watson was saying. She also knew that he was extremely busy so she did not ask for a clearer explanation. Mrs Adeyemi was depressed when she left the doctor's office and this feeling intensified when she went home and started to read the written material. 'I don't understand any of this', she thought despairingly, 'I must be stupid'. Later, her daughter helped her search the internet but a query for 'breast cancer treatment' came up with 87 million results. Many of the internet sites contained confusing and contradictory information.

These challenges early in Mrs Adeyemi's cancer journey continued. She chose to have neoadjuvant chemotherapy but had trouble managing her symptoms. She experienced several side effects but seldom told her oncologist about them because she felt these were to be expected and that she should just put up with them. Mrs Adeyemi spent many more months suffering from physical and emotional distress without adequate support from her healthcare team.

Patient risk factors for low health literacy

As we noted earlier, current conceptualizations of health literacy allocate responsibility to both the individual seeking health information/services and to the individuals providing the health information/services. Thus, in our scenario, one could argue that Mrs Adeyemi was at fault for not asking more questions and clarifying any points of confusion, and equally, that missteps occurred on the part of the health professional and the health system. For example, Dr Watson could have been more sensitive to his patient's non-verbal cues, and he may have wrongly assumed an adequate level of health comprehension and potential decision-making based on Mrs Adeyemi's English proficiency and educational/professional background. Health literacy research suggests that Mrs Adeyemi possesses several demographic characteristics or risk factors that are associated with limited health literacy including:

Age

Health literacy scores tend to decrease as we age (Willms and Murray 2007) and only 12% of adults over age 65 in Canada have adequate health literacy skills (Canadian Council on Learning 2007). The extent of low health literacy in senior populations is especially troubling, as older people often require additional information related to chronic health problems and medications.

Ethnicity/immigration status

Ethnicity is another factor associated with health literacy challenges. In the US, members of non-White ethnic groups and people whose first language is not English often exhibit limited levels of health literacy (US Department of Health and Human Services 2010). In Canada, the Aboriginal population and immigrants—regardless of length of residence—experience more literacy problems than the Canadian-born population (Canadian Public Health Association 2006). Ethnic minority individuals may not know how to seek out and utilize available information in unfamiliar healthcare contexts, or they may encounter barriers to accessing and/or understanding the information (Zanchetta and Poureslami 2006).

Foreign-born immigrant women

This particular population may have acute health literacy concerns. Canadian research found that approximately one-third of foreign-born women have extreme difficulty with printed materials, compared to one-fourth of foreign-born men and about one-tenth of Canadian-born men and women (Rootman and Gordon-El-Bihbety 2008).

Language

People who are not proficient in the resident country's official language(s) may be disadvantaged in health contexts (Zanchetta and Poureslami 2006). Even when individuals are competent in everyday (social) English, their language skills may not be sufficient to handle complex health-related tasks, such as understanding medical assessment, diagnosis, treatment, and care (Garrett *et al.* 2008). For ethnically diverse populations, language barriers may negatively impact cancer care by delaying diagnosis and treatment, and influencing communication about treatment options and prognosis (Karliner *et al.* 2011).

Shame

People with limited health literacy often feel shame or embarrassment about their skill level (Wolf *et al.* 2007) and hide their struggles with reading or comprehension, even from their own families (Parikh *et al.* 1996). Difficulties tend to be 'invisible' to healthcare professionals, and may lead to the providers overestimating patient comprehension (Kelly and Haidet 2007).

Distress from illness

People face additional challenges of processing health information when they are sick, or are stressed about being sick (Sentell *et al.* 2013). Patients with a new cancer diagnosis are often confronted with critical decisions regarding treatment and care during a time of heightened emotionality (Thorne *et al.* 2014).

Other demographic factors

Associations with limited health literacy have also been found for employment status, education, and poor social support, among other factors. People who are unemployed are more likely to have lower health literacy levels than people who are employed (Canadian Council on Learning 2008). Although individuals with fewer years of education are likely to have inadequate health literacy, educational achievement is not a good predictor of health literacy skills (Kutner *et al.* 2006). Research also suggests that having positive social support can buffer and alleviate adverse health impacts of low health literacy (Lee *et al.* 2004).

Clinician/context factors—amplifying health literacy challenges

We noted earlier that assumptions made by the oncologist in our scenario could have led to a suboptimal interaction with his patient and potentially long-lasting health consequences for her. Other factors of the clinician and healthcare context can also create or amplify communication challenges when dealing with individuals with limited health literacy:

Using medical jargon

A common complaint by patients is that healthcare providers use complex medical terms during interactions, making it difficult for lay people to understand the information (Sentell *et al.* 2013). This issue is exacerbated if the technical terminology is transmitted rapidly by physicians (Schillinger *et al.* 2004). When information is not provided in a way that is sensitive to people with limited health literacy—especially those from minority ethnic groups—patient trust is diminished and the relationship with the healthcare professional can be damaged (Song *et al.* 2012). For example, an Australian Aboriginal patient said, 'Instead of talking high and mighty to a person … they should sit down and relax and actually talk English to that person instead of using big words, fancy words, making themselves look good, and making themselves feel proud that they can, you know, "I know what this word is, but you don't because you are small" ' (Shahid *et al.* 2013).

Not checking for patient understanding

Healthcare providers may not take the time to guide the patient through the information in written materials, explaining the content as they follow along. They also may not ensure that patients have understood verbal information. When physicians fail to check for comprehension, patients may perceive this as being disrespectful and it can reinforce patient assumptions that they should not ask questions or seek further explanations, despite their lack of understanding (Sentell *et al.* 2013).

Dealing with ethnically diverse populations

Healthcare professionals may inadvertently be less patient-centred with certain ethnic groups (Shahid *et al.* 2013). For example, studies with African American patients have found that healthcare providers are more verbally dominant with them, see them as less effective communicators, and treat them more contentiously compared to White patients (Johnson *et al.* 2004; Street Jr. *et al.* 2007). Patient language proficiency can also influence clinician communication. Oncologists in a California study were more likely to simplify discussions of risks and benefits of treatment approaches and be more directive regarding treatment recommendations when consulting with a limited-English patient than with an English-proficient patient (Karliner *et al.* 2011).

Complexity of print materials

Patient education often relies on printed health information, yet the reading level of many pamphlets, brochures, etc. exceeds the reading ability of the intended audience (Rudd *et al.* 2000). Patients also complain of the lack of written information that is available in 'plain English' and that an overwhelming amount of information is given to them (Sentell *et al.* 2013; Thorne *et al.* 2014). Even health information available on the internet can be problematic for the average reader, as it is often written at high school reading levels (grade 10 or higher) (Hochhauser 2002), and may not always be accurate.

Recommendations/interventions

Many of the patient factors that impact health literacy (e.g. educational level, language skills, or previous health-related experiences) are not under the control of healthcare providers. However, clinicians and healthcare facilities can implement certain strategies that help mitigate the effects of limited health literacy during medical encounters (see www.ucalgary.ca/bejoythomas/health-literacy for examples and resources). As low health literacy is a society-wide problem, taking a 'universal precautions' approach

(Baker 2006) and applying strategies for **all** patients may result in improved information comprehension and uptake.

Pre-screen patients for health literacy

Although there is no comprehensive measure that assesses all domains of health literacy, screening tools have been created to quickly identify people who struggle with limited health literacy. Pre-screening alerts the clinician to possible challenges so that they can tailor the communication to individual patient needs and capacities. For example, the Newest Vital Sign (NVS) (Weiss *et al.* 2005) can be administered in three minutes and is moderately predictive of individuals with limited literacy and numeracy skills (Baker 2006). Another brief measure (Chew *et al.* 2004) assesses patients' self-reported difficulty in understanding healthcare providers and written materials, such as appointment slips or instructions.

Use question prompt lists

These structured lists of questions are designed to improve the quality of communication in clinical encounters. Question prompt lists enable patients to consider critical issues (e.g. diagnosis, treatment-related decisions, symptom management, etc.), acquire specific information that they need, and provide a framework for them to state any concerns to their healthcare providers (McJannett *et al.* 2003). Questions for discussion between patient and oncologist might include: 'Will I have side effects for the rest of my life?', 'Can I take vitamins or other supplements?', and 'For how many months or weeks will I have treatment?' (Eggly *et al.* 2013).

Schedule extra time

Patients with limited health literacy may require longer appointments, particularly on the initial or critical visits (new to clinic, treatment planning, etc.). This ensures that the patient has sufficient time to ask questions (especially in conjunction with a question prompt list) and get clarification on anything that is unclear. Also, in many cultures, taking one's time in an interaction and 'not feeling rushed' is a sign of respect on the part of the healthcare provider.

Improve verbal communication

Talking to patients in simple everyday language is very important (Sentell *et al.* 2013). Healthcare providers should limit the amount of verbal information given to patients and should also ensure that instructions are repeated (Davis *et al.* 2002). Audio-recording the interaction allows the patient to review what was said at a later time. Clinicians could also encourage patients to bring family or friends to appointments, both for social support and for assistance in understanding medical information (Lee *et al.* 2004).

Make written materials easy to understand

Printed materials provided to patients should be accessible and engaging with limited use of medical jargon. The writing style should utilize 'plain language' principles, but avoid being simplistic or condescending. Educational material for use with ethnically diverse populations should be carefully translated and culturally sensitive, with input from target audiences. Ideally, physicians or their staff should walk through any handouts with the patient at the time of consultation.

Provide information using other media

Health professionals could use show-and-tell, videos, and pictures to supplement written materials (Sentell *et al.* 2013). If such additional materials are used for ethnically diverse populations, they should also be pretested by patients and members of the target communities to ensure comprehension and cultural appropriateness.

Assess comprehension using 'teach back' or 'show me' approaches

Healthcare providers should avoid asking the question, 'Do you understand?' (as the answer will usually be affirmative, due to the stigma attached to limited health literacy) (Davis *et al.* 2002). Instead, experts suggest using a 'teach back' or 'show me' approach where the patient is asked to repeat the information or instructions to assess comprehension (Baker 2006; Davis *et al.* 2002).

Using community navigators and interpreters to assist patients

Language barriers in the healthcare system could be addressed by providing paid or volunteer interpreters from the relevant communities (Rootman and Gordon-El-Bihbety 2008). Community navigators can help patients with paperwork, appointment reminders, social support and advocacy (Hendren *et al.* 2011). Evidence strongly supports the clinical benefit of using professional interpreters who are trained in medical terminology and cultural brokerage (Karliner *et al.* 2011). Using family members of patients as ad hoc interpreters is problematic (Thomas *et al.* 2010) and not recommended.

Now, having taken these strategies and recommendations into consideration, let us re-imagine the consultation between Dr Watson and Mrs Adeyemi:

> Before the appointment, Dr Watson's staff had elicited information about Mrs Adeyemi's level of health literacy using a brief screening questionnaire. The nurse offered to have an interpreter present but when this offer was declined, booked a longer-than-usual appointment with Dr Watson.
>
> During the consultation, Dr Watson discussed treatment options in simple language and showed Mrs Adeyemi the location of her tumour using a three-dimensional model of a breast. He used a question prompt list to make sure that questions commonly asked by breast cancer patients were covered. This made Mrs Adeyemi feel that it was normal for people in her situation to have questions, so she felt comfortable seeking clarification if something was not clear to her. Dr Watson also had Mrs Adeyemi repeat her diagnosis and treatment options back to him until he was confident that she understood the information. Although upset by a cancer diagnosis, Mrs Adeyemi was very satisfied with the consultation.
>
> Mrs Adeyemi left the office with an audio recording of the meeting, a booklet and several pamphlets describing the treatment options and available services and resources. Dr Watson encouraged her to go over the materials with her daughter and write down any questions they might have for him. The booklet and pamphlets were in plain, easy-to-understand language, and Mrs Adeyemi found them very helpful in making her decision to have neo-adjuvant chemotherapy. When she experienced several side effects, she discussed symptom relief with her oncologist. Importantly, Mrs Adeyemi continued to have a sense of self-efficacy in navigating the healthcare system, and even accompanies other members of her community to medical appointments as an interpreter and patient navigator.

Conclusions

Improving health literacy for all individuals, and using more accessible approaches for including ethnically diverse populations, will be an increasing health priority in coming years. However, this endeavour will require sustained and targeted initiatives. As one researcher notes: 'To be a health literate society, we need a health literate public, health literate health professionals, and health literate politicians and policy-makers' (Kickbusch *et al.* 2005).

Acknowledgements

The authors thank the Canadian Breast Cancer Foundation and the Prairie Metropolis Centre for their generous support of our research. We also thank Drs John Robinson and Lauren Walker for their helpful comments on the manuscript.

References

Baker DW, Wolf MS, Feinglass J, Thompson JA, Gazmararian JA, Huang J (2007). Health literacy and mortality among elderly persons. *Arch Intern Med* **167**, 1503–9.

Baker D (2006). The meaning and the measure of health literacy. *J Gen Int Med* **21**, 878–83.

Berkman ND, Dewalt DA, Pignone MP, *et al.* (2004). *Literacy and health outcomes. Evidence Report, Technology Assessment No. 87.* Rockville, MD: Agency for Healthcare Research and Quality. (Publication # 04-E007-2).

Canadian Council on Learning (2008). *Health Literacy in Canada: A Healthy Understanding.* [Online] Available at: http://www.ccl-cca.ca/CCL/Reports/HealthLiteracy/index.html [Last accessed June 10, 2015].

Canadian Council on Learning (2007). *State of Learning in Canada: No Time for Complacency.* [Online] Available at: http://www.ccl-cca.ca/pdfs/SOLR/2007/NewSOLR_Report.pdf [Last accessed June 10, 2015].

Canadian Public Health Association (2006). *Increasing understanding of the impact of low health literacy on chronic disease prevention and control: Final report.* Canadian Public Health Association, Ottawa, ON, Canada.

Chew LD, Bradley KA, Boyko EJ (2004). Brief questions to identify patients with inadequate health literacy. *Family Medicine* **36**, 588–94.

Davis TC, Dolan NC, Ferreira MR, *et al.* (2001). The role of inadequate health literacy skills in colorectal cancer screening. *Cancer Investig* **19**, 193–200.

Davis TC, Williams MV, Marin E, Parker RM, Glass J (2002). Health literacy and cancer communication. *CA Cancer J Clin* **52**, 134–49.

Eggly S, Tkatch R, Penner LA, *et al.* (2013). Development of a question prompt list as a communication intervention to reduce racial disparities in cancer treatment. *J Cancer Educ* **28**, 282–9.

Eichler K, Wieser S, Brugger U (2009). The costs of limited health literacy: a systematic review. *Int J Public Health* **54**, 313–24.

Garrett PW, Dickson HG, Whelan AK (2008). Communication and healthcare complexity in people with little or no English: the Communication Complexity Score. *Ethn Health* **13**, 203–17.

Hendren S, Chin N, Fisher S, *et al.* (2011). Patients' barriers to receipt of cancer care, and factors associated with needing more assistance from a patient navigator. *J Nat Med Assoc* **103**, 701–10.

Hochhauser M (2002). Patient education and the Web: what you see on the computer screen isn't always what you get in print. *Patient Care Manag* **17**, 10–12.

Johnson RL, Roter D, Powe NR, Cooper LA (2004). Patient race/ethnicity and quality of patient-physician communication during medical visits. *Am J Public Health* **94**, 2084–90.

Karliner LS, Hwang ES, Nickleach D, Kaplan CP (2011). Language barriers and patient-centered breast cancer care. *Patient Educ Couns* **84**, 223–8.

Kelly PA, Haidet P (2007). Physician overestimation of patient literacy: a potential source of health care disparities. *Patient Educ Couns* **66**, 119–22.

Kickbusch I, Wait S, Maag D (2005). *Navigating health: the role of health literacy.* [Online] Available at: http://www.ilcuk.org.uk/images/uploads/publication-pdfs/pdf_pdf_3.pdf [Last accessed June 10, 2015].

Kutner M, Greenberg E, Jin Y, Paulsen C (2006). *The Health Literacy of America's Adults: Results From the 2003 National Assessment of Adult Literacy.* NCES 2006–483. US Department of Education, National Center for Education Statistics, Washington DC, WA.

Lee SY, Arozullah AM, Cho YI (2004). Health literacy, social support, and health: a research agenda. *Soc Sci Med* **58**, 1309–21.

Lindau ST, Tomori C, Lyons T, Langseth L, Bennett CL, Garcia P (2002). The association of health literacy with cervical cancer prevention knowledge and health behaviors in a multiethnic cohort of women. *Am J Obstet Gynecol* **186**, 938–43.

McJannett M, Butow P, Tattersall MH, Thompson JF (2003). Asking questions can help: development of a question prompt list for cancer patients seeing a surgeon. *Eur J Cancer Prev* **12**, 397–405.

Nielsen-Bohlman L, Panzer AM, Kindig DA (2004). *Health Literacy: A Prescription to End Confusion.* National Academies Press, Washington DC, WA.

Parikh NS, Parker RM, Nurss JR, Baker DW, Williams MV (1996). Shame and health literacy: the unspoken connection. *Patient Educ Couns* **27**, 33–9.

Public Health Agency of Canada (2014). *What is Health Literacy?* [Online] Available at: http://www.phac-aspc.gc.ca/cd-mc/hl-ls/index-eng.php#tabs-2 [Last accessed June 10, 2015].

Rootman I, Gordon-El-Bihbety D (2008). *A Vision for a Health Literate Canada: Report of the Expert Panel on Health Literacy.* Canadian Public Health Association, Ottawa, ON, Canada.

Rudd RE, Colton T, Schacht R (2000). *An Overview of Medical and Public Health Literature Addressing Literacy Issues: An Annotated Bibliography.* NCSALL Reports# 14. National Center for the Study of Adult Learning and Literacy, Cambridge, MA.

Schillinger D, Bindman A, Wang F, Stewart A, Piette J (2004). Functional health literacy and the quality of physician-patient communication among diabetes patients. *Patient Educ Couns* **52**, 315–23.

Sentell T, Dela Cruz MR, Heo HH, Braun KL (2013). Health literacy, health communication challenges, and cancer screening among rural native Hawaiian and Filipino women. *J Cancer Educ* **28**, 325–34.

Shahid S, Durey A, Bessarab D, Aoun SM, Thompson SC (2013). Identifying barriers and improving communication between cancer service providers and Aboriginal patients and their families: the perspective of service providers. *BMC Health Serv Res* **13**, 460.

Song L, Hamilton JB, Moore AD (2012). Patient-healthcare provider communication: perspectives of African American cancer patients. *Health Psychol* **31**, 539–47.

Street RL Jr, Gordon H, Haidet P (2007). Physicians' communication and perceptions of patients: is it how they look, how they talk, or is it just the doctor? *Soc Sci Med* **65**, 586–98.

Sudore RL, Yaffe K, Satterfield S, *et al.* (2006). Limited literacy and mortality in the elderly: the health, aging, and body composition study. *J Gen Int Med* **21**, 806–12.

Thomas B, Lounsberry J, Carlson L (2010). Challenges in communicating with ethnically diverse populations. (Ch. 32) In: Kissane DW, Bultz BD, Butow PM, Finlay IG (eds). *Handbook of Communication in Oncology and Palliative Care.* Oxford University Press, Oxford, UK.

Thorne S, Hislop TG, Kim-Sing C, Oglov V, Oliffe JL, Stajduhar KI (2014). Changing communication needs and preferences across the cancer care trajectory: insights from the patient perspective. *Support Care Cancer* **22**, 1009–15.

US Department of Health and Human Services (2010). *National Action Plan to Improve Health Literacy.* US Department of Health and Human Services, Office of Disease Prevention and Health Promotion, Washington DC, WA.

Weiss BD, Mays MZ, Martz W, *et al.* (2005). Quick assessment of literacy in primary care: the newest vital sign. *Ann Fam Med* **3**, 514–22.

Willms DJ, Murray TS (2007). *Gaining and Losing Literacy Skills over the Lifecourse.* 89-552- MWE2007016. Ottawa, ON, Canada: Statistics Canada.

Wolf MS, Davis TC, Tilson HH, Bass PF 3rd, Parker RM (2006). Misunderstanding of prescription drug warning labels among patients with low literacy. *Am J Health Syst Pharm* **63**, 1048–55.

Wolf MS, Williams MV, Parker RM, Parikh NS, Nowlan AW, Baker DW (2007). Patients' shame and attitudes toward discussing the results of literacy screening. *J Health Commun* **12**, 721–32.

World Health Organization (2013). *Health Literacy: The Solid Facts*. WHO Regional Office for Europe, Copenhagen, Denmark.

Zanchetta MS, Poureslami IM (2006). Health literacy within the reality of immigrants' culture and language. *Can J Public Health* **97**(Suppl 2), S26–30.

CHAPTER 42

Communication and cancer-related infertility

Zeev Rosberger, Sylvie Aubin, Barry D. Bultz, and Peter Chan

'Your sperm is healthy but it's no gold medal winner. And it won't make up for her deficiencies' said our fertility specialist to my husband as I sat next to him. 'I'd give you a 2 per cent chance of falling pregnant. 10 per cent with IVF.'

Tracy Gillett

Reproduced with permission from Raised Good, '*How I survived the emotional rollercoaster of infertility*,' Copyright © Raised Good 2016, available from http://raisedgood.com/how-i-survived-the-emotional-rollercoaster-of-infertility/

Introduction to communication and cancer-related infertility

The quote presented above may or may not be typical of the types of communication prospective patients receive when seeking treatments for idiopathic origins of infertility. The multiple issues at the intersection of emotional pain, hope, and technological innovation in this setting are complex at best, and should never be treated with other than the highest levels of dignity and respect. In the present chapter, we will review the evidence and best practices regarding fertility preservation (FP) in young men and women of reproductive age who are at risk of infertility because of the systemic impact of a cancer, or more likely from the illness course and treatments. More specifically, we will review and summarize the communication skills, tools, and resources necessary to facilitate the critical role that healthcare professionals (HCPs) should play across all cancer settings.

When infertility is a consequence of a cancer diagnosis and/or its treatments, this complexity is of a higher order and the sensitivity required by the healthcare professional in interacting with a patient and/or his partner begins at a different point in the illness trajectory. This is particularly true for those who require cancer treatment comprised of high dose chemotherapy, combination chemotherapy, radiation therapy to the pelvis, and/or surgical removal of the reproductive organs as part of their cancer treatment.

Initially, while the challenges of prognosis, survival, and treatment regimen decisions assume prime importance, the communication of fertility-related risk information is usually presented in the context of other potential cancer treatment side effects. Patients are asked to assimilate much complex information that may present with both immediate and potentially long-term consequences. Ideally, the potential for cancer treatment to negatively impact a patient's fertility should be thoroughly addressed during the treatment planning process. However, research suggests that the dialogue regarding this issue between physician and patient occurs neither uniformly nor routinely (Schover *et al.* 2002; Duffy *et al.* 2005).

While the timing of discussion regarding fertility issues may not necessarily be viewed as paramount at the time of diagnosis, fertility will become increasingly important over time in cancer survivorship (Thewes *et al.* 2003; Achille *et al.* 2006). Parenthood for many cancer patients is a fundamental goal of cancer survivorship. Studies documenting the attitudes of young cancer survivors have revealed that parenthood is viewed as a positive and important life experience. Survivors have also expressed that their experience with cancer would make them better parents. Additionally, 60% of young cancer survivors reported they would attempt to achieve the role of being a parent as an important life goal, even if they were to die young (Schover *et al.* 2002). Low levels of accurate knowledge and comfort with communication, timing, and other factors have been found to contribute to poor fertility risk communication (Schover *et al.* 2002). Nevertheless, the introduction of the topic of fertility risk and FP early in the illness trajectory may or may not occur uniformly nor does it always result in timely implementation of FP. A recent study highlights current issues facing young (ages 15–39) cancer patients regarding availability and use of fertility preservation measures prior to treatment. Only 33% of the 550 young adult survivors who were surveyed reported taking steps to preserve fertility (Bann *et al.* 2015). While fertility preservation techniques have been more widely available, there remain gaps in geography (more likely to use FP in the US northeast vs. the south), cost, and whether the patient received chemotherapy. Men were still more likely than women to participate in FP, likely due to the higher invasiveness, complexity, risks along with the higher cost of oocyte harvesting procedures and banking.

Evolving research into follicular biology has opened new possibilities for FP in women. While still not fully developed, this research promises to provide women with new options beyond hormonal stimulation, particularly in young women with breast cancer.

Male fertility

Potential risks of infertility due to treatment include:

1. surgery (e.g. orchiectomy);

2. radiation (e.g. to the pelvis); or

3. gonadotoxic chemotherapy regimens.

The most prevalent cancers in young men include testicular cancer, lymphoma (Hodgkin's and non-Hodgkin's) and leukaemia. While five-year survival rates have improved significantly in recent years (95% for testicular and approximately 80% for the lymphomas), fertility presents as an important issue for these men. It has been fairly well established that the systemic effects of the disease process prior to diagnosis may already compromise spermatogenesis significantly, resulting in subnormal semen parameters and hormonal profiles. As a result, as many as 12% of men may be azoospermic at time of diagnosis. Current treatment regimens for testis cancer include surgical removal of the affected testis. For advanced and metastatic diseases, additional surgery (retroperitoneal lymph node dissection) may be necessary for diagnostic and therapeutic considerations. This procedure often results in additional sexual side effects including dry ejaculation (anejaculation) and erectile dysfunction. Adjuvant chemotherapy and radiation may affect sperm production and quality (e.g. motility, DNA integrity), further limiting future fertility (Dohle 2010). Current data suggests that these cancer therapies will result in impaired fertility in virtually all men either temporarily (with recovery in up to two years) or perhaps permanently for 15–30% of men.

Reproductive options

Modern assisted reproduction techniques (ART), such as intracytoplasmic sperm injection (ICSI) in which only a single living sperm is required to inject directly into an oocyte to achieve fertilization, make it feasible for cancer survivors who have significant impairment in semen profile post-treatment to father genetic children. Even for cancer survivors who have no spermatozoa found in semen (azoospermia), microsurgical retrieval of sperm within the testes is feasible in about half of these patients to have sperm usable for procreation. These techniques are highly technical and may not be widely available. Given the availability of these and other modern ART and cryopreservation technologies, sperm banking prior to treatment in cancer patients is currently the most important fertility preservation approach. Gonadal stem cell retrieval and testis tissue preservation are currently in experimental stages of research and have not yet demonstrated efficacy in fertility preservation in human. Sperm cryopreservation remains the primary method, but innovative methods of including embryonic stem cell research, though perhaps in early stages, remain promising (Zhou *et al.* 2016). It is estimated that among male cancer survivors, approximately 15% used their preserved sperm and have resulting offspring (Dohle 2010). A recent study suggested that when using cryopreserved sperm, the success rate among cancer survivors appears to be at least comparable to that in non-cancer populations (Garcia *et al.* 2015).

Female fertility

For the female cancer patient undergoing treatment with obvious direct effect (i.e. surgery) to the reproductive organs, discussions about fertility issues may be more readily addressed, but still many remain surprised by unexpected premature menopause. One recent study demonstrates that childhood cancer survivors who experience spontaneous menstruation five years or more after their cancer diagnosis are at 13-fold increased risk of non-surgical premature menopause in comparison to siblings (Chemaitilly *et al.* 2006). Young breast cancer survivors also have been found to be at increased risk of premature menopause. Many factors have been shown to be associated with chemotherapy induced premature menopause, including an individual's age at the time of treatment, the type of chemotherapy regime, and the number of months since completion of treatment (Petrek *et al.* 2006).

Loss of fertility as the result of their cancer treatment has been shown to cause persistent feelings of sadness and grief lasting more than a year post-treatment in female cancer survivors (Carter *et al.* 2005). Qualitative research suggests that fertility and menopause are important for young cancer survivors. Chemotherapy places women at risk of premature menopause and infertility. Oestrogen deprivation can cause other side effects (i.e. hot flashes, sexual dysfunction) (Thewes *et al.* 2003; Duffy *et al.* 2005). Premature menopause/or loss of reproductive function has been shown to be associated with poorer emotional functioning and greater risk for sexual difficulties (Ganz *et al.* 2003). Concerns about fertility have been reported, especially among younger women and survivors without children following stem cell transplant. Stem cell transplant (SCT) survivors indicated persistent fertility-related concerns even 10 years post-treatment (Hammond *et al.* 2007). Wenzel and colleagues also evaluated the relationship between infertility and long-term quality of life in female cancer survivors and found reproductive concerns were of great importance, and centrally linked to psychosocial outcomes (Wenzel *et al.* 2002). Interestingly, even those individuals who undergo fertility-preserving surgery have been noted to experience persistent emotional distress and reproductive concerns over time post-operatively (Carter *et al.* 2007). Importantly, young women with breast cancer who are referred early after diagnosis to a reproductive specialist may have the opportunity to undergo more than one cycle of ovarian stimulation with the possibility of having more oocytes available for FP and increasing the chances of successful progeny outcomes (Lee *et al.* 2010).

Reproductive options

As medical technology advances, survivors of cancer diagnosed during childhood or young adulthood not only have an improved likelihood of survival, but may also be able to access emerging assisted reproductive techniques. In some cases, individuals may be eligible for conservative fertility-preserving surgical treatment, as is the case for specific types of early stage gynaecological cancers (Nick *et al.* 2012). For other types of cancers, such as breast cancer, leukaemia, and lymphoma, cryopreservation of gametes (ooyctes) and/or embryos (Sonmezer and Oktay 2004) can be a viable option for biological offspring when concerns exist about premature menopause and sterility. However, upon completion of treatment, this option would require a functional uterus and no contraindications to pregnancy, which can be complex issue in individuals with hormone receptive cancers. Otherwise, family building may require the assistance of another individual or third party. Third-party parenting (i.e. the involvement of a third person beyond the parenting couple or single parent) in order to create a child is possible in the case of individuals where treatment causes gonadal toxicity. Techniques can include egg (oocyte) donation, sperm donation, embryo donation, in vitro fertilization (IVF) with or without a gestational carrier (surrogacy), and/or adoption. When possible, preservation of the ovaries offers the possibility of a biological child through assisted reproduction with egg retrieval.

Many young cancer patients will be faced with treatment options that may require surgical removal of some or all reproductive organs. For these individuals, family building options will require the assistance of an egg donor or surrogate. Adoption is another alternative for family building in cancer survivorship. It should be noted that for some individuals this process presents both difficult and emotional challenges. Some survivors not only must confront their loss of reproductive function, but also question the possibility of a hostile legal environment towards being a parent after cancer. Also, when adoption is being considered, 'open adoptions' may represent a hurdle not experienced in normal birthing. It is also possible that adoption agencies may be reluctant to consider cancer survivors as potential parents due to possible late health risks after cancer treatment. The legal environment on possible legal disputes are not yet clear from a jurisprudence perspective in Canada, for example (Feldstein 2014).

Guidelines and standards of practice for the clinician

In 2006, The American Society of Clinical Oncology (ASCO) formally published guidelines on fertility preservation in cancer patients and called attention to issues of reproductive knowledge and access (Lee *et al.* 2006). This important summary of the critical issues and recommendations has spurred a wider discussion regarding the clinical and research agenda, for not only the development of innovative fertility preservation techniques, but also the epidemiological and public health efforts to both understand the facilitators and barriers to FP, and the communication challenges that FP presents in the clinical situation. Essentially, the clinical goals set out in the guidelines for both the patient and healthcare provider should include discussions of reproductive health issues not only **prior** to treatment but also **throughout** the continuum of their care, to ensure the assimilation of information and to address evolving questions regarding fertility.

The ASCO recommendations also include the following:

1. Oncologists discuss risk of infertility as early as possible.

2. Referral to reproductive specialist as early as possible.

3. Encourage patients to enrol in clinical trials to advance knowledge in the field.

The ASCO guidelines also point to important potential barriers to fertility preservation, including:

1. Lack of knowledge about infertility risk and possible alternatives for future fertility (i.e. cryopreservation, third-party parenting and/or adoption).

2. Failure to discuss/consider options with the patient prior to treatment.

3. Limited discussion due to concerns about insurance coverage and high cost.

4. Investigational status of many of the techniques available, in particular for women.

Since the publication of these guidelines, additional guidelines for FP in adolescent and young adult cancer patients have been published worldwide. A systematic review of these guidelines (Jakes *et al.* 2014) points to the fact that, in spite of inconsistencies in the quality and process of these guideline's development, the results obtained did not affect the general conclusions arrived at and more importantly, the recommendations made, which generally reflect the ASCO position.

Loren *et al.* (2013) have more recently updated the ASCO guidelines by reviewing the over 200 publications since the Lee *et al.* (2006) ASCO guidelines were made public (Loren *et al.* 2013, Lee *et al.* 2006). While no new, major changes were made to the 2006 guidelines from this extensive review, some additional comments were added and clarifications made. In summary:

1. All healthcare professionals (HCPs) engaged in the care of young cancer patients (including oncologists, paediatricians, nurses, psychosocial oncologists, etc.) should be knowledgeable and have the ability to engage patients at risk for infertility.

2. HCPs should discuss FP with patients and/or their significant others or parents/guardians depending on their age. This includes early, pre-treatment discussion of the parameters of FP, risks, referring to fertility specialists as necessary and psychosocial oncology specialists, if distress is encountered.

3. In adult males, sperm cryopreservation is the standard method now available and the only one with proven efficacy. All other methods remain uncertain or are being studied empirically (e.g. testicular tissue cryopreservation). In addition, there is an increased risk of DNA damage in sperm collected after initiation of chemotherapy.

4. In adult females, it is now well established that both oocyte and embryo cryopreservation are effective tools in FP. Other methods (e.g. ovarian transposition, hormonal ovarian suppression are still unreliable).

5. In children who are post-pubertal, sperm cryopreservation and oocyte cryopreservation are available with parental permission, if under the age of consent which varies widely across jurisdictions.

These guidelines are further reinforced by the National Comprehensive Cancer Network (NCCN) directive that adolescent and young adult cancer patients should be considered a distinct group with needs and treatment approaches that may be different from those of adult cancer patients and should be treated at centres specializing in this age group (Coccia *et al.* 2012). They recommend that this age group requires unique focus, not only because they face a life threatening illness; they are also in the developmental stage of their lives where relationships, family building, job-seeking, and stability are evolving goals. Thoughts of childbearing and rearing may not yet be on their minds, but must be brought forward nevertheless to avoid possible disappointment and regret later on. Indeed, referral to a fertility specialist or team is recommended within 24 hours of a diagnosis of cancer.

Focus on practical strategies

1. Oncologists and other healthcare professionals (e.g. reproductive specialists) should be well informed of the available evidence for risk of infertility (both short and long term) depending on tumour type, staging, and treatment options and duration (Lee *et al.* 2006; Achille *et al.* 2006).

2. As stated strongly in both sets of ASCO guidelines, discussions concerning fertility risks must take place prior to the initiation of systemic therapies, as even one chemotherapy infusion may significantly affect sperm production and quality. Patients have indicated in numerous studies that open discussion and dialogue between the oncologist and patient will enhance trust and facilitate communication (Achille *et al.* 2006). Sperm preservation methods and cost should be discussed, with sperm banking (cryopreservation) encouraged and insisted upon by the physician for possible later use in ART, if necessary. Safety of preserved sperm (e.g. transmission for increased risk of cancer and/or teratogenic effects in offspring) should be discussed.

3. Age and relationship status of the patient is critical. Patients should be encouraged to involve partners/spouses in decision-making, as data suggests that their involvement facilitates sperm banking agreement. Younger patients (of age for personal health decision-making) may wish parents to be either involved or uninvolved, while those below age of consent will require parental consent to produce and bank sperm.

4. Desire for fatherhood and/or current fatherhood status is variable (and age dependent) but should be explored with future-oriented thinking around fatherhood, even if the patient is currently not in a relationship.

5. This discussion will also improve adherence to banking, even if morbidity and especially mortality, are of current primary concern to the patient.

6. Reassurance should be given regarding concerns about damaged sperm or transmission of increased cancer risk to progeny, for which there is no current evidence.

7. Referral to a fertility specialist should be encouraged.

8. Some consideration should be given to the related issues of sexuality, intimacy, body, self-image, etc. (Aubin and Perez 2015).

Key communication skills

1. Clear concise factual information provided both verbally and written, reinforced by more detail on numerous reputable websites regarding fertility risk and preservation methods in the context of diagnosis and treatment prior to initiation of treatment.

2. Including significant others in discussions as appropriate, including consultation with spiritual leaders where appropriate.

3. Direct, firm directions on cryopreservation where clearly indicated (e.g. sperm banking for men).

4. Ongoing continuous discussion of fertility issues through treatment and survivorship stages.

The oncofertility (r)evolution

There has been an explosion of educational resources (books, pamphlets, and websites) to assist cancer patients, their families, and HCPs in better understanding reproductive health issues related to cancer and its treatments. In particular, an edited book (Woodruff *et al.* 2014) entitled *Oncofertility Communication: Sharing Information and Building Relationships Across Disciplines*, covers all of the intricacies and complexities described in this chapter in greater depth. Furthermore, several websites have been developed by medical professionals that include comprehensive and multidisciplinary approaches to FP in cancer patients. These include: The Oncofertility Consortium at Northwestern University (http://oncofertility.northwestern.edu/resources/about-fertline), which includes a fertility hotline, links to more information, local expertise, education, lectures, both for professionals and through a portal, for patients and families, etc. The use of multimedia apps and other communication tools facilitates communication by providing access on multiple modalities. As the target population is relatively young and peri-millennial, the use of these new approaches to interactive communication has broken down important access barriers (LaBrecque *et al.* 2014). This consortium has spread its messages globally. In addition, the website is a hub for clinicians and researchers to enhance collaborations that will move the field ahead. Other websites include Fertile Hope (http://www.fertile-hope.org) and the American Cancer Society (http://www.cancer.gov/), to name just two. Fertile Hope also offers a national referral list of reproductive specialists, which can be extremely helpful in addressing the survivorship issues of cancer patients, as does the Cancer Knowledge Network, which includes an oncofertility network with links for professionals and patient resources.

Innovative multidisciplinary, multimodal, and multimedia approaches to a serious public health problem such as cancer-related infertility should have great impact over the coming decades in improving outcomes and quality of life.

Case examples

Females

Breast cancer

Lucy is a 36-year-old women with a history of breast cancer treated with lumpectomy surgery, chemotherapy, and radiation. She also completed a five-year trial of tamoxifen therapy. Lucy reported that discussions regarding treatment-related fertility risks took place the day after her diagnosis and it was considered as an important factor in her treatment decision-making. She obtained valuable information about fertility preservation methods, which helped her decide to undergo oocyte harvesting procedures immediately in order to assure cryopreservation prior to initiating treatment. Although she did not experience any communication problems with her care team during this process, she reported that issues arose after she completed treatment, more specifically about her ability to conceive. She described obtaining vague and inconsistent answers that varied from one specialist to another, in addition to feeling that her distress regarding her difficulties to conceive was perceived as secondary since she was doing very well from a disease standpoint.

Key communication issues

1. Timely discussions made regarding fertility post-diagnosis leading to FP.

2. Lack of consistent follow-up with a fertility specialist in the survivorship phase.

Hodgkin's lymphoma

Rebecca is a 24-year-old women diagnosed with Hodgkin's lymphoma treated with a two-year trial of chemotherapy. Rebecca reported that based on the severity of diagnosis, she was urged to start treatment as quickly as possible. Communications with her care team thus focused on treatment course, outcome, and symptom management. Rebecca reported that at no point during these conversations was fertility mentioned, nor was she given any information. While attending a young adult survivorship conference, Rebecca described the shock she felt at learning that her fertility may have been compromised.

Key communication issues

1. Missed opportunity for timely initial FP discussions; should have been referred immediately to a specialist for consultation.

2. Once discovering possible fertility challenges during post-treatment phase, discussion should be initiated and efforts made to inform and educate the patient as to her current risks and possible risk reduction strategies.

Males

Hodgkin's lymphoma

Bernard was a previously healthy 30-year-old man who was diagnosed a week ago with Hodgkin's lymphoma and was scheduled to undergo chemotherapy. He had one child with his 32-year-old wife through IVF two years previously due to his wife's infertility. As they had planned to have more children in the future, Bernard asked his haematologist about the risk of infertility after his chemotherapy. His haematologist informed him that since they required IVF due to his wife's reproductive status, even if his sperm count drops in the future, IVF would still be a feasible option. Upon initiation of his chemotherapy, he developed significant adverse events including nausea, vomiting, diarrhoea, and tiredness. Further, he discussed his concerns with future fertility with other oncologists and was left with the impression that chemotherapy could have significant negative impact on his sperm production. He then requested sperm banking for fertility preservation. Although he was informed that motile sperm were found and stored, he is now concerned that because sperm banking was done when he was not in his 'top-shape', after chemotherapy had already begun, this may have negatively impacted on sperm that he has stored. Throughout his chemotherapy, he was feeling angry, anxious, and regretful (for not initiating sperm banking earlier).

Key communication issues

1. Missed opportunity for early FP through sperm banking.

2. Need for feedback and education regarding current worries regarding sperm viability from fertility specialist.

3. Psychosocial referral to help him deal with regret, anger, and anxiety.

Testicular cancer

A 19-year-old college student was newly diagnosed with testicular cancer. He is a foreign student who is on a temporary visa for his undergraduate study. After surgical removal of his left testis and further evaluation, he was advised to undergo chemotherapy and might require further surgery to resect the lymph node in the retroperitoneum close to the nerves controlling ejaculation. His urologist counselled him that his cancer treatment could negatively impact his fertility and he was told to undergo sperm banking for FP. He has a limited social network and, due to the urgency of his illness, he had to make all decisions independently and promptly. Due to cultural and religious reasons, he has limited experience with masturbation and was unsure whether he could produce an ejaculated semen sample for banking. To complicate the situation further, although his health insurance covers his cancer treatment, no coverage is provided for fertility management. He has limited personal financial means. Although his oncologist reassured him of his good prognosis with regard to his testis cancer treatment, he experienced despair with regards to his future fertility. Though he was given appropriate counselling and clinical information with regard to his cancer treatment and fertility risks, he felt helpless with regards to his options.

Key communication issues

1. Timely information given post-diagnosis.

2. Limited social network—referral to psychosocial oncology specialist with cross-cultural training, who could possibly help him deal with his spiritual and financial concerns, and feelings of helplessness.

3. Possible referral to a clergy who could discuss issues related to sperm harvesting or any form of assisted reproductive technology.

Conclusion

In the presence of a cancer diagnosis and the treatment of the disease, it is critical to remember that we must treat the 'whole patient' and not just the cancer. Cancer is an illness that affects the patient and the family and it is a chronic illness which, though highly treatable, will have consequences likely to remain part of the patient's experience for many years. Communication about fertility issues and best practices associated with good clinical care can play a positive role in reducing the emotional burden of fertility risks.

References

Achille MA, Rosberger Z, Robitaille R, et al. (2006). Facilitators and obstacles to sperm banking in young men receiving gonadotoxic chemotherapy for cancer: The perspective of survivors and health care professionals. *Hum Reprod* **21**, 3206–16.

Aubin S, Perez S (2015). The clinician's toolbox: Assessing the sexual impacts of cancer on adolescents and young adults with cancer (AYAC). *Sex Med,* **3**, 198–212.

Bann CM, Treiman K, Squiers L, et al. (2015). Cancer survivors' use of fertility preservation. *J Womens Health (Larchmt)* **24**, 1030–7.

Carter J, Rowland K, Chi D, et al. (2005). Gynecologic cancer treatment and the impact of cancer-related infertility. *Gynecol Oncol* **97**, 90–5.

Carter J, Sonoda Y, Abu-Rustum NR (2007). Reproductive concerns of women treated with radical trachelectomy for cervical cancer. *Gynecol Oncol* **105**, 13–16.

Chemaitilly W, Mertens AC, Mitby P, *et al.* (2006). Acute ovarian failure in the childhood cancer survivor study. *J Clin Endocrinol Metab* **91**, 1723–8.

Coccia PF, Altman J, Bhatia S, *et al.* (2012). Adolescent and young adult oncology. Clinical practice guidelines in oncology. *J Natl Compr Canc Netw* **10**, 1112–50.

Dohle GR (2010). Male infertility in cancer patients: Review of the literature. *Int J Urol* **17**, 327–31.

Duffy CM, Allen SM, Clark MA (2005). Discussions regarding reproductive health for young women with breast cancer undergoing chemotherapy. *J Clin Oncol* **23**, 766–73.

Feldstein L (2014). *Legal Considerations before Freezing Embryos* [Online]. Available at: https://cancerkn.com/legal-considerations-freezing-embryos/ [Last accessed April 25, 2016].

Ganz PA, Moinpour CM, Pauler DK, *et al.* (2003). Health status and quality of life in patients with early-stage Hodgkin's disease treated on Southwest Oncology Group Study 9133. *J Clin Oncol* **21**, 3512–19.

Garcia A, Herrero MB, Holzer H, Tulandi T, Chan P (2015). Assisted reproductive outcomes of male cancer survivors. *J Cancer Surviv* **9**, 208–14.

Hammond C, Abrams JR, Syrjala KL (2007). Fertility and risk factors for elevated infertility concern in 10-year hematopoietic cell transplant survivors and case-matched controls. *J Clin Oncol* **25**, 3511–7.

Jakes AD, Marec-Berard P, Phillips RS, Stark DP (2014). Critical review of clinical practice guidelines for fertility preservation in teenagers and young adults with cancer. *J Adolesc Young Adult Oncol* **3**, 144–52.

LaBrecque SF, Wallach H, Waimey KE (2014). Oncofertility communication: tools for professionals and the public. In: Woodruff TK, Clayman ML, Waimey KE (eds). *Oncofertility Communication-Sharing Information and Building Relationships across Disciplines*. Springer-Verlag, New York, NY.

Lee S, Ozkavukcu S, Heytens E, Moy F, Oktay K (2010). Value of early referral to fertility preservation in young women with breast cancer. *J Clin Oncol* **28**, 4683–6.

Lee SJ, Schover LR, Partridge AH, *et al.* (2006). American Society of Clinical Oncology recommendations on fertility preservation in cancer patients. *J Clin Oncol* **24**, 2917–31.

Loren AW, Mangu PB, Beck LN, *et al.* (2013). Fertility preservation for patients with cancer: American Society of Clinical Oncology clinical practice guideline update. *J Clin Oncol* **31**, 2500–10.

Nick AM, Frumovitz MM, Soliman PT, Schmeler KM, Ramirez PT (2012). Fertility sparing surgery for treatment of early-stage cervical cancer: open vs. robotic radical trachelectomy. *Gynecol Oncol* **124**, 276–80.

Petrek JA, Naughton MJ, Case LD, *et al.* (2006). Incidence, time course, and determinants of menstrual bleeding after breast cancer treatment: a prospective study. *J Clin Oncol* **24**, 1045–51.

Schover LR, Brey K, Lichtin A, Lipshultz LI, Jeha S (2002). Knowledge and experience regarding cancer, infertility, and sperm banking in younger male survivors. *J Clin Oncol* **20**, 1880–9.

Sonmezer M, Oktay K (2004). Fertility preservation in female patients. *Hum Reprod Update* **10**, 251–66.

The Oncofertility Consortium at Northwestern University, Chicago, IL. Available at: http://oncofertility.northwestern.edu/resources/about-fertline

Thewes B, Meiser B, Rickard J, Friedlander M (2003). The fertility- and menopause-related information needs of younger women with a diagnosis of breast cancer: a qualitative study. *Psychooncology* **12**, 500–11.

Wenzel L, Berkowitz RS, Newlands E, *et al.* (2002). Quality of life after gestational trophoblastic disease. *J Reprod Med* **47**, 387–94.

Woodruff TK, Clayman ML, Waimey KE (2014). *Oncofertility Communication-Sharing Information and Building Relationships Across Disciplines*. Springer-Verlag, New York, NY.

Zhou Q, Wang M, Yuan Y, *et al.* (2016). Complete meiosis from embryonic stem cell-derived germ cells in vitro. *Cell Stem Cell* **18**, 330–40.

CHAPTER 43

Communicating about sexuality in cancer care

John W. Robinson, Joshua J. Lounsberry, and Lauren M. Walker

Introduction to communicating about sexuality in cancer care

Extensive research has shown that cancer, and its treatment, can interfere with healthy sexual functioning. Indeed, sexual dysfunction is frequently cited as one of the top adverse effects of cancer treatment (Hampton 2005). However, while healthcare providers routinely discuss quality of life issues with cancer patients, the literature suggest that too often this does not include an assessment of sexual concerns. One study reported that 96% of healthcare providers stated that discussing sexuality was part of their job, while only 2% said that they regularly spoke to patients about sexuality (Hautamaki *et al.* 2007). When questions incorporating sexual functioning were included in routine patient assessments, approximately 41% of patients indicated problems with sexual function (Baker *et al.* 2005). However, if patients are not asked specifically about sexual functioning, less than 10% will raise sexual concerns (Driscoll *et al.* 1986). Clearly, the responsibility to initiate discussion about sexuality rests with the healthcare provider.

Establishing the sexuality information needs of the cancer patient can sometimes be difficult, and it becomes more so when healthcare providers make erroneous assumptions concerning sexuality. Healthcare providers often hold the belief that cancer patients are, and should be, most concerned with treating their cancer and that other considerations are tangential. Indeed, many patients do choose life-prolonging treatment despite the loss of sexual function; however, these patients likely still struggle to cope with sexual side effects of treatment. In contrast, some patients are willing to trade years of life to maintain sexual function. Individual differences about the value of sexual function need to be considered.

In cancer care there is a prevalent diffusion of responsibility, whereby healthcare providers believe that someone else will discuss sexuality with patients, resulting in no one assuming the task of assessing sexual concerns (Fitch *et al.* 2013). Even when healthcare providers do accept responsibility, there are myriad reasons for not initiating the conversation, including: limited time; a lack of education or experience; provider or patient embarrassment; and a host of possible religious, gender, cultural, or language barriers. Healthcare providers may also make assumptions regarding: the sexual orientation of the patient; the patient preference for same-gender consultation; sexuality not being part of the presenting problem; or that sexuality is not a concern for the very young patient, the older patient, or the single patient (Julien *et al.* 2010). However, there is a wealth of evidence that patients have unmet sexuality needs, irrespective of age, sex, partnership status, culture, disease status, or cancer type (Sporn *et al.* 2014).

Unresolved sexual problems can have devastating effects on the lives of both the patient and their partner and range from: mild embarrassment, unhappiness, and frustration; to profound humiliation, shame, loss of self-esteem, and complex mental health issues; to an erosion of the relationship bond. These facts suggest that conversations about sexuality should be a routine part of cancer care (Fitch *et al.* 2013).

Where to begin: The PLISSIT model

While there are several different models of intervention for patients suffering from sexual difficulties, the PLISSIT model is frequently used in cancer care and can easily be adapted to various types of practice (Robinson 1998). The model describes four progressive levels that can be used to guide assessment and intervention (Annon 1976).

- ◆ PERMISSION. Raise the topic of sexuality so that patients feel that they have permission to talk about sexual concerns.

- ◆ LIMITED INFORMATION. Provide information to address the sexuality concerns of the patient, including sexual sequelae common to their situation.

- ◆ SPECIFIC SUGGESTIONS. Taking into consideration their sexual history and current context, provide specific strategies for dealing with problems and maintaining sexuality.

- ◆ INTENSIVE THERAPY. Patients with premorbid sexual concerns, mental health problems, long-standing relationship difficulties, and those with more complex sexual issues should be referred to a specialist.

While the model is designed with a hierarchical structure, in practice it is rarely used in a linear fashion. There are many areas of overlap between each of the levels and, as different issues develop, the healthcare provider may be required to move back and forth between levels.

Permission

Raising the subject of sex during the first meeting grants patients Permission to talk about their concerns and serves to legitimize sexuality in the context of cancer. Granting Permission should be standard practice so the choice of pursuing this topic is left open to the patient.

Ignoring sexual dysfunction can lead to erosion in the spousal bond, self-concept, and social relationships. Additionally, early intervention can lead to the resumption of sexual activity, which has been shown to enhance quality of life and to increase the chances of optimal recovery of sexual function. Incorporating a generic question about sex into an initial history or follow-up visit can be an effective first step. While the therapeutic benefit of the mere disclosure of personal information to a trusted healthcare provider has long been recognized, some patients/couples may not want further discussion, so the issue should not be forced. The patient may wish to concentrate on their primary treatment or may not yet have concerns regarding sexuality. However, by granting Permission, the healthcare provider has let the patient know that such conversations are welcome, should concerns arise in the future.

Questions to initiate discussion:

- What impact has cancer had on your sex life?

- Are you experiencing any changes in sexual function?

- Many patients feel differently about themselves sexually as a result of their cancer. How has it been for you?

Patient sexuality is more often overlooked when the sexual organs are not directly involved; however, there are a number of sexual side effects associated with treatments common to most cancers. Patients often struggle sexually because of incontinence, hygiene, fatigue, pain, changes in life roles, loss of independence, loss of earning power, and changes in their body image. In many cases the impact of treatment clearly disrupts a sense of sexuality (e.g. weight gain/loss, alopecia, disfigured, lost breast, ostomy, surgical scars, laryngectomy). In other cases, the loss is less obvious but nonetheless significant: loss of body hair, uterus, rectum, and decreased physical strength or stamina. Few patients are unaffected by such challenges, and thus the majority require information on sexuality regardless of the cancer site or type of treatment.

Chemotherapy commonly affects sexual functioning. For females, chemotherapy-induced menopause creates many challenges including vaginal thinning and dryness, sexual pain, and loss of interest in sex. Women who have permanent ovarian failure after chemotherapy are at high risk of sexual dysfunction after treatment. Chemotherapy can also result in hypogonadism and damage to pelvic nerves in men, resulting in erectile dysfunction, disrupted blood flow, and reduced arousal. Surgery and radiation therapy can result in altered blood flow to the pelvic organs, nerve damage, and atrophy to genital tissue.

Some patients may be too young at the point of diagnosis or treatment to be engaged in sexual activity; however, given the ever increasing survival rates for cancer, the patient will likely wish to become sexually active at some point in their lives.

On the other end of the spectrum are those who may be thought of as 'too old' or 'too sick' to care about their sexuality. The healthcare provider must remain aware of the fact that couples in their 70s and 80s may still want to be sexually active and that even patients who are palliative find comfort in sexual intimacy.

> **Box 43.1** Clinical example illustrating the PLISSIT Model
>
> **Permission:** Chris and Patti, a Canadian couple in their late forties, had been married for 25 years and had become caught up in their busy life. Then, Patti was diagnosed with cancer and underwent an allogeneic stem cell transplant.
>
> Everything was going well with regard to Patti's physical recovery when I saw them at their nine-month follow-up. In a routine manner, I asked how things were going in their relationship. They cautiously confided that there had been some changes in their relationship. Both Chris and Patti reported having never felt closer than during the crisis of initial diagnosis and primary treatment. However, now that Patti was out of the hospital and was doing better physically, things had begun to deteriorate in the relationship. They had become frustrated with one another and had begun bickering over the smallest things.
>
> I informed the couple that it is common for issues to arise once the threat of cancer subsides. Sometimes this uprising of issues can be related to the disruption in the level of sexual intimacy in the relationship and the uncertainty about resuming sexual relations. As it turned out, Patti was having concerns that Chris was no longer attracted to her, while Chris was patiently waiting for Patti to let him know when she was ready to resume their sexual relationship. Patti also reported being a bit fearful of initiating sexual activity because she was unsure how Chris might respond to her.
>
> As we talked, the couple began to realize that the tension they had been feeling in the relationship was coming from the pent-up feelings they both had about this issue. The couple expressed relief and gratitude about finally breaking the silence around sexuality.

Relationship status is another important consideration when discussing sexuality. Whether or not the patient is currently engaged in a romantic relationship has a bearing on the types of concerns that they are likely to have and also their degree of comfort in expressing specific concerns. It should be noted that single patients are a particularly vulnerable population. Also, it is incumbent upon the healthcare provider to inquire about the sexual orientation of the patient, rather than assuming them to be heterosexual.

Finally, ethnic or religious diversity can be a factor. The healthcare provider should always remain aware of patient cultural/religious assumptions, as well as their own, with regard to sexuality. That being said, while there are likely to be many differences in the desired method of communication, the types of sexual dysfunction after cancer are common to patients from all ethnic or religious groups (Box 43.1).

Limited Information

The next level of intervention is the provision of information pertinent to patient concerns. Although the healthcare provider may need to warn the patient that cancer treatment can impair sexual functioning, it is crucial to convey the message that sexual activity need not come to an end. Patients may wonder if they can continue sexual relations during treatment or they may have concerns about satisfying their partner. Failure to provide information may lead the patient to expend needless emotional energy worrying about

Box 43.2 Resources

- Schover L (2015). *Sexuality and cancer: for the woman with cancer and her partner*. American Cancer Society, New York, NY. Available at: http://www.cancer.org/acs/groups/cid/documents/webcontent/002912-pdf.pdf

- Schover L (2015). *Sexuality and cancer: for the man with cancer and his partner*. American Cancer Society, New York, NY. Available at: http://www.cancer.org/acs/groups/cid/documents/webcontent/002910-pdf.pdf

- Canadian Cancer Society (2012). *Sexuality and cancer: a guide for people with cancer*. Canadian Cancer Society, Toronto, Canada. Available at: http://www.cancer.ca/~/media/cancer.ca/CW/publications/Sexuality%20and%20cancer/Sexuality-and-cancer-2016-EN.pdf

- Katz A (2010). *Man, Cancer, Sex*. Hygeia Media, Pittsburgh, PA.

- Katz A (2010). *Woman, Cancer, Sex*. Hygeia Media, Pittsburgh PA.

concerns that could easily have been allayed. It is also important to remember that the patient will likely feel overwhelmed when initially diagnosed with cancer and may forget much of the sexual information provided at the time of diagnosis and treatment. Therefore, during follow-up visits, patients will benefit from being asked again about their sexual concerns.

Following primary treatment, the patient should be provided with resources outlining the lasting effects of cancer treatment in general, as well as specifics for their particular situation. Written information can be particularly helpful because it allows the patient to work with the material on their own time. Numerous reliable sources of written information are available for patients (see Box 43.2).

Sexual response cycle

The sexual response cycle is a helpful model for explaining both sexual functioning and the ways in which various treatments will likely affect sexual functioning. In addition to the diagram outlining the sexual response cycle (Fig. 43.1), patients often find three-dimensional (3D) models, or drawings of pelvic anatomy helpful when trying to understand the changes that are taking place at the various stages of the cycle.

The sexual response cycle, first described by Masters and Johnson, is presented as a linear series of phases beginning with Desire. Desire is commonly experienced as sexual thoughts/fantasies or spontaneous physical sexual urges. When a person acts upon their desire, they move to the Arousal phase. Lingering in a state of sexual arousal is referred to as the Plateau, from which the sexual tension that is built up in the Arousal phase can, with further stimulation, be released with Orgasm. The Resolution phase refers to the period during which the body returns to physiological norms.

Revised sexual response cycle

Basson's (2005) refinement of the sexual response cycle can be particularly useful in helping patients understand the changes they are experiencing (Fig. 43.2). It is applicable to both female and male cancer patients. This model differentiates between 'spontaneous' sexual desire and 'responsive' sexual desire. The concept of 'spontaneous desire' corresponds to the aforementioned Masters and Johnson conceptualization of 'desire'. In contrast, Basson theorizes that 'responsive sexual desire' follows arousal, rather than precedes it. Responsive sexual desire may come after an invitation for sexual activity is presented, or after sexual stimulation begins and arousal unfolds.

Basson also suggests that there are other benefits that come from sexual experiences that serve to motivate sexual activity. For example, a person might find sexual activity rewarding for the closeness and intimacy it provides between the couple. If a patient is motivated to engage in sexual activity and if they begin to feel sexually aroused, desire will often follow. The importance of enhancing motivation and understanding the patient's fears about engaging in sexual activity are highlighted in Basson's revised conceptualization as motivators serve to reinforce desire in future sexual encounters. The revised model, also highlights the role that thoughts and emotions play in sexual response and motivation (Box 43.4).

The PRISM model (**P**hysical Pleasure—**R**elational **I**ntimacy Model of **S**exual **M**otivation) is a useful clinical tool for helping patients clarify their own motivations for sexual activity. As a sexual values exercise, this tool can help couples better understand their own 'motivators', and those of their partner (Beck *et al.* 2013). The model predicts that placing value on sex for relational intimacy, rather than focusing only on physical pleasure, contributes to couples' sexual resiliency.

Resuming sexual activity

The sexual response cycle can be used to help the patient understand that the absence or impairment of one aspect of sexual

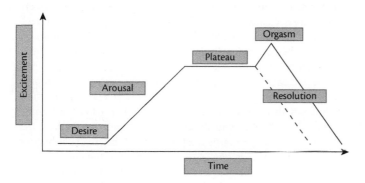

Fig. 43.1 Sexual response cycle.

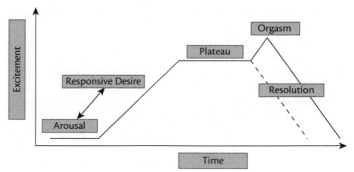

Fig. 43.2 Revised sexual response cycle.

functioning does not preclude satisfying sexual experiences. For example, after radical prostatectomy, sexual desire, pleasurable genital sensation, and the ability to orgasm often are not impaired, even though the patient may experience erectile difficulties and loss of ejaculate. For a man, arousal is usually palpable in that there is a direct association between the sight or sensation of an erection building and a report of subjective arousal. Thus, when there is a loss of erectile function, the man may overlook more subtle sensations of arousal (e.g. increased heart rate, breathing, and skin sensitivity), and assume that arousal is unattainable. Often, men find it helpful to learn about the physiology of orgasm, particularly the fact that the nerves that are involved in erectile function are different from those involved in sensation and orgasm. Analogies, such as those described in Box 43.3, are one way of providing Limited Information, and can be an effective way of simplifying complicated concepts.

Box 43.3 Helpful analogies

Appetite comes as we eat analogy

Just as cancer patients commonly lose their spontaneous appetite for food, so too do they lose their appetite for sexual relations. When the appetite is weak, the idea of eating a four-course meal is sure to stifle any willingness to begin the first course. Likewise, for a person lacking spontaneous sexual desire, considering engaging in intercourse can be unappealing. The French axiom, 'L'appetit vient en manegeant' or the 'appetite comes while we eat' is one that captures this concept and resonates with the cancer patient's experience. If patients are gently encouraged to taste some food knowing that they can just nibble the bits that they find appealing, and feel free to stop without question when they are satiated, there will often be an enjoyment of the food, and a concomitant awakening of appetite. Similarly, many patients are more willing to engage in sexual touching when there is no pressure to reach climax or alternatively, to proceed to intercourse. Granting patients Permission to engage in sexual activity without the expectation of intercourse or orgasm can be liberating for patients experiencing sexual changes.

Orgasm/sneeze analogy

It can be instructive for patients to think of orgasms as pelvic sneezes. The tension in the face and the tickle in the nasal passages indicate that a sneeze is building. Likewise, for orgasm there is a build-up of muscle tension and congestion which we call arousal. A sneeze releases facial tension and an orgasm is the pleasurable release of sexual tension. Of course, sneezes can be stifled and the tension allowed to dissipate, just as arousal can be allowed to dissipate without orgasm. The point being that orgasms are not mandatory. Another related concept is that erections are not required for orgasms, orgasm will result from sexual stimulation of any kind that produces sufficient arousal.

To carry the metaphor further, we can have a wet sneeze if there is mucus in the nasal passages and dry sneezes if there is none. Similarly, men have wet orgasms—ejaculate—if they have a functioning prostate that produces seminal fluid, and dry orgasms if their prostate was removed or irradiated. Wet and dry sneezes may feel different but they are both, unmistakably, sneezes.

Box 43.4 Clinical example

Limited Information

Chris and Patti did have questions and concerns about resuming sexual intimacy. Patti brought up the common concern of changes in how her body responds sexually and wondering why she wasn't experiencing the same level of sexual desire she had before her treatment. I informed the couple that changes in sexual response and a loss of spontaneous desire are particularly common. When the idea that 'our appetite develops as we eat' was presented to the couple, they both found that it applied well to their situation. I also informed the couple that while women do have an awareness of the physiological sensations of arousal, it is the thoughts and emotions that she experiences that determine her level of subjective arousal. If Patti were to embrace her perceptions of sexual feelings and thoughts, her arousal might be reinforced. Normalizing the situation reduced the couple's anxiety and allowed Patti to look for solutions, rather than concentrate on the bodily changes. I also provided the couple with a booklet that contained an explanation of the changes that were likely following cancer treatment, so that they might review things on their own. While the couple was provided with the tools to resolve their issues, the door was left open to take the conversation further, if the couple so desired.

Issues of fertility

Although fertility issues are most pressing for patients who wish to have children, the ability to procreate can be an important part of a positive sexual image, independent of the wish to reproduce. The loss of fertility can exacerbate the struggle to maintain a positive body image after cancer and can result in the feeling of being 'damaged goods'. Given that chemotherapy and broad irradiation are likely to affect fertility, it is incumbent upon the healthcare provider to inform the patient about options for preserving fertility. Research suggests that, unless the healthcare provider takes the initiative to refer patients to a fertility specialist, it is unlikely that patients will go of their own accord (Achille et al. 2006) (Box 43.4). For more information on this issue see Chapter 34.

Specific Suggestions

Attention to patient context is always important, but it is even more so when providing Specific Suggestions. While people across cultures, religions, and sexual orientations are more alike than they are different, it is important to remain aware that there may be issues specific to particular groups. Resources are available to help healthcare providers become more sensitive to diversity issues; however, patients themselves are often happy to explain how their background and upbringing informs their sexuality. The key is not to make assumptions about patients, because there are likely unknown influencing factors.

It is important to include partners in the conversation when providing Specific Suggestions. Partners often have concerns of their own, but can also play a vital role in helping the patient overcome any difficulties. The couple should choose together which of the suggested strategies are of interest to them. A brief sexual history can be helpful in understanding the dynamics of the couple's intimate relations and the beliefs and attitudes that they have about sexual activity (Box 43.5). The sexual history will also help to reveal

Box 43.5 Questions to guide the assessment of sexual function

Desire phase

Are there times when you spontaneously experience desire for sexual activity? How frequently?

If your partner approaches you sexually, how do you usually respond?

Arousal phase

How easy or difficult is it for you to, become sexually aroused or excited?

Men: Do you ever experience difficulties obtaining or maintaining an erection?

Women: Do you experience a sense of pelvic fullness and find that your labia become engorged? Do you have any difficulty becoming naturally lubricated or wet?

Do you ever experience pain with sexual activity?

Orgasm phase

On most occasions, when you wish to, are you able to reach orgasm?

Do you sometimes find that you reach orgasm faster than you want, or that it takes longer than you would like?

Everybody is different in the types of stimulation that feels pleasurable or that is most likely to help them reach orgasm. What types of stimulation work best in helping you reach orgasm?

Resolution

When you reflect back on your recent sexual experiences, how do you usually feel?

Are you concerned with any aspect of how your body responds sexually, with your sexual relationship, or your ability to be a good lover?

the specific nature of the sexuality problem facilitating successful intervention. For example, if the patient reports loss of sexual desire, but the healthcare provider is unaware that they are experiencing dyspareunia (painful intercourse), the root cause will have been missed and any suggestions to improve desire will likely fail.

Another important contextual factor is the use of medications that interfere with sexual functioning. For example, depression is strongly associated with sexual dysfunction and the use of antidepressants often exacerbates the problem. More than half of those who take antidepressant medications, especially selective serotonin reuptake inhibitors, experience decreased desire, difficulties becoming aroused, and problems reaching orgasm. However, there are antidepressants (mirtazapine, moclobemide, nefazodone, reboxetine) that have been found to have limited negative effects on sexual functioning. Bupropion, in particular, has been reported to improve sexual function for women treated for breast cancer (Mathias et al. 2006) and for men experiencing erectile dysfunction or delayed ejaculation (Clayton and Shen 1998).

Be aware of the most common sexual problems

In order to become effective in the provision of Specific Suggestions, the healthcare provider will need to acquaint themselves with the

sexual sequelae for the patient population in question. Describing the approaches to treating the sexual difficulties for all of the specific cancer sites is beyond the scope of this chapter; however, there are sequelae that are common to most cancers. It is important to remember that it is rarely cancer itself that directly interferes with sexual functioning; rather, it is the treatment that most often causes the problems. At the very least, healthcare providers should be knowledgeable concerning the most common sexual sequelae; vaginal dryness and dyspareunia, loss of desire, and erectile dysfunction.

Vaginal dryness and dyspareunia

Vaginal dryness and female dyspareunia are common after chemotherapy and pelvic radiotherapy. Estrogen replacement therapy (ERT) can be an effective treatment (Collaborative Group on Hormonal Factors in Breast Cancer 1997). Some findings suggest that localized forms of ERT, such as vaginal creams (e.g. premarin, vagifem), or rings (estring, estrace) can be effective in reducing vaginal dryness and improving the health of vaginal tissue without significantly increasing serum levels of estrogen in hormonally sensitive cancer survivors (Ponzone et al. 2005). However, combining: (i) pelvic floor muscle relaxation exercises to reduce vaginal tightness or tension; (ii) water- or silicone-based lubricants during sexual activity; (iii) vaginal moisturizers (which are used daily or every other day); and (iv) vitamin E (100–600 IU/day orally or locally) is as effective in improving vaginal health as hormonal treatment options (SOGC Clinical Practice Guidelines 2005). Some studies (Juraskova et al. 2013) even demonstrate that natural products such as coconut oil or olive oil are helpful as sexual lubricants. Non-hormonal polycarbophil moisturizer (e.g. Replens®), or vaginal moisturizers containing hyaluronic acid (e.g. Gynatrof®, Repagyn®) have also been shown to improve vaginal health and sexual function for some women.

Loss of desire

Another common problem is loss of sexual desire. Many consider androgen as a first line treatment for men and women experiencing a loss of sexual desire; however, the role of androgens in sexual response is complex and controversial. A comparison of women with hypoactive sexual desire disorder with controls showed no differences between the groups of women in testosterone levels (Basson et al. 2010); this remains to be tested in cancer patients. Improvements in sexual response have been shown with the supplementation of testosterone to high physiologic levels (Buster et al. 2005). While androgen replacement is considered safe by some—even in women with hormone sensitive tumours—many caution against its use (Stahlberg et al. 2004) as the long-term implications of androgen supplementation are unknown. Contextual and relationship factors were found to be more important than hormonal ones in a study of women who underwent surgical menopause (Kotz et al. 2006) and behavioural interventions, especially those addressing motivational issues, have shown promise, even for women with low androgen levels (Basson 2005).

Men also commonly experience a loss of sexual desire following certain cancer treatments. Androgen-deprivation therapy, a treatment for prostate cancer, often results in a loss of sexual desire and difficulties with arousal because of castrate levels of testosterone. However, hormonal explanations for loss of sexual desire are overly simplistic in men as well, because the factors that influence motivation for sexual activity and spontaneous or responsive sexual desire are broad. Psychosocial variables are equally, if not more, important than hormonal variables in the subjective experience of sexual desire. For example, there does appear to be some evidence that men are capable of a full sexual response despite castrate levels of testosterone (Wassersug 2009).

Erectile dysfunction

Erectile dysfunction is the most common sexual problem for which men seek treatment. The majority of men treated for prostate cancer will lose the ability to naturally obtain an erection sufficient for intercourse (reviewed in Walker *et al.* 2015). Men having pelvic surgeries, such as cystectomy or anterior–posterior resection, and those receiving pelvic radiotherapy for prostate, colorectal, or bladder cancer, may experience erectile dysfunction as well. Healthcare providers should be aware of the most effective interventions for promoting erectile function in men and for helping couples maintain sexual intimacy despite erectile dysfunction (Beck *et al.* 2009; Walker *et al.* 2015). A variety of medical options to improve erectile function exist (e.g. vacuum erection device, intracavernous injections, oral medications), each with varying effectiveness for patients. For example, oral medications such as phosphodiesterase-5 inhibitors may be helpful for men with erectile dysfunction with psychogenic causes, but may be less helpful for men experiencing physiological changes in nerve and vascular function (see Walker *et al.* 2015 for suggestions on optimizing the medical treatment of erectile dysfunction). Penile rehabilitation—the practice of using pro-erectile aids soon after prostatectomy to preserve penile oxygenation with the hope of promoting nerve recovery and preventing smooth muscle changes—is recommended to patients by many clinicians, even though the evidence supporting its effectiveness is weak (Mulhall *et al.* 2013).

Sensate focus: An effective intervention to promote sexual recovery

Sensate focus exercises provide a safe and comfortable framework through which couples can begin to explore sexuality with sensual touch. Couples learn to focus on the feelings that arise as they are pleasuring their partner and are being pleasured, without the expectation or pressure to become aroused or engage in activities that are anxiety provoking. Special consideration must be given to the cancer patient because they are sometimes self-conscious about bodily changes and their sense of sexual appeal or attractiveness. The patient is encouraged to start with what is comfortable for them, and to proceed at their own pace. Such activity helps to facilitate rewarding experiences of physical touch and reduce negative experiences associated with pain, pressure, fear, or resentment. Mindfulness may work well in conjunction with sensate focus. Brotto and colleagues (Brotto and Basson 2014) have found that training in mindfulness helps women stay focused on sensual feelings and improves their sexual function. There are materials available to help healthcare providers to become familiar with, and implement, this strategy (Schover 1997) (Box 43.6).

Intensive Therapy

Approximately 80% of cancer patients' sexual concerns can be managed by intervention at the first three levels of the PLISSIT model. Nonetheless, the healthcare provider should be able to recognize the point at which the patient/couple should be referred to a specialist. Intensive Therapy is needed for patients with more complex medical problems or if there are relationship or attitudinal factors that impede their ability to use the Limited Information or the

---

Box 43.6 Clinical example

Specific Suggestions

The tone of the conversation suggested that both Chris and Patti would be open to moving beyond Limited Information into the provision of Specific Suggestions. I provided the couple with instructions on the use of sensate focus and I encouraged them to try the exercise at home. If they started slow, with no intention of sexual intercourse, just as in the metaphor of eating an appetizer, Patti's appetite might slowly begin to develop. If her desire did not appear, there was no pressure or expectation that their sexual touching lead to intercourse. Both Patti and Chris agreed that this would be a good solution.

I informed the couple that following a stem cell transplant, labial or vaginal dryness, and atrophy of the vaginal tissue is common (Spiryda *et al.* 2003). I provided the couple with a silicone-based lubricant. I told them that arousal would likely take longer to emerge than they were used to, and suggested that using the lubricant would facilitate pleasurable sexual stimulation and reduce friction and/or pain.

When I saw the couple at follow-up, I could immediately see the difference in how they were relating to one another. When I commented on the change, they explained that the sensate focus exercises had provided them with a comfortable way of reconnecting physically and emotionally. They had come to the realization that while sexuality is not the glue that holds them together, it is the lubricant that helps smooth out the rough patches.

Specific Suggestions. A history of poor psychological coping, sexual or physical abuse, substance dependence, or longstanding history sexual dysfunction is also associated with an increased propensity for major sexual difficulties.

The healthcare provider may also be faced with compliance issues following the provision of Specific Suggestions. It has repeatedly been shown that merely recommending that women use vaginal dilators to prevent vaginal stenosis after pelvic radiotherapy results in very low compliance rates. Likewise, the advent of phosphodiesterase-5 inhibitor medications have led some to believe that erectile dysfunction is easily treated. However, 50% of men stop using the aid within a year (reviewed in Walker *et al.* 2015). Most concerning are the patients who, when medical treatments do not seem to work, withdraw from all intimate contact and physical affection with their partners. Use of strategies such as motivational interviewing (Miller and Rollnick 2013), or values clarification (Beck *et al.* 2013) can help couples find motivation to sustain behavioural changes and persist through the process of sexual recovery. These types of interventions are best left to those who have been professionally trained in their use, therefore, knowledge of appropriate referral pathways is important (Box 43.7).

Reflecting on practice

Just as patients have a right to know if treatments will result in hair loss or nausea, so too do they have a right to know the ramifications of treatment on their sexuality. Rather than perpetuating the culture of silence around sexuality, healthcare providers can work to help patients improve or maintain good sexual health. Most patients'

Box 43.7 Clinical example

Intensive Therapy

Although it was unlikely that Chris and Patti needed Intensive Therapy, I made sure that they were aware that seeing a specialist was possible and not out of the ordinary. I pointed out that, if left to their own devices, couples often avoid talking about sensitive issues because they are afraid of making matters worse. Couples who do seek professional counselling improve their chances of maintaining or improving sexual intimacy because it can help couples to have meaningful discussions about difficult issues and to express pent-up feelings.

needs are easily met by establishing an environment in which their sexual concerns can comfortably be discussed with their healthcare provider through the normalization of thoughts and feelings, the presentation of accurate information, and the provision of appropriate suggestions. Proficiency in communicating about sexuality with cancer patients requires little more than a basic understanding of the most common sexual sequelae of cancer treatments and a willingness to initiate a conversation. For more complex issues, the healthcare provider simply refers the patient to a specialist.

Clearly, healthcare providers endeavour to provide the best possible care to their patients. Thus, as conscientious healthcare providers, we must ask why sexuality is so often overlooked when its importance is repeatedly demonstrated. Our intent in these pages was to provide a tool to facilitate communication, while inviting a critical appraisal of the healthcare provider's beliefs, assumptions, and stereotypes. The hope is that healthcare providers will reflect on the manner in which their context affects practice; that is, to base practice on evidence rather than assumption, and to assign priority to the patient's well-being.

References

Achille MA, Rosberger Z, Robitaille R, *et al.* (2006). Facilitators and obstacles to sperm banking in young men receiving gonadotoxic chemotherapy for cancer: the perspective of survivors and health care professionals. *Hum Reprod* **21**, 3206–16.

Annon JS (1976). *Behavioral Treatment of Sexual Problems: Brief Therapy.* Harper & Row, Oxford, UK.

Baker F, Denniston M, Smith T, West MM (2005). Adult cancer survivors: how are they faring? *Cancer* **104**, 2565–76.

Basson R (2005). Women's sexual dysfunction: revised and expanded definitions. *CMAJ* **172**, 1327–33.

Basson R, Brotto LA, Petkau AJ, Labrie F (2010). Role of androgens in women's sexual dysfunction. *Menopause* **17**, 962–71.

Beck AM, Robinson JW, Carlson LE (2013). Sexual values as the key to maintaining satisfying sex after prostate cancer treatment: the physical pleasure-relational intimacy model of sexual motivation. *Arch Sex Behav* **42**, 1637–47.

Brotto LA, Basson R (2014). Group mindfulness-based therapy significantly improves sexual desire in women. *Behav Res Ther* **57**, 43–54.

Buster JE, Kingsberg SA, Aguirre O, *et al.* (2005). Testosterone patch for low sexual desire in surgically menopausal women: a randomized trial. *Obstet Gynecol* **105**, 944–52.

Clayton DO, Shen WW (1998). Psychotropic drug-induced sexual function disorders: diagnosis, incidence and management. *Drug Saf* **19**, 299–312.

Collaborative Group on Hormonal Factors in Breast Cancer (1997). Breast cancer and hormonal replacement therapy: collaborative reanalysis of individual data from 51 epidemiological studies of 52.705 women with breast cancer and 108.411 women without breast cancer. *Lancet* **350**, 1047–59.

Driscoll CE, Garner EG, House JD (1986). The effect of taking a sexual history on the notation of sexually related diagnoses. *Fam Med* **18**, 293–5.

Fitch MI, Beaudoin G, Johnson B (2013). Challenges having conversations about sexuality in ambulatory settings: part II—health care providers perspectives. *J Cancer Oncol Nurs* **23**, 182–96.

Hampton T (2005). Cancer survivors need better care: new report makes recommendations. *JAMA* **294**, 2959–60.

Hautamaki K, Miettinen M, Kellokumpu-Lehtinen PL, Aalto P, Lehto J (2007). Opening communication with cancer patients about sexuality-related issues. *Cancer Nurs* **30**, 399–404.

Julien JO, Thom B, Kline NE (2010). Identification of barriers to sexual health assessment in oncology nursing practice. *Oncol Nurs Forum* **37**, E186–90.

Juraskova I, Jarvis S, Mok K, *et al.* (2013). The acceptability, feasibility, and efficacy (Phase I/II Study) of the OVERcome (Olive Oil, Vaginal Exercise, and MoisturizeR) intervention to improve dyspareunia and alleviate sexual problems in women with breast cancer. *J Sex Med* **10**, 2549–58.

Kotz K, Alexander JL, Dennerstein L (2006). Estrogen and androgen hormone therapy and well-being in surgically postmenopausal women. *J Women's Health* **15**, 898–908.

Mathias C, Cardeal Mendes CM, Ponde de Sena E, *et al.* (2006). An open-label, fixed-dose study of bupropion effect on sexual function scores in women treated for breast cancer. *Ann Oncol* **17**, 1792–6.

Miller WR, Rollnick S (2013). *Motivational Interviewing: Helping People Change*, 3rd edition. The Guilford Press, New York, NY.

Mulhall JP, Bivalacqua TJ, Becher EF (2013). Standard operating procedure for the preservation of erectile function outcomes after radical prostatectomy. *J Sex Med* **10**, 195–203.

Ponzone R, Biglia N, Jacomuzzi M, Maggiorotto F, Mariani L, Sismondi P (2005). Vaginal oestrogen therapy after breast cancer: is it safe?. *Eur J Cancer* **41**, 2673–81.

Robinson JW (1998). Sexuality and cancer: Breaking the silence. *Aust Fam Physician* **27**, 45–7.

Schover LR (1997). *Sexuality and Fertility After Cancer.* Wiley, New York, NY.

SGOC Clinical Practice Guidelines (2005). The detection and management of vaginal atrophy. *Int J Gynecol Obstetics* **88**, 222–8.

Spiryda LB, Laufer MR, Soiffer RJ, *et al.* (2003). Graft-versus-host disease of the vulva and/or vagina: diagnosis and treatment. *Biol Blood Marrow Transplant* **9**, 760–5.

Sporn N, Smith KB, Pirl WF, Lennes IT, Hyland KA, Park ER (2014). Sexual health communication between cancer survivors and providers: how frequently does it occur and which providers are preferred?. *Psychooncology*, Epub.

Stahlberg C, Pedersen AT, Lynge E, *et al.* (2004). Increased risk of breast cancer following different regimens of hormone replacement therapy frequently used in Europe. *Int J Cancer* **109**, 721–7.

Walker LM, Wassersug RJ, Robinson JW (2015). Psychosocial perspectives on recovering sexual recovery after prostate cancer treatment. *Nature Rev Urology* **12**, 167–76.

Wassersug RJ (2009). Mastering emasculation. *J Clin Oncology* **27**, 634–6.

SECTION E

Communication issues across the disciplines

Section editor: Simon Noble

Screening for distress: A communication tool that highlights patient concerns and facilitates psychosocial programme development

Barry D. Bultz, Paul B. Jacobsen, and Matthew Loscalzo

Introduction to screening for distress

Psychosocial programmes that may intuitively be in the best interest of our patients, even those supported by clinical observations and good science, are often subject to resistance. These programmes represent a change in health delivery culture and we know that, in general, change of any kind is met with resistance.

The practice of psychosocial oncology is seen as a somewhat 'soft' area and one that, in the minds of some, takes a lower priority. This is a problem, in that psychosocial professionals know clearly that our area of practice does change patient outcomes. The question becomes how to communicate these benefits and thereby change the culture to be one of greater acceptance and support.

To change the culture in health service delivery, we must learn to effectively communicate who we are, what we do, and how our practice will improve healthcare outcomes in a biopsychosocial world and in an economical way. In all of medicine and particularly in care today, we are seeing an increase in awareness of cancer care for the whole patient through the implementation of standardized screening for distress across the care continuum.

In psychosocial oncology, communication issues are ubiquitous. From primary treatment centres, to academic/tertiary care facilities and rural settings, patients face many of the same psychosocial and supportive care needs. In economically developing countries, psychosocial care delivery faces an even greater challenge because of the need to compete with basic primary cancer treatments. Even basic treatments, such as chemotherapy and radiation therapy, are limited and underfunded.

The goal of this chapter will be to discuss the impact and prevalence of biopsychosocial distress, the opportunities 'screening for distress' brings to the clinical teams' awareness of the whole patient, and why screening for distress should be considered as a key aid in communication with the patient and the multidisciplinary team. Also, this chapter will highlight why screening for distress is a simple communication tool that might prove helpful in the development of psychosocial oncology programmes.

Background

In the brief history of specialized cancer care, recognition of whole patient care and the specialty of psychosocial oncology (Rehse and Pukrop 2003; Stanton 2006; Zimmermann et al. 2007) have gained the attention of healthcare system administrators, providers, patients, and the advocacy community.

The growth and development of psychosocial oncology was triggered by the landmark text On Death and Dying (Kubler-Ross 1969). Prior to Kubler-Ross's book, talking about death and dying had been a subject that not only received little attention, but also had been conspicuously avoided in an attempt to spare the patient depression, anxiety, and loss of hope.

Kubler-Ross's book was a catalyst to change oncology practice. It rapidly caught the attention of healthcare providers, the academic community, and popular press, filling a gap in our knowledge about whole person and end-of-life care. In so doing, Kubler-Ross inspired a new discipline in healthcare—palliative care and psychosocial oncology. Since her pioneering work, there has been an exponential increase in many facets of pain and complex symptom management in the care of all patients, and particularly cancer patients. So transformational was the pioneering work of Kubler-Ross that it resulted in a cultural shift in medical education to include a science of caring applied to those facing a diagnosis of cancer and terminal illness.

Since the popularization of On Death and Dying, academic medicine, including psychology, psychiatry, social work, pastoral/ spiritual care and nursing, began researching and teaching healthcare providers how best to treat physical pain, have a conversation about emotional distress, and improve the patient experience for those imminently facing death. Through research, psychosocial oncology and palliative care, professionals investigated new intervention strategies to improve quality of life, and reduce multifactorial suffering.

Today, a cultural shift in healthcare is taking place, whereby patients are better informed. Difficult topics we avoided in the past are more likely to surface, stimulated by patients, or the frank reality of the limitations of medicine. As a result, we see the importance of effective communication not only as something we must do, but something we must do well.

Branding distress the 6th Vital Sign

Despite the compelling research indicating high prevalence rates of distress in cancer patients (Zabora *et al.* 2001; Carlson *et al.* 2004), communicating these findings seems to have little consequence in facilitating adequate patient–staff ratios when establishing psychosocial oncology programmes, or in healthcare payment plans. Nonetheless, sharing the magnitude of the problem with administrators and colleagues is critical in creating a better understanding of the place of psychosocial oncology in each institution. In fact, the prevalence of patient distress has begun to garner the attention of policy makers with the branding of distress as the 6th Vital Sign in cancer (Bultz and Carlson 2005, 2006; Holland *et al.* 2007; Bultz and Johansen 2011). Starting from the endorsement of distress as the 6th Vital Sign by the Canadian Strategy for Cancer Control (Rebalance Focus Action Group 2005), a cultural shift is taking place.

In 2010, the International Psycho-Oncology Society (IPOS) endorsed the significance of whole patient care with its standards, stating that:

◆ Quality cancer care must integrate the psychosocial domain into routine care; and

◆ Distress should be measured as the 6th Vital Sign after temperature, blood pressure, pulse, respiratory rate, and pain.

Following the declaration of these guiding principles in oncology, 75 cancer care organizations and societies including the Union for International Cancer Control (UICC) have now endorsed the IPOS standards. Furthermore, the American College of Surgeons Commission on Cancer, an accreditation body, emphasized the need to develop and implement a process to integrate and monitor on-site psychosocial distress screening and referral for the provision of psychosocial care (American College of Surgeons Commission on Cancer 2012). As well, Taiwan mandated screening for distress as the 6th Vital Sign in 2013 and the UICC stated in Target 8 of the World Cancer Declaration that *effective pain control and distress management services will be universally available* by 2025 (http://www.uicc.org/world-cancer-declaration). These endorsements more than opened the door for whole patient care and indeed mandated and legitimized the role of psychosocial oncology within cancer care programmes.

Role of screening for distress

There is general agreement that the percentage of cancer patients who initiate a request for psychosocial care represent a small fraction of those who are distressed (Carlson *et al.* 2004). Consequently, psychosocial programmes face the challenge of identifying the larger population of patients who are distressed, but have not sought help. To address this challenge, a number of governmental and professional organizations have recommended that cancer patients be routinely screened for the presence of heightened distress (National Comprehensive Cancer Network 1999; National Institute for Clinical Excellence (NICE) 2004; Rebalance Focus Action Group 2005).

Several arguments can be made for implementation of routine screening for distress. First, evidence suggests that heightened distress is associated with a number of negative outcomes, such as poorer adherence to treatment recommendations (Kennard *et al.* 2004), worse satisfaction with care (Von Essen *et al.* 2002), and poorer quality of life (Skarstein *et al.* 2000). Second, heightened distress is highly treatable. Numerous randomized controlled trials show that psychological distress, including anxiety and depression, can be alleviated by pharmacological and non-pharmacological interventions (Jacobsen *et al.* 2006). Third, heightened distress is common. Prevalence estimates derived from large-scale studies typically exceed 30% (Zabora *et al.* 2001; Carlson *et al.* 2004). A fourth, and perhaps most important reason to screen routinely is evidence that heightened distress often goes unrecognized, and therefore untreated, by oncology professionals (Fallowfield *et al.* 2001).

Although routine administration of a screening measure would address the problem of underrecognition of distress, clinicians seem reluctant to use these tools (Mitchell 2007). The format and length of many existing tools may be a barrier; the time required for administering, scoring, and interpreting these measures favours use of more informal but less reliable methods. To address this, several ultra-short screening tools have been developed, such as the single-item distress thermometer (National Comprehensive Cancer Network 1999). A systematic review concluded that these ultra-short tools have psychometric properties that favour their use for screening purposes (Mitchell 2007). There is recognition, however, that physical symptoms (e.g. pain and fatigue) are major contributors to psychological distress (Carlson *et al.* 2004; Graves *et al.* 2007). Therefore, multisymptom approaches to screening, such as the Edmonton Symptom Assessment System (ESAS) (Watanabe *et al.* 2011) have been recommended (Canadian Partnership Against Cancer 2009) and are being used in many settings as part of a broader approach to routine distress screening that may have greater clinical utility (Bower *et al.* 2014).

It is tempting to believe that greater recognition of distress through implementation of routine screening will lead directly to less psychological suffering. Unfortunately, the evidence does not support this view. For example, a randomized trial found no differences in health-related quality of life between cancer patients whose care providers did and did not receive the results of a quality of life assessment (Rosenbloom *et al.* 2007). These and others' studies (McLachlan et al. 2001; Boyes *et al.* 2006) have taught us that information about heightened distress provided to treating clinicians must be accompanied by specific actions on their part for screening to make a difference. For example, a recent study compared a usual practice condition in which oncology care providers rated their patients' distress and decided if referrals were indicated, versus a screening condition in which providers received information about whether a patient's level of distress exceeded a cut-off, suggesting referral to psychosocial care (Bauwens *et al.* 2014). Findings showed that 5.5% of distressed patients in usual care vs. 69.1% of distressed patients in the screening condition received referrals, and that 3.7% of distressed usual care patients vs. 27.6% of screened distressed patients ultimately accepted the referral.

The importance of referrals in improving patients' emotional well-being is underscored by a seminal study conducted by Carlson and colleagues that compared cancer patients randomized to receive: minimal screening plus usual care; full screening with report to care providers; or full screening plus triage with referral to resources (Carlson *et al.* 2010). Findings showed that patients in the last group were more likely to receive a referral and more likely to score below the cut-off for high distress on the distress thermometer at follow-up than patients in the other two groups.

The evidence that screening alone does not improve quality of life outcomes, points to the importance of linking screening activities to referrals with psychosocial oncology professionals. Patients identified as distressed need to be referred to professionals who have the requisite skills to identify the source(s) of patient distress and apply the appropriate interventions in a timely manner. This view is consistent with conclusions of a recent US Institute of Medicine report (Adler *et al.* 2008) on meeting the psychosocial health needs of cancer patients. The report identified three components as being fundamental to the delivery of effective care:

1. the identification of psychosocial needs through activities such as routine screening;

2. the development and implementation of a plan that links patients with needed psychosocial services, and coordinates psychosocial and biomedical care; and

3. follow-up and re-evaluation.

Clearly, this model of care will need to be operationalized in different ways given the resources available and the volume of patients seen in any particular setting. Nevertheless, it serves as a useful model for planning a new psychosocial oncology programme or evaluating the adequacy of existing programmes, and may lead to a better understanding of staffing ratios required to address patient needs.

Strategies for psychosocial programme development

The primary factor contributing to the successful development/expansion of a psychosocial oncology programme is institutional support that builds from the need being articulated from front-line nursing staff, physicians, and clinical team leaders to administrator decision makers. Regardless of how the development process is initiated, it is incumbent on those involved to identify the goals of the proposed programme, provide support based on patient's screening data and enumerate the resources necessary to achieve those goals.

The most important resource for programme development is personnel. Consideration of the programme's goals, which are to reduce multifactorial patient distress along the cancer trajectory, enhance patient's quality of life and improve patient reported outcomes, should guide selection of the disciplines to be represented in the programme (e.g. psychiatry, psychology, social work, and/or spiritual/pastoral care). For example, programmes that seek to offer a comprehensive array of psychosocial services and assist all patients identified as 'distressed' will require a greater number of professionals from a greater number of disciplines, than programmes that are more narrowly focused.

Given the limited resources generally available for development of psychosocial programmes, it is essential to maximize their use. A key objective must be to have all psychosocial professionals working together in a collaborative fashion. Toward this end, the roles and responsibilities of each professional are defined, in part, by their areas of expertise and professional training, which need to be clearly outlined. Often, this begins with an initial evaluation of programme needs in order to determine what mental health disciplines and support services need to be involved in patient care. In addition to limiting duplication of effort across disciplines, this approach maximizes the utilization of each professional's skill set.

Communicating advances

All cancer care must be evidence-based. Fortunately, there have been many studies demonstrating interventions that are effective in helping patients and their families cope with the diagnosis and treatment of cancer. With continued research in psychosocial care, there is an ever-increasing body of knowledge outlining the benefits to patients and the cost-offsets for healthcare systems. Part of the role of psychosocial oncology must be to share these findings with medical colleagues and the public. Within the academic institution, formal channels exist in the form of rounds, grand rounds, internship and residency training, and advisory and board meetings. Being 'at the table' with administrators and other decision makers presents this opportunity. Speaking to colleagues and other health providers at local, national, and international meetings can be seen as essential in the development of psychosocial oncology. Educating patient groups and the media is another effective tool to promote the value and impact of psychosocial oncology.

Making the business case

Psychosocial programme development may be easier to accomplish within the not-for-profit sector, where the goal is generally to create value by enhancing the social good (Collins 2005). In this sector, funding for psychosocial programmes almost always comes from institutional resources, philanthropy, or billing for services. Given that in private healthcare systems, mental health professionals are reimbursed for services at significantly reduced rates when compared to medical or surgical services, strong institutional support and philanthropy are usually essential if a programme is to develop. In nationalized health systems, a number of factors need to be raised to support the importance of these services. Importantly, when reporting on the prevalence of distress, the research and clinical value of the multidisciplinary team, the accreditation requirements, and the cost-efficacy case is all-critical, and need to be constantly articulated to build up support for the service.

In the for-profit sector, making the ethical/compassionate case should be one of the main drivers, rather than a typical business model where profit is the primary metric. Effective arguments should include: hospital/cancer centre accreditation; patient safety; risk management; cost savings to the institution; quality patient care; and patient satisfaction. Perceived competitiveness becomes more an issue in for-profit settings. These points represent the most compelling motivations for institutions to core fund the development of psychosocial programmes. However, given funding constraints, fundraising and philanthropy should be considered a viable supplemental option.

In the American system, most, if not all, hospital-based psychosocial oncology programmes are often poorly reimbursed and are, therefore, seen as a cost centre for the institution. However, evidence suggests that timely and appropriate psychosocial care can, in fact, reduce costs (Adler *et al.* 2008). Therefore, in developing a psychosocial programme, a strong business plan is necessary to demonstrate credibility in the domains of service, research, and education. But even the strongest business case will not be adequate to fund a programme if there is a lack of leadership, vision, and teamwork. Great psychosocial programmes grow because they provide relevant, targeted, and highly visible services that are helpful to the cancer experience of the patient and add prestige to specific key constituents.

Engage stakeholders

Regardless of the particular constituency, it is necessary to understand what motivates stakeholders as they relate to psychosocial care. In simple terms, why should other stakeholders care about psychosocial oncology? What do they have to gain, or lose, with the implementation of a psychosocial oncology programme? How can these programmes enhance patient care, improve compliance, and perhaps even enhance survivorship? It is always important to remember that a new or evolving psychosocial oncology programme is extremely vulnerable to resistance or opposition. While it takes a great deal of time and effort to create a new programme, it takes very little effort to undermine one. Therefore, it is essential at the outset to build bridges with other programme leaders and to highlight the value added by the psychosocial programme; it is essential to understand the perspectives of those who can support these programmes. This starts with knowing what these individuals value most in the present climate, then clearly identifying specific benefits to them as professionals and if possible, to them personally (e.g. bonuses for performance) and finally delineating specific performance outcomes (e.g. enhanced patient experience, more new patients seen, efficiencies, and quality). General statements about compassionate care are seldom adequate to engage highly stressed, busy colleagues. This is where working as an integrated, interdisciplinary team with one unified message can almost always be the difference between success and failure. When all team members think like a programme with an aligned, unified message, there is a stronger likelihood of a culture shift that is essential for programme implementation and growth (Loscalzo *et al.* 2011).

Communication strategies with nursing

Psychosocial teams that do not engage with the nursing team from the beginning do so at their own peril, and simultaneously lose powerful allies. The psychosocial team can easily build meaningful relationships with nursing by evaluating what they value. Nurses at the bedside care about making patients feel safe and comfortable, and about reducing suffering. They are also committed to ensuring that patients and their family members get the best medical and psychosocial services possible. Research is beginning to demonstrate the benefits of 'screening for distress' as a valuable tool for identifying patients with varying levels of distress, so that a conversation between nurse and patient can take place. It is well known that screening by itself is not enough. Screening followed by a conversation about key concerns and referral to the appropriate professional for treatment can in fact be facilitated in a timely way and can make the difference in better outcomes for the patient and heathcare team. As screening becomes standard practice, it therefore will become necessary to teach and train the healthcare team how to effectively and efficiently use findings from screening questionnaires.

What physicians want from the psychosocial programmes

Physicians want to be sure that patients receive the best services possible, in the most efficient and cost-effective way possible; therefore, it is important that the psychosocial programmes focus on these areas. Physicians who are clinically focused are much more concerned with the quality of direct services to patients and families. All professionals would like to see a smooth-flowing and organized clinic, where patients and families are supported, and distress is prospectively managed by the interdisciplinary team.

Psychosocial services have become highly specialized and are tailored to the changing treatment regimes. Therefore, it is best to have an assigned psychosocial oncology professional with expertise in the specific cancers working in a particular clinic. This ensures that psychosocial interventions are evidence-based and state-of-the-art. This model also supports the highest levels of team functioning. Because cancer clinics tend to be high stress and emotionally charged environments, it is a great benefit to the patients, physicians, and nurses to have a team member who is knowledgeable about that setting and is built into the system of caring. Despite the recommendations by the Institute of Medicine and accreditation bodies, physicians may not have the time or the skills necessary to diagnose and or manage complex psychosocial problems. They may see these issues as a distraction and as a misuse of their time. This reluctance on the part of physicians provides a unique opportunity for the psychosocial team to introduce distress screening to facilitate whole patient care into the interdisciplinary team. While physicians seldom hold the unrealistic expectation that the psychosocial team will 'fix' the distressed patient or family member, they do expect that the psychosocial professional will improve the patient experience within the healthcare setting, benefiting all stakeholders.

A necessary role of the psychosocial team is educating physicians about the psychosocial perspective in an ongoing disease process. By far, most of the education will be as result of case-based role modelling by the mental health professional. For example, the mental health professional can demonstrate the ability to enable the patient and their family members to focus their distress to meaningful communication, which under the best circumstances can be replicated by the physician. Mental health professionals can demonstrate to physicians, through role modelling with actual situations in the clinic, the process of engaging emotionally upset patients by:

1. taking the time to listen and to allow for emotional ventilation;

2. repeating back what you think you heard, so the patient or family member can fill in key areas;

3. giving emotional support and praise for putting concerns into words;

4. focusing on defining with maximum clarity the problem situation;

5. developing a meaningful plan of action with the patients, family, and healthcare team; and

6. clearly defining a follow-up plan and evaluation of effectiveness.

What hospital administrators want from the psychosocial team

The pressures on hospital administrators are constant and intense, as they are charged with managing many complex problems on a daily basis. Having acknowledged this fact, we also know that hospital administrators are essential partners in creating a successful psychosocial programme. They see themselves as caring individuals who bring order and fiscal discipline to institutions, and it is in this context that psychosocial professionals must help them see the significant benefits this area of practice can bring. For psychosocial programmes to be successful, there needs to be a clear and understandable rationale as to why they should exist and a compelling argument as to why resources must be diverted from other areas. Screening for distress data can be significantly influential since it comes from the home institution (it is 'their' data), impacts patient care, the bottom line, and many other variables that matter deeply to hospital administrators. An added value of screening is that it encourages professionals to align and to use scarce resources wisely. Therefore, the psychosocial team must be able to communicate with administrators about the psychosocial benefits to patients and the institution. Benefits about public image, being a compassionate facility, and cost savings are some of the key discussion points that serve to attract administrators' attention. Any programme without clear objectives, benefits, and identified liabilities will raise the suspicion of administrators. Since psychosocial care may be seen as a 'soft' science by some, it is necessary to ensure that goals and objectives are clearly stated, and that benefits to the institution are repeatedly communicated.

Hospital administrators need to understand how 'screening for distress' and the psychosocial programme can support the vision and mission of the institution. The psychosocial oncology programme must be seen as the 'connective tissue' of the healthcare system and must be perceived as essential for the institution to reach its goals. Increasingly, accreditation standards are recognizing this important area, and certainly hospital administrators are concerned about the accreditation of their facility. Effectively identifying and addressing barriers to medical care is a key role. Through systematic screening and the management of patient distress, the psychosocial team can work to improve patient reported outcomes. This is an environment where the psychosocial team can clearly demonstrate to administrators and others the value of psychosocial management of complex problems. The benefits to the patient, family, healthcare staff, and to the system overall are many and are objectively measurable.

Summary and conclusions

Cancer will affect at least 40% of our population over the course of their lifetime and 35–45% of affected individuals will suffer from clinically significant distress (Zabora *et al.* 2001; Carlson *et al.* 2004). These figures, combined with ever-increasing survival rates and life expectancies, make quality of life a salient issue for cancer patients and survivors. Thus, the need for psychosocial care to help patients adjust and cope and live with the sequelae associated with cancer and its treatments has never been greater.

Despite significant advances in clinical care, research and education programme development in psychosocial oncology still has a 'hard row to hoe'. Given the 'soft science' argument waged against psychosocial oncology, it becomes increasingly imperative to communicate clearly about the relevance of screening for distress and the benefits of psychosocial care from an evidence-based perspective, focusing on the value added in the care of the patients, the benefits to the healthcare team and the institution. However, with the increased attention to the patient experience, ability to cope, and quality of life over the past three decades, psychosocial oncology has begun to play an increasingly central role in comprehensive cancer care. Clinicians, researchers, and educators must continue to work diligently to demonstrate the benefits of screening patients for distress. They must also ensure the appropriate referral to the right professional in a timely way as an important strategy in reducing patient burden, enhancing quality of life, and reducing healthcare costs. Like Sisyphus from Greek mythology continually struggled to push a boulder uphill, psychosocial oncology continues to face challenges in gaining a place as a core service in cancer care.

References

Adler NE, Page A, Institute of Medicine (US) (2008). Committee on Psychosocial Services to Cancer Patients/Families in a Community Setting, National Institue of Medicine (US) and Committee on Psychosocial Services to Cancer Patients/Families in a Community Setting. *Cancer Care for the Whole Patient: Meeting Psychosocial Health Needs*. National Academies Press, Washington, DC, WA.

American College of Surgeons Commission on Cancer, 2012. Cancer Program Standards: Ensuring Patient-Centered Care. [Online] Available at: https://www.facs.org/~/media/files/quality%20programs/cancer/coc/programstandards2012.ashx [Last accessed August 31, 2015].

Bauwens S, Baillon C, Distelmans W, Theuns P (2014). Systematic screening for distress in oncology practice using the Distress Barometer: the impact on referrals to psychosocial care. *Psychooncology* 23, 804–11.

Bower JE, Bak K, Berger A, Breitbart W, *et al.* (2014). Screening, assessment, and management of fatigue in adult survivors of cancer: an American Society of Clinical oncology clinical practice guideline adaptation. *J Clin Oncol* 32, 1840–50.

Boyes A, Newell S, Girgis A, McElduff P, Sanson-Fisher R (2006). Does routine assessment and real-time feedback improve cancer patients' psychosocial well-being? *Eur J Cancer Care* 15, 163–71.

Bultz BD, Carlson LE (2006). Emotional distress: the sixth vital sign—future directions in cancer care. *Psychooncology* 15, 93–5.

Bultz BD, Johansen C (2011). Screening for distress, the 6th vital sign: where are we, and where are we going? *Psychooncology* 20, 569–71.

Bultz BD, Carlson LE (2005). Emotional distress: the sixth vital sign in cancer care. *J Clin Oncol* 23, 6440–1.

Canadian Partnership Against Cancer (2009). Guide to Implementing Screening for Distress, the 6th Vital Sign. [Online] Available at: https://www.gem-measures.org/Public/DownloadDocument.aspx?LinkID=71 [Last accessed August 31, 2015].

Carlson LE, Angen M, Cullum J, *et al.* (2004). High levels of untreated distress and fatigue in cancer patients. *Br J Cancer* 90, 2297–304.

Carlson LE, Groff SL, Maciejewski O, Bultz BD (2010). Screening for distress in lung and breast cancer outpatients: a randomized controlled trial. *J Clin Oncol* 28, 4884–91.

Collins JC (2005). *Good to Great and the Social Sectors: Why Business Thinking is Not the Answer: A monograph to accompany good to great: why some companies make the leap—and others don't.* HarperCollins, Boulder, CO.

Fallowfield L, Ratcliffe D, Jenkins V, Saul J (2001). Psychiatric morbidity and its recognition by doctors in patients with cancer. *Br J Cancer* **84**, 1011–15.

Graves KD, Arnold SM, Love CL, Kirsh KL, Moore PG, Passik SD (2007). Distress screening in a multidisciplinary lung cancer clinic: prevalence and predictors of clinically significant distress. *Lung Cancer* **55**, 215–24.

Holland JC, Bultz BD, National Comprehensive Cancer Network (NCCN) (2007). The NCCN guideline for distress management: a case for making distress the sixth vital sign. *JNCCN* **5**, 3–7.

Jacobsen PB, Donovan KA, Watson IS (2006). *Management of Anxiety and Depression in Adult Cancer Patients: Toward an Evidence-Based Approach*. Springer, New York, NY: pp. 1552–79.

Kennard BD, Stewart SM, Olvera R. *et al.* (2004). Nonadherence in adolescent oncology patients: preliminary data on psychological risk factors and relationships to outcome. *J Clin Psychol Medical Settings* **11**, 31–39.

Kubler-Ross E (1969). *On Death and Dying*. Macmillan, New York, NY.

Loscalzo M, Clark KL, Holland J (2011). Successful strategies for implementing biopsychosocial screening. *Psychooncology* **20**, 455–62.

McLachlan SA, Allenby A, Matthews J, *et al.* (2001). Randomized trial of coordinated psychosocial interventions based on patient self-assessments versus standard care to improve the psychosocial functioning of patients with cancer. *J Clin Oncol* **19**, 4117–25.

Mitchell AJ (2007). Pooled results from 38 analyses of the accuracy of distress thermometer and other ultra-short methods of detecting cancer-related mood disorders. *J Clin Oncol* **25**, 4670–81.

National Comprehensive Cancer Network (1999). NCCN practice guidelines for the management of psychosocial distress. *Oncology (Williston Park)* **13**, 113–47.

National Institute for Clinical Excellence (NICE) (2004). *Guidance on Cancer Services: Improving Supportive and Palliative Care for Adults with Cancer*. National Institute for Clinical Excellence, London, UK.

Rebalance Focus Action Group (2005). A position paper: Screening key indicators in cancer patients: Pain as a 5th vital sign and emotional distress as a 6th vital sign. *Can Strategy Cancer Control Bull* **7** (Suppl), 4.

Rehse B, Pukrop R (2003). Effects of psychosocial interventions on quality of life in adult cancer patients: meta analysis of 37 published controlled outcome studies. *Patient Educ Couns* **50**, 179–86.

Rosenbloom SK, Victorson DE, Hahn EA, Peterman AH, Cella D (2007). Assessment is not enough: a randomized controlled trial of the effects of HRQL assessment on quality of life and satisfaction in oncology clinical practice. *Psychooncology* **16**, 1069–79.

Skarstein J, Aass N, Fossa SD, Skovlund E, Dahl AA (2000). Anxiety and depression in cancer patients: relation between the Hospital Anxiety and Depression Scale and the European Organization for Research and Treatment of Cancer Core Quality of Life Questionnaire. *J Psychosomatic Res* **49**, 27–34.

Stanton AL (2006). Psychosocial concerns and interventions for cancer survivors. J Clin Oncol **24**, 5132–7.

Union for International Cancer Control (UICC) (2013). World Cancer Declaration. Available at: http://www.uicc.org/world-cancer-declaration [Online].

Von Essen L, Larsson G, Oberg K, Sjoden PO (2002). 'Satisfaction with care': associations with health-related quality of life and psychosocial function among Swedish patients with endocrine gastrointestinal tumours. *Eur J Cancer Care* **11**, 91–9.

Watanabe SM, Nekolaichuk C, Beaumont C, Johnson L, MYERS J, Strasser F (2011). A multicenter study comparing two numerical versions of the Edmonton Symptom Assessment System in palliative care patients. *J Pain Symptom Manage* **41**, 456–68.

Zabora J, Brintzenhofeszoc K, Curbow B, Hooker C, Piantadosi S (2001). The prevalence of psychological distress by cancer site. *Psychooncology* **10**, 19–28.

Zimmermann T, Heinrichs N, Baucom DH (2007). "Does one size fit all?" moderators in psychosocial interventions for breast cancer patients: A meta-analysis. *Ann Behav Med* **34**, 225–39.

CHAPTER 45

Social work support in settings of crisis

Carrie Lethborg and Grace H. Christ

Introduction to social work support in settings of crisis

A diagnosis of cancer as a lived experience is universally stressful. Improvements in anti-cancer treatments and early detection programmes have meant that cancer is a chronic, rather than terminal illness for many. But the initial expectation for most patients is that cancer is life threatening. As a result, this disease provokes fear in many areas of patient's lives, such as fear of uncontrolled pain, isolation, loss of control, and loss of self. Indeed, a significant proportion (15–40%) of people living with a cancer diagnosis experience clinical levels of distress (Zabora *et al.* 2001). The prevalence of such distress can fluctuate throughout each experience as treatments, support, and physical factors change.

Social work has a long history of providing support to people living with cancer and their families. The overall objective of the social worker in this setting is to support and equip the patient and those close to them to navigate and adjust to the impact of the disease on their lives (Christ 1991). However, the very nature of social work as a profession makes it somewhat complex to describe operationally. The International Federation of Social Workers characterizes the profession thus:

- The social work profession promotes social change, problem solving in human relationships and the empowerment and liberation of people to enhance well-being.

- Utilizing theories of human behaviour and social systems, social work intervenes at the points where people interact with their environments.

- Principles of human rights and social justice are fundamental to social work.

This definition highlights the breadth of the social work focus, whereby the conceptualization of a problem may involve a political and policy perspective, a gender perspective, understanding of life stage and roles, and the client-described lived experience. In addition, the profession aims to focus on the strengths and resources a person brings to their life experiences. Interventions may involve the mobilizing of resources, family counselling, teaching problem-solving skills, and multidisciplinary team consultation. This multisystem and multimodal focus is, in many ways, unique to social work (Hepworth *et al.* 2002).

The focus of this chapter will be on the social work role during the crisis periods of the cancer experience.

The importance of context, situation, and meaning model

The social work perspective views living with cancer as an experience accompanied by a series of challenges as treatment decisions are made, side effects are endured, and relationships strained. For most patients, these challenges are managed with support from loved ones and their healthcare team. However, any one of these difficulties can develop into a crisis or a situation where customary methods of coping do not work and the person living with the disease feels overwhelmed (Roberts 2000).

The starting point, when working with a person experiencing a crisis, is to understand what is happening for this individual. While a crisis by its very nature requires efficient action, it is also important to clarify the issue(s) that have brought about the crisis; sometimes they differ from the presenting problem (Parad 1971; Scheyett 2002). Acute responses to crisis include helplessness, confusion, anxiety, shock, anger, sadness and panic (Golan 1978; Lillibridge and Klukken 1978). These responses can occur due to the difficulty exceeding the person's current resources and coping mechanism (James and Gilliland 2001).

The model used here considers three broad aspects of a case: context, situation, and meaning. Here, the context includes the specific factors that make up the individual and their life experience, the situation is the reason or trigger for the crisis, and the meaning is how the individual experiences the situation. This model can be used in both assessment and intervention in the clinical setting.

The context, situation, and meaning model in assessment

Context

The social work assessment considers cancer in relation to the many factors that make up each individual patient's life. It is acknowledged that a person brings to their cancer experience a number of factors that make this experience uniquely theirs, such as:

- their age and the particular challenges of their life stage;

- their gender;

- the roles they play in their social and working lives;

- the relationships they have and how supportive or burdensome they are;

◆ their assumptive world (Janoff-Bulman1989), including general world views and beliefs and cancer specific beliefs;

◆ the amount and efficacy of their social support;

◆ their psychosocial history, including past losses, trauma and other significant experiences;

◆ their cultural background, including beliefs, customs, roles;

◆ their socioeconomic background, including the resources and choices available to them and their political and power status in their community.

The patient is also viewed from within their family context (where family is defined by the client themselves) with a family-centred approach being crucial to comprehensive care (Quinn and Herndon 1986; Pederson and Valanis 1988; Zabora *et al.* 1990). Indeed, cancer is viewed as a 'family experience', whereby family members are reciprocally affected by illness in each other (Northouse 1984).

Situation

In any assessment, the situation that has brought about the crisis is an obvious concern. However, the presenting problem is not always the actual cause of the crisis and thus assessing the underlying problem(s) is important. Crises in the setting of cancer are seen by the social worker as fluid and ongoing throughout each individual experience of living with the disease. More recently, illness stages or crisis points have been conceptualized as transition points that present the patient and family with new coping tasks. Typically these stages relate to diagnosis, treatment induction and side effects, treatment completion, recurrence/metastasis, advanced illness, terminal illness, and family bereavement.

Particular stresses can be predicted during transitions from one phase of illness/treatment to another. Some of these transitions and their demands are obvious, (e.g. diagnosis, terminal illness) but others are less expected, such as the stresses associated with the successful completion of a treatment process.

As medical advances alter the course of the illness/treatment trajectory, the illness stages also change in intensity, duration, and expected outcome. Thus the psychosocial challenge to the patient and family is altered. For example, the ability to control some disease metastases for many months or even years creates more hope for extended life, but also more treatment, side effects, and late effects; this requires that patients learn to live with greater ambiguity of outcome.

In the cancer setting, the presenting situation causing a crisis for the patient and/or their family is often triggered by a transition point. A patient who feels they 'coped well' with their initial diagnosis may struggle greatly with a recurrence, for example. However, the stress of the cancer experience may also trigger relational issues or concerns about finances or work situations that have been a problem for some time. Assessing the situation is thus central to focusing on an intervention.

Meaning

The stress of living with cancer becomes a crisis when the experience is intolerable to the person living with the disease. An important aspect of this experience is the meaning that it has for the individual. Crises can thus be self-defined; whereby what is a crisis for one person may not be a crisis for another.

Within the assessment, understanding the meaning given to the event enhances the appreciation of why the situation has caused distress and assists in the development of the intervention. This is not to say that the patient is the cause of the distress, but it acknowledges that the way they view the situation is key to understanding their crisis. To give an example, one person might see their diagnosis as a battle they are going to fight with hope and much support around them; they may see themselves as lucky that they have the love and care that they have. Another person, with the same diagnosis and the same resources, might see this as yet another bad thing that has happened to them, a challenge they could never face and feel quite 'beaten' down by their cancer. The difference is partly due to the meaning they give to their cancer diagnosis.

The context, situation, and meaning model in the clinical encounter

In the cancer setting, the following clinical goals are important (Christ 1993):

◆ To understand the individual's unique lived experience of the illness and treatment process.

◆ To identify the strengths embodied by the client.

◆ To identify the resources available to the client.

◆ To identify the specific concerns of the client at this stage.

◆ To prioritize concerns with the client into manageable components, so that the most distressing aspects can be dealt with quickly.

◆ To identify an agreed upon outcome goal(s).

◆ To develop a strategy or strategies to achieve this goal(s).

These goals are achieved using the following processes that are informed by the situation, context and meaning model:

◆ Developing a therapeutic relationship.

◆ Problem identification and the development.

◆ The implementation of strategies to manage concerns.

Each process will be described separately.

Developing a therapeutic relationship

The first of these processes is the same for any clinical encounter. A therapeutic intervention cannot occur without the development of a relationship of understanding between the clinician and the client. Such a relationship, often formed in times of stress and with short timelines, requires the use of effective and empathic communication and relational skills.

Communication is a two-way process, whereby both parties hear and understand what each other is trying to say. This requires active listening, with the social worker asking the client to describe their perception of the situation and noting their verbal and non-verbal responses. In order to check that they have actually heard this information as the client stated, the social worker feeds back their understanding throughout the encounter. In addition to understanding what the client is saying, the social worker aims to understand the meaning that situation has for each individual.

In order for communication to occur most effectively, it is important that the setting is as comfortable as possible. In general, this requires that there are few distractions, is private, comfortable, and that the discussion occurs at a time most conducive to open communication. Clearly, within the hospital or the outpatient setting these factors can be difficult to achieve, but they should remain an aim for each encounter.

Use of self is another communication skill important in joining with the client. The clinician monitors verbal and non-verbal cues and is cognizant of their 'tone'. If the client is angry and loud, for example, the social worker needs to reflect this energy while maintaining a sense of calm. If the client is tearful and withdrawn, then a more subdued response is required. The client's reactions and behaviours are not judged as pathological or wrong, but understood as efforts to cope with a highly stressful situation until proven otherwise.

Problem identification

Within the therapeutic relationship, the clinician is able to discuss the specific source of the client's concerns. However, this can be a complex process. In the setting of cancer it is often assumed that the client is anxious because they have cancer and, indeed, this is often the case. However, identifying what it is about the cancer that is upsetting, how this is impacting on their life, and what specific factors are contributing to their distress is more involved. This is where the therapeutic relationship moves into a counselling relationship. The aim of counselling is to move a person from a state of unease (such as distress, sadness, anger, and so on) to a state of coping (Ragg 2001). This requires first understanding the problem at hand and interpreting it to the client in a way that permits the provision of strategies to address this/these problems. The context, situation, and meaning matrix are crucial at this stage.

The development and implementation of strategies

In the setting of a crisis, it is important to ensure the safety of the client first, and then to define the priority issues to focus on in an intervention. The model below offers three broad steps useful in this process:

◆ Step 1. Ascertain safety of client. Rule out any safety issues for the client or others (e.g. clinical depression, domestic violence, medical concerns).

◆ Step 2. Assessment. The assessment process aims to understand, not only the presenting problem, but also the wider aspects of the crisis. One of the most powerful skills available to the social worker in assessment is that of questioning. During the clinical encounter there are three kinds of questioning that can be helpful (with examples to illustrate):

• Questions to gain information:

  ▪ Can you tell me more about that?
  ▪ Can you tell me what happened?

• Questions to check understanding:

  ▪ So, what you're saying is you feel …?
  ▪ Can I just check with you, did you say your mother accompanied you to the doctor?

• Questions to encourage further understanding of the situation or to test a theory about the situation:

  ▪ You mentioned that you have been the carer for everyone in your family and that you are not used to needing help. I wonder how this impacts on the way you and your husband have interacted?
  ▪ It is interesting to me that you describe yourself as 'not coping' when you have just told me the things you accomplish in a week. Do you see a discrepancy between these two things?

◆ Step 3. Intervention development.

• Break down the crisis into smaller issues that can be addressed separately.

• Work with client to develop strategies to address the issues identified.

• Identify barriers and strengths to carry out these strategies.

These steps offer a framework for the clinical encounter that can be used in a crisis. An example of such a crisis in the setting of cancer is that of treatment completion; this framework will be illustrated below using a case example of this particular transition in the cancer experience.

The context, situation, and meaning model—a clinical example

Treatment completion is a phase of common distress in the cancer experience. While there is often a sense of relief when anti-cancer treatment is completed, a crisis at the completion of treatment is not uncommon. The assessment of the cancer patient who is in crisis at the treatment completion phase requires an understanding of their unique context and the meaning they give to treatment completion. However, the situation of treatment completion can differ from patient to patient also. Thus, it is important to begin with an understanding of treatment completion and the range of issues involved with this transition.

The patient's reaction to the end of treatment can vary depending on the reason for completion. It may have been a successful course of treatment, or it may have induced toxic reactions that had meant they had been unable to continue. Even when treatment has clearly been successful, patients may report feeling apprehensive about the decreased contact with medical staff and returning to normal living. Because they expect to feel more positive emotions, patients often think this anxiety is abnormal (Lethborg and Kissane 2003).

Families and partners also may expect the patient to return to normal life quickly following treatment, not realizing that psychosocial recovery often takes much longer than physical recovery. Finally, the healthcare system itself at times has unknowingly contributed to this anxiety by not clearly defining a patient care plan that specifies the terms of follow-up and ongoing access to knowledgeable medical and psychosocial care.

At treatment completion the client may need to:

◆ recognize the fear of having less medical surveillance and develop ways to cope with ambiguity and uncertainty, for example by creating a specific care plan with clear access to experts;

◆ recognize the need to re-negotiate expectations of support from family and friends;

◆ normalize the stressful process of redefining self and family following confrontation with a life-threatening condition.

The case study in Box 45.1 is from a real clinical situation, using different names and some details to maintain the client's anonymity. Having said this, the crisis situation being presented is not uncommon for people living with cancer.

Using the steps described previously, working with Marcie would begin in the following way.

Box 45.1   Case study

Marcie is a 45-year-old woman. She is the mother of two teenage children: a daughter aged 15 and a son aged 17. She has been married to Steve for 20 years. Prior to her cancer diagnosis, Marcie worked as a writer for a women's magazine. Steve is an arts accountant.

Marcie completed treatment for early stage breast cancer five weeks ago. She was diagnosed almost 12 months ago and has undergone surgery and chemotherapy.

Aside from a two-week period, when her treatment had to be delayed due to a chest infection, Marcie describes her experience of diagnosis and treatment as 'hard but manageable'.

However, she has recently been having trouble sleeping, having headaches, and feeling tearful. She has been fighting with Steve more and more, and wanting to retreat, and be on her own. She believes she is not coping. She has asked to see the social worker urgently as she is concerned that her marriage is going to end.

Step 1: Ascertain safety in a crisis situation

In the first instance, it was important to ascertain if this situation puts her at risk at all. If she describes an inability to get to sleep and early waking, feelings of hopelessness and helplessness, and a loss of appetite over a four-week period, for example, then the possibility of depression requiring treatment must be considered. However, if Marcie is still managing most aspects of her life, then the clinician can pursue the context/situation/meaning aspects of this referral.

Step 2: Assessment

In talking with Marcie, the social worker asked about her life experiences in general, her family, the support she receives from people in her life, and so on. She also asked some general questions about Marcie's cancer experience, how she felt, what she thought, what she did in response to her diagnosis and treatment. The assessment then focused on the specific issue, of 'marital distress' and her feelings, thoughts, and actions in relation to this. Using various kinds of questioning, the information from Marcie's assessment is summarized in Table 45.1. Thus, Marcie's situation can be described in the following way:

The context of her crisis involves the setting of a cancer diagnosis 12 months ago and the completion of treatment within the past five weeks. In addition, the period of mid-life for a professional woman, mother, wife, and friend. Marcie has a history of mild anxiety.

In relation to the situation of this case, Marcie's identified problem relates to marital discontent. The broader assessment of this situation includes post-traumatic stress following treatment completion, role confusion, managing uncertainty, and withdrawal from social support. Marcie also described a number of psychological and physical manifestations of distress. However, she did not have clinical levels of depression or anxiety.

For Marcie, the meaning of this crisis is that cancer has 'beaten her'. She described this crisis as a 'failure' and stated that she has never failed before. Pre-cancer, Marcie states that she always succeeded in whatever she took on and, though being a working mother at times took its toll, she had enjoyed the challenge and felt she did it well. She also described common feelings relating to living with uncertainty, feeling that her husband doesn't understand the ongoing nature of her cancer experience and not being sure about her life direction.

Table 45.1 Information from Marcie's assessment

Context		Situation	Meaning
Gender	Female	Voiced concerns about loss of femininity due to cancer and challenges to her self-image	'I don't know how to be around others right now, I feel anxious and unattractive.'
Roles	Mother	Reduction of energy, need to discuss role changes within family	'I was always able to manage the juggle of all these roles in the past, and I was proud of it.'
	Wife	Tension within marriage in relation to life threat and role change	
	Friend	Some friends have been there for Marcie but some have not	
	Professional	Reintegrating back to work is causing anxiety	
Life stage	Mid-life	Teenage children becoming independent Identity restructuring after confrontation with life threat	'I am not sure who I am right now, I don't know this "me" and I don't know what is around the corner.'
Health	Cancer diagnosis 12 months ago	Treatment completed, but full recovery takes more time for patient and family This was not what Marcie expected she is surprised that she is still experiencing stress related to her cancer	'I thought it (the stress of cancer) would be over when treatment was over.'
Psychological State	History of mild anxiety	Tearfulness, insomnia, worry about the future, describes withdrawing from family and friends However, clinical depression ruled out at this point	'Breaking down now means I am a failure, cancer has finally beaten me.'
		Fear of the unknown	'I don't know what my future holds—I feel like I have lost control.'
Client identified problem	Fighting with husband		'We seem further apart than ever—he has no idea what I am going through.'

Marcie is still managing most aspects of her life but describes difficulty in knowing how to live with uncertainty, feeling that her husband doesn't understand the ongoing nature of her cancer experience, not being sure about her life direction, and the need to re-define self and family after her traumatic confrontation with mortality.

Step 3: Intervention development

Marcie's assessment illustrates how a presenting problem can reveal a range of concerns and issues. It is important to break down these into smaller issues and to work with the client to identify what are the most pressing and urgent concerns at that time. This is necessary both for practical reasons (most social workers have high case loads) and so that the action taken can be done in a manageable way, with the client as a partner in the process.

When these issues were separated for the development of an intervention plan, the following points were agreed between Marcie and the social worker:

- Marcie is in no immediate danger to herself or others.

- Marcie describes feeling anxious about the future and doesn't know how to 'stop worrying'.

- Marcie feels that her husband is impatient for her to 'get back on with life' and that he doesn't understand her.

- Marcie is re-thinking her vocation as the time for her to resume work draws closer.

Prioritizing these issues, the problems, along with the identified barriers and strengths brought to this case, were identified in planning this intervention (see Table 45.2).

While couple therapy could have been offered to Marcie as an initial intervention, given the wider context and meaning it becomes clear that a range of interventions would be beneficial. It was likely that an effective intervention could involve counselling that focuses on cognitive, psychological, and social aspects of managing uncertainty and post-traumatic response, as well as some couple counselling.

Table 45.2 Issues considered in planning intervention

Identified issues	Focus of intervention
Anxiety about uncertainty	Normalizing reaction to uncertainty. Cognitive skills to challenge automatic negative thoughts.
Marital tension	Couple counselling to enable a sharing of the experience of living with cancer and of caring for someone with cancer.
Life review	Goal-setting/meaning-based intervention to review life goals and begin to plan for future goals.
Barriers to action plan	Marcie describes herself as a 'worrier' for as long as she can remember and as having to have control over her life. She feels it will be hard to learn to 'let go' of these tendencies.
	Marcie describes her marriage as being 'strong' in the past and that this is a surprise to her that they would be fighting now. She is sure her husband will come to counselling. She has been a successful woman in all roles in her life and is willing to learn how to overcome the current difficulties she is having.

Table 45.3 Intervention provided

Session One	Aimed to develop the therapeutic relationship, whereby Marcie felt safe enough to share her concerns and to identify the situation that had caused the crisis and the severity of her experience. It also aimed to assist Marcie to make sense of her situation in order to 'normalize' her distress.
Session Two	Aimed to work with the specific issues identified and in this case included teaching some cognitive skills, such as challenging automatic negative thoughts, problem-solving and relaxation techniques.
Session Three	Aimed to work on goal setting for the future, including identifying life goals and purpose, and to review the use of skills developed to date.
Session Four	A joint session with Marcie and her husband to discuss both their 'journeys' through cancer and for each other to hear the differences in their experiences and perceptions. This session resulted in a better understanding of each other's experiences and a joining together to begin to re-consider goals and future plans.

In fact, the intervention with Marcie took four sessions in total, although she rated a drop in her level of distress by half after session one. Marcie attributed her reduced distress to being able to better understand the process both she and her husband had been through since diagnosis, and feeling that her current stress was normal and did not mean she had 'failed'. The sessions with Marcie are shown in Table 45.3.

It is important to point out that, while each step in the social work clinical encounter has been described here in detail, the process itself can occur quite quickly. The social worker aims to develop a realistic timeline to manage the identified problems that take into account both social work resources and extent of the crisis. In Marcie's case, she was seen on the same day as her concerns were raised during a routine follow-up medical consultation.

This clinical encounter has been illustrated in this chapter as proceeding from the development of a therapeutic relationship to problem identification and intervention development. Of course, this process is not always linear, and the skills used to join with the client are required throughout the clinical encounter. However, the model presented illustrates the need for a comprehensive assessment before intervention development can begin. Interventions that are clinician-led and do not adequately take into account the client's perspective are going to be less effective than those that include the client as a 'partner' in the therapeutic relationship. Equally limiting are interventions that focus on the client as separate to their context (i.e. family, cultural background, gender, life stage, and so on).

The social work intervention in the setting of a crisis brought about by the cancer experience aims to fully understand the client and their specific concerns, and to tailor interventions accordingly. Such an approach requires ongoing communication throughout the clinical encounter and an understanding of the complexity involved with living with this disease.

References

Christ G (1991). Principles of oncology social work. In: Holleb A, Fink D, Murphy G (eds). *American Cancer Society Textbook of Clinical Oncology*. pp. 594–605. American Cancer Society, Atlanta, GA.

Christ G (1993). Psychosocial tasks throughout the cancer experience. In: Stearns N, Herman J, Lauria M, Fogelberg P (eds). *Oncology Social Work: A Clinician's Guide*. pp. 79–99. American Cancer Society, Atlanta, GA.

Golan N (1978). *Treatment in Crisis Situations*. Free Press, New York, NY.

Hepworth D, Rooney R, Larson J (2002). *Direct Social Work Practice: Theory and Skills*, 6th edition. Books/Cole, Pacific Grove, CA.

James KJ, Gilliland BE (2001). *Crisis Intervention Strategies*. Brook/Cole, Pacific Grove, PA.

Janoff-Bulman R (1989). Assumptive worlds and the stress of traumatic events: applications of the schema construct. *Social Cognition. Special Issue: Stress, Coping, and Social Cognition* 7, 113–36.

Lethborg C, Kissane D (2003). 'It doesn't end on the last day of treatment': a psycho-educational intervention for women who have completed adjuvant treatment for early stage breast cancer. *J Psychosoc Oncol* **21**, 25–41.

Lillibridge EM, Klukken PG (1978). *Crisis Intervention Training*. Affective House, Tulsa, OK.

Northouse L (1984). The impact of cancer on the family. *Int J Psychiat Med* **14**, 215–42.

Parad H (1971). Crisis intervention. In: Morris R (ed). *Encyclopedia of Social Work*, 16th edition. pp. 196–202. National Association of Social Workers, New York, NY.

Pederson LM, Valanis BG (1988). The effects of breast cancer on the family: a review of the literature. *J Psychosocial Oncology* **6**, 95–118.

Quinn WH, Herndon A (1986). The family ecology of breast cancer. *J Psychosoc Oncol* **4**, 95–118.

Ragg D (2001). *Building Effective Helping Skills: The Building Effective Helping Skills: The Foundation of Generalist Practice*. Allyn and Bacon, Boston, MA.

Roberts A (2000). An overview of crisis theory and crisis intervention. In: Roberts A (ed.). *Crisis Intervention Handbook: Assessment, Treatment, Research*. Oxford University Press, New York, NY.

Scheyett AM (2002). Approaching complex cases with a crisis intervention model and teamwork: a commentary. *J Genet Counsel* **11**, 377–82.

Zabora JR, Smith-Wilson R, Fetting JH, Enterline JP (1990). An efficient method for psychosocial screening of cancer patients. *Psychosomatics* **31**, 192–6.

Zabora J, BrintzenhofeSzoc K, Jacobsen P, *et al.* (2001). A new psychosocial screening instrument for use with cancer patients. *Psychosomatics* **42**, 241–6.

CHAPTER 46

Communication in cancer radiology

Kimberly Feigin and Donna D'Alessio

Introduction to communication in cancer radiology

Diagnostic radiologists are often the first to know of a patient's medical diagnosis, disease progression, or response to treatment. Traditionally, radiologists have been primarily consultants to referring physicians, reporting results of imaging examinations to ordering physicians, who then relayed the information to patients. In recent years, radiology has evolved to include more procedures that bring radiologists into direct contact with patients. This is particularly true in certain subspecialties of radiology, such as interventional radiology and breast imaging. This chapter will explore current concepts in communication in cancer radiology, using the subspecialty of breast imaging as a model.

Communicating results of radiologic examinations

Communication with referring physicians

Communication with referring physicians is the most common type of communication a radiologist undertakes, usually in the form of a written report. In the age of PACS (picture archiving and communication systems), wherein diagnostic images are readily available to all caregivers, a radiologist's interpretive report must be accurate, clear, meaningful, and timely in order maximize the radiologist's contribution to patient care. Descriptions of radiologic findings must be accompanied by the radiologist's opinion of their significance, such as a specific or differential diagnosis, and the radiologist's level of certainty, so that the implications for patient management are clear to the referring physician (Schwartz et al. 2011). While the American College of Radiology (ACR), in its *practice parameter for communication in diagnostic radiology*, recommends that a radiology report should suggest 'follow-up or additional diagnostic studies to clarify or confirm the impression … when appropriate' (American College of Radiology 2014), such a suggestion must be carefully considered and worded in order to prompt appropriate management without exposing the patient to unnecessary investigations or constraining the referring physician.

In breast imaging, the need for uniformity and clarity in radiology reporting, along with the need for consistency of management recommendations, resulted in the creation of a standarized lexicon. The ACR's Breast Imaging Reporting and Database System (BI-RADS) is a lexicon and reporting format created to 'standardize (breast imaging) reporting, reduce confusion in breast imaging interpretations and management recommendations, and facilitate outcome monitoring' (American College of Radiology BI-RADS Committee 2013). All BI-RADS reports conclude with an overall assessment that assigns a precisely defined numerical classification to any breast imaging examination and recommends the most appropriate course of action (see Table 46.1). Studies have shown significant improvement in interpretive skills and interobserver agreement among radiologists following training in the proper use of BI-RADS. More radiology subspecialties now benefit from similar standardization of reporting, including lung cancer screening (Lung-RADS) and hepatocellular carcinoma assessment (LI-RADS).

Table 46.1 Breast imaging reporting and data system (BI-RADS) assessment categories

Numeric code	Category	Typical management recommendation
0	Incomplete—need additional imaging evaluation and/ or prior mammograms for comparison	Recall for additional imaging and/or comparison with prior examination(s)
1	Negative	Routine mammography screening
2	Benign	Routine mammography screening
3	Probably benign	Short-interval (six-month) follow-up or continued surveillance mammography
4	Suspicions	Tissue diagnosis
5	Highly suggestive of malignancy	Tissue diagnosis
6	Known biopsy—proven malignancy	Surgical excision when clinically appropriate

In addition to routine reporting of imaging findings, the *ACR practice parameter for communication of diagnostic imaging findings* outlines steps that a radiologist must take when an imaging finding suggests a need for immediate or urgent intervention, when s/he discovers a finding that, if not acted on, may eventually result in an adverse patient outcome, or when there is a discrepancy between a preceding interpretation of the same examination and where failure to act may adversely affect patient health. In such cases, in addition to a routine written report, the radiologist must directly communicate these findings to the referring clinician or his or her representative 'in a manner most likely to reach the attention of the treating or ordering physician/healthcare provider in time to provide the most benefit to the patient', and document the communication (American College of Radiology 2014). In the United States, these requirements are also a part of the Joint Commission on Accreditation of Healthcare Organizations (JCAHO) Hospital National Patient Safety Goals published in 2015. The European Association of Radiologists and the United Kingdom's Royal College of Radiologists have adopted similar guidelines (Wallis and McCoubrie 2011; European Society of Radiology 2013), emphasizing their global importance.

Communication errors or delays in radiology reporting may result in substantial patient morbidity and mortality, and are costly. Such errors are among the top three reasons radiologists are sued for medical malpractice. In an analysis of medical liability cases in the United States from 1999 to 2003, radiologist defendants were held responsible for communication failures in 25 cases, over which the average indemnification (shared by co-defendants) was US $1.9 million (Kushner and Lucey 2005).

Occasionally, clinicians will request an informal verbal 'kerbside' radiology consultation. These types of consultations may expedite patient care; however, the radiologist should engage with prudence. Verbal consultations are frequently requested when prior studies and reports are not available, patient history is incomplete, and viewing conditions are suboptimal. They require additional skills on the part of the radiologist, including effective time management and the ability to summarize pertinent findings quickly, yet the time and effort to perform these types of consultations are not financially compensated. Verbal consultations should be documented whenever possible to protect the radiologist from any potential inaccuracies recorded by the recipient (Kushner and Lucey 2005; American College of Radiology 2014).

Communication with patients

Partially in response to malpractice lawsuits alleging failure to communicate urgent or significant radiographic abnormalities, a trend has emerged for radiologists to communicate results directly to patients. In several legal cases since the 1990s, courts ruled that, occasionally, a radiologist has a duty to communicate abnormal findings directly to the patient (Berlin 2009). The *ACR practice parameter for communication of diagnostic imaging findings* states that 'in certain situations, the interpreting physician may feel it is appropriate to communicate the findings directly to the patient' (American College of Radiology 2014). This is particularly true when a patient is self-referred or is referred by a third party, such as an insurance company, employer, or federal benefit programme, and unexpected or serious findings result (American College of Radiology 2014).

This trend of direct radiologist–patient communication has dovetailed with patients' increasing desire to participate in their own healthcare decision-making processes. Many patients prefer to hear radiology results from their radiologists upon completion of imaging procedures, rather than waiting to hear their results at another time or from their own referring physicians, whether the results are normal or abnormal.

Additional advantages of directly communicating radiology results to patients include timelier reporting and the presence of a safeguard, should the referring physician fail to receive or respond to the written report. A radiologist is the physician in the best position to understand the meaning of the radiology test result in the context of the test's limitations and to suggest alternate imaging tests or follow-up, if warranted. Furthermore, radiologists' direct communication with patients may improve radiologists' relationships with patients and elevate the stature of radiologists in the healthcare system.

Disadvantages of direct radiologist–patient communication are also numerous. Radiology departments are typically not ideal places for delivering bad news, providing few supports for patients in such circumstances. In fact, the radiologist is often physically isolated from the patient in a reading room or clinical workstation. The extreme example of this is in transcontinental teleradiology. Also, time spent in consultation with patients detracts from time available to interpret imaging exams and is limited and expensive, yet studies show that patients are not willing to pay additional fees for this service.

Patients are only temporarily in the care of radiologists, who may not know relevant parts of the patient's history or other clinical findings. Radiologists are not usually responsible for clinical management and may not even know what should, or can, be done to treat a given patient, despite patient expectations of immediate therapeutic recommendations. Referring physicians may not be adequately forewarned of the results and of their disclosure to the patient, and therefore may not be prepared to receive an urgent call from a distressed patient. Many referring physicians, therefore, want to know of a disclosed abnormal result as soon as possible and prefer to tell the patient themselves. Studies have shown that patients' understanding of radiology results is imperfect and that wording of such discussions is important. For all of these reasons, some patients prefer to hear test indications and results from their own physicians, with whom they generally have an established relationship (Cabarrus *et al.* 2015; Thornton *et al.* 2015).

Reporting of mammography results is a model for direct radiologist–patient communication. Many patients are self-referred for screening mammography, so that the radiologist must assume responsibility for communicating results to patients and for arranging appropriate follow-up. By 1999, the United States Congress's Mammography Quality Standards Act mandated written notification of mammography results directly to patients within 30 days of the examination. Radiologists who interpret mammograms, and patients themselves, generally prefer direct reporting of mammography results, and most patients prefer immediate in-person reporting of results of screening mammography to mailed written reports (Raza *et al.* 2001). Most patients (78%) are willing to wait an additional 30–60 minutes at the time of screening mammography for an immediate result, but the majority (89%) are not willing to pay extra for this service (Raza *et al.* 2001). Most women are willing to accept delayed reporting for screening mammograms if double interpretation is to be performed, suggesting that if patients understand that there is an advantage to be gained in waiting for results, they will better tolerate a delay.

When radiologists give results directly to patients, they must do so in a compassionate, yet unequivocal, manner. Physician affect is important and should accurately reflect the seriousness of the situation, while remaining as encouraging and optimistic as possible. Radiologists should use plain terms in place of medical jargon and disclose information at a pace commensurate with the patient's ability to absorb it. Clarity of reporting is crucial for patient satisfaction, to guarantee patient understanding, and to ensure appropriate follow-up. Studies have shown that patient-reported results are least likely to agree with radiologist-documented results when results are abnormal (Karliner *et al.* 2005; Jones *et al.* 2007).

Communicating with patients about image-guided interventional procedures

Radiology has evolved to include minimally invasive image-guided diagnostic and therapeutic interventional procedures that bring radiologists into direct contact with patients in a dynamic similar to that of surgeons. Interventional oncology, in particular, is an arena in which the use of imaging has revolutionized the performance of image-guided biopsy and tumour ablation. In breast imaging, percutaneous image-guided breast biopsy performed by radiologists has become a mainstay of breast diagnosis. Radiologists who perform interventional procedures must be prepared to obtain informed consent for image-guided interventions, to discuss their potential complications, and to discuss results of biopsies with patients.

Obtaining informed consent for an interventional radiology procedure entails discussing details of the proposed treatment, possible additional interventions that might be required during the course of the planned procedure, common and serious side effects, the probability of success, and alternative treatment options. Additionally, patients are interested specifically in what to expect in terms of pain, and they want to know when they can expect to receive the results of the procedure. Periprocedural anxiety can be reduced if the patient is properly informed about the procedure in advance, and to this end many institutions provide patients with access to websites that describe common procedures in detail. Clinic nurses and/or patient navigators can be very helpful in providing information, scheduling appointments, and giving emotional support to patients undergoing interventional radiology procedures.

Principles for discussing biopsy results with patients are similar to principles for discussing complications or suboptimal outcomes of image-guided procedures. The United States Health Insurance Portability and Accountability Act (HIPAA) requires that results must be discussed directly and privately with patients, unless a patient has explicitly requested that results be given to a designated representative. Delivering biopsy results to patients is ideally done in person, but logistical considerations, including patient distance from their medical facilities, and the burden of scheduling return appointments for both patients and radiology facilities, often preclude this. In breast imaging, telephoning biopsy results is often more expeditious and has been shown to be well-tolerated by patients, whether results are positive or negative (Purnell and Arnold 2010). Telephoning results is preferable to mailing written results, as it is faster; women are more likely to understand the results (Karliner *et al.* 2005); and women have an immediate opportunity to ask questions. Also, the patient can absorb results in private and prepare additional questions for subsequent appointments. Disadvantages

of telephoning results are that the call may come at an unexpected or inconvenient time, and that non-verbal communication cues are not available to either the patient or the radiologist. When radiologists discuss news with patients over the phone, therefore, they must first confirm that the patient is receiving the call at a time and place in which he or she can speak freely. As patients' emotional reactions may be difficult to discern without the benefit of non-verbal cues, radiologists must also ask patients to verbalize their responses and must be aware of emotional cues provided via paralanguage, such as tone, speech pattern, pauses, and pitch (Reisman and Brown 2005).

Whether or not a biopsy result is positive for cancer, the patient's understanding of the results must be optimized. Radiologists should give results in the patient's preferred language with the assistance of medical interpreters if needed (Harvey *et al.* 2007) and use unambiguous lay terms. For example, patients may confuse the meaning of 'positive' (abnormal) and 'negative' (normal) findings, since in medicine the meanings of these words are the opposite of their colloquial connotations. Radiologists should establish the patient's expectation of the result before giving information, and they must ask patients to verbalize their understanding of results to confirm their comprehension, and continue to present information to patients in alternate ways until the process of checking back confirms that adequate understanding is achieved.

When a biopsy yields cancer, clear and supportive communication is particularly important. Among breast cancer patients, for example, this diagnostic consultation is a highly memorable event (Mager and Andrykowski 2002). In one study of breast cancer patients, patients' perceptions of a physician's emotional supportiveness during the diagnostic consultation correlated with better later psychological adjustment to their illness, as measured by fewer cancer-related post-traumatic stress disorder symptoms, less depression, and less general distress (Mager and Andrykowski 2002). Patients perceive radiologists to be supportive when their manner is unhurried, they invite and attend to patients' comments and questions, affirm patients' feelings, respect patients as individuals, focus on the positive, and are available to patients (Wright *et al.* 2004). Radiologists must offer hope, but avoid false reassurances. Specifically, they should mention any good prognostic features of a given lesion, but should not mislead the patient, as this may ultimately undermine trust (Wright *et al.* 2004; Harvey *et al.* 2007). The radiologist should give the patient an idea of what to expect in the future and an immediate concrete plan, such as a referral to a surgeon with a phone number. The radiologist should conclude the consultation by providing his or her own contact information and, if possible, contact information for an additional support staff member in case questions or problems arise.

When a biopsy yields benign results, the radiologist should convey the good news first to relieve anxiety, so that patients will be better able to concentrate, and then explain the results in more detail. Patients desire clear information about the future implications of a benign result, particularly with respect to cancer risk (Schonberg *et al.* 2014).

Special considerations in communicating radiology results

Cultural and sociodemographic factors

Physician–patient communication in radiology should be tailored to meet the needs of the individual patient, and cultural and sociodemographic factors must be considered. Radiologists should familiarize themselves with cultural beliefs among patients in their practices and with findings in the literature that may help guide communications. Relatively less well-educated women, for example, have been found to experience greater levels of anxiety prior to breast biopsy (Steffens *et al.* 2011) and to demonstrate persistent anxiety and lack of reassurance following benign diagnosis of breast symptoms, suggesting that these women may benefit from more detailed consultations or additional support services (Meechan *et al.* 2005). It is unclear why certain minority populations have been shown to demonstrate relatively poor understanding of radiology results. In breast imaging, studies have shown a trend that African Americans, Latinos, and Asians are more likely than white referents to report receipt of confusing or conflicting information at breast imaging encounters, even when language barriers and socioeconomic factors are taken into account (Zapka *et al.* 2004; Karliner *et al.* 2005; Jones *et al.* 2007; Miller *et al.* 2013). African American women, whose breast cancers are diagnosed at a later stage on average than their white counterparts' breast cancers with consequent relatively high breast cancer mortality rates, were found to be more than 2.5 times more likely to complete timely and appropriate follow-up of abnormal mammograms when they reported that clinic staff informed them of what was to happen after the mammogram (Kerner *et al.* 2003), confirming that clear communication with patients is crucial for screening efficacy. Younger women are also less likely to report a complete understanding of mammography results than older women (Zapka *et al.* 2004) and are more likely to report experiencing significant stress upon receipt of an abnormal mammography result (Steffens *et al.* 2011). Older women are more likely to require information regarding how to manage medications and chronic medical conditions prior to and during an image-guided biopsy procedure and are less likely to have an emotional support network. Special care must be taken to consider patients' specific needs, to ensure their understanding of results, and to eliminate barriers to compliance, in order to improve healthcare outcomes.

Uncertainty in radiology

Uncertainty is a frequent issue in physician–patient communication and is particularly relevant in radiology, with imaging examinations often having limited specificity and sensitivity. Patients often value their physicians' expertise above other characteristics and skills (Wright *et al.* 2004), so a great challenge for physicians is to explain what they do not know, while still inspiring their patients' trust.

The discovery of imaging findings of questionable clinical significance is common in radiology, particularly on screening examinations. Non-specific radiology results often lead to the performance of additional diagnostic tests, potentially fostering patient anxiety and/or confusion. An empathetic explanation of the limitations of a given radiology examination is often required.

In breast imaging in particular, false-positive screening mammograms may lead to elevated levels of distress and anxiety. Such false-positive examinations may breed less anxiety for patients undergoing mammographic screening when patients have been forewarned of the possibility of a false-positive result, when radiologists use false-positive examination encounters with patients as 'teachable moments' to personally educate patients, and when follow-up examinations can be performed promptly. Some authors

suggest that this anxiety reduction in turn may lead to improved future compliance with follow-up recommendations (Kerner *et al.* 2003).

Not infrequently, limited radiological specificity results in the need for delayed follow-up imaging to assess for change over time in a relatively benign-appearing lesion. For example, a breast lesion on imaging may receive a BI-RADS assessment category of '3: probably benign' when a radiologist judges it to have a less than approximately 2% probability of malignancy. According to BI-RADS guidelines, the radiologist may recommend imaging surveillance of such a lesion over time, instead of an immediate biopsy in an attempt to avoid performing a biopsy that is likely to be benign, thereby limiting attendant morbidity and cost. Patients may suffer adverse psychological consequences from waiting for follow-up; however, at least one study suggests that stress levels are lower among women undergoing short-interval follow-up mammography, than among women undergoing immediate core biopsy for probably benign breast lesions (Steffens *et al.* 2011). Radiologists may clarify patients' results and allay anxiety by explaining how their imaging findings fit known criteria for categorizing lesions as probably benign, and by emphasizing the safety and effectiveness of radiologic surveillance as an alternative to core biopsy or other interventions for such lesions.

Imaging examinations often have limited sensitivity, and radiologists must convey this concept to patients, lest patients be inappropriately reassured by a falsely negative test. For example, the sensitivity of mammography is decreased in women with dense breasts, so that if a patient has a palpable breast mass or other salient sign or symptom suggestive of breast cancer, and a mammogram is negative, the radiologist must stress to both the patient and her referring physician the need to continue to pursue a diagnosis. Many US states have even enacted legislation requiring radiologists to directly inform mammography patients of their breast density and of the reduced sensitivity of mammography among dense-breasted women.

Recent initiatives and future directions in radiology communication

Technology-based distribution of radiology results

Improving communication in radiology requires increasing efficiency in the distribution of results to referring physicians and patients. The adoption of speech-recognition software that provides contemporaneous computer-generated transcription has improved timeliness in report turnaround in many radiology facilities. In some centres, PACS and related technology have been helping to facilitate efficient routine and non-routine reporting by automating two-way communication between radiologists and referring physicians. Thus electronically, a significant imaging finding may be directly linked with relevant report text, the referrer promptly alerted, receipt verified, and the communication archived. Findings of different levels of severity may be variously tracked, with different physicians, or patients themselves, notified at specified intervals, in order to optimize patients' safety and outcomes. Some authors advocate the use of secure HIPAA-compliant internet-based access of radiology reports and images for both referring physicians and patients in order to expedite and ensure their availability (Cabarrus *et al.* 2015; Henshaw *et al.* 2015).

Standardization of reporting

Improving communication in radiology also requires increasing accuracy and consistency of reporting (Schwartz *et al.* 2011). An evolution has taken place from free-text (prose) radiology reports toward a structured report format with a standardized language and content, much like the BI-RADS lexicon, but now increasingly in use throughout all imaging modalities. The Radiological Society of North America has developed a unified imaging terminology resource called RadLex and provides standardized report templates on the internet for radiologists' use.

The goals for standardized reporting are not only to improve uniformity in language and report structure and thereby limit result ambiguity, but to also improve clinical outcomes. Standardized reports permit the formation of a radiology database, a platform from which quality of care metrics can be assessed. For example, by linking to other clinical data in a patient's electronic medical record, a radiology database may not only trigger electronic communication of results, but also track patient compliance with follow-up recommendations and facilitate peer review. Such a reference database is also invaluable for developing clinical decision support and assisting research.

Patients want access to their radiology reports and medical images (Cabarrus *et al.* 2015), and automation and innovation will eventually allow for radiologist–patient communication to be customized and expanded. In the future, a technologically savvy patient could have imaging results delivered electronically to his or her smartphone with options for electronic follow-up reminders and scheduling, and links to related information. Such a communication method could easily incorporate images into textual correspondence, potentially mitigating some of the language and educational barriers to patient comprehension of radiology test results.

Promoting improvement in radiologists' communication skills

Finally, improving communication in radiology requires refining radiologists' competence in interpersonal and communication skills. The US Accreditation Council for Graduate Medical Education (ACGME) mandated in 2002 that residents must demonstrate competency in interpersonal and communication skills. In radiology, this is defined as the ability to 'communicate effectively with patients, colleagues, referring physicians and other members of the healthcare team concerning imaging appropriateness, informed consent, safety issues, and results of imaging tests or procedures'. This type of training involves didactic instruction, supervised practice, and skills evaluations. Performance measures include evaluations of residents' written reports and written evaluations by residents' superiors, peers, and subordinates in addition to self-assessment.

After training, radiologists must continue to demonstrate maintenance of their communication skills. In 2007, in order to align their goals with those of the ACGME and the American Board of Medical Subspecialties, the Joint Commission on the Accreditation of Healthcare Organizations (JCAHO) published new guidelines for medical credentialing and privileging that require ongoing practitioner-specific data collection in several 'general competencies', one of which is practitioners' interpersonal and communication skills (Donnelly 2007). In 2009, the JCAHO implemented guidelines requiring continuous data-based evaluation and monitoring of physician practice performance. Some university radiology departments have instituted initiatives to promote professionalism and effective communication, and to document compliance with the JCAHO standards (Donnelly 2007), such as eliciting patient input and educating radiologists in standards of customer service. Further adoption of such initiatives will likely foster widespread quality improvement in radiology communications.

Conclusion

Radiologists' communications with referring physicians must be accurate, meaningful, and timely, and therefore measures that improve uniformity and consistency of radiology reporting and prompt distribution of results are of paramount importance. The evolution of radiology to include more procedures that bring radiologists into direct patient contact has prompted the need for direct radiologist–patient communication, which is likely to increase with continuing advances in medical imaging. It is essential that patients perceive these interactions as compassionate and comprehensible, and this is optimally achieved when radiologists tailor their communications to the needs of individual patients. For radiologists, improved communication with referring physicians and patients alike will ultimately result in timelier diagnoses, enhanced professional relationships, and superior healthcare outcomes.

References

American College of Radiology (2014). ACR practice parameter for communication of diagnostic imaging findings. Available at: http://www.acr.org/~/media/C5D1443C9EA4424AA12477D1AD1D927D.pdf [Online].

American College of Radiology Bi-Rads Committee (2013). *ACR BI-RADS Atlas: Breast Imaging Reporting and Data System.* American College of Radiology, Reston, VA.

Berlin L (2009). Communicating results of all outpatient radiologic examinations directly to patients: the time has come. *AJR Am J Roentgenol* **192**, 571–3.

Cabarrus M, Naeger DM, Rybkin A, Qayyum A (2015). Patients prefer results from the ordering provider and access to their radiology reports. *J Am Coll Radiol* **12**, 556–62.

Donnelly LF (2007). Performance-based assessment of radiology practitioners: promoting improvement in accordance with the 2007 joint commission standards. *J Am Coll Radiol* **4**, 699–703.

European Society of Radiology (2013). ESR communication guidelines for radiologists. *Insights Imaging* **4**, 143–6.

Harvey JA, Cohen MA, Brenin DR, Nicholson BT, Adams RB (2007). Breaking bad news: a primer for radiologists in breast imaging. *J Am Coll Radiol* **4**, 800–8.

Henshaw D, Okawa G, Ching K, Garrido T, Qian H, Tsai J (2015). Access to radiology reports via an online patient portal: Experiences of referring physicians and patients. *J Am Coll Radiol* **12**, 582–6 e1.

Jones BA, Reams K, Calvocoressi L, Dailey A, Kasl SV, Liston NM (2007). Adequacy of communicating results from screening mammograms to African American and White women. *Am J Public Health* **97**, 531–8.

Karliner LS, Patricia Kaplan C, Juarbe T, Pasick R, Perez-Stable EJ (2005). Poor patient comprehension of abnormal mammography results. *J Gen Intern Med* **20**, 432–7.

Kerner JF, Yedidia M, Padgett D, *et al.* (2003). Realizing the promise of breast cancer screening: clinical follow-up after abnormal screening among Black women. *Prev Med* **37**, 92–101.

Kushner DC, Lucey LL (2005). Diagnostic radiology reporting and communication: the ACR guideline. *J Am Coll Radiol* **2**, 15–21.

Mager WM, Andrykowski MA (2002). Communication in the cancer 'bad news' consultation: patient perceptions and psychological adjustment. *Psychooncology* **11**, 35–46.

Meechan GT, Collins JP, Moss-Morris RE, Petrie KJ (2005). Who is not reassured following benign diagnosis of breast symptoms? *Psychooncology* **14**, 239–46.

Miller LS, Shelby RA, Balmadrid MH, *et al.* (2013). Patient anxiety before and immediately after imaging-guided breast biopsy procedures: impact of radiologist-patient communication. *J Am Coll Radiol* **10**, 423–31.

Purnell CA, Arnold RM (2010). Retrospective analysis of communication with patients undergoing radiological breast biopsy. *J Support Oncol* **8**, 259–63.

Raza S, Rosen MP, Chorny K, Mehta TS, Hulka CA, Baum JK (2001). Patient expectations and costs of immediate reporting of screening mammography: talk isn't cheap. *AJR Am J Roentgenol* **177**, 579–83.

Reisman AB, Brown KE (2005). Preventing communication errors in telephone medicine. *J Gen Intern Med* **20**, 959–63.

Schonberg MA, Silliman RA, Ngo LH, *et al.* (2014). Older women's experience with a benign breast biopsy-a mixed methods study. *J Gen Intern Med* **29**, 1631–40.

Schwartz LH, Panicek DM, Berk AR, Li Y, Hricak H (2011). Improving communication of diagnostic radiology findings through structured reporting. *Radiology* **260**, 174–81.

Steffens RF, Wright HR, Hester MY, Andrykowski MA (2011). Clinical, demographic, and situational factors linked to distress associated with benign breast biopsy. *J Psychosoc Oncol* **29**, 35–50.

Thornton RH, Dauer LT, Shuk E, *et al.* (2015). Patient perspectives and preferences for communication of medical imaging risks in a cancer care setting. *Radiology* **275**, 545–52.

Wallis A, McCoubrie P (2011). The radiology report—are we getting the message across? *Clin Radiol* **66**, 1015–22.

Wright EB, Holcombe C, Salmon P (2004). Doctors' communication of trust, care, and respect in breast cancer: qualitative study. *BMJ* **328**, 864.

Zapka JG, Puleo E, Taplin SH, *et al.* (2004). Processes of care in cervical and breast cancer screening and follow-up—the importance of communication. *Prev Med* **39**, 81–90.

CHAPTER 47

Communication in surgical oncology

Amanda Tristram

Introduction to communication in surgical oncology

As in every field of oncology, the importance of communication for the surgical oncologist cannot be overstated. The surgeon may become involved with the cancer patient at almost any point in the disease process. It is not possible to cover all possible consultations types in one chapter, so they will be considered within three broad settings: pre-operative, post-operative, and follow-up. In many instances, the surgeon performs the biopsy that diagnoses the cancer and needs to be able to appropriately convey not only the diagnosis, but also its implications. In other instances, surgery itself is the main treatment for the disease and the surgeon becomes the primary caregiver for these patients. Finally, the surgeon may become involved in a palliative setting, in which the main objective is to communicate the limitations of the role of surgery in a way that allows a patient to come to an informed decision.

Several studies have indicated that patient satisfaction and trust in the treating physician are based upon their perceptions of appropriate communication (Costantini *et al.* 1998; Detmar *et al.* 2001; Fallowfield *et al.* 2002, 2003; Razavi *et al.* 2003). In each study, a patient-centred approach with excellent communication of information was found to be important (Jenkins and Fallowfield 2002). While some situations are unique to each surgical subspecialty in surgical oncology, many aspects of the surgeon's daily life are common to all subspecialties. In order to properly address the patient's needs and to communicate effectively, it is helpful to have a framework to approach these common situations.

Before the operation

As with any oncology specialty, the first meeting with a surgical oncologist is of paramount importance. In this consultation, the patient will look to the surgeon for information, about both the surgical procedure and the cancer. During this visit the patient will make judgements about their surgeon. Honesty, clear language and a kind manner will provide an excellent base for all that follows. It is helpful to provide the patient with a short synopsis of what one hopes to accomplish during this first appointment. Additionally, assuring the patient that there will be an opportunity to ask questions and voice concerns will also be welcome. Be aware of the varying degrees of understanding the patient may have of the disease process and that some may require more or less explanation of any given aspect. Due to time pressures, it is easy for the consultation to become a one-way information-giving event. Establishing a basic framework that avoids this can be helpful. Bear in mind that there may have been a long wait to see you in an overcrowded waiting room and the patient may need to let of some steam before you can make any progress. This is true for any consultation, but particularly so for the first visit. Not knowing who you are going to see, what they are going to tell you, or anxious anticipation of the surgical procedure ahead can all heighten the sense of unease. Allowing patients an opportunity to vent any frustrations and acknowledging these can help get the consultation under control. This has been described as 'exercising the chimp' in the book *The Chimp Paradox* (Peters 2012). The chimp will then need to be put back in its box. Outlining the plan for the consultation can be a good way of achieving this.

A possible framework for the consultation would be as follows:

- Explain to the patient what the plan for and the purpose of the visit is.

- Find out what the patient knows already and what their main concerns are. An overview of the information that is already known regarding this patient's cancer can then be given in this context.

- Be clear about how much is already known and what still needs to be established regarding the patient's condition.

- Explain the different treatment options, including the consequences of no treatment.

- Indicate your (the surgeon's) role in the treatment of the cancer.

- Describe the surgical procedure(s), including possible consequences of the procedure and variations in approach that could be considered.

- Indicate other healthcare providers who may be involved in the care of the patient, either now or at a later date.

- Establish lines of communication for the patient and review the next steps. Where possible, ensure the patient has a date for the next step.

- Give an opportunity for the patient to ask questions and raise concerns.

Studies have clearly shown the amount of information processed at an initial consultation is variable and that physicians can overestimate the ability of the patient to retain information (Dunn et al. 1993). It can therefore by very helpful to suggest how the patient might communicate questions or concerns in the future. For example, providing the patient with written information and indicating where questions can be written down to be asked at future visits. Further consultation may well be necessary for a patient to reach an informed decision about surgery. This may be with another member of the team, for example a specialist nurse. Ensure the patient has contact details for how to contact the team if needed.

When trying to be kind and soften the blow of a cancer diagnosis, surgeons often use words such as: worrying, sinister, benign, mass, and tumour. Often the patient does not know what these mean and rather than being reassured, the patient is left confused and unable to ask the simple question 'is it cancer?' Using precise language always keeps the conversation honest. If you do not think the patient has understood that word or phrase you have used, then explain it and check they have understood.

Diagnosis and staging

Diagnosis and staging usually fall within the remit of surgical oncology. The proposed treatment will often depend on precise histological diagnosis and clinical or radiological staging being discussed within a multidisciplinary meeting. Explaining the rationale for the time this takes to the patient is important, as patients are often keen to undergo surgery to remove the tumour as quickly as possible. It may be appropriate to explain that the small risks from delaying treatment will be far outweighed by ensuring that the most appropriate treatments and prognosis can be discussed (Christakis 1999; Piccirillo et al. 2004).

Pre-operative discussion

Once it is has been agreed that surgery is the next step, discussion of its various aspects is required, not only for the patient to be able to give informed consent, but also so that they and their families know what to expect. The key components are: pre-operative preparation; the procedure; anaesthetic and pain management; risks and side effects; post-operative communication plan.

Pre-operative preparation

The information a patient needs pre-operatively can be complex, from how long to fast for, whether to take medications, and where and when to turn up. Many units will have specific written information available and pre-operative clinics to ensure this is covered correctly. Many units now incorporate an enhanced recovery approach to surgical admissions. An essential part of this is ensuring patients know, prior to admission, what their likely time course for recovery and discharge will be.

The procedure

There are two main aspects to this, which can get confused in an era where there are multiple surgical approaches. This first is to establish what the surgery is likely to achieve and might include exactly what will be examined or removed. There may be some procedures which are definitely planned and some that are only planned in certain circumstances. This should all be explained to the patient and documents. Consent forms now have space for this detailed information to be included and provision for the patient to have a copy. What might not be performed should also be explained, for example, if the cancer turns out to be more widespread than anticipated on imaging. Although it may seem harsh to explain this pre-operatively, it will be invaluable for the patient to have covered this, if it turns out to be the case.

The second aspect is what approach will be taken. For example, will it be laparoscopic surgery? Will it be an open procedure? If it is to be robotic, it is probably advisable to explain exactly what this entails to the patient and reassure them that the surgery is not actually being performed by a robot.

Anaesthetic and pain management

Although patients will generally have an opportunity to speak with the anaesthesic team regarding the type of anaesthesia and its associated risks, it is helpful in the pre-surgical discussion for the surgeon to briefly mention the options available, as well as post-operative pain management. For example, discussing the possibility of having surgery 'awake' in advance allows the patient to think about this, rather than having to make a snap decision on the morning of surgery. Knowing that post-operative discomfort will be addressed and that they will have opportunities to discuss all these issues further with the anaesthetist can be very reassuring to patients.

Risks and side effects

Discussing the potential risks of a procedure may provoke anxiety and having strategies to deal with this can make the conversation more productive. For example, a blood clot in the legs or lungs is a potentially serious complication, so it is worth explaining that they will need to wear anti-thrombotic stockings and receive injections to reduce the risk. Additionally, they will be encouraged to mobilize early, reducing the risk of blood clots as well as other complications, such as infection. Knowing the risks of a given procedure is essential for a patient in order to give informed consent, and giving some thought about how this can be done in a positive light is worthwhile. Risks also need to be put into context—explaining there is a risk of damaging the ureter will mean little to most patients. Explaining what the ureter is, that a second operation might be needed to repair this, as well as how common injuries are, will all give meaning to the statement. Patients can also be helped by distinguishing between short-term and long-term effects with an idea about the potential for recovery. For example, lymphedema may be a permanent complication of a groin node dissection, but without explicitly stating this, a patient might be forgiven for assuming this would improve as they recovered from the operation. It is often worthwhile asking directly if there is anything that they are particularly concerned about.

Post-operative communication plan

Prior to any procedure, explain when you will see them afterwards and when they will get any results. For example, you might say that you will see them immediately after the operation and be able to explain what was found and what procedures were carried out, but that they will have to return to get results of any biopsies. This ensures that the patient has appropriate expectations and an opportunity to be involved in planning when they might get any bad news. There are choices to be made about whether a patient would like to know immediately or perhaps wait until the next day. This might be particularly appropriate if major surgery is planned, or if the patient would like a relative to be present. Waiting until afterwards and then trying to guess whether they would like to be told immediately or to wait for a relative is likely to have only a 50% chance of being appropriate.

After the operation

Whether on the ward or in clinic, there are two aspects to post-operative visits: operation-centred and disease-management centred. It may be helpful to deal with the surgical post-operative aspects first, such as wound healing, as this can break the ice and then allows the full focus to be on disease management. If results are to be given, it is essential to ask the patient their date of birth and then to check this and the date of the procedure before continuing. It may be helpful to go through the pathology report with the patient and the family members, in order to confirm what you are saying.

There are four broad possibilities from a disease management point of view and it is helpful for the patient to know which of these applies in order to give context:

1. The surgery appears to have removed all the tumour and no further adjuvant treatment is needed. In this setting, the focus will be on future follow-up plans.

2. The surgery appears to have removed all the tumour, but further adjuvant treatment needs to be considered. This will require explaining the basics of the further treatment options and ensuring that the patient knows what to expect next. It is optimal to be able to tell them who they will see next, where, and when.

3. The surgery has not removed all the disease and adjuvant treatment with curative intent needs to be considered. Although difficult, it is essential to be honest with the patient, in order for them to make informed decisions about treatment options. As above, they will need to know who, when, and where they are to be seen next.

4. The surgery has not removed all the disease and palliative care options, perhaps including palliative adjuvant treatment need to be considered. This is perhaps the hardest setting for the surgical oncologist; however, without honesty at this point, the patient will not be able to make decisions about what their priorities for further treatment are. At this point, there will probably be multi-disciplinary input and it essential the patient knows who to contact and how.

Giving results by phone is always difficult. Although from a practical point of view this may seem helpful, it should be agreed in advance. The patient should be aware that it might be bad news and agree that being told this during a telephone conversation is acceptable. It is important that there is time for any questions arising during such a call to be addressed and that the patient is in an appropriate setting at the other end of the phone.

Further follow-up

Explain why the patient is coming, what symptoms they should look out for between visits and what they should do if they experience any. Further follow-up appointments are opportunities for patients to discuss issues that may have arisen since, or that they have felt unable to ask before. Patients often hold surgeons who have cured their cancer in high regard and do not like to trouble them with difficult questions. The surgeon may need to give permission for the patient to raise potentially awkward issues, such as sexual dysfunction or aetiological concerns, for example, which may derive from news reports they have seen regarding head and neck cancer and sexual contact.

Written communication

Communication skills do not end when the patient leaves the room or the ward. Comprehensive written records allow accurate ongoing communication with the patient, their GP, and other healthcare professionals. At the end of the consultation a summary of what has been explained to the patient should be documented and communicated to all those involved with their care. A patient will often see their own GP following a consultation about cancer and it is vital for the GP to know what the patient is aware of. This is also true for the rest of the oncology team. Those without direct access to a copy of your medical records will need a formal letter written. Try to stick to the salient points: diagnosis; treatment so far; the plan (and rationale for this); and how much the patient knows. Some practitioners and units have a policy of copying the patient in on all letters. This can be very helpful to reinforce the rationale behind decision-making and helps other health professionals to know that the patient is aware of the same information as they are. The patient can be asked whether they would like this in advance and the letter might be dictated while the patient is present. This provides a summary of the consultation and an opportunity to correct misunderstanding that might become apparent.

Conclusion

Communication in surgical oncology can be extremely challenging, but also extremely rewarding. It will not always be possible to be perfect, especially in complicated situations. Two basic principles will help here, as in most encounters: be honest and be kind.

References

Christakis N (1999). *Death Foretold—Prophecy and Prognosis in Medical Care*. The University of Chicago Press, Chicago, IL.

Costantini M, Foley K, Rapkin B (1998). Communicating with patients about advanced cancer. *JAMA* **280**, 1403–4.

Detmar S, Muller M, Wever L, *et al.* (2001). The patient-physician relationship. Patient–physician communication during outpatient palliative treatment visits: an observational study. *JAMA* **285**, 1351–7.

Dunn SM, Butow PN, Tattersall MH, *et al.* (1993). General information tapes inhibit recall of the cancer consultation. *J Clin Oncol* **11**, 2279–85.

Fallowfield L, Jenkins V, Farewell V, *et al.* (2002). Efficacy of a Cancer Research UK communication skills training model for oncologists: a randomised controlled trial. *Lancet* **359**, 650–6.

Fallowfield L, Jenkins V, Farewell V, *et al.* (2003). Enduring impact of communication skills training: results of a 12-month follow-up. *Brit J Cancer* **89**, 1445–9.

Jenkins V, Fallowfield L (2002). Can communication skills training alter physicians' beliefs and behavior in clinics? *J Clin Oncol* **20**, 765–9.

Peters S (2012). *The Chimp Paradox: The Mind Management Programme to Help You Achieve Success, Confidence and Happiness*. Vermilion, London, UK.

Piccirillo J, Tierney R, Costas I, *et al.* (2004). Prognostic importance of comorbidity in a hospital-based cancer registry. *JAMA* **291**, 2441–7.

Razavi D, Merckaert I, Marchal S, *et al.* (2003). How to optimize physicians' communication skills in cancer care: results of a randomized study assessing the usefulness of posttraining consolidation workshops. *J Clin Oncol* **21**, 3141–9.

CHAPTER 48

Communication in non-surgical oncology

Lai Cheng Yew and E. Jane Maher

The importance of cancer

There are 2.5 million people living after a diagnosis of cancer in the United Kingdom, rising to four million in 2030 (Maddams *et al.* 2012). It is now estimated that by 2020 almost one in two people will develop some form of cancer during their lifetime. The risk of cancer increases with age and 60% of those living with and beyond cancer are more than 65 years old, with many cancer patients having two or three additional co-morbidities, including sensory impairments such as deafness and cognitive issues, affecting communication. Cancer remains the commonest cause of death, but median survival has improved from less than two years 40 years ago, to a median of six years, with 38% of cancer patients now dying from a cause other than cancer.

The importance of cancer is reflected in the enormous media interest that it attracts. For example, when the UK charity, Macmillan Cancer Support, surveyed mainstream national newspapers over a six-month period a decade ago, it found 500 articles (almost three articles per day) mentioning the word 'cancer' (Macmillan Cancer Support 2001). There are thousands of websites about cancer, which provide easy access to a wealth of unfiltered information; this can be useful but also amplifies some of the myths that surround the illness. The perception of cancer is hugely influenced, not only by the scale of the media attention, but also the language used in situations involving cancer. Patients with cancer are often described as 'victims', 'fighting' a 'battle', and 'surviving' because of a 'positive attitude'. Cancer is perceived as a feared disease because of both the mortality and pain associated with it. Similarly, while in the past the diagnosis of metastatic disease implied a rapid demise, many patients with metastatic breast and prostate cancer may have several years of good quality life. Public opinion has not kept up with these changes. The way in which cancer is portrayed by the media creates a frame of reference on which patient–clinician communication is based.

Cancer as a complex illness

There are over 200 different types of cancer with very different illness trajectories and communication challenges, and it is helpful to consider them in three groups (McConnell *et al.* 2014). The first group includes cancers such as lung, pancreatic, and glioblastoma, where currently the majority of patients still die within a year, and the priority is a focus on earlier diagnosis and the need for good palliative care for most patients from the time of diagnosis. In a second group, which includes common cancers such as breast and stage 1 squamous cell cancers, most patients will live at least a decade. In this group, there is an increasing need to focus on recovery and survivorship, including lifestyle change, to reduce the impact of cancer treatment on the incidence and complexity of other chronic illness, months or years later. Then, there is a third group of largely 'incurable but treatable' cancers including hormone sensitive metastatic breast and prostate cancer, where disease emerges years after apparently successful treatment and several haematological malignancies. In this group, survival is typically more than a year but less than five years (although it can be much longer), but with multiple decisions as to the balance between cancer treatment and palliative care, and challenges in deciding the right time to move to hospice care. As new drugs emerge, this type of 'chronic cancer' is becoming more common but it is largely invisible in the public discourse about cancer, where the public view cancer more simply as being 'cured and restored to normal' or 'incurable and dying quickly'. In newspaper and magazine articles, the words 'cure' and 'treatment' are often used interchangeably.

Breast, lung, colorectal, and prostate cancer account for over half of all new cases. Different types of cancer have very different illness trajectories, defined not only by the natural history and stage of the cancer, but also patient characteristics and treatment options available. There is considerable variation between different cancer types, such as pancreas versus breast; but, in the majority of cases, cancer care involves numerous clinicians and healthcare professionals throughout the patient's cancer journey. In addition, treatments are becoming much more complex, often involving a combination of surgery, chemotherapy, radiotherapy, and biological agents. For all these reasons, communication in cancer is particularly challenging for both the patient and the clinician.

The role of non-surgical oncology

The non-surgical oncologist is involved in almost every patient's cancer journey—either at diagnosis, during treatment, at follow-up, at recurrence, through survivorship, and even at the end of life. The main treatment options offered by this group are chemotherapy, radiotherapy, and biological therapies, all of which can be used in the radical or palliative setting. There are significant acute and late toxicities associated with these treatments, some of which are life threatening (e.g. neutropenic sepsis).

Many of the treatment regimes in current use have been studied in a much younger population than the typical patients, who are older and with more co-morbidity than in the clinical trials, which provide the evidence base for their use. Treatment-related morbidity is high during and immediately after cancer treatments, but some problems do not emerge until months or years later. Therefore, the non-surgical oncologist does not just provide a particular treatment, but has a much more involved role in monitoring toxicities during treatment and in long-term follow-up. Because they can also offer palliative treatments, they will often diagnose and/or treat a recurrence and initiate palliative care.

Communication issues will arise at all these stages of a patient's cancer illness, and the non-surgical oncologist must be aware of the complexities of the relationship with the patient. There are key communication points when patients shift from different health states (e.g. diagnosis of cancer; completion of initial anti-cancer treatment; recurrence; each time treatment is no longer 'working' and disease is progressing; diagnosis of significant, irreversible, treatment-related effects; moving from living with incurable cancer to dying with cancer). Recent modelling work with common cancers enables prediction of the number of key decision points expected in populations of patients with different cancers (Maher and McConnell 2011).

Frameworks linking communication and outcome

The communication between patient and clinician can be better understood using the framework defined by the US National Institutes of Health (NIH) (Epstein and Street 2007). This links six key functions and seven pathways of communication with measurable health and quality of life outcomes. More effective patient–clinician communication can improve health outcomes.

Functions of communication

1. Fostering healing relationships

2. Exchanging information

3. Responding to emotions

4. Managing uncertainty

5. Making decisions

6. Enabling self-management

The six core functions of communication overlap and interact to produce communication that affects health outcomes—primarily survival and quality of life. There is little research on the relationship between communication and health outcomes, but the NIH monograph proposes a number of pathways, which help to understand this link. This is based on the idea that the proximal outcomes of communication, essentially immediate outcomes on the functions of communication listed above, and intermediate outcomes such as adherence to advice and patient empowerment, contribute to the third set of outcomes—those related to health (i.e. survival and quality of life).

For most patients, the outcomes of greatest relevance are the health outcomes—survival and quality of life. The relationship between communication and health outcomes can be mediated by the proximal and intermediate outcomes (Fig. 48.1). For example, a patient who has been given clear information about tamoxifen (effective information exchange—proximal outcome) by a clinician with whom she has developed a rapport (good patient/clinician relationship—proximal outcome) is more likely to take the tamoxifen for the recommended time period (adherence—intermediate outcome), which results in improved survival (health outcome). However, communication can directly affect health outcomes; for example, a clinician can inform a patient of a normal test result,

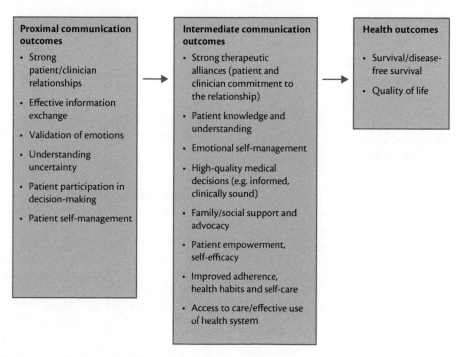

Proximal communication outcomes

- Strong patient/clinician relationships
- Effective information exchange
- Validation of emotions
- Understanding uncertainty
- Patient participation in decision-making
- Patient self-management

Intermediate communication outcomes

- Strong therapeutic alliances (patient and clinician commitment to the relationship)
- Patient knowledge and understanding
- Emotional self-management
- High-quality medical decisions (e.g. informed, clinically sound)
- Family/social support and advocacy
- Patient empowerment, self-efficacy
- Improved adherence, health habits and self-care
- Access to care/effective use of health system

Health outcomes

- Survival/disease-free survival
- Quality of life

Fig. 48.1 The influence of effective communications on health outcomes.

Pathways of communication- A-G

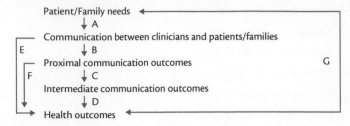

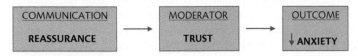

Fig. 48.2 The interrelation of communication and health outcomes.

Fig. 48.3 The central role of trust.

resulting in reduced anxiety, and improved quality of life. Thus, the pathways linking communication with health outcomes are complex and may or may not involve the proximal and intermediate outcomes as mediators. The flow diagram (Fig. 48.2) shows how these pathways of communication are thought to be interrelated.

The importance of different communication functions, pathways, and outcomes will vary between cancers, patients, and even during the cancer journey, as the experience of patients and their families is complex and dynamic. For example, at diagnosis, a patient may prioritize information gathering and participation in decision-making (functions 2 and 5), but at the end of life, the patient may need more empathy and a strong relationship with the clinician (functions 3 and 1). The differing communication needs will determine which pathways are more relevant to the appropriate health outcome.

There are a number of factors which moderate the relationship between communication and health outcomes. Moderators interact with an independent variable to predict an outcome; for example, if a patient trusts his/her doctor, then if the clinician expresses reassurance, the patient will be less anxious than a less trusting patient (Fig. 48.3).

Moderators can be intrinsic or extrinsic to clinicians, patients, and their relationship. Intrinsic moderators are individual or relationship characteristics that affect cognitive and affective processes of the patient/clinician (e.g. the patient's emotional state, knowledge about the illness, motivation, and health literacy). Extrinsic moderators include cultural beliefs, social support, access to care and disease factors (e.g. stage, type of cancer). These moderators vary in their susceptibility to change, and this is important as those factors which are more easily modified can be targeted in order to improve communication.

The key functions of communication are linked to proximal and intermediate communication outcomes, and distal health outcomes via a number of complex pathways. The relationship between communication and health outcomes is moderated by several factors. Focusing on the modifiable moderators should lead to improved health outcomes.

Communication at the time of diagnosis of cancer

The key communication issues at the time of diagnosis of cancer are breaking bad news, giving information, making decisions about future management, explaining prognosis, and providing emotional support to patient and families. Effective communication is essential at this stage of the cancer journey, as often further diagnostic tests are required to formulate the management plan, and these need to be performed quickly to minimize delay before treatment starts. However, patients are often highly emotional at this time, which makes it difficult for them to retain and assimilate information, and make rational decisions. This problem is further compounded if the initial bad news is poorly communicated, resulting in increased levels of anxiety and a weak patient–clinician relationship.

Aligning perspectives of a patient–clinician interaction

Communication between patient and clinician can be improved if there is some shared understanding of each other's perspective, and the purpose of the interaction is defined. Clinicians often misjudge patients' perspectives, preferences, and beliefs about health, particularly when there are racial/ethnicity differences (Balsa and McGuire 2003). This creates bias and leads to misunderstandings. In some cultures, it is very difficult to accept a diagnosis of cancer. In a recent study by Lords and colleagues (2013), 48% of South Asian patients agreed with the statement on a questionnaire, 'I don't believe I have cancer', 15 weeks after diagnosis, compared with 31% of white patients. If there is no word for cancer as in Gujarati or Hindi, understanding this illness is even more difficult. As well as cultural differences, mismatches in health literacy (understanding health in general and the care process) can be a major barrier to communication (Davis *et al.* 2002).

Information sharing

The information given at diagnosis is particularly important as it sets the scene for the patient's cancer journey. Inadequate information can lead to significant anxiety. The majority of patients with cancer want as much information as possible (Jenkins *et al.* 2001). In the United Kingdom, access to timely, high-quality information is very dependent on cancer site; for example, 90% of patients with breast cancer received written information at diagnosis compared with only 67% of patients with prostate cancer (National Audit Office 2005). On the other hand, patients can feel that too much information is given at this time, and this is often difficult to interpret, making it even harder to make decisions. The clinician has to judge how much detail a patient wants about diagnosis, prognosis, and treatment options. This will vary considerably even between patients who have cancer of the same site. In addition, some cancers may result in cognitive impairment (e.g. brain tumour, brain metastases). For these patients, communication can be improved by providing information in small chunks, repeating key points, summarizing and checking for understanding, and giving written materials and/or audio recordings.

Decision-making

Patients must feel that they have had sufficient information to make a decision. For the clinician, it is important that a clinically sound decision is made and that it is consistent with recommendations. However, patients may not want as much information as the clinician gives, and sometimes they prefer a lack of choice (Salmon and Hall 2004). Participation in the decision-making process can be an unwarranted burden and patients frequently do not want to take responsibility for the final decision (National Breast Cancer Centre

> **Box 48.1** Patient perceptions of probability
>
> In a study investigating consent into a hypothetical trial, 50 patients with cancer were asked to correctly interpret the following statement:
>
> 'A particular type of cancer responds to radiation treatment in 10% of cases'
>
> - The radiation treatment is about 10% effective in an individual patient: 22%
> - On average, for 10 out of 100 patients, the tumour will decrease in size after radiation treatment: 46%
> - There is a 10% chance of survival: 10%
>
> Adapted from Sutherland HJ *et al.*, 'Are we getting informed consent from patients with cancer?', *Journal of the Royal Society of Medicine*, Volume 83, Issue 7, pp. 439–443, Copyright © 1990 The Royal Society of Medicine, by permission of SAGE.

> **Box 48.2** Patient perceptions of randomization in trials
>
> In a study investigating consent into a hypothetical trial, 50 patients with cancer were asked to correctly interpret the following statement:
>
> 'A process called randomization is used to select your treatment in this clinical trial'
>
> - The process will select the best treatment for me: 14%
> - Each individual patient has exactly the same chance of receiving the drug, or not receiving the drug, as any other participating patient: 66%
> - One treatment is given one time, another is given another time: 0%
> - The doctor decides which treatment is the right one for me: 19%
>
> Adapted from Sutherland HJ *et al.*, 'Are we getting informed consent from patients with cancer?', *Journal of the Royal Society of Medicine*, Volume 83, Issue 7, pp. 439–443, Copyright © 1990 The Royal Society of Medicine, by permission of SAGE.

and National Cancer Control Initiative 2003). Some patients are more concerned with the personal individual relationships that they form with their clinicians than the provision of information (Burkitt-Wright *et al.* 2004). Whether the patient feels heard and trusts the clinician to act on their behalf may be more important than the degree to which the patient feels they have participated in the decision. Improving the quality of the interaction with the clinician in this way leads to increased satisfaction and reduced anxiety.

Prognosis and uncertainty

Discussing prognosis can be especially challenging, as it raises issues of probabilities and uncertainties. The availability of online prognostic tools; for example, Adjuvant Online has made it easier to avoid words such as 'small', 'large', and 'rare'. However, percentages are often confusing (e.g. quoting 30% of patients with your specialty cancer will be alive in 10 years leads to uncertainty, as the patient does not know which group they will be in). Understanding statistics is difficult for patients, particularly those who have low literacy levels. The example in Box 48.1 illustrates how statistics can be misinterpreted.

The issue of uncertainty is a particular problem for patients with cancer of unknown primary. These patients generally have a poor understanding of their disease and its causes, prognosis, and treatment (Boyland and Davis 2008).

Discussing randomized controlled trials

Discussing randomized controlled trials is one of most problematic areas of cancer communication. Some 52% of senior UK clinicians attending communication skills training acknowledged that providing complex information and seeking consent for clinical trials was their primary communication problem surpassing breaking bad news (Fallowfield *et al.* 2002). Currently only one in three patients approached about clinical trials will consent to randomization. Trials with a 'no treatment arm' are especially difficult to recruit for.

The discussion of clinical trials requires specific skills and understanding of a complex language. Increasingly, the responsibility for giving patients information about trials falls on specialist research nurses. In a clinical trial discussion, the healthcare professional must include an explanation of the standard therapy, reason for the

trial, uncertainty about novel drugs/procedures, the concept of randomization, and defining terms such as 'double-blind' or 'placebo-controlled'. If communication is inadequate, patients may fail to understand the experimental nature of the trial and be unclear about treatment options, and, therefore, be unable to give truly informed consent (Fallowfield and Jenkins 1999).

Randomization is a difficult concept for patients to understand, as the example in Box 48.2 illustrates. Jenkins and colleagues surveyed 200 patients, 200 oncologists, and 341 people without cancer and gave them seven descriptions of randomization. The most favoured description of randomization by patients and members of the public was a computer, and not the doctor or patient who would decide which treatment was given. The most disliked description (and the one used by more than a quarter of the oncologists) was 'a computer will perform the equivalent to tossing a coin to allocate you to one of two methods of treatment'. This was seen as trivializing the situation and was particularly upsetting in the context of life-threatening disease (Jenkins *et al.* 2005).

Communication during treatment

Once a diagnosis has been made and a management plan decided, it is essential that good communication continues throughout treatment, not least to pick up potentially life-threatening side effectsi such as neutropenic sepsis. Perhaps more importantly, especially for palliative treatments, some idea of quality of life must be ascertained during treatment, as this will be the primary endpoint. Patients must feel comfortable enough to voice their concerns during treatment in order to fully assess their experience. Clinicians are often unable to elicit patients' most important concerns, which usually relate to quality of life. Multiple studies have shown that radiotherapy and chemotherapy toxicity scores are a poor measure of quality of life and patient function.

Validated measures of health-related quality of life have been shown to be of use in guiding treatment choices. In a randomized study conducted by Brundage and colleagues (2007), 'surrogate' lung cancer patients were presented with quality of life information in addition to survival and toxicity data, and their preference for chemotherapy was recorded. If there was a benefit in quality of life, more patients changed their decision about chemotherapy, and this number increased if the quality of life difference was larger. This study shows how health-related quality of life data can influence patients' choices.

Quality of life data can also be used to show the effect of interventions in communication. Velikova *et al.* (2004) conducted a three-arm randomized trial to look at whether an assessment of quality of life along with an intervention (feedback from the doctor after review of the quality of life results) could improve patient outcome. EORTC QLQ 30 questionnaires were used to measure quality of life at baseline and subsequently over a period of six months. There was a significant difference in quality of life between patients who completed questionnaires and those who did not. The difference was even larger for those who had feedback from the doctor. This study clearly shows that a simple intervention, which can easily be performed in clinic, can significantly improve communication, and lead to improved health outcomes.

Another intervention shown to improve quality of life is the use of prompts in conversations between healthcare professionals and patients. Aaronson *et al.* (2007) compared the quality of life in two cohorts of patients. The first group completed quality of life questionnaires at the beginning and end of the study period, but did not receive an intervention. The patients in the second cohort were prompted by the nurses in a series of outpatient visits. These prompts influenced the subjects discussed in the consultations (e.g. symptoms, sexuality). Validated scores of quality of life showed improvement in the group of patients whose conversations were changed by prompts.

Psychosexual functioning

Clinicians are generally good at giving information about diagnosis and treatment (>90% of patients in one study) but less frequently discuss sexual functioning (38%). Patients also may deliberately avoid discussing or responding to questionnaire items about sexual well-being. The group most at risk of sexual dysfunction are those patients who have had pelvic surgery/radiotherapy and/or hormone manipulation. In one study, 82% of women under 50 years old who had surgery and radiotherapy for gynaecological cancer suffered sexual dysfunction (Basen-Engquist and Bodurka 2007). Many of these women are depressed or anxious because of chronic sexual problems. When interviewed in one study, women who had undergone major surgery for carcinoma of the cervix or vulva in the previous five years reported that they would have liked more information on physical, sexual, and emotional after-effects of treatment (Corney *et al.* 1993). They also wanted their partners to have been included in the discussions and a quarter of the partners themselves would have liked more information. It is, therefore, very important to identify patients who have psychosexual needs. This subject must be discussed in a suitably private environment (e.g. examination rather than consulting room, and questions should be asked in a sensitive manner). Quality of life prompts can help to stimulate relevant discussion, as can the introduction of non-threatening subjects, such as sleep.

Communication and survivorship

Communication skills training tends to concentrate on the issues discussed previously—breaking bad news, giving information about diagnosis, prognosis, and treatments, monitoring toxicities from treatment and, to a lesser extent, assessing quality of life. However, as cancer incidence rises and survival rates improve, there are an increasing number of patients living with and surviving cancer, who have a specific set of needs that is frequently neglected by clinicians. In the year transition between completion of primary treatment and 'living with cancer', patients often feel abandoned by the hospital system (Cardy *et al.* 2006). This may have a detrimental effect on recovery rates, as patients and carers often feel unsupported.

In order that patients feel less abandoned once treatment is complete, it is important that they have some understanding of the purpose of follow-up. Currently, most cancers are followed up by a hospital team for around 2–10 years after completion of treatment. However, few recurrences are found by routine surveillance; in breast cancer, most recurrences are self-detected and are usually incurable. Patients also find it difficult to manage the uncertainty aspect of survivorship. While the primary treatment may have 'cured' them or at least put them into remission, not knowing whether the cancer will return is a continuing cause for anxiety.

The move to living with a chronic illness can be a difficult adjustment to make, as patients are more likely to be in poor health and have psychological and functional disability. Many patients have to live with the late side effects of treatment, which may present some years after initial treatment and can be debilitating. The emotional and psychological burden of cancer can persist long after treatment has finished, which may be a contributing factor to patients not being able to work. People younger than 65 years with a cancer diagnosis are six times more likely to not be able to work because of their health than those without a cancer diagnosis, according to a US study comparing 5,000 cancer survivors and 90,000 people without cancer (Hewitt *et al.* 2003). This places an additional financial burden on patients surviving cancer.

Another issue that becomes relevant to survivorship is teaching new health behaviours to not only improve general health, but also reduce the risks of specific consequences of cancer treatment. Weight gain after treatment is a recognized problem, which can result in obesity. The benefits of exercise during and after treatment have been clearly shown (Kirshbaum 2007). Once treatment has finished, interventions to increase physical activity and improve diet can be used to reduce the long-term sequelae of obesity. Another example of reducing late complications of treatment is smoking cessation after chest radiotherapy, in order to preserve remaining lung function. Lifestyle modification only becomes an issue for patients who survive cancer.

Post-primary treatment support programmes have been shown to improve health outcomes including quality of life and psychological functioning, and also reduce disability from cancer (Rehse and Pukrop 2003; Coulter and Ellins 2006). The emphasis is on helping people to manage their own care. Interventions include giving patients information on recurrence and late side effects; an assessment of support needs (say at three months post-treatment); and communication with the GP, summarizing treatment and any ongoing needs. These measures provide patients with self-management strategies that lead to improved knowledge, better coping behaviour, adherence to treatments, and self-efficacy in symptom management. However, the most effective intervention is participation in self-help and support groups, which provide an environment where patients can share information and experiences.

Communication in end-of-life care

Raising the issue of approaching end of life is difficult for patients and clinicians. Many patients find it hard to ask difficult and sensitive questions about prognosis without prompting (Street 1991), and clinicians often wait to be asked (Parker *et al.* 2006). A recent randomized controlled trial found that the use of questionnaire prompts resulted in longer consultations, twice as many questions being asked by patients, more end-of-life discussions but also fewer unmet needs (Clayton *et al.* 2007). If prognosis is estimated, clinicians tend to be overoptimistic (Glare *et al.* 2003). A systematic review showed that physicians are generally poor at predicting prognosis in terminally ill patients, with errors (more than double or less than half of actual survival) in 30% of cases. Two-thirds of these errors were overestimates.

One of the reasons why discussing end-of-life issues is so difficult is that many patients are having active cancer treatment in the last few months of life, with as many as 10% receiving active treatment in the last few weeks (Earle *et al.* 2004). For these patients there is no clear cut off between not having active treatment and the start of end-of-life care. End-of-life discussions are often still linked in with the stopping of active treatment, which is too late for effective advance care planning. Oncologists rarely initiate discussions with patients about possibly being in the last year of life (so-called 'what if' conversations) during active treatment. This leads to confusion about prognosis and supportive care options for patients. Primary care teams tend not to refer patients for community support until they have received the appropriate signal from the specialist (Lamont and Christakis 2002). Palliative care and hospice staff may only be peripherally involved in patients' care. Site-specific nurses may be more closely involved with patients, but they often do not see end-of-life discussions as part of their role (Maher *et al.* 1992; Gattellari *et al.* 1999; Grunfeld *et al.* 2001).

Treatment is often initiated in the last few months of life as a way of 'giving hope' to patients. A recent study of the use of second line palliative chemotherapy in breast cancer found that 'giving hope' was one of the most important aims for oncologists in offering treatment (Grunfeld *et al.* 2001; Grunfeld *et al.* 2006). Thus, treatment is acting as a substitute for communication about end-of-life issues. In some countries, in particular the United States, oncologists prefer to use anti-cancer therapy rather than supportive care alone in advanced disease (Maher *et al.* 1992). Less than half of European radiotherapists and only 15% of American radiotherapists participated in the terminal care of their patients, according to a survey of the management of non-small cell lung cancer (NSCLC) patients. Many oncologists are not involved in the supportive care of their patients and consequently there are fewer end-of-life discussions.

The lack of opportunities to discuss the implications of being in the last year of life can seriously affect quality of life for patients and their carers, and place an unnecessary burden on the NHS. According to the 2004 report, *Unclaimed Millions*, over half of patients who die from cancer are not receiving the benefits they are entitled to (Disability Living Allowance and Attendance Allowance). This has a significant financial impact on terminally ill patients. Quality of life may also be affected by inappropriate prolongation of active cancer treatment. Delaying the 'what if' discussion may leave patients and carers without the emotional support and information needed to make adequate preparations for death (Goldstein *et al.* 2004; Fried *et al.* 2005). Carers often lack understanding of prognosis and also support for themselves, which can result in inappropriate and avoidable hospital admissions of patients with advanced cancer (Higginson *et al.* 1994).

It is, therefore, of great importance that patients with incurable cancer are given multiple opportunities to discuss their possibly being in the last year of life. End-of-life discussions should not be associated only with the withdrawal of treatment or dying, but should be initiated at the start of palliative treatment and regularly reviewed (e.g. every three months). Patients who may be approaching the last year of life can be identified more effectively if the 'surprise' question is asked (i.e. whether the physician would be 'surprised' if the patient died within a year). 'What if' discussions can then take place at the appropriate time and adequate support for end-of-life needs can be provided.

Medical well-being and its impact on communication

Effective communication between doctor and patient is dependent on the well-being of the doctor. Taylor *et al.* (2005) surveyed doctors from various different specialties in the United Kingdom in 1994 and 2002, and found that there was an increase in psychological morbidity over time, which was more pronounced in clinical oncologists compared with doctors in other specialties. The decline in mental health was due to increased job stress without a comparable increase in job satisfaction. Increased stress and burnout can have a negative impact on communication with patients.

Communication skills training can improve the mental health of physicians. In a survey conducted by Ramirez *et al.* (1996), consultants who lacked communication skills training were more likely to suffer burnout. Physicians should also have training, which includes coping strategies to help them deal with their own emotions. Stress often lasts beyond the consultation itself; and therefore, it is essential that physicians develop self-awareness and monitor their own well-being.

References

Aaronson NK, Hilarius DL, Kloeg P, Detmar SB, Gundy CM (2007). The use of Health-Related Quality of Life (HRQL) assessments in daily clinical oncology nursing practice: a community hospital-based intervention study. In: Proceedings of the International Psych-Oncology Society 9th World Congress of Psycho-Oncology, London, September 16–20, 2007.

Balsa AI, McGuire TG (2003). Prejudice, clinical uncertainty and stereotyping as sources of health disparities. *J Health Economics* **22**, 89–116.

Basen-Engquist K, Bodurka DC (2007). Medical and psychosocial issues in gynaecological cancer survivors. pp. 1838–45. In: Patricia Ganz (ed.). *Oncology: An Evidence-Based Approach*. Springer, New York, NY.

Boyland L, Davis C (2008). Patients' experience of carcinoma of unknown primary site: dealing with uncertainty. *Palliat Med* **22**, 177–83.

Brundage MD, Feldman-Stewart D, Leis A, Bezjak A (2007). The importance of quality of life information to a lung cancer (NSCLC chemotherapy treatment decision—results of a randomized evaluation. In: Proceedings of the International Psycho-Oncology Society 9th World Congress of Psycho-Oncology. London, September 16–20, 2007.

Burkitt-Wright E, Holcomb C, Salmon P (2004). Doctor's communication of trust, care and respect. Qualitative study. *BMJ* **328**, 864–7.

Cardy P, Corner J, Evans J, Jackson N, Shearn K, Sparham L (2006). Worried sick: the emotional impact of cancer, Macmillan Cancer Support. Available at: http://www.macmillan.org.uk/Documents/GetInvolved/Campaigns/Campaigns/Impact_of_cancer_english.pdf [Online].

Clayton JM, Butow PN, Tattersall MH, *et al.* (2007) Randomized controlled trial of a prompt list to help advanced cancer patients and their caregivers to ask questions about prognosis and end-of-life care. *J Clin Oncol* **25**, 715–23.

Corney RH, Crowther ME, Everett H, Howells A, Shepherd JH (1993). Psychosexual dysfunction in women with gynaecological cancer following radical pelvic surgery. *Br J Obstet Gynaecol* **100**, 73–8.

Coulter A, Ellins E (2006). *Patient-Focused Interventions*. Picker Institute Europe.

Davis TC, Williams MV, Marin E, Parker RM, Glass J (2002). Health literacy and cancer communication. *CA Cancer J Clin* **52**, 134–49.

Earle CC, Neville BA, Landrum MB, Ayanian JZ, Block SD, Weeks JC (2004). Trends in aggressiveness of cancer care near end of life. *J Clin Oncol* **22**, 315–21.

Epstein RM, Street RL Jr (2007). *Patient-Centered Communication in Cancer Care: Promoting Healing and Reducing Suffering*. National Cancer Institute, NIH Publication No. 07-6225. Bethesda, MD.

Fallowfield L, Jenkins V (1999). Effective communication skills are the key to good cancer care. *Eur J Cancer* **35**, 1592–7.

Fallowfield L, Jenkins V, Farewell V, Saul J, Duffy A, Eves R (2002). Efficacy of a Cancer Research UK communication skills training model for oncologists: a randomised controlled trial. *Lancet* **359**, 650–6.

Fried TR, Bradley EH, O'Leary JR, Byers AL (2005). Unmet desire for caregiver-patient communication and increased caregiver burden. *J Am Geriatr Soc* **53**, 59–65.

Gattellari M, Butow PN, Tattersall MH, Dunn SM, MacLeod CA (1999). Misunderstandings in cancer patients. *Ann Oncol* **10**, 39–46.

Glare P, Virik K, Jones M, Hudson M, Eychmuller S, Simes J, Christakis N (2003). A systematic review of physicians survival predictions in terminally ill cancer patients. *BMJ* **327**, 195–8.

Goldstein NE, Concato J, Fried TR, Kasl SV, Johnson-Hurzeler R, Bradley EH (2004). Factors associated with caregiver burden among caregivers of terminally ill patients with cancer. *J Palliat Care* **20**, 38–43.

Grunfeld EA, Ramirez AJ, Maher EJ, *et al.* (2001). Chemotherapy for advanced breast cancer: what influences oncologists decision-making. *Br J Cancer* **84**, 1172–8.

Grunfeld EA, Maher EJ, Browne S, *et al.* (2006) Perceptions of palliative chemotherapy: the view of advanced breast cancer patients. *J Clin Oncol* **24**, 1090–8.

Hewitt M, Rowland JH, Yancik R (2003). Cancer survivors in the United States: age health and disability. *J Gerontol* **58**, 82–91.

Higginson I, Webb D, Lessof L (1994). Reducing hospital beds for patients with advanced cancer. *Lancet* **344** (ii), 409.

Jenkins V, Fallowfield L, Saul J (2001). Information needs of patients with cancer: results from a large study in UK cancer centres. *Br J Cancer* **84**, 48–51.

Jenkins GP, Aronsky D (2005). A feasibility study for the computerized recruitment of subjects for research studies. *AMIA Annu Symp Proc* **996**.

Kirshbaum M (2007). A review of the benefits of whole body exercise during and after treatment for breast cancer. *J Clin Nurs* **16**, 104–21.

Lamont EB, Christakis NA (2002). Physician factors in the timing of cancer patient referral to hospice palliative care, *Cancer* **94**, 2733–7.

Lord K, Ibrahim K, Kumar S, *et al.* (2013) Are depressive symptoms more common among British South Asian patients compared with British White patients with cancer? A cross-sectional survey. *BMJ Open* **3**, e002650. doi:10:1136/bmjopen-2013-002650

Macmillan Cancer Support (2001). Cancer in the Media; May—October 2000. Report prepared for Macmillan Cancer Support by BMRB Information Services.

Maddams J, Utley M, Moller H (2012). Projections of cancer prevalence in the United Kingdom, 2010–2040. *Br J Cancer* **107**, 1195–202.

Maher EJ, Coia L, Duncan G, Lawton PA (1992). Treatment strategies in advanced and metastatic cancer: differences in attitude between the USA, Canada and Europe. *Int J Radiat Oncol Biol Phys* **23**, 239–44.

Maher J, McConnell H (2011). New pathways of care for cancer survivors: adding the numbers. *Br J Cancer* **105**, S5–S10.

McConnell H, White R, Maher J (2014). Understanding variations: Outcomes for people diagnosed with cancer and implications for service provision. European Network of Cancer Registries Scientific Meeting and General Assembly. Available at: http://www.encr.eu/images/docs/Conference_2014/poster_presetations/Hanna_McConnell.pdf [Online].

National Audit Office (2005). *Tackling Cancer: Improving the Patient Journey*. National Audit Office, HC 288 session 2004–2005, February 25, 2005.

National Breast Cancer Centre and National Cancer Control Initiative. (2003) Clinical practice guidelines for the psychosocial care of adults with cancer. Camperdown, Australia: National Breast Cancer Centre (Last accessed November 20, 2007). Available at: http://www.nhmrc.gov.au/publications/symposes/files/cp90.pdf [Online].

Parker SM, Clayton JM, Hancock K, *et al.* (2006). A systematic review of prognostic/end-of-life communication with adults in the advanced stages of a life-limiting illness: patient/caregiver preferences for the content, style and timing of information. *J Pain Symptom Manage* **34**, 81–93.

Ptacek JT, Fries EA, Eberhardt TL, Ptacek JJ (1999). Breaking bad news to patients: physicians' perceptions of the process. *Support Care Cancer* **7**, 113–20.

Ramirez AJ, Graham J, Richards MA, Cull A, Gregory WM (1996). Mental health of hospital consultations: the effect of stress and satisfaction at work. *Lancet* **347**, 724–8.

Rehse B, Pukrop R (2003). Effects of psychosocial interventions on quality of life in adult cancer patients: meta-analysis of 37 published controlled outcome studies. *Patient Educ Counsel* **50**, 179–86.

Salmon P, Hall G (2004). Patient empowerment or the emperor's new clothes? *J R Soc Med* **97**, 53–6.

Street RL (1991). Information giving in medical consultations: the influence of patients' communicative styles and personal characteristics. *Soc Sci Med* **32**, 541–8.

Sutherland HJ, Lockwood GA, Till JE (1990). Are we getting informed consent from patients with cancer? *J R Soc Med* **83**, 439–43.

Taylor C, Graham J, Potts HW, Richards MA, Ramirez AJ (2005). Changes in mental health of UK hospital consultants since the mid-1990s. *Lancet* **366**, 742–4.

Velikova Booth L, Smith AB, *et al.* (2004). Measuring quality of life in routine oncology practice improves communication and patient well-being: a randomized controlled trial. *J Clin Oncol* **22**, 714–24.

CHAPTER 49

Palliative medicine: Communication to promote life near the end of life

Nicola Pease

When is 'end of life'? When does a patient become a palliative care patient?

End of life often means different things to different people; for some patients, carers, and healthcare professionals, it will mean the last few days or weeks of life. However, to others, it might mean the last 6–12 months of a patient's life. Within the United Kingdom, General Medical Council guidance indicates that patients should be considered as 'approaching the end of life' when they are thought likely to die within the next 12 months (General Medical Council 2010).

For many healthcare professionals, policy makers, and the general public, end-of-life care is synonymous with palliative care (Twycross 2003). For this reason, it is important that the two classical models of transition to palliative care are acknowledged (Twycross 2003; Murray *et al.* 2005; see also Figs 49.1 and 49.2).

Figure 49.1 illustrates the 'older more traditional model' where patients with a life-limiting illness suddenly transitioned from primary medical specialty (e.g. oncology/respiratory medicine or cardiology) to palliative care, abruptly moving from 'active treatments' into palliative/hospice care. A more modern model of care (Fig. 49.2) illustrates an integrated service where palliative care works alongside the primary medical specialty to deliver a more collaborative patient-centred service and has proven beneficial for

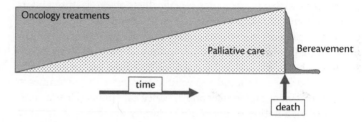

Fig. 49.2 Transition between palliative and active treatments is linked to the patients' fluctuating condition, occurs at any time and represents integrated services (Murray 2005).

Adapted with permission from Lynn J and Adamson DM, *Living well at the end of life: Adapting health care to serious chronic illness in old age*, Rand Health, Washington, USA, Copyright © 2003 RAND.

patient outcomes in terms of quality of life, patient mood, and even a survival time advantage (Temel *et al.* 2010). With this more collaborative approach the patient and their family are less likely to feel 'handed over' or abandoned by the primary medical team plus the 'sharing' of care between primary medical specialty and supportive/palliative care will allow mutual support in terms of education, teamworking, and communication with the patient. Often these different models of patient care can co-exist, depending on the primary physician's understanding of the role of palliative care.

Identifying when to involve specialist palliative care can seem difficult to predict. Some specialists may feel that the mention of palliative care will mean that the patient gives up hope, or is less compliant with treatment. On the contrary, evidence indicates that palliative care involvement results in better patient satisfaction, symptom control, and reduced hospital admissions (Brumley *et al.* 2007).

Predicting an individual patient's disease trajectory is notoriously difficult. Prognostic indicator 'tools', as illustrated below, have been developed to provide some guidance and can be used irrespective of the patient's care setting. Twycross (2003) states for cancer patients where no reversible cause is identified: '... if deteriorating month by month, the prognosis is likely to be months, if deteriorating week by week, the prognosis is likely to be weeks, if deteriorating day by day, the prognosis is likely to be days' (Twycross 2003, p. 30).

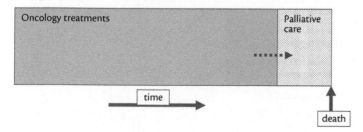

Fig. 49.1 The transition to palliative is abrupt. For example, the patient may have to alter financial insurance cover to obtain the service (Murray 2005).

Adapted with permission from Lynn J and Adamson DM, *Living well at the end of life: Adapting health care to serious chronic illness in old age*, Rand Health, Washington, USA, Copyright © 2003 RAND.

The Gold Standard Prognostic Indicator (Thomas 2011) is a straightforward three-part tool, which uses a combination of the 'intuitive surprise question?'—'*Would you be surprised if this patient were to die in the next few months?*' in combination with general and disease specific indicators of decline. The combined answers to these questions provide a prognostic guide, which in turn gives the clinician increased confidence in initiating end-of-life discussion with the patient/carers.

Perhaps the single most important predictive factor in cancer patients is functional ability—if patients spend more than 50% of their time in bed/lying down, prognosis is likely to be three months or less (Thomas 2011).

In many ways, end-of-life discussion can be thought of as planning for the worst while hoping for the best. 'Life near the end of life' will mean different things to different people. Patients will have highly individual goals and priorities. For some patients, the priority may be length of life, but for many patients 'life' may mean something completely different; for example, the ability to put their affairs in order, plan a 'healthy death', or to achieve something important which has resonance specifically to them. Without information about their condition, their treatment options, and possible outcomes, patients cannot make informed choices/decisions about how/where they might want to live in the last phase of their lives.

Although there is both evidence and consensus that patients with a terminal diagnosis should and want to be offered opportunities to discuss treatment preferences and advance care plans (Health 2008; GMC 2010), a national survey of UK family doctors found that in practice, patients and healthcare professionals rarely discussed end-of-life plans in the last months of life (Abarashi and Echteld 2011).

A large systematic review (Hancock *et al.* 2007) relating to truth-telling regarding prognosis to adult patients with progressive, advanced, life-limiting disease, identified that although the majority of healthcare professionals felt that patients should be told the truth regarding prognosis, in clinical practice, many clinicians avoid discussing the topic or withhold information. Reasons for this included perceived lack of training, uncertainty about prognostication, insufficient time, requests from family members to withhold information, a feeling of inadequacy or hopelessness regarding the unavailability of further curative treatment, and fear of a negative impact on the patient. Interestingly, studies within this same review identified that patients can discuss prognosis without it having a negative impact on them.

Transition/referral to palliative care

Having identified that the patient is probably entering the last 12 months of their life, how should this information be offered to patients? How should one share that treatments are no longer effective and the disease is progressing?

Each of these situations is of course breaking bad news. Breaking bad news is defined as information that seriously and adversely affects the patient's view of their future (Buckman 1984). Often patients with a cancer diagnosis will recall receiving bad news at the time of the initial diagnosis; however, for patients with advanced end organ failure, the initial diagnosis may not have been perceived as a life-limiting illness. As the disease slowly progresses, often with periods of exacerbation/relapse of symptoms and recovery, if the topic of an overall downwards trajectory is not raised, patients may believe that there will always be treatment options which will rescue

them from periods where they are highly symptomatic and sometimes critically unwell. It is therefore important that the clinician ascertains what the patient already understands about their illness.

Much is written about breaking bad news, and several strategies exist (Baile and Parker 2010); these include 'SPIKES' (Baile and Buckman 2000), a protocol adapted from Buckman's six-step protocol, or 'breaking bad news: a ten-step approach' (Kaye 1996). Whichever strategy is used, a key principle in breaking bad news is 'ask before you tell'. Find out what the patient already knows. What is their understanding of their illness? Having ascertained what the patient knows, one needs to elicit 'how much information/detail do they want to know?' These steps are crucial as they identify a starting point and direction of information sharing (guided by what the patient wants to know). Inherent in gaining this information is permission from the patient that they wish to proceed.

Having a strategy for breaking bad news is useful; however, in a busy clinic, where a patient has been attending regularly and their consultation has fallen into a predictable pattern, when is the right time? How should one make a start? Who should do it?

These are very real and valid questions. Surveys of clinicians have found that they report lack of knowledge, skills and confidence in how to initiate end-of-life conversations with patients and difficulties in knowing the right time to raise such topics (Almack *et al.* 2012). Acknowledging these difficulties, in 2007 the Cardiff six-point toolkit was developed (Noble *et al.* 2010).

The toolkit (Box 49.1) breaks down the bare essentials of any palliative consultation and specifically offers tools which can be refined by clinicians, such that they become more comfortable using them. The toolkit is not offered as a further protocol for breaking bad news but supports and facilitates other breaking bad news strategies. Within the toolkit, aside from 'comfort', which one would expect used at the start of any consultation and maintained throughout, there is no specific 'order' of use. See Table 49.1 as an example of the toolkit in action. It can be applied to any consultation (e.g. information gathering, collusion, denial, and so on).

Tool 1: Comfort

The concept of comfort encompasses many aspects of any consultation. Comfort includes the setting of the consultation (an area conducive to sensitive exchange of information), the lighting of the room (recognizing that a significant proportion of communication is non-verbal) and the physical/psychological comfort of those involved.

Bad news is inherently upsetting to the patient/relatives and can evoke strong emotions such as tears or sobbing. Bad news should

---

Box 49.1 The Cardiff six-point toolkit

1. Comfort
2. Question style
3. Language
4. Listening/use of silence
5. Reflection/acknowledge
6. Summarizing

Reproduced courtesy of Dr Nikki Pease and Professor Ilora Finlay.

Table 49.1 Illustrates the toolkit in action—breaking bad news

Tool	Doctor	Patient
Comfort	Good morning Ms K. Are you comfortable on that chair or would you prefer the higher seat?	
		Yes, thank you. A higher chair would help.
Non-verbal	Looking serious	
Question—open	How have things been?	
		Oh, not so good.
Reflection	(pause) … not so good?	
		No, I've been tired all the time and my appetite has gone again.
Reflection	Tired all the time?	
		Yes, I just don't have any energy and I don't think the new tablets suit me; the ache in my back is worse some nights and stops me sleeping.
Question—focused	Does anything else stop you sleeping?	
		No … well maybe a bit of worry, but that's to be expected.
Question—focused	What sort of things do you worry about?	
		Everything!
Reflection	Everything?	
		Yes, what will happen if this does not work, what I should do if things get worse?
Reflection	Things get worse?	
		Yes, the cancer, I am worried about it getting worse.
Acknowledge	I can see that this has been a difficult time for you	
		Yes, it has.
Summarizing (followed by checking back that patient agrees with the summary)	You have mentioned that you're tired, your backache is worse, your appetite has gone, and your worries are stopping you sleeping. Is that right?	
		Yes, I do worry a lot. So do you think the cancer is getting worse?
Partial reflection	I'm sorry to say I share your worries.	
Listening—use of silence		Oh …
Non-verbal (confirms the bad news)	Uh huh (nodding slightly)	… (at this point on starting to realize that this is bad news patients frequently look down /avoid eye contact). The silence here may seem long but be mindful that the bad news to the patient may have far reaching implications and many questions/ thoughts maybe going through their minds. It is essential that you allow this silence as interruption here will stop patients processing information.
		Mmmm … (patient makes eye contact again). So what can be done?
Acknowledge/ summarizing followed by a hypothetical question	This can be a difficult time (pause) would it help if I summarized where I think we are. We both think things might have got worse. You've mentioned tiredness, have back pain, and aren't eating well. (pause) Have you ever thought that this might happen?	
Silence		
		Well … yes … I suppose it is always in the back of your mind. In a way with the pain getting worse I have thought about it yes. What do you suggest doctor?

(continued)

Table 49.1 (continued)

Tool	Doctor	Patient
Non-verbal	Nods …	
Combination of reflection and summarizing used to spell out a plan	Ah yes, with everything that you have told me and the fact that we both feel that things might have got worse; I feel it would be wise to 'take a break' from chemotherapy until we know more. For the back pain I would like to request a fairly urgent scan to help find out the cause. We can review your painkillers today however I would like to refer you to my palliative care colleagues who have expertise in controlling symptoms.	
		Ok doctor … I was worried that I would have to live with the pain but it seems there is something that you can do. I'll be guided by what you think is best.

always be sensitively given; however, be mindful that if patients do show emotions, not to attempt 'to make bad news good news'. Saying things like 'there, there it will be ok' or feeling compelled (due to your own unease) to say something to 'make it better', may temporarily improve the situation, but it will give false reassurance and ultimately promote patient distrust. At times where patients are tearful/upset, other aspects of the toolkit such as 'acknowledging' or 'use of silence' are better used.

Tool 2: Question style

The question style of any consultation is crucially important. As a general rule, the more open the question, the more information is obtained. Open questions are questions that give no indication as to the answer. Open questions, such as 'How have things been?' allow the patient to talk about anything that has been happening and thereby to prioritize to their agenda. A recent systematic review of 'How to communicate with patients about future illness progression and end of life' (Parry *et al.* 2014) concluded that 'open' questions are useful and non-threatening. However, when used alone they are often insufficient in encouraging patients to explore future planning, as they can make it particularly easy for both patient and healthcare professional to avoid engaging in difficult conversation. That said, if a patient does opt to answer in terms of difficult future topics (end of life, disease progression, and so on), it clearly indicates their willingness and wish to talk about these topics.

Focused questions do just as the name suggests: they focus down on a particular area, for example 'Tell me more about your vomiting?' or 'you mentioned you weren't really coping … tell me more about that'. Hypothetical questions are a type of focused question which involves a possibility or probability for the future; for example, 'Have you ever wondered what might happen if the chemotherapy stopped working?' (Table 49.2). Recent evidence concluded that hypothetical questions are a highly effective tool in encouraging patients to engage with difficult issues (Parry *et al.* 2014).

Direct questions, which narrow matters down further, are often used to clarify. For example, 'Do you vomit after every meal?' are of limited use in encouraging open communication.

Table 49.2 Introducing end-of-life topics—the toolkit in action (linking the review evidence (Parry *et al.* 2014) to the toolkit)

Tool	Doctor	Patient
Comfort	Hello Mr A, I am sorry I have kept you waiting.	
		Oh that's ok doctor, I know how busy these clinics are. I have my son with me today is that ok?
Open question	Yes, that's absolutely fine. I am pleased to meet you (son). How you are Mr A?	
		Oh not too bad.
Reflection	(pause) Not too bad?	
		Well my appetite has gone, I am sleeping a lot more and I have a new problem which I am worried about.
Reflection	A new problem?	
		Yes, for the past three weeks I have had pain just under my right ribs in the front here (points to right upper quadrant), I have also been sick a few times, just suddenly sick with very little warning.
Listening /Acknowledge	Mmm … I'm sorry to hear this. Do you mind if I examine you? (examination identifies large hepatomegaly).	

Table 49.2 (continued)

Tool	Doctor	Patient
		No doctor, you carry on, sorry but I haven't been able to do my trousers up as my tummy is swollen.
Comfort (recheck)	Ok thank you. (completes examination) Mr A, please sit up, are you comfortable?	
		Yes thank you, it is better sat up. What do you think is going on doctor?
Summarizing cues/ information from patient	Well from examining you and what you have said in that you have been sick a few times, your tummy is swollen, and you have pain. I am concerned that things are not normal.	
		Not normal?
Summarizing	Yes, I am worried that the swelling of your abdomen, the vomiting, and on examining you, I am fairly certain that your liver is enlarged.	
		Oh, that's not a good sign is it?
Reflection	Well … no, I'm afraid it is not a good sign, although we would need to confirm it with a scan, all these things together would mean that the hormone tablets are not really working.	
		Ah, um, I see (patient often loses eye contact here as is assimilating the new bad news).
Silence (allowing patient time to think)		
		So what next doctor?
Hypothetical question	Well had you ever thought this might happen … that there might be a time when the treatment stops working so well?	
		Well yes I suppose, we had talked about it my wife and I.
Reflection	Talked about it?	
		Yes, we talked that if that time came, you know when the treatment wasn't really helping me … that we would want to go off and see the grandchildren and have a bit of quality time together.
Reflect/acknowledge	Yes … quality time together.	
		Yes, I would want to look at my priorities and sort stuff out.
Summarizing	Well I think as things are that would be sensible. If it is ok with you I will request a scan to confirm things but we need to start to plan with you so that you can achieve what is important to you. With regard to the vomiting and the pain and in fact to help you 'sort stuff out' about future plans I would like to refer you to my palliative care colleagues.	
		Ok but will that mean that I don't see you again … because I wouldn't want that.
Developing a management plan	No not at all. I will see you after the scan. The reason I want to refer you to my colleagues is that they work both in hospital and in the community. They have expertise in helping with symptoms you have and planning with you for the future.	

Multiple questions (often a series of short questions rolled into one sentence) and leading questions are best avoided. Multiple questions can confuse the patient, who will usually choose to answer the last question asked and miss the previous questions. Leading questions often lead to the wrong answer; for example, 'since starting the painkillers how much better is your pain?'

Tool 3: Language

Language is far more than the spoken word. People communicate by the way they look or dress, their demeanour, body posture, and facial expressions. In fact, up to 60% of communication is non-verbal, 33% the tone that we use, and only approximately 7% the spoken word. We can all perhaps recall people saying 'pass me my spectacles, I can't hear you properly'—this isn't a mistake, it acknowledges the significant part of communication that is non-verbal. Much can be transferred by gesture, facial expression, or touch.

In considering the words spoken, endeavour to use vocabulary familiar to the patient, acknowledging that at times of stress (e.g. receiving bad news), the processing of information may be slower. Be mindful to use straightforward words and short sentences. Keep it simple. All healthcare professionals must avoid using medical jargon or unnecessarily complex words as a barrier.

Tool 4: Listening use of silence

Key tools in communicating are not only listening but the use of silence. Communication studies have indicated that doctors do not listen to their patients enough and often interrupt the patient's dialogue prematurely, in a desire to problem solve or follow their own agenda (Beckman and Frankel 1984).

Silence

- Allows the patient time to assimilate information, react to that information, and frame questions.
- Demonstrates that the patient is being listened to.
- Can encourage patients to engage in difficult topics and conversations.
- Used in combination with appropriate touch can display sensitivity.

People have a low tolerance for silences in conversations, and thus silence can work to encourage talk. A recent systematic review (Parry et al. 2014) found evidence that when a difficult topic was broached, when the healthcare professional remained silent, the patient engaged in the topic.

Tool 5: Reflection/acknowledge

Reflection involves the listener (healthcare professional) repeating back a patient's word or short phrase, such that the patient is encouraged to continue.

Reflection

- Demonstrates that the patient is being listened to.
- Encourages patients to continue with their 'story' or difficult topic.
- Allows clinicians to pick up on patients' cues and sometimes prioritize.

Acknowledgement is achieved by using a short sentence to demonstrate empathic recognition of the patient's situation/ distress. It is very useful when patients make comments to which there is no straight forward answer. For example, a patient who is so distressed by starting to receive bad news:

Patient: *'It's bad isn't it doctor, it's bad; am I going to die?'*

Doctor: *'That is a very difficult question to ask, what makes you ask it now?'*

This acknowledges Mrs S's distress while not answering the question she posed. The acknowledgement avoids the doctor giving a banal answer and may defuse some of the high emotion/ distress while encouraging the patient to be more explicit.

Tool 6: Summarizing/recapping

Summarizing is the process of taking the salient information given by the patient and recapping this back during the consultation.

Summarizing

- Demonstrates to the patient that they have been listened to.
- Allows the clinician to check that all the information important to the patient is included.
- Is very useful to clinicians if they feel lost in a consultation or if indeed the consultation has lost direction in that it allows one to recap what has been understood thus far.
- Can be very useful to introduce difficult topics when used with a hypothetical question (Parry et al. 2014).

Communicating about the end of life can sometimes be challenging. In stressful situations, patients or relatives can display various emotions including anger, denial, hopelessness, or collusion. The toolkit can facilitate better communication in these consultations.

Anger

Irrespective of the cause of the anger, the aim of the consultation is to defuse the situation. To achieve this, one needs to identify why the patient/relative is angry, being mindful not to assume reasons.

Comfort

Ensure a safe environment, and encourage the angry person to sit down with you, preferably with your eye level at or below theirs. Sitting over someone can appear dominating and worsen the situation.

Question styles

Use open questions to explore the situation and identify the person's agenda. Avoid immediate problem solving until you are reasonably certain you have ascertained their real concerns. Avoid 'answering back'.

Non-verbal language

Keep calm with an open body posture and good eye contact to convey that you are taking the situation seriously.

Language

Language should be kept straightforward, avoid complicated terminology. Often angry patients/relative will speak quickly; endeavour to slow the pace of the consultation by speaking slowly and clearly.

Listening/use of silence

Give the situation your full attention; listening is your most effective tool. When they are speaking, engage in active listening.

Table 49.3 Discussing death—the toolkit in action

Tool	Doctor	Patient
Question—open	How have you been?	
		Terrible, I'm fed up with it all.
Reflection	Fed up?	
		Yes, you wouldn't let a dog die like this.
Question—focused	Do you feel as if you are dying?	
		Of course I do and I just want to get it over with quickly.
Reflection	Over quickly?	
		Well, you know, end it all.
Reflection	So can you tell me the specific things that make you feel life is so awful that you want to end it all?	
		Well I can't do what I used to, don't feel like the person I was.
Reflection	Don't feel like the person you were?	
		No, look at me now. I'm a burden. And it frightens me.
Reflection	It frightens?	
		Yes. I'm frightened of being a burden, frightened of what tomorrow holds and frightened of losing my independence and my dignity.
Acknowledge /Reflection	I am sorry that things are difficult, is there anything you can think of that would help you feel more independent and with more dignity?	
Silence (listening)	…	
		What if my wife cannot cope?
Reflection	Cope?	
		With my toilet needs.
Focused question /clarification	Have you spoken about this with her?	
		No, you see we're pretty private about stuff like that.
Summarize	So can I summarize what I think I've heard: you feel so wretched that you want to die, you are frightened of being a burden, frightened that your wife can't cope and worried about some of the intimate aspects of care such as the toilet. Is that about right?	
		Yes.
	And is there anything else?	
		No that's the main things.
Summarize the plan and check back on it (active listening, observing patient comfort)	So, could we try to make sure your privacy is maintained, get support for your wife and look at ways to increase your sense of control over your own care?	
		That would be really helpful.

Reflection/acknowledge

Acknowledge this is a difficult time/situation for them. Perhaps reflect back key words or phrases to complement active listening and gently clarify possible misconceptions.

Summarize

Summarize or recap the points heard as it will not only allow a little breathing space, but reinforces that the patient has been heard.

Endeavour to recap the agreed management plan towards the end of the consultation.

Denial

Although denial may not be seen as harmful to the patient, it prevents shared decision-making and planning for the future. Where children or dependents are involved, it can be crucial that denial is addressed to ensure appropriate future planning. That said, denial is a coping strategy and as such it can be harmful to suddenly shatter this wall of defence. It is psychologically safer for patients to gradually help them (or family) recognize that their understanding of the illness/treatments does not match the reality of the situation.

Using open questions, hypothetical questions, reflection, summarizing, and other elements of the toolkit are extremely useful. Open questions allow for information gathering, which can then be summarized and followed by a hypothetical question. For example: 'May I just recap on what I understand … you mentioned that your breathing is more difficult, you've lost quite a bit of weight and are struggling to manage the stairs … Have you ever wondered what might be causing these problems?'. Another useful hypothetical question in encouraging end-of-life discussions is 'Have you thoughts on what you would want if things didn't go as well as we all hope?'

Collusion

Significant triggers to collusion are when treatment options fail, the patient becomes palliative, or the end of life is approaching. Collusion is defined as a secret agreement or understanding for purposes of trickery or fraud; underhand scheming or working with another; deceit, fraud, or trickery (Oxford English Dictionary 2015). Within healthcare collusion may be explicit, where families or 'decision makers' seek to protect their loved one by asking doctors not to tell; or it may be more covert. Recently, the concept of the 'recovery plot' has been described (The et al. 2000) where the focus of communication is on treatment and recovery issues rather than distressing symptoms, possibility of relapse or recurrence, long-term disability, and death. The recovery plot allows healthcare professionals and relatives to focus on the treatment calendar and interventions rather than exploring patient's information wishes and planning for the future.

Collusion is a universal phenomenon present in varying degrees within most cultures. Importantly, within healthcare, collusion is frequently partial, in that healthcare professionals are 'permitted' to share some information (e.g. diagnosis) with the patient but not all information (e.g. prognosis). 'Collusion is not always a conspiracy of silence; it may be a conspiracy of lopsided communication' (Chaturvedi et al. 2009). In the presence of collusion, the communication toolkit is invaluable. Focused questions such as 'Are you the type of person who wants me to speak to you directly or would you prefer me to speak to your family beforehand?' can clarify a patient's wishes and avoid later accusations from their family.

Addressing collusion is often a two staged process—the toolkit being used throughout.

Stage 1: Talking with the family

Use open questions to ascertain their understanding of the illness. Listen to them explain why they do not wish their loved one to be told, pick up on cues, and reflect back to let them know they are being listened to. Acknowledge the families' situation and that they know the patient far better than you. Acknowledge their wish to protect the patient. It can be helpful to stress to the family that you are 'not here to make the situation more difficult than it already is'. You are not here to take away hope. Summarize the information gathered to explain that the patient knows that they are ill—for example 'You have mentioned your wife has lost weight, is eating very little, and is tired a lot of the time. I just wonder what she must

be thinking?' (hypothetical question) … followed by silence, to allow the family time to think.

Reflect 'you mentioned your wife worked as a … she is clearly an intelligent person who I suspect has questions about her illness'. Explain that you would want to answer such questions with gentle honestly, you would not suddenly announce devastating information. Once reassured, families are often relieved not to have to maintain the collusion.

Stage 2: Talking with the patient and the family

Often this stage involves breaking bad news, usually in the presence of the family (see Table 49.3).

The toolkit, as described above for breaking bad news, can be very useful.

Life at the end of life will mean different things to different patients. You will by now have a sense of how the toolkit can be used to facilitate any palliative care consultation. As clinicians we increasingly have the knowledge and training to recognize when patients are deteriorating and are probably entering the last phase of life, whether days, weeks, or months. As healthcare professionals, we have a duty to compassionately offer information to patients, to encourage them to ask questions such that they are empowered and able to share the decision-making. It is only then that patients will have sufficient information to make plans for life at the end of life.

References

Abarashi E, Echteld M, Donker G, Van den Block L, Onwuteaka-Philipsen B, Deliens L (2011). Discussing end-of-life issues in the last months of life: a nationwide study among general practitioners. *J Palliat Med* **14**, 323–30.

Almack K, Cox K, Moghaddam N, Pollock K, Seymour J (2012). After you: conversations between patients and healthcare professionals in planning for end of life care. *BMC Palliative Care* **11**, 15. Available at: http://bmcpalliatcare.biomedcentral.com/articles/10.1186/1472-684X-11-15 [Last accessed Feb 2015].

Baile W, Buckman R, Lenzi R, Glober G, Beale EA, Kudelka AP (2000). SPIKES a six-step protocol for delivering bad news: Application to the patient with cancer. *Oncologist* **5**, 302–11.

Baile W, Parker P (2010). Breaking bad news. In: Kissane D, Bylund C, Butow P, Bultz B, Noble S, Wilkinson S. *Handbook of Communication in Oncology and Palliative Care*. Oxford University Press, Oxford, UK.

Beckman H, Frankel R (1984). The effect of physician behavior on the collection of data. *Ann Intern Med* **101**, 692–6.

Brumley R, Enguidanos S, Jamison P, et al. (2007). Increased satisfaction with care and lower costs: results of a randomised trial of in-home palliative care. *J Am Geriatr Soc* **55**, 993–1000.

Buckman R (1984). Breaking bad news: why is it still so difficult? *BMJ* **288**, 1507–9.

Chaturvedi S, Loiselle C, Chandra P (2009). Communication with relatives and collusion in palliative care: A cross-cultural perspective. *Indian J Palliat Care* [online] **15**, 2–9. Available at: http://www.ncbi.nlm.nih.gov [Last accessed: Feb 2015].

Department of Health (2008). End of life care strategy: promoting high quality care for adults at the end of life. Available at: http://www.gov.uk [Last accessed: Feb 2015].

General Medical Council (2010) Treatment and care towards the end of life. Available at: http://www.gmc-uk.org/guidance/ethical_guidance/end_of_life_care.asp [Last accessed: Jan 2015].

Hancock K, Clayton J, Parker S, et al. (2007) Truth-telling in discussing prognosis in advance life-limiting illness: a systematic review. *Palliat Med* **21**, 507–17.

Kaye P (1996). *Breaking Bad News: A Ten-Step Approach*. EPL Publications, Northampton, UK.

Murray S, Kendall M, Boyd K and Sheikh A (2005). Illness trajectories and palliative care. *BMJ* **330**, 1007–11.

Noble S, Pease N, Finlay I (2010). The United Kingdom general practitioner and palliative care model. In: Kissane D, Bylund C, Butow P, Bultz B, Noble S, Wilkinson S. *Handbook of Communication in Oncology and Palliative Care*. Oxford University Press, Oxford, UK.

OED Online (2015). Collusion, n. In: *Oxford English Dictionary* [Online]. Available at: http://www.oxforddictionaries.com/definition/english/collusion [Last accessed February 5, 2016].

Parry R, Land V, Seymour J (2014). How to communicate with patients about future illness progression and end of life: a systematic review. *BMJ Support Palliat Care* **4**, 331–4.

The A, Hak T, Koeter G, van Der Wal G (2000). Collusion in doctor-patient communication about imminent death: an ethnographic study. *BMJ* **321**, 1376–81.

Temel JS, Greer JA, Muzikansky A, *et al.* (2010). Early palliative care for patients with metastatic non-small-cell lung cancer. *N Engl J Med* **363**, 733–42.

Thomas K (2011). Prognostic indicator guidance. The Gold Standards Framework Centre In End of Life Care CIC. Available at: http://www.goldstandardsframework.org.uk/cd-content/uploads/files/General%20Files/Prognostic%20Indicator%20Guidance%20October%202011.pdf [Last accessed: Jan 2015].

Twycross R (2003) *Introduction to palliative care*. Radcliffe Medical Press, Oxford, UK.

CHAPTER 50

Communication issues in pastoral care and chaplaincy

Peter Speck and Christopher Herbert

Introduction to communication issues in pastoral care and chaplaincy

The diagnosis of a life-threatening disease can trigger a variety of reactions in the recipient of such news. In addition to a range of emotional and psychological responses, there will come a time when questions of a more existential nature will arise. These may relate to causality, to the possible meaning and purpose of the illness, or what the future may hold in terms of the individual's beliefs about what happens when we die. These questions may be difficult to voice or for others to hear and respond to, but they are very much the concern of pastoral and spiritual care.

If we are to be able to discern and respond appropriately to the questions that arise in the minds of patients, families, and staff, it is important that those responsible for the provision of spiritual care can develop a relationship with the person who is ill to enable the airing of such issues and the exploration of appropriate responses which will support the person at various stages in the progression of the disease. The UK guidance for supportive care in adult cancer (NICE 2004) made it clear that all staff in a palliative care setting share a responsibility for spiritual care, even if there are specially designated people appointed to provide for the range of discerned need. This applies whether the setting is within a hospital, a hospice, or the community. The implication of this is that the level of communication skills held by all staff should be sufficient to facilitate conversations and exploration of responses to the illness, to enable assessment of need and referral to appropriate people at various times in the illness journey. Assessment tools can be lengthy or insensitive and directive, restricting the ability of the patient to set the agenda. An effective assessment will highlight the issues that are important to the patient and may begin with a question such as 'What are the things that are really important to you now?' Answers may include the person's family, their treatment options, the extent to which they can maintain some control over what happens, and so on. The conversation may move to an exploration of what has helped the person cope when life has been difficult in the past. This may reveal the person's own strengths, those of significant people in their life, or their beliefs (religious or otherwise). By inviting the patient to explore what is important to them and review their strategies for coping, the caregiver is indicating a willingness to listen and respond to non-clinical issues. Such a conversation may reveal strong and healthy beliefs that are significant for the patient and from which they gain ongoing strength and support. The conversation may also expose distress and anxieties

that may lead to an intervention by a psychologist, social worker, or spiritual care provider (Speck 2004). Sometimes it is more appropriate for a chaplain/spiritual caregiver to work and support the staff member in continuing the conversation, rather than to take over and replace the staff member. The decision as to who should provide for the identified need will depend on the resources available, the patient's choice as to how they wish to continue the conversation, and whether the patient is cared for at home or in an inpatient setting.

The inpatient setting

Much of chaplaincy in a hospital or hospice is concerned with assessing and meeting the needs of patients, staff, and families, whether they are religious or not. Chaplains come from a faith tradition but are usually able to work with people who are within and outside of their faith group. Because they are used to reflecting on existential issues in a broad way, they should be able to work creatively with many of the questions and concerns raised by people adjusting to a life-threatening illness. This does not mean that they will have easy and ready answers, but by their training and their experience should be able to stay with the tensions, uncertainty, and anger voiced by people.

Pastoral care is concerned with enabling people to grow, to learn, to be sustained, and to achieve healing that is more than physical wellness in the context of their beliefs. For those whose belief contains an understanding of a deity or God, then the communication is not only interpersonal, but also with that sense of 'otherness' we frequently term 'the divine or the sacred'. In the context of a religious belief, this means that the individual may seek support in terms of prayer, sacrament, or other ritual, and counselling for specific areas of concern. Each faith tradition will have its own specific rituals appropriate to times of illness and these may be conducted privately with the sick person, or corporately with other believers by the bedside or place set aside for religious worship in the hospital or hospice.

This may range from specific acts of prayer, the laying on of hands for healing, strengthening, and blessing, or anointing with oil. There may also be specific rituals appropriate at the time of approaching death, and those used as the body is subsequently prepared for the funeral of the deceased (Speck 2003; Cobb 2005). In addition, the individual may wish to explore their belief, their understanding of the deity or what happens after death, and to seek help for areas of doubt or conflict in their faith. It is important not to assume that believers will have no doubts even after years of faith. It is also important to respond to the patient's own agenda and to avoid proselytizing.

Spiritual caregivers also need appropriate training and supervision to remain sensitive within pastoral relationships, as well as dealing with issues in their own agenda, which arise out of the nature of their work. It is essential that pastoral care givers maintain their own spiritual life in order to be able to 'journey' with others—sometimes into very dark places.

Alice was a 33-year-old married woman and mother of two young children. She developed pancreatic cancer with metastatic spread. On admission she was both frightened and very angry. When the chaplain met her, in the course of a general visit to her ward, she was very scathing about what the chaplain represented. After her verbal attack Alice was surprised that the chaplain re-visited the following day, and she asked how the chaplain could represent a God who 'allowed such terrible things to happen'. This began an exploration of the nature of God, the problem of suffering, and the seeming unfairness of much that happens to us. No easy answers were offered, but neither did the chaplain duck the issues or run away. A mutually respectful relationship developed and Alice realized that the chaplain was able to stand 'the heat' and was not going to offload a religious framework onto her. She began to use these encounters as a safe space, not only to ventilate feeling, but also to explore her fears and review options for her family and their future. As it became clear that her prognosis was very poor, she was also able to use the chaplain to help her, and later her husband, to plan her funeral, and how best to prepare her children for her death. This latter need led to a member of the child psychology team joining the chaplain to work with the family as a unit. Alice was still not sure if she really believed in God or could trust God to ensure that in the end it would all work out, but she did feel she could trust the chaplain to conduct her funeral in a way that would not compromise her views and wishes. Alice also created a narrative of her life in which she recorded significant incidents and people who had shaped her and made her what she was. In particular, she talked of the love she had for her husband and children, as well as some of her hopes for their future. In particular she wrote out recipes for dishes that she knew the family enjoyed so that they could continue to make and enjoy them. In one section, she acknowledged her ambivalence about God, together with the hope that there would be some continuity beyond death so that she might know her husband and children again. When Alice died, the chaplain conducted the funeral and was joined by the local vicar from the area where Alice and her family lived. This provided an opportunity for the community clergy to relate meaningfully with the family and provide ongoing support over the months following the funeral.

In this example it is significant that the chaplain was not affronted by the negativity expressed at the first meeting, but felt able to return later and sensitively see whether they could relate, or if the patient really did not wish any further contact. Palliative care is frequently provided by members of a multiprofessional team and it is essential that there is good communication between the members of that team. The chaplain/spiritual caregiver should be a member of that team, known, respected, and trusted by them, so that each can draw on the skills of others in the best interests of the patient and family. In the case of Alice, it was important that the other members of the team did not assume the chaplain was upsetting Alice when they observed some of her angry interchanges. The ventilation and working through of fears, anxieties, and anger can be an important feature of pastoral care—as recognized in other forms of therapeutic work. It was also important that the chaplain collaborated with other members of the multiprofessional team and the appropriate faith leader in the community.

The community or home setting

Historically, pastoral care developed as part of the role of community clergy who sought to support, educate, and provide for the needs of their people in a whole range of life crises. The more specialist pastoral care in hospitals, hospices, and other institutions grew out of this background.

Christian churches and other faith groups in the United Kingdom have been providing pastoral care in the community for centuries. In the seventeenth-century *Book of Common Prayer*, for example, a specific order of service was created entitled 'The Visitation of the Sick'. This service is prefaced with the rubric: 'When any person is sick, notice shall be given thereof to the Minister of the Parish; who, coming into the sick person's house, shall say …'.

Two hundred years later, manuals for Church of England parish priests written in the early nineteenth century, as well as encouraging a sacramental ministry to the sick, exhorted clergy to carry out pastoral work with appropriate decorum:

> The assistance given by the minister to his sick parishioners should not be confined to prayer and conversation; much aid may be afforded them through books. There are many small tracts he [sic] may give away, and some larger works he may lend, when occasion calls for them (Bodemer and Gaissmaier 2015, p. 11).

This manual does not reveal what the reactions of any possible beneficiary of such earnest endeavours might have been.

Over a century later, in the 1960s, a series of influential books on the provision of pastoral care were produced. Among them were *The Pastoral Care of the Dying* (Autton 1996) written by a highly regarded hospital chaplain, and *Sick Call*, a handbook on visiting the sick for the newly ordained by Kenneth Child (1965), a former hospital chaplain and parish priest.

In the 1980s, a new series of books providing advice on pastoral care were produced. Among them was *Letting Go: Caring for the Dying and Bereaved* (Ainsworth-Smith and Speck 1982) and *Being There: Pastoral Care in Illness* (Speck 1988). While these volumes were designed as practical texts, they were addressed, significantly, not only to clergy but also to laypeople, and marked a significant shift in the perception of who actually offered pastoral care.

In 1992, Christopher Moody questioned previous pastoral role models for the clergy, the professionalism of the nineteenth century, and the counselling and community worker models of the twentieth century. While acknowledging that such models in the last decades of the twentieth century continued to exist, he nevertheless championed a view of the church, which saw its *raison d'être* as interacting with local communities, but in ways that were more culturally sensitive:

> … the contemporary situation of cultural diversity requires us to travel light … There is a great danger otherwise that we [the book is addressed to the Church] will become increasingly estranged in a cultural ghetto, sustained only by our own sense of exile, rather than reviving a sense of being on pilgrimage towards something new (Moody 1992).

Text extract reproduced from Christopher Moody, *Eccentric Ministry: Pastoral Care and Leadership in the Parish*, Darton, Longman & Todd, London, UK, Copyright © 1992, with permission from Darton, Longman & Todd.

Three years after Moody's book was published, David Stoter, then the Manager of the Chaplaincy Department and Bereavement Centre, Queen's Medical Centre, Nottingham, gave voice to a concept in pastoral care which had become increasingly popular: spirituality. He wrote:

> Spiritual care was, until recent years considered to be mainly the responsibility of the hospital chaplain or a minister of religion, priest or religious leader and requests for help were usually referred to the appropriate person for attention, and the matter was then thankfully left in their hands ... Things are now changing radically, however, and there is currently a surge of interest in caring for the whole person and looking after their physical, emotional, social and spiritual needs (Stoter 1995).

This echoes earlier work, which differentiated spirituality from religion, while recognizing their interrelatedness (Speck 1988). It is interesting to note the delightful tension between the job description of the chaplain as 'manager' (a word which can conjure up a mechanistic, task-orientated occupation) and the content of the book, which emphasizes the necessity for a truly holistic, patient-centred approach to pastoral care.

> Healing ... [is] concerned with whatever is happening within the person who is in the process of being cured, or who is beginning the journey of coming to terms with deteriorating health or with the prospect of death. Healing is about journeying towards wholeness of mind, body and spirit as an entirety (Stoter 1995).

Spiritual care, a central theme of Stoter's book, is defined as

> '... that integrating power or force in total patient care which signals the overwhelming need to recognise the person who is suffering and, by extension, to recognise the suffering in family, among friends and indeed for the professionals involved as well' (Stoter 1995).

In such a scenario, the key component is the creation of good partnerships between everyone involved in the accompaniment of the patient on his or her 'journey'.

A similar concern is articulated in the work of Professor John Swinton and Dr Harriet Mowat, albeit about spiritual care in dementia, but echoes much thinking about spiritual care in wider settings. They write:

> Spiritual care is driven by a belief that life is purposeful and that shared human experiences and relationships is one vital way of living with purpose in the midst of a very difficult condition. Spiritual care implies that we are all the same; we need meaning and purpose in our lives ... [t]he Spiritual task is to offer friendship, comfort and hope to each other in ways that are **meaningful to the individuals** concerned (Swinton and Mowat 2014, p. 10).

This very brief survey of the literature surrounding Christian pastoral care, from the sixteenth to the twenty-first century, reveals that the language brought to our understanding of care is constantly changing, influenced deeply by culture and context. The major metaphors of the sixteenth century, for instance, were about illness as God's 'visitation' in which sickness was seen as being for the trying of patience, for an example to others, for the testing of faith or as a sign that things needed to be corrected. In the twentieth century the metaphors changed; the notion of sickness as a journey, a pathway, or a pilgrimage became paramount. In the twenty-first century, one of the most recent Christian liturgical expressions of how sickness is understood includes the word 'wholeness'. The title of these services is 'A Celebration of Wholeness and Healing' (Common Worship 2000), but while it focuses on the needs of the individual, it also points out that prayer for healing ... *needs to take seriously the way in which individual sickness and vulnerability are often the result of injustice and social oppression* (Common Worship 2000). In brief, then, the language used to describe sickness and pastoral reactions to it, and the struggle to discern whether or not any sickness might have some kind of moral purpose or outcome, has undoubtedly changed across the centuries in the United Kingdom. However, the central questions for the patient, as has been argued at the beginning of this chapter, have remained essentially the same: 'Is there any purpose?' 'What is my destiny?' 'What am I here for?' 'Is hope of any kind a chimera or a reality?'

In a hospital setting, these questions can be very sharp, not least because the normal mundane matters of getting on with life are suddenly stripped away. In these circumstances, the sensitivity of chaplains and all the medical staff need to be of a high order. While the questions themselves may be stark, the actual setting in which they can be addressed, the hospital ward, for example, may not be immediately conducive to the patient opening up his or her soul to someone who will listen. But it is the quality of listening which is absolutely vital; giving serious, uncluttered attention to the patient is so important. Within many hospitals, the staff and patients come from a variety of ethnic and faith backgrounds. Pastoral care has been a mainly Christian understanding; however, other faith leaders have begun to widen their religious and teaching role in order to offer wider support to their people who are sick. Rabbis, Imams and others have recognized a need to listen to, and support, patients who are asking deep questions arising out of their experience of illness. To this end, many non-Christian faith leaders are joining chaplaincy teams and attending training courses to develop skills in this aspect of care.

Unfortunately, this kind of attentive listening seems to be in short supply across the professions. If I (CH) may be anecdotal for a moment, I recently visited a friend in hospital. The nurse came to the bedside to take blood pressure and temperature readings. The equipment used was state-of-the-art, but the nurse gave the patient not a single moment of attention. Not a single word was exchanged. The eyes of my friend pleaded for attention but the nurse, not having looked at the patient, did not register the unspoken questions. It was pitiful—but apparently not untypical in that particular hospital.

Communication skills begin not at 'skills' level but much deeper, with the basic attitude of one human being to another. The message, unspoken but of intense power, which the nurse gave to my friend was that she did not matter. It was very hurtful. If the attitude is wrong, then clearly real communication is going to be difficult. Had the nurse actually given the patient undivided attention, even if only briefly, the levels of stress would have been alleviated.

The setting where this event happened was in an orthopaedic ward; how much more sensitivity is required when the patient is receiving palliative care. Then total and compassionate attention will be among the most important gifts to be offered. Following the Francis report into the lack of care for some patients at the Mid-Staffordshire NHS Foundation Trust (Francis 2010), compassion and communication are now buzzwords within healthcare.

The best forms of pastoral care, therefore, require the caregiver to regard the other person as having absolute worth and to give that person absolute attention. Vilalta *et al.* (2014) suggest being recognized and valued as a person is the foundation requires us:

- to listen deeply, not only to what is said, but also to what is unsaid;
- to discern when it is right to keep silence, and not talk endlessly to the patient;

◆ to discern when it is right to speak, and what might or might not be said.

This can sometimes be easier in the context of the person's own home, without some of the distractions or interruptions that can occur in the busy inpatient unit.

If pastoral care and communication skills are thought of as being like a quarry face in which various geological layers are exposed, the bottom layer should be the largest one, that is, the basic attitude towards the other person; above that lies the layer of listening with attention; then should come the ability to judge when silence is best; and only near the top should words themselves feature. Where such layered communication skills are exercised and where the fundamental attitude towards the patient is one in which that patient's human value is treated with absolute respect, as happens in many hospices, then true pastoral care and deep human learning can and does take place—and the effect on patients, staff, and patients' families can be transformative.

At the heart of the pastoral encounter is the sense of 'presence', which has been captured well in the writings of Nolan (2011) who has identified four developmental moments, or ways, in which the pastor may be present with the patient. The arrival of the chaplain, whose uniform often indicates a particular faith perspective, triggers an *evocative* presence in which the patient may respond in a welcoming or dismissive way. How the chaplain responds is important if the encounter is to continue and enable the second *accompanying* presence to develop. This requires an ability to 'be with' the patient and for the encounter to move into that of the *comforting* presence. Nolan states that:

Typically, chaplains build trusting relationships in which existentially urgent questions may be asked and given honest, occasionally unorthodox, replies that allow the patient to find their own authority and satisfying answers. Equally typical is the chaplain's preparedness to remain with the authenticity of the patient's experience, often in a place beyond where words are effective (Nolan 2011, p. 24).

This can eventually lead into the chaplain becoming a *hopeful* presence, which may enable the patient to re-discover hope in their situation.

There is a paucity of quality research to describe, or evaluate, the interaction between chaplains and patients. A recent Cochrane Review highlights the need for better quality research to inform best practice (Candy *et al.* 2012). While Nolan offers a helpful intervention model that may assist chaplains/pastoral care givers, he also acknowledges that the study drew on the experience of chaplains alone, and needs to be explored further to gain a patient perspective.

Conclusion

Pastoral care, wherever it is offered, requires the caregiver to focus on, and relate to, the whole person who is before them. It is to be distinguished from counselling since the encounter takes place within the context of a belief system held by the pastoral carer, and which may or may not be shared by the recipient of care. The essence of the communication is the creation of a safe space within which the person can explore such issues as: personal worth and value; the possible purpose of what is being experienced; the

opportunity to access strength and power to rise above (transcend) the here and now experience, thereby sustaining hope in a future. Being a recipient of palliative care is but one life event for which pastoral care can be a resource, complementary to other aspects of care, and requiring careful attention to the sensitive use of communication skills.

Acknowledgements

Text extracts from Stoter D, *Spiritual Aspects of Health Care*, Mosby, London, UK, Copyright © 1995 reprinted with permission from Elsevier.

Text extract reproduced from Swinton J and Mowat H, *What is spiritual care?*, The Purple Bicycle Project, University of Aberdeen, UK, Copyright © 2014, with permission of the authors.

References

Ainsworth-Smith I, Speck P (1982). *Letting Go: Caring for the Dying and the Bereaved*. SPCK, London, UK.

Autton N (1966). *The Pastoral Care of the Dying*. SPCK, London, UK.

Candy B, Jones L, Varagunam M, Speck P, *et al.* (2012). Spiritual and religious interventions for well-being of adults in the terminal phase of disease. *Cochrane Database Syst Rev* **5**, CD007544. DOI:10.1002/14651858.

Child K (1965). *Sick Call: A Book on the Pastoral Care of the Physically Ill*. SPCK, London, UK.

Cobb M (2005). *The Hospital Chaplain's Handbook: A Guide For Good Practice*. Canterbury Press, Norwich, UK.

Common Worship: Pastoral Services (2000). Wholeness and Healing. pp. 8-99. Church House Publishing, London, UK.

Elder Brother (1882). *A Manual for the Parish Priest, being a few hints on the pastoral care, to the younger clergy of the Church of England; from an elder brother*. 2nd edition. FC & J Rivington, London, UK.

Francis R (2010). *Independent Inquiry into Care Provided by Mid-Staffordshire NHS Foundation Trust. January 2005–March 2009*. HMSO, London, UK.

Moody C (1992). *Eccentric Ministry: Pastoral Care and Leadership in the Parish*. Darton, Longman & Todd, London, UK. pp. 130–1.

Nolan S (2011). Hope beyond (redundant) hope: how chaplains work with dying people. *Palliat Med* **25**, 21–5.

NICE: National Institute for Clinical Excellence (2004). *Improving Supportive and Palliative Care for Adults with Cancer*. Available at: https://www.nice.org.uk [Online].

Speck P (1988). *Being There: Pastoral Care in Time of Illness*. SPCK, London, UK.

Speck P (2003). Spiritual/religious issues in care of the dying. In: Ellershaw J, Wilkinson S (eds). *Care of the Dying: A Pathway to Excellence*. Oxford University Press, Oxford, UK.

Speck P (2004). Spiritual issues in palliative care. In: Doyle D, Hanks G, MacDonald N (eds). *Oxford Textbook of Palliative Care*, 2nd edition. Oxford University Press, Oxford, UK.

Stoter D (1995). *Spiritual Aspects of Health Care*. Mosby, London, UK.

Swinton J, Mowat H (2014). What is spiritual care? *The Purple Bicycle Project* University of Aberdeen. Available at: https://www.ac.uk/sdhp/purple-bicycle-project-538.php [Online].

Vilalta A, Valls J, Porta J, Viñas J (2014). Evaluation of spiritual needs of patients with advanced cancer in a palliative care unit. *J Palliat Med* **17**, 21–5.

CHAPTER 51

Communication in oncology pharmacy: The challenge of treatment adherence

Bethan Tranter and Simon Noble

Introduction to communication in oncology pharmacy

As with other professions, pharmacists have experienced a change from traditional drug-oriented services, including distribution and preparation, towards patient-oriented services (Liekweg *et al.* 2004). Many professional organizations and societies believe that pharmacists have a pivotal role in the provision of information in oncology, hospice, and palliative care; that pharmacists should be integral members of interdisciplinary teams (Lipman 2002). High-quality cancer care requires both traditional and expanded pharmacist and pharmacy technician activities, including a variety of leadership, clinical, educational, administrative, and support responsibilities. In this chapter, we describe the pharmacy professions' roles and responsibilities in the provision of care to patients with cancer, with a particular emphasis on communication and the promotion of patients' treatment adherence.

Professional knowledge and skills

Pharmacy staff practising oncology and palliative care require a broad, integrated knowledge, and a strong commitment to optimally meet patients' needs. The scope of this knowledge extends far beyond that of pharmaceutical knowledge and covers a breadth of field from the laboratory to the bedside and even the wider societal population (CAPHO 2009).

The skills required of an oncology pharmacist are likewise considerable and include good communication, collaboration, problem identification, and resolution. As lifelong learners, pharmacists will need to develop the analytic skills necessary to evaluate evidence through systematic and critical analysis. Subsequent reflection on the data will facilitate problem solving in daily practice, as well as enhancing their ability to make informed decisions based on the strongest evidence. Use of retrieval techniques to access necessary information is vital. In communicating information about medications, pharmacists need to structure the material in systematic categories, avoid jargon, and carefully go through the rationale, dose, mode and timing of administration and potential side effects for each medication (CAPHO 2009). Pharmacy staff need to be part of the multidisciplinary team with strong professional relationships to ensure a cohesive patient-focused approach to care. Thus pharmacists and pharmacy technicians are responsible for their continuing competence in this specialty practice area.

Pharmaceutical care

It is well accepted that the professions have made the paradigm shift from traditional distribution services towards patient-oriented and clinical pharmacy services, which for oncology include central services for compounding systemic anti-cancer therapies.

In 1990, in recognition of the numerous risks to patients associated with complex and multiple medication therapies, Hepler and Strand introduced the concept of 'pharmaceutical care' to advance the development of the profession and improve patient safety (Liekweg *et al.* 2004). Pharmaceutical care is defined as the 'direct, responsible provision of drug therapy for the purpose of achieving definite outcomes that improve a patient's quality of life' (Lipman 2002). It continues to be considered best practice today and sits alongside the newer concept of medicines optimization (NICE 2015).

Medicines optimization, like pharmaceutical care, is a patient-focused approach to improving the outcomes that patients achieve from their medicines. Decisions are made jointly between patients and healthcare professionals, using the best available evidence and taking into account the individual's needs and wishes. Within oncology, given the side effects profile of most of the systemic anti-cancer therapy (SACT) agents, the focus needs to be on maintaining a patient's quality of life, during and after chemotherapy, while balancing the likelihood and duration of disease response. Consequently, patients need to be offered an appropriately indicated, effective, safe, and convenient drug therapy. To limit therapy-associated toxicity, supportive care has become an integral part of anti-cancer systemic therapy with many supportive care medications prescribed prophylactically. Meanwhile, in the palliative setting, medication therapy is the cornerstone of most symptom control management. Hence the role of the pharmacy team in educating and supporting patients within these settings is fundamental.

The care process

Pharmaceutical care can be structured according to the SOAP method, in which **S**ubjective information and **O**bjective parameters for the patient are **A**nalysed to create an individual care **P**lan.

In collaboration with the prescribing physician and the patient, the goals of the individual's drug therapy are defined and added to the plan. To ensure continuous review of the care plan, regular appointments with the pharmacist are established throughout treatment. This plan needs to be re-evaluated and adjusted according to the patients' response and needs (Liekweg *et al.* 2004).

Treatment of a cancer patient is complex and the selection of therapy—chemotherapy, hormone, and other therapies—belongs to the prescribing physician in consultation and agreement with the patient. The medication record, if complete, provides an overview of the drug history of the patient and is required to discern the patient's situation. For this reason, it is quite appropriate that the oncology pharmacist takes a medication history from the oncology patient (CAPHO 2009). A comprehensive medication history should contain information relating to:

- adverse drug reactions, including allergies;
- past and currently prescribed medication therapy, including the names of the medications, doses, frequency of administration, indications and duration of therapies;
- non-prescription medication use;
- alternative or complimentary therapies being used;
- compliance issues;
- details of prescribers of medication and where dispensed (CAPHO 2009, p. 38).

The oncology pharmacist also has a key role in the prevention, identification, and resolution of drug-related problems. These may include

- taking medicines that are not indicated;
- lack of anticipatory prescribing of supportive drugs needed for predictable toxicities;
- receiving incorrect doses of medication;
- taking an inappropriate dose of an indicated medication;
- experiencing an adverse drug reaction or interaction;
- poor compliance for whatever reason;
- failure to fill a prescription due to lack of money;
- drug dependency (CAPHO 2009, p. 38).

A number of these problems can be detected just from reviewing the patient health record. This information provides a realistic picture and assessment of the patient.

Pharmaceutical care in oncology is a continuous process. The oncology pharmacist should evaluate the patient throughout their cancer journey for the development of drug-related issues or difficulties. In particular, they should assess:

- response to treatment including symptom control medicines;
- drug-related adverse events with particular attention to life-threatening of serious chemotherapy related toxicities;
- changes in the patient's clinical condition that may require dosage adjustment (e.g. changes in absorption, drug transport of weight adjusted dose);
- changes in clinical condition that necessitates discontinuation of therapy;
- patient hospitalization (CAPHO 2009, p. 38).

Target populations for pharmaceutical care

As a consequence of limited resources, it is unlikely that pharmacists will be able to provide pharmaceutical care to all oncology and palliative care patients. Those patients with complex drug regimens, chronic diseases, and who need to be frequently hospitalized, benefit most from pharmaceutical care. These characteristics apply to many oncology patients (Liekweg *et al.* 200). Patients most likely to benefit from pharmaceutical care include (CAPHO 2009):

- patients with drug absorption difficulties;
- those with hepatic or renal insufficiency that may affect chemotherapy drug metabolism or elimination;
- patients with other co-morbidities which may impact on chemotherapy dosing such as renal, hepatic, or cardiac impairment;
- patients with other co-morbidities, which may be affected by chemotherapy;
- patients receiving significant polypharmacy for non-cancer indications;
- patients on drugs commonly associated with drug–drug interactions with oncology medications;
- patients on drugs with a narrow therapeutic window;
- patients receiving drugs within a clinical trial setting;
- patients receiving medication in doses outside those recommended for their licensed indication (CAPHO 2009, p. 37).

Communication to achieve seamless pharmaceutical care

In the ambulatory setting, the continuous monitoring of medication use is helpful, given the number of medical practitioners that cancer patients tend to see (Liekweg *et al.* 2004). Seamless pharmaceutical care helps when patients are transferred from one clinical service or setting to another. When a cancer patient is discharged from the hospital or ambulatory care facility to the community, the oncology pharmacist should ensure a medication summary is provided, as well as communicating with primary care practitioners about any specific outcomes they need to be aware of. Electronic linkages facilitate this communication via an electronic health record. Through good communication, it is hoped that there will be improved seamless care, fewer adverse drug events, and improved overall experience and outcomes for the patient (CAPHO 2009).

The multidisciplinary team—a triangle of care

Good working relationships with physicians, allied healthcare providers, nurses, and community healthcare providers are fundamental. Sharing information appropriately ensures patient safety and optimal treatment outcomes. A fundamental feature is that pharmacists accept responsibility for the patient's pharmacotherapeutic outcome alongside physicians. This ensures that the patient and their medication needs are at the apex and the main focus of these efforts (Liekweg *et al.* 2004).

In oncology, the goal of treatment is either cure or slowing disease progression, while palliating symptoms and reducing the incidence of adverse effects, organ toxicity, and drug resistance (Liekweg *et al.* 2004). Ideally a site-specific pharmacist dedicated to particular tumour types will facilitate this focus. The specific practice of pharmacists on healthcare teams can be defined within a scope-of-practice document or a similar tool or protocol developed by the healthcare organization. This document can include referral and communication guidelines, including the documentation of patient encounters and the methods and processes for sharing patient information with appropriate members of the multidisciplinary team (Lipman 2002). The visible presence of pharmacists during inpatient care rounds and close by ambulatory clinics, in interdisciplinary team conferences and in informal discussions, is vital (CAPHO 2009).

Alongside other healthcare professions, oncology pharmacists are now practicing as independent prescribers. Independent prescribers are responsible for the patients in their care and will work closely with the patient's physician and other team members to ensure good quality care and an excellent patient experience. Roles vary across organizations, with pharmacists typically reviewing patients prior to their next treatment cycle, assessing the patient for drug therapy-related toxicities, making dose adjustments and prescribing supportive care as necessary (NLIAH 2012).

Medication safety and quality

SACT are well established as being high-risk medicines in terms of patient safety. The widely reported incidents involving the incorrect administration of vincristine have acted as learning tools across medical, nursing, and pharmacy professions alike and highlight the importance of multidisciplinary roles within the patient safety arena (NPSA 2008). In 2010, a themed analysis of patient safety incidents involving anti-cancer medicines over five years was published. Out of nearly 5,000 reported incidents, 25 were recorded as resulting in death, and serious or moderate patient harm. The report made a number of recommendations to include the necessary processes and procedures to facilitate the correct prescribing, monitoring, and administering of SACTs, which are still considered best practice (NPSA 2010).

Over time, cancer chemotherapy has evolved from being delivered primarily in inpatient settings to outpatient clinics because of greater convenience and lower cost. Each organization should establish a minimum acceptable level of pharmacist responsibility for outpatients. This should include prospectively reviewing orders, screening laboratory test results, providing drug information and counselling patients. Investigational drug protocols should only be initiated at sites where comprehensive pharmaceutical services are available (Cohen 2007).

The generally narrow therapeutic range of anti-cancer drugs means a particular risk for the patient with respect to drug safety. Institutions should establish dosage limits for anti-neoplastic agents, set up dose-verification procedures that stress multiple independent checks, and work to standardize the prescribing vocabulary (Cohen et al. 1996). The use of validated electronic prescribing systems for SACT is similarly considered a core standard. Pharmacists have a key role within their implementation, ensuring that SACT regimens and technical pharmacy aspects are configured as per local practice. Organizations should consider the introduction of electronic prescribing systems as essential to support safe services (NPSA 2010). Hiring specific 'safety pharmacists' ensures that safety checks and quality system processes are incorporated into all pharmacy procedures. The ultimate focus of any medication safety pharmacist is the safety of each individual patient (Turple 2008).

Poor communication among physicians, pharmacists, nurses, and other healthcare providers can lead to medication errors. Alert and knowledgeable patients who know that they can contact a pharmacist for advice can be the last line of defence against medication errors. Failure to heed patient concerns has led to serious errors, which could have been prevented (Cohen 2007). All healthcare providers should cooperate in identifying potential problems and solutions. Multidisciplinary discussions should take place after a medication error and routinely as part of quality improvement efforts. If caregivers work together as a team, most errors can be contained. A system of reporting all errors ensures that practitioners learn from their mistakes; each error should be reviewed by a multidisciplinary team with the ultimate goal of system-wide improvements (Cohen 2007).

Treatment guidelines and evidence-based care

Clinical practice guidelines (CPGs) provide evidence-based recommendations regarding the treatment of different diseases and symptoms. Proper selection and application of the guidelines require an understanding of their purpose, rationale, development methods, critical evaluation, potential implementation strategies, and their limitations.

The implementation of CPGs can contribute to improving patients' quality of life and can reduce unnecessary drug costs (Liekweg et al. 2004). CPGs, especially those of high quality, are a key component in a practice model that integrates evidence with clinical expertise and the patient's values (Gaebelein and Gleason 2007). Therapeutic or CPGs involving medications should be elaborated through a multidisciplinary team approach with physicians, pharmacists, and other healthcare professionals. However, no matter how CPGs are developed, they are meant to be a guide to healthcare decisions and not dictate them.

Many potential barriers exist that preclude oncology practitioners from implementing such recommendations into their practice. These barriers include:

- lack of familiarity or awareness that a CPG exists;
- disagreement with the guideline recommendations;
- fear of cookbook medicine and loss of autonomy;
- time constraints or lack of personnel to implement the CPGs effectively;
- lack of input into CPGs during their development or adaptation for use.

To overcome the first barrier—a lack of familiarity and awareness—the pharmacist must make every effort to be familiar with available CPGs and where to locate them. Various sources exist, including peer-reviewed journals, which are searchable through MEDLINE, EMBASE, Google, or Yahoo.

In the event that oncologists are unaware of particular CPGs, strategies such as academic detailing (a process by which the pharmacist visits a physician to provide a 10 to 15-minute educational intervention on a specific topic) or in-service education should be instituted. Algorithms outlining specific treatment protocols should be made easily accessible, so that physicians can consult them while providing care.

When a physician disagrees with a guideline recommendation, the pharmacist could locate, evaluate, and share the evidence that supports the improvement in patient outcomes or lowering of the cost. For instance, Dranitsaris *et al.* showed prospectively that implementation of evidence-based anti-emetic guidelines, with the support of pharmacists, promoted more clinically appropriate use of 5-HT3 antagonists, which improved patient care, outcomes and reduced costs (Liekweg *et al.* 2004). While there is great uniformity in the CPGs developed to date, there is more diversity in the specifics of the clinical pathways that can be used to realize a guideline. Clinical pathways, such as specific chemotherapy regimens, drug doses, and schedules, schedules for imaging studies and follow-up parameters, provide a more comprehensive approach to patient management.

Direct patient care consultations and counselling

Oncology pharmacists should be available for the patients, families, and other healthcare professionals within both the inpatient and outpatient setting. These consultations typically involve information gathering with particular focus on medication history, evaluation of medications being taken or initiated, and patient education. The communication of educational information throughout anti-cancer therapy includes side effect counselling and management, and proper handling techniques. With a growing armoury of oral anti-cancer medicines being licensed, community pharmacies will become frequently involved in the dispensing of such medicines. The skills noted above are equally as valid for oral anti-cancer medicines and as such the community pharmacist shares equal responsibility with the oncology pharmacist to ensure that no matter where a patient receives their medication, they have the same standard of care.

Cancer chemotherapy drugs have a considerable risk of toxicity and patients should be made aware of anticipated side effects as well as serious toxicities, which would necessitate medical assessment. It is recommended that a specialist pharmacist review all oncology patients at least once (CAPHO 2009). Consultations should aim to address any anxieties patients may have by providing understandable and relevant information about their medicines, including advice on how to prevent and manage recognized side effects (CAPHO 2009). In doing this, the pharmacist must be mindful that the patient will receive the information within the context and anxieties which surround their overall cancer journey. They must therefore be sensitive to the patients' emotions and provide empathic support as the conversation unfolds. Discretion is important in discussing adverse events—ask the patient how much information they desire and tailor the content to each individual's needs. The goal is to adequately educate patients to render treatment safe, without creating fear.

Wherever possible, verbal information may be supported by additional communication aids including written information, and visual aids such as charts, DVDs, or website details. The ideal information leaflet will contain written information which should cover the following details of each medicine:

♦ The medication's name, its dose, and what it is for (specific to the patient's treatment regimen);
♦ How it should be stored;
♦ How it should be taken and for how long;

♦ Potential side effects;
♦ What to do if they forget to take a dose;
♦ How to minimize potential adverse events;
♦ Potential interactions with:
  • other drugs
  • foods
  • over the counter supplements and herbal medicines
♦ When to seek emergency medical care;
♦ Any other information regarding access or coverage of the medication (CAPHO 2009, p. 40).

In the event that the patient is receiving cancer chemotherapy in the home using ambulatory infusion pumps, they should be informed of procedures for handling cytotoxics and waste products, and made aware of the expected length of the infusion. In addition, home spill kits should be provided to these patients (CAPHO 2009).

A follow-up meeting or telephone consultation is often beneficial and a way to evaluate the impact of medication counselling on the patient's knowledge and understanding. This also provides an opportunity, if required, to reinforce important information. All medication consultations should be documented by the pharmacist in each patient's health record (CAPHO 2009). With new oral anti-cancer therapies, the pharmacy team are ideally placed to take lead roles in not only patient education, but also by undertaking remote reviews of biochemical monitoring parameters and assessing patients' SACT-related toxicities via a telephone assessment to determine suitability of treatment continuation. Such a service can be considered to maximize the multidisciplinary team's skill mix, as well as improving job satisfaction and patient experience of those involved.

Medication order review (triage)

Whenever medication is to be dispensed, the pharmacist should verify the outgoing drugs against the treatment protocol, the patient's medication history, and past medical history. If no treatment protocol exists, it is recommended the pharmacist check the prescription against two independent literature sources (CAPHO 2009, p. 16).

The oncology pharmacist should check the following:

♦ the patient's name, diagnosis, and unique identification details (e.g. hospital number and date of birth);
♦ history of drug allergy and adverse events;
♦ weight, height, and body surface area for all chemotherapy patients;
♦ prescriber signature (written or electronic);
♦ serum blood values necessary for safe drug prescribing (e.g. full blood count, electrolytes and liver function tests and dose modifications where needed);
♦ the name of the medication, formulary status, and chemotherapy protocol;
♦ drug dosage, number of planned doses/cycles, and interval between doses;
♦ mode, frequency of administration, and complete directions for use;

- planned stop date, dependent on treatment duration;
- cumulative doses of selected drugs;
- when and by whom prescription was written;
- when treatment is planned;
- compatibility of drug with any co-morbidities (e.g. renal, cardiac, or hepatic disease);
- significant interactions of medicines with other drugs, food, or any self-medications (e.g. herbal or complementary therapies);
- planned use of supportive therapies (e.g. anti-emetics, hydration, and so on);
- ensure any medicines planned for home use are charted (e.g. oral chemotherapy, corticosteroids, anti-emetics, haematopoietic-stimulating factors);
- for parenteral drugs: correct intravenous fluid, volume concentration, and drug stability;
- if drug is part of a clinical trial: name of drug regime, trial protocol, and patient identification numbers (CAPHO 2009, pp. 16–17).

Time may be needed to resolve any questions regarding the chemotherapy order with the prescriber and document the resolution in the patient's health record. Telephone or verbal orders for chemotherapy should not be allowed or accepted (CAPHO 2009). Effective and comprehensive medication order review can detect potential medication errors and ensures increased patient safety.

Medication use evaluation

The aims of medication use evaluation (MUE) is to ensure the best possible patient outcomes and quality of life through alignment with the overarching objectives of drug use evaluation (DUE). The ongoing evaluation of medications should be a coordinated process between medical and pharmacological committees (e.g. Oncology Drug Advisory Committee (or equivalent) and/or the Pharmacy and Therapeutics committee). Ideally, the amalgamation of such committees at a local level will ensure seamless and consistent practice (CAPHO 2009). In the past decade, DUEs have been focused on expensive and new chemotherapy agents. MUE involves the following:

- the promotion of optimal therapy through the development of criteria for the use of specific cancer drugs;
- evaluation of approved oncology drugs against predetermined criteria;
- identification of problem areas (e.g. overuse of expensive anti-emetics);
- promotion of appropriate drug use through education programmes and subsequent evaluation of their impact on practice;
- compliance with recognized quality standards, such as professional practice regulations, legal requirements, and local accreditation programmes.

Results of DUEs should be communicated to the MUE team or programme, and any problems identified should be resolved. The frequency of evaluation depends on the need and economic impact (CAPHO 2009).

Research initiatives

Initiation of, and participation in, clinical and/or health services research is appropriate for the oncology pharmacist's practice. Such research improves the knowledge base and expertise of oncology pharmacy practice (CAPHO 2009). To facilitate research initiatives, it is useful to have working knowledge research methodology and be able to evaluate the current literature. Dissemination of outcomes through the presentation and/or publication of results are an integral component of the research process (CAPHO 2009). In a well-designed clinical trial, the oncology pharmacist will be an integral member of the trial management group and should have a working knowledge of all aspects including trial design, approval, and implementation methodology at their practice site (CAPHO 2009).

There are specific recommendations for oncology pharmacists working in clinical environments that conduct clinical trials in therapeutic medicinal products (CTIMPs). These include:

- Following local policies and standard operating procedures (SOPs) for clinical trial management. Oncology CTIMPs may differ from other clinical trials in their expected toxicities and number of early-phase studies. Involving the pharmacist in a thorough review of each protocol is helpful, while some operational issues within the pharmacy may be undertaken by a technician.
- Confirming that, prior to administration of study medication or placebo, informed consent has been provided according to the study protocol.
- Ensure SOPs for breaking patient treatment identification codes are available where necessary.
- Provision of written information/data sheets for all drugs being evaluated within the studies.
- Maintenance of accurate records of receipt, storage, and dispensing of trial drugs provided by the institutional pharmacy.
- Use of pharmaceutical patient care model to monitor compliance, concomitant drug use, and adverse effects.
- Maintenance of easily accessible trial data and information (manual, binder, or digital).
- Participation in pharmacy societies that are associated with the relevant clinical trials consortium (CAPHO 2009, p. 42).

The enrolment of patients into clinical trials is an integral part of the most tertiary cancer centres, of which the oncology pharmacist is an essential component. Many tertiary centres will conduct a significant amount of activity in community-based sites and the pharmacist will need to ensure continuity of care between sites (CAPHO 2009). Inevitably, support of clinical trial activity will impact on the pharmacist's time. In certain centres, a formalized process through resource impact committees exists to evaluate the effect of clinical trials clinical care, education, and training.

Other specialty pharmacy practices

Paediatric oncology

The pharmacist working in a paediatric setting will face several unique challenges. First of all, paediatric oncology encompasses the care of all children below adult age. As such there will be a diverse patient group of varying physical, emotional, and physiological characteristics. Communication with a five-year-old will differ considerably to one with a fifteen-year-old patient. Furthermore, paediatric oncology raises challenges beyond the immediate toxicities, which need to be addressed in adult oncology. Consideration of long-term toxicities and late effects are of the utmost importance (CAPHO 2009). The majority of paediatric cancer patients (approximately 75%) will be cured. Consequently, issues arising from long-term survival, such as health-related quality of life and late effects like the development of second malignancies, cardiomyopathy, and endocrine dysfunction are important. In addition, it is custom and practice that wherever possible most paediatric chemotherapy is delivered within the context of a clinical trial.

It is inevitable that a child's family will be involved in their treatment and will wish to be included in all discussions, particularly when the child is below the legal age of consent. Therefore, families will be important partners with healthcare providers in ensuring paediatric cancer patients have the best possible outcomes from their medicines (CAPHO 2009). As with adults, seamless care is very important between community, clinic, and hospital settings over the course of the treatment programme. Communication between pharmacists regarding the paediatric patients care plan is crucial.

Pharmaceutical care in these children is aimed at maximizing both short and long-term outcomes. The pharmacist contributes by ensuring correct drug dosages, delivery techniques, formulations, and routes of administration. Accurate dosing is essential, particularly in the growing child. The pharmacist should ensure all drug orders are triaged according to dosing guidelines and track the cumulative doses of cytotoxics (CAPHO 2009).

The paediatric pharmacist should be aware of how parameters like age and organ function influence both acute and long-term toxicities. Dose setting also affects complications like nausea, infection, constipation, and so on. Care plans are adjusted to reflect these organ functions (CAPHO 2009).

Clinical pharmacy practice in community oncology

Cancer patients may be geographically resident in rural communities, where community oncology programmes provide treatment closer to home. Such outreach programmes may operate via the concept of 'shared care'. A cancer centre oncologist may retain overall responsibility, while care is delivered by the multidisciplinary team (family physicians, surgeons, nurses, pharmacists, and support staff) in the rural or community setting. Here the role of, and communication from, the community liaison pharmacist (who is usually at the tertiary centre) to the team in the community is crucial. He or she can be directly involved in the triage of orders, which, if electronically entered at the tertiary centre, ensures the highest level of patient safety and seamless care.

Conclusion

With the knowledge that has accumulated within their discipline, pharmacists have expanded their clinical role to offer enhanced pharmaceutical care to cancer patients. The implementation of this pharmaceutical care improves the communication between healthcare providers to enrich the function of the multidisciplinary team. Beneficial outcomes include increased treatment adherence and optimal care for patients, with ultimately satisfaction enjoyed by the whole healthcare system.

References

Canadian Association for Pharmacy in Oncology (2009). Standards of Practice for Oncology in Canada, Version 2 1–55. Available at: https://www.capho.org [Online].

Cohen MR (2007). Preventing medication errors in cancer chemotherapy. In: Cohen MR. *Medication Errors*, 2nd edition. American Pharmacists Association, Washington DC, WA.

Cohen MR, Anderson RW, Attilio RM, *et al.* (1996). Preventing medication errors in cancer chemotherapy. *Am J Health Syst Pharm* **53**, 737–46.

Gaebelein CJ, Gleason BL (2007). Evaluating and implementing practice guidelines. In: *Contemporary Drug Information: An Evidence-Based Approach*. Lippincott, Williams & Wilkins, New York, NY.

Liekweg A, Westfeld M, Jaehde U (2004). From oncology pharmacy to pharmaceutical care: new contributions to multidisciplinary cancer care. *Support Care Cancer* **12**, 73–9.

Lipman AG (2002). ASHP statement on the pharmacists' role in hospice and palliative care. *Am J Health Syst Pharm* **59**, 1770–3.

National Institue for Health and Care Excellence (NICE) (2015). Medicines optimisation: the safe and effective use of the best possible outcomes (NG5). Available at: http://www.nice.org.uk/guidance/ng5 [Online].

National Patient Safety Agency (NPSA) (2008). Using Vinca Alkaloid Minibags (Adults/Adolescent Units) (NPSA 2008/RRR04). Available at: http://www.npsa.nhs.uk/patientsafety/alerts-and-directives/rapidrr [Online].

National Patient Safety Agency (NPSA) (2010). A themed review of patient safety incidents involving anti-cancer medicines, November 1, 2003–June 30, 2008. Available at: http://www.nrls.npsa.nhs.uk/resources/?entryid45=75475 [Online].

NHS Wales Award Winners 2012 (2012). Available at: http://www.wales.nhs.uk/sitesplus/829/news/23413 [Online].

Turple J (2008). Practice spotlight: medication safety pharmacist. *Can J Hosp Pharm* **61**, 273–4.

CHAPTER 52

Communication challenges with the elderly

Ronald D. Adelman, Michele G. Greene, and Milagros D. Silva

Introduction to communication challenges with the elderly

With the present explosive growth of the elderly population and its extensive use of health services (Adelman *et al.* 2000), it is important to know about how physicians communicate with older patients. This chapter first highlights some distinct aspects of the physician–older patient encounter that influence communication. The authors then describe a range of communication issues that may have particular meaning for health professionals caring for older patients who are diagnosed with cancer or life-threatening disease, undergoing treatment for this, or requiring palliative care for symptom relief.

There is a controversy about when 'old age' begins; that is, nothing magical occurs at the chronologic age of 65 that marks an individual as older. The age of 65 was not derived from a biologic process; it was defined by social demographic data. Even so, the age of 65 is generally perceived as the beginning of old age. However, it is clear to gerontologists that the process of ageing starts decades earlier in life, before reaching the age of 65, and an individual's chronologic age often is not an accurate predictor of function.

If one conceptualizes the ageing population to include individuals from 65 years of age to death, old age may encompass a span of as many as 35 years or more. Thus, some gerontologists view the elderly patient population as being composed of several age cohorts: the young-old (individuals 65 to 74 years old); the middle-old (individuals 75–84 years old); and the old-old (individuals 85 years and over). Each of these age groups has its own unique historical perspective and may have different social support and psychological needs, as well as different types of medical problems. For instance, the old-old are more likely to have cognitive impairments, poorer physical health, fewer financial and social resources, and are less likely to be consumer-oriented than the young-old cohort (Adelman *et al.* 1991). In addition, the majority of older patients have below-basic literacy levels and significant problems with health literacy (Gazmararian *et al.* 2003). The combined effect of greater consumerism and a higher level of health literacy among the young-old compared to the old-old, are likely to result in different interactions with physicians. Given the heterogeneity among elderly individuals, it is difficult and, indeed, hazardous to make generalizations about older patients (Haug and Ory 1987). By utilizing geriatric assessment instruments (e.g. measuring cognitive, psychological, functional status), an older patient can be evaluated for his or her unique level of function (Extermann and Hurria 2007).

Also, with improved health status and recent more positive social perceptions of ageing, many in the field of ageing consider individuals in their sixties and early seventies to be in late middle age. Compared to younger adult patients, however, communication with the older patient is likely to be complicated by ageist attitudes, sensory deficits, cognitive impairment, functional limitations, and the frequent presence of an accompanying relative or caregiver in the medical visit.

Aspects of the physician–older patient encounter

Geriatric medicine

Older patients often have multiple medical problems that mask one another or make the treatment process for any one disease more difficult. Common diseases often present atypically in older people, yet many physicians have not been taught specific diagnostic skills for evaluating the geriatric patient. For example, classic signs of coronary artery disease, such as chest pain or shortness of breath on exertion, may be more difficult to track in an older person with severe osteoarthritis, who has trouble with ambulation.

Older patients have usually accumulated longer medical histories than younger patients. Considerable expertise is required to distinguish important and pertinent clinical problems in an initial evaluation. Many geriatricians acknowledge that it may take two or three visits to assess the geriatric patient adequately. The tasks of geriatric medicine are quite challenging; not only is it important to obtain a comprehensive medical history, but it is essential to secure a social and psychological history as well. This task can be daunting given the time constraints of contemporary medicine. To be able to access the personhood of the older patient amid all this data collection requires exemplary interpersonal skills on the part of the physician. Additionally, accessing the patient's perspective on goals of care and their wishes, including advance decision-making, is an important task of the geriatric medical encounter.

Treatment of the older patient is made more complex by the co-existence of multiple medical problems, the increased risk of adverse drug effects in older people, and the risks inherent in polypharmacy and seeing multiple physicians. Communication problems can result in adverse drug events. Mira *et al.* (2013) reported that only one-third of older patients stated their physicians asked about medications from other physicians. Moreover, complementary and alternative medicine (e.g. discussing non-vitamin supplements and massage) are infrequently discussed in older patients' medical visits (Koenig *et al.* 2012).

One of the major differences in the care of older patients is the decrease in reserve in the older patient should something go wrong. Homeostatic reserve has a much wider breadth in younger patients, compared to their older counterparts (Hazzard 1994). As some frail elderly patients may be homebound and have difficulty returning for routine follow-up office visits, evaluation of ongoing treatment, and the early recognition of new problems become much more compelling.

Finally, setting goals for treatment and care may be more challenging with the elderly patient. Many of the problems encountered in geriatric medicine cannot be solved. For example, many cancers will become chronic care issues. However, the inevitable decline of the elderly patient spells a need for balanced and realistic goals for the physician, patient, and the patient's family, or other designated healthcare proxy. As mentioned earlier, knowing the patient's wishes and establishing a dialogue that enables discussion and revision of approaches to care with time are pivotal to the rendering of holistic care.

The aggressive curing instinct that develops in medical training is not always appropriate in geriatric practice. The physician instead must be able to recognize the time at which more treatment is perhaps unjustified, and must help patients and families come to terms with this difficult reality. However, symptom relief is always critical at any stage of an older patient's illness. Palliative care encompasses symptom relief for any stage of illness; that is, strategies to relieve multidimensional symptoms from chronic illness, from life-prolonging therapy such as radiation and chemotherapy, as well as for symptoms at the end of life. Acceptance of death and skills in helping a patient die comfortably, and attend to the affected significant others, are prerequisites for the physician caring for older patients. These abilities require special insight, self-awareness, and training and will be discussed in greater detail later in this chapter.

Attitudes toward age and ageing

Ageism, defined as the system of destructive false beliefs about older people, is one of the last 'isms' to be acceptable in Western society. It is pervasive in the medical care system (Greene *et al.* 1986). In a qualitative study, Higashi *et al.* (2012) identified physicians'-in-training perspectives on elderly patients. They stated that caring for older patients was 'frustrating' and 'boring' and that social work more than medical care was needed.

Ageism in the medical encounter may result in the disregard of medical problems of older people and inappropriate misattributing their problems to 'normal' ageing (Greene *et al.* 1987). Physicians may be less likely to recommend preventive regimens or treat medical problems or psychiatric problems aggressively when the patient is older (Greenfield *et al.* 1981; Cobbs *et al.* 1999). Some physicians spend less time with older patients or may be inattentive to older patients. Physicians may consider elderly patients more 'difficult' to deal with than their younger counterparts (Adelman *et al.* 1991).

The origins of ageist beliefs are multifactorial. Our fears of our own ageing and death, a subject still taboo in many societies, play a major role in the development of ageist attitudes. In Western societies, preoccupied with productivity and youth, fears of obsolescence, and physical and mental losses foster an ageist perspective. Distinct from other 'isms', such as sexism and racism, ageism has a dangerously personal focus; we all become old—that is, if we are fortunate enough to survive. If an individual has become old and has incorporated significant dislike for ageing or older people, this older person then becomes the object of his or her own discrimination. This self-directed prejudice has ominous implications for successful ageing; that is, older people themselves may be ignorant about normal ageing or have preconceived ageist attitudes that affect medical care. For example, when an older individual believes that depression or impaired memory is part of normal ageing, s/he will not readily seek medical attention, and possible treatment will not be pursued.

Ageist bias is relevant especially in the context of medical care, as these attitudes may cause health providers and patients to discount or deny needs for care. It may be that healthcare professionals are more susceptible than the layperson to the development of ageist attitudes (Greene *et al.* 1986). By definition of their work, physician trainees are primarily exposed to the most vulnerable elderly populations: the ill, the frail, the confused, the demented, and the hospitalized. Robust older people are generally not in the patient sample they are exposed to. Ageism, therefore, may be an occupational hazard of the health professional and can undermine medical care. For example, one study documented how older women with breast cancer are treated less aggressively than their younger counterparts (Greenfield *et al.* 1981). Still, little is known about how subtle negativism about older patients by health providers' influences their medical care.

Sensory deficits

Hearing is obviously an important component of communication. Presbycusis, or decreased hearing of higher frequency sounds, is one of the most common and significant sensory changes that affect older people. The incidence of sensorineural hearing loss increases each decade so that by the seventh and eighth decades 70–80% of older adults are affected (Cobbs *et al.* 1999). This prevalence makes hearing loss a significant factor to address in older patient–physician communication. In the office setting, amplification with a microphone and headset can enhance communication. Establishing good visual contact, reducing background noise (as listening is more difficult with competing sounds), rephrasing rather than repeating misunderstood phrases, and pausing at the end of a topic may also facilitate communication. To optimize verbal communication, it is helpful for the physician to stand two to three feet away from the patient and to speak at normal to slightly louder levels (Cobbs *et al.* 1999). Hearing loss is an important predictor of function for older people, with far greater implications than the immediate inability to communicate in the medical encounter. Recognition and discussion of this fact in the medical visit are important elements of comprehensive geriatric care. For those older patients who use hearing aids, it is important to remind patients to always wear them to medical visits. Perhaps, most importantly, the physician should ask the patient the best strategies for communicating within the clinical setting.

Vision loss also has a considerable impact on patient–physician interaction, because visual dues are vital in communication. After the age of 65, there is a decrease in visual acuity, contrast sensitivity, glare intolerance, and visual fields. Older patients who experience visual loss are twice as likely to have difficulty with basic activities of daily living (ADL) and instrumental ADLs, as compared with those who have normal vision (Cobbs *et al.* 1999). Because a large percentage of elderly people are visually compromised, effective communication strategies for these individuals need to be addressed in the medical visit. Sitting close to the older patient with visual loss is one such strategy. The medical office can help compensate for visual loss through environmental supports, such as improved illumination, and the use of contrasting colours in décor and signage. Also, paying attention to the size of print in patient information handouts or any other communication, such as appointment cards and letters, can make a significant difference for the visually impaired older patient.

Functional deficits

Many older patients have functional limitations and problems with basic and instrumental ADL. These limitations may make the logistics of a medical consultation difficult (e.g. getting to the room, moving from chair to examination table, and so on). Indeed, in a healthcare system where domiciliary visits are not undertaken, these frail older patients may be seen so infrequently that visits to the doctor are emotionally and physically taxing, and the patient may have generated an extensive agenda to be addressed during the visit.

Allowance for functional deficits may extend the duration of the medical encounter (i.e. helping the patient move onto an examination table, or assisting with undressing and dressing). Few consulting rooms are equipped with appropriate equipment to help patients manoeuvring in a small examining room and there is little research that examines whether and how physicians make allowances for functional deficits. Yet, it is clear that those patients with functional deficits, who visit the doctor unaccompanied, do require special provision from the service.

By contrast, when a domiciliary visit is undertaken, a great deal of information can be gleaned from seeing the patient's home and how she or he lives and functions there.

Cognitive impairment

A common myth about old age is that ageing is synonymous with cognitive decline. The incidence of dementia among older people in their sixties is low (e.g. the rate of moderate to severe dementia is about 2% among persons 65–69 years of age); however, the incidence of cognitive dysfunction progressively increases with age (Costa *et al.* 1996).

There is a broad range of cognitive loss among individuals with dementia and unless the physician is trained to uncover this problem, it can be missed in those patients with mild or even moderate loss. Obtaining an accurate assessment of the patient's cognitive status is essential to assure optimal communication and medical treatment. At times, geriatricians perform a brief mental status examination as part of an initial assessment. As most patients are sensitive about such testing, it is imperative to prepare the patient before performing the examination. Stating that these tests are performed for all patients or, 'it's only a screen, don't worry about getting the answers correct' can be reassuring. Incorporating the mental status examination into the physical examination so that these questions appear as a routine part of the neurological examination may make the test less threatening for the older patient.

If a patient has some cognitive impairment, the physician's approach to the older patient must be modified. Unfortunately, some health providers falsely assume that a diagnosis of mild cognitive impairment or dementia means that the patient's capacity is impaired in all dimensions of human intellect, emotion, and behaviour. This might be termed 'dementiaism'; that is, inappropriately stereotyping patients with any cognitive impairment as being incompetent and incapable of participating in their care (Adelman *et al.* 1991). All dementias are not the same: major differences exist between mild and severe dementias, and the type and range of losses among individuals varies widely. Each patient with mild cognitive impairment (MCI) or dementia requires careful evaluation and an individually tailored approach and treatment plan.

Patients who have early dementia often are concerned or upset about their cognitive problems and are more sensitive to the physician's responsiveness and attitude. Attending to the patient's perspective is important. When a cognitively impaired patient is upset with mental status testing during the first visit, it is wise to abandon the test and focus on developing a relationship with the patient. The physician can always return to testing in future visits when a greater degree of trust has been established. Communication skills with cognitively impaired individuals require knowledge of how the disease progresses for individual patients and the changing needs of individuals over time. As communication with the patient becomes more difficult, the physician must establish a solid relationship with the patient's family or significant other to provide the most appropriate and sensitive care for the patient.

Physicians' communication skills with cognitively impaired elderly patients can affect patient satisfaction and compliance with treatment recommendations. In the setting of sensory deficits and MCI, it is key to provide information to patient and family in a language that they understand by checking understanding and paraphrasing. On an individualized basis, providing written information at an appropriate level can be helpful. Also when discussing a topic with a patient with MCI, use simple phrases, and make frequent breaks to clarify the plan. During triadic conversations, it is important to obtain the patient's perspective by considering interviewing the patient alone, remaining neutral by listening to all concerns, and requesting assistance from other disciplines, including social work. It is important to ensure that appropriate informed consent is obtained before proceeding with interventions or treatments in cognitively impaired patients.

Orange and Ryan (2000) state there is no concise list of strategies to facilitate communication with dementia patients, as this would reflect an oversimplification of the complexity of communication. Such a perspective also downplays the role of individual variability, which is the hallmark of older adults in general and individuals with dementia in particular. Physicians require significant patience when communicating with patients with dementia. Patients' individual traits such as verbosity, muteness, or the lack of meaning in their language can test the patience of even the most empathetic physician. Of course, productive time spent listening to patients, often with their well-informed caregivers present, is an essential step toward understanding the patient and the context of the visit.

Accepting that patients' needs vary widely and adjusting communication to suit individual needs is essential. Box 52.1 (adapted from Orange and Ryan 2000) shows general strategies that may be useful with patients with dementia.

> **Box 52.1** Strategies for communication with individuals with dementia
>
> **Language**
> - Use simple active declarative sentences
> - Use yes/no questions or closed-ended questions
> - Avoid ambiguous and indefinite terms and non-specific pronouns
> - Avoid technical terms and jargon
> - Avoid giving instructions or information over the phone, as understanding over the phone is usually much poorer than in person
>
> **Cognition**
> - Be the memory trigger for patients
> - Use patients' personal, long-term memory (i.e. autobiographical memory) as a source for topics for discussion
> - Maintain patients' attention by using their name, asking them specific questions, using gestures or light touch
>
> **Speech**
> - Use pauses and stress important words to highlight information
> - Speak clearly and slowly at a slightly low pitch and at a slightly louder volume
> - Use calm, soothing speech which captures and maintains attention
>
> **Non-verbal**
> - Use calm facial expressions, body movements, and posture; becoming angry or overexcited may alarm and confuse patients
> - Use slow and deliberate movements; quick ones can appear threatening
> - Get patients' attention first before talking; get close but not too close to minimize distraction and help focus attention
> - Touch slightly on hand to (re) gain attention and to reassure
> - Maintain eye contact, unless not appropriate based on the patient's cultural norms
>
> **Conversation**
> - Focus on information exchange rather than the patients' accurate use of words
> - Introduce yourself at each new contact and call patients by their full name
> - Learn and use patients' personal history to make conversation meaningful and relevant
>
> - Explain what you are doing as you are doing it
> - Do not interrupt patients; it is confusing and may cause them to forget what they want to say
>
> **Emotions**
> - Acknowledge patients' emotions
> - Use an empathetic tone of voice and responses, which signals that you understand patients' feeling of loneliness, anxiety, helplessness, and so on
> - Ignore patients' sudden verbal outbursts, do not respond in an agitated manner
>
> Adapted from *Clinics in Geriatric Medicine,* Volume 16, Issue 1, JB Orange and EB Ryan, 'Alzheimer's Disease and Other Dementias: Implications for Physician Communication', pp. 153–173, Copyright © 2000, with permission from Elsevier, http://www.sciencedirect.com/science/journal/07490690

Third persons in the medical encounter

One major characteristic that distinguishes the geriatric medical consultation from other encounters is that often the older patient is accompanied by a third person (e.g. spouse, adult child, or professional caregiver); various studies have found that 20–57% of elderly patients are accompanied by a third person to a medical visit (Prohaska and Glasser 1996).

The third person (or additional persons) may either facilitate or inhibit the development and maintenance of a trusting physician–patient relationship. The third person probably plays multiple roles during the visit depending, for example, on the duration of the encounter, the particular content of the interaction, the health status of the patient, and the needs of the accompanying individual.

Three major roles for the third person have been conceptualized, the advocate, the passive participant, and the antagonist (Adelman *et al.* 1987). When the third person is supportive of the patient, that person is considered an advocate. This person actively encourages and empowers the patient. The passive participant is a third person who is present but minimally involved in the encounter. With scant knowledge about the patient, the passive participant is generally disengaged from the interactional dynamics of the visit. The antagonist is a third person who works against the patient on either overt or covert levels. This individual may be openly hostile and rude to the patient, and the patient's agenda is either discounted or ignored. The antagonist tries to take advantage of the patient or the physician or both. These potential roles have not yet been empirically validated. To examine the dynamics of dyadic versus triadic visits, Greene *et al.* (1994) compared a matched sample of two-person and three-person encounters. It was noted that, although the content of physician talk was not different in dyads or triads, patients in triads were frequently referred to as 'she' or 'he' by physicians; patients raised fewer topics overall in triads than in dyads; patients were less responsive to topics they raised themselves and were less assertive in triads than in dyads; and less shared laughter and joint decision-making took place in triadic than in dyadic encounters. This study demonstrates that the presence of a third person in the medical encounter with an older person and his or her physician is likely to influence the interactional dynamics of the encounter. Indeed, no matter how minor the involvement of the third person during the visit, his or her presence may change the basic content and process of the encounter. Many geriatricians believe it essential to spend some time in every encounter alone with the patient, which may occur during the physical examination part of the visit. This enables private time for a patient to reveal important issues that may not be raised in multiperson encounters.

Strategies for improving the physician–older patient relationship

How can an effective and empathic relationship develop between an older patient and his or her physician? What specific components of communication help to create such a relationship? In this section, the authors describe some approaches that physicians and patients may employ to improve communication. These strategies are derived from the authors' analysis of the empirical literature to date and clinical experience in geriatric care (RA). Few data exist correlating interactional processes with health outcomes for older patients; therefore, these recommendations represent the authors' perspectives on how physicians and older patients can develop a positive relationship at the present level of understanding.

Understanding the patient's perspective

A non-ageist approach is critical for the development of the physician–older patient relationship (Adelman et al. 1991), and must recognize the remarkable heterogeneity of the elderly population (Haug and Ory 1987). Each patient (whether older or younger) must be seen as an individual with specific needs and different concerns and beliefs. A physician is non-ageist when he or she pays attention to issues such as health promotion for the older patient (indicating optimism about the older patient's future), and anticipatory care (i.e. allowing planning for an active future) covering prevention of falls, ensuring safe prescription-writing to prevent side effects or drug-related problems, and decreasing caregiver stress.

Getting to know the older patient as a person is the best antidote to ageist behaviour. When a physician perceives the older patient as a person with a defined history of accomplishments as well as future goals, ageist stereotypes are likely to be abandoned. An excellent method to incorporate this framework into practice is to conduct a life review (Haight and Webster 1995; Haigh and Haight 2007). Often this oral history gives a fascinating glimpse into the patient's world and the patient's identity, encompassing the history of many decades, as well as providing a means of determining what is important to the patient. Accessing this narrative history to the patient's story may be time-consuming initially, but it is worth the extra time because it gives a formidable jump-start to the development of trust, which is unfortunately missing so often in the medical encounter. The simple act of listening can be poignant for the patient, as well as the physician. Indeed, through the very act of listening to an older patient's life history, the physician comes to understand the patient's present life, value system, achievements and failures, and this knowledge assists in the diagnosis and treatment of current problems. Allowing for, and supporting, the patient's presentation of self, that is, the patient's disclosure of his or her identity, undoubtedly improves the relationship (Greene et al. 1994). To reiterate, the more one knows the patient as a person, the less the patient is relegated to a stereotype.

A physician who makes a house call and sees the severely functionally impaired or hospice patient in his or her own environment has an added opportunity to cement their relationship. The effort of making a home visit, which is relatively unusual in contemporary practice, is likely to have special meaning for a homebound older person. The home visit gives the physician a unique opportunity to examine family dynamics, functional status, living conditions, and gain a glimpse at the patient's identity. The physician may see photographs, paintings, and memorabilia that invite the physician to learn more about the patient's life. Being a visitor or a guest in another's home changes the power dynamics of the medical visit and allows the patient to exert more control in the encounter. This levelling of the interactional playing field may make it easier for the patient to discuss socioemotional issues and express his or her perspectives about medical care and treatment, and perhaps enable more joint decision-making.

Studies show that physicians often do not give patients a chance to introduce their concerns (Marvel et al. 1999), and patients' questions are given low priority in medical encounters (West 1984; Frankel 1990). In one study, Greene and Adelman (1996) found that physicians were more responsive to the topics they raised themselves, as compared to the topics that older patients raised. Furthermore, when older patients are able to initiate discussion of their issues, they are not addressed as thoroughly as when physicians raise the issue. Moreover, there is a lack of concordance between the older patient agenda for the visit and the physician agenda for the visit (Greene et al. 1989), even though a focus on patient-raised issues or the 'patient-centred' approach is essential to establishing rapport (Stewart et al. 1995).

Patients need encouragement to participate fully in the consultation, although not all older patients feel comfortable in this role. Before seeing the physician, patients should be asked to list and prioritize their problems and their questions. Patients should consider whether they wish to have a trusted family member or friend accompany them and, during the consultation, ask for clarification of any aspects that are unclear. After the visit, telephone follow-up can facilitate understanding and will expose difficulties with, or intolerance of, medication or other concerns.

Integrating the psychosocial into medical decision-making

The psychosocial domain is a core element of geriatric medical decision-making, because older patients tend to have multiple medical and psychosocial problems. Some of these problems may be embarrassing and uncomfortable for the patient to raise, so the physician must create an environment in which patients feel safe to raise difficult subjects such as loneliness, depression, anxiety, abuse and neglect, caregiver burden, fears about death, concerns about family members, advance directives, memory loss, incontinence, sexual dysfunction, or addiction (e.g. alcohol, drugs, gambling). These highly personal topics will only be raised when the patient feels the physician can be trusted with such disclosures. It is important to emphasize that the physician need not have the expertise to treat these problems—it is, however, essential that the physician make the appropriate referral to a professional with the appropriate skills to assist the patient.

How does the physician create the safe atmosphere in a consultation? First, physicians must assure patients that all information is confidential; when patients understand that their privacy will be preserved, they are likely to be more disclosing. In addition, physicians must strive to be non-judgemental, which is no easy task when patients' attitudes differ significantly from those of the physician.

Physicians should provide continued support and encouragement to patients as they reveal their embarrassing or emotionally taxing concerns, allowing the patient to talk without interruption, verbally acknowledging distress, and being attentive to such nonverbal cues as tear-filled eyes, voice alterations, or trembling hands. The physician's duty is to try to assist the patient by providing informational, instrumental, and/or emotional support. This support may be as basic as letting the patient know that the physician is available to listen again at the next visit. The experienced physician realizes that intimate questions may be revisited over time. By raising unresolved issues over time, the physician reveals his or her engagement with the patient's ongoing story, which may be clinically and interpersonally useful. Sensitive timing in raising personal issues is part of the art of medicine; for example, asking an older patient about do-not-resuscitate orders during a first medical visit may not be appropriate for many patients.

Obviously, the physician alone cannot provide all the support needed to meet psychosocial needs, so appropriate referral to a social worker or other health professional becomes an important component of geriatric medicine.

Attention to sensory and functional limitations

All medical premises must accommodate wheelchairs and those who accompany the patient, and have suitably adapted toilets for disabled patients. The physical environment of a practice sends powerful messages to older people; particularly those with functional deficits, and many doctors' offices are not designed with older patients' needs in mind. Older patients' needs must be considered in the planning, construction, furnishing, and equipping of all medical environments. On a domiciliary visit, the physician can observe whether the apartment or house accommodates the older patient's functional limitations and can spot how adapting the environment to a patient's functional status could allow a patient to continue to live independently.

Communication between older patients and their providers about cancer

Cancer has a disproportionately high incidence and toll on the elderly population. Sixty per cent of all cancers and 70% of all cancer deaths occur in people aged 65 and over (Yancik 1997). Middle-old and old-old patients grew up in the era in which cancer was almost always a death sentence and, for some, the word 'cancer' denotes pain and certain death. Because of this history, older patients may have an inordinate fear of cancer, which can result in denial, lower attendance for cancer screening and, possibly, non-adherence to cancer treatment regimens. Thus, it is important for the clinician to determine older patients' beliefs about cancer. The clinician may specifically ask the patient: what do you know about the disease? What are your concerns/fears/beliefs about treatment? What are your short-term and long-term goals for care? The notion that each type of cancer is different and that many cancers are treated like a chronic disease may be a revelation for older patients and needs to be discussed.

Ageism and cancer

There is an extensive literature that documents the occurrence of ageism in the treatment and care of older patients with cancer, manifested in a variety of ways. Older patients are frequently excluded from clinical trials, despite the recommendation of the Food and Drug Administration (FDA) in 1989 to include older patients (Townsley et al. 2005). This exclusion means that clinicians do not have sufficient data to determine whether to treat or how to treat older patients with cancer. Many in the medical profession assume that life-prolonging treatment is more a priority for younger than older patients. They assume that older cancer patients cannot tolerate aggressive surgery or chemotherapy. However, research demonstrates no significant differences in outcomes for older and younger patients who participate in clinical trials (Townsley et al. 2005).

Ageism in the medical profession often guides diagnostic and treatment decisions. For example, Litvak and Arora (2006) found that older women with breast cancer are 'understaged, underdiagnosed, and undertreated' in comparison to younger women; Faiella and Gulden (2007) concur that women with breast cancer are treated less aggressively; and Bouchardy et al. (2003) found that older patients with breast cancer less frequently receive breast-conserving surgery, axillary node dissection, and adjuvant radiation therapy, chemotherapy, and hormone therapy. Thus overall, older women with breast cancer are not given optimal treatment. With respect to other cancers, Fuchshuber (2004) reported that older patients are less likely to receive surgery for lung, liver, pancreas, oesophagus, and gastric and rectal cancer. Peake et al. (2003) found that older patients with lung cancer are undertreated. Chemotherapy is less likely to be offered to older patients with stage III colon cancer or to older women with ovarian cancer (Elkin et al. 2007).

What is it about ageing and cancer that results in prejudicial management and treatment? Bouchardy et al. (2003) suggest that patients' co-morbidities, lesser life expectancy, and poorer functional status may affect physicians' decisions. Penson and colleagues (2004) consider the assumptions that clinicians make about older patients, like the belief that older patients value symptom relief over life-prolonging treatment, will not tolerate chemotherapy well (Faiella and Gulden 2007), despite literature to the contrary (Peake et al. 2003), or that risks associated with surgery and treatment are too high, or lack long-term benefits (Fuchshuber 2004).

Diagnosis of cancer

The communication literature on diagnosis of cancer focuses most frequently on the delivery of bad news to patients. This literature describes communication between physicians and patients of all ages. We do not know if older patients have different needs at this crucial time, although there is some indication that older individuals cope psychologically with the diagnosis of cancer as well, if not better, than their younger counterparts (Adelman et al. 1991; Extermann and Hurria 2007). While some suggest that older patients are less interested in knowing their diagnosis than younger patients (Greene et al. 1994), others note that patients still desire information, but do not want to be as actively involved in decision-making about treatment (Extermann and Hurria 2007). In one community sample, 88% of older individuals wanted to be told whether they have cancer (Marvel et al. 1999). Because of these differences in attitude and knowledge, physicians need to evaluate each older patient's understanding and expectations about the disease.

Regardless of age, individual patient preferences for information and support need to be ascertained. As previously mentioned, since many cancers have become chronic diseases, communication skills are needed to support a long-term relationship between the older cancer patient and the physician. Caring for a patient with cancer occurs in stages; it is a dynamic process and patient needs will change over time. A longitudinal perspective on communication about cancer is likely to be the most effective and realistic; recognizing that communication must continue from the delivery of bad news, through what may be difficult treatments to either survivorship or death. Of note, Hagerty *et al.* (2005) recognize that communicating prognosis involves more than the delivery of bad news. Consideration must be given to how much information to provide and whether to present statistically-derived survival data and anticipated life expectancy. The patient's health literacy and socioemotional state must be taken into account.

Treatment of cancer

Although treatment for cancer should be based on physiologic rather than chronologic age (West 1984), older patients receive substantially less aggressive or appropriate cancer treatment than younger patients (Adelman *et al.* 1991; Greene and Adelman 1996). Breast cancer patients older than 70 years are less likely to receive appropriate surgery for their condition than patients aged 50–69 years (Greene *et al.* 1989). Elderly patients with non-Hodgkin's lymphoma, and those with breast cancer, are much less likely to receive sufficient chemotherapy doses to promote the best chances for survival (Stewart *et al.* 1995). Nordin *et al.* (2001) discuss the age-based inequality of care in gynaecologic oncology, which results in poorer prognosis for older women. Furthermore, there is evidence that older cancer patients in nursing homes receive less adequate pain-management than younger cancer patients (Yancik 1997).

There is no difference in younger and older patients' desire for surgery that will offer a possibility of cure from cancer (Nordin *et al.* 2001). Getting the most effective treatment is equally important to older and younger women with breast cancer (Greenfield *et al.* 1981; Adelman *et al.* 1991; Nordin *et al.* 2001). Older women, like their younger counterparts, wish to be involved in decision-making about treatment (Adelman *et al.* 1991).

Although treatment for many cancers may be different in an older population because of the course of the disease, co-morbidity, and the toxicity of regimens, treatment decisions must be individually tailored and take into account the older patient's lifestyle, preferences, and concerns about quality of life (Hurria *et al.* 2006). While there is some indication that older patients prefer a less active role in medical decision-making (Townsley *et al.* 2005) and consider their visits less participatory than younger patients (Penson *et al.* 2004), physicians must ascertain older patients' desire for involvement in treatment decisions (Greene *et al.* 1994; Hurria *et al.* 2006).

Patients may not be known well by the surgeon or oncologist who is recommending life-altering treatment. Communication about patients' values, preferences, and life circumstances needs to be integrated into decisions about appropriate treatment and care. Given the extended period of treatment, ample time exists to develop a supportive relationship. In some practices, the bulk of care during treatment may be delegated to non-physician staff, such as nurses and physician assistants. A full-scale research agenda regarding communication between these health professionals and older patients is needed.

Older cancer patients may be concerned about becoming a burden to their family; their caregivers may be elderly themselves and thus require significant informational and instrumental support. If the caregiver has functional impairments or limited vision or hearing, the role may be more challenging and impact on both the patient's and caregiver's own health. The physician needs to be open to discussions about the burden of care and approaches for alleviating these stressors. Communication about referrals to social work and other social service agencies may be key at this time. For more frail older patients, it may be important to make certain that follow-up plans are clearly understood and organized in advance, for example, arranging for post-chemotherapy phlebotomy in the home (Yancik 1997).

Cancer survivorship

As previously mentioned, the notion of surviving cancer may not be one that is seriously considered by those older patients who may conceptualize the diagnosis as meaning the end of life. Therefore, to think about being a cancer survivor and living a full and meaningful life after diagnosis and treatment may require negation of a firmly held belief of many years. The physician must be prepared to communicate the realities of a good prognosis (as well as a poor one) to the older cancer patient.

The dearth of research investigating health professional–older patient communication about cancer is partially explained because such study requires grounding in multiple disciplines (including communication, sociology, psychology, and medicine). Many of the research questions require a multidisciplinary approach. The following reflects some of the research questions that require investigation:

1. How do different age cohorts of older individuals perceive cancer? For example, do young-old cancer patients have a more optimistic and consumerist approach than their old-old counterparts? What are older patients' perceptions and fears about treatment and prognosis? How do these perceptions influence the identification of symptoms, coping with the disease, and adherence to treatment regimens?

2. How does health literacy of older individuals affect communication with health professionals and older patients' ability to follow recommended treatment regimens?

3. Are there ageist biases in cancer screening, detection, and treatment? How do these biases affect screening recommendations, diagnosis, care, and physician–older patient communication?

4. What are older patients' preferences regarding the amount and type of information they receive about a diagnosis of cancer and subsequent treatment? How can physicians identify older patients' preferences for participation in decision-making about cancer treatment?

5. What are the emotional, instrumental, and informational supports needed by older individuals? How can physicians best respond to these needs?

6. How does physician specialty (i.e. primary care, oncology, and surgery) influence the quality of communication with older cancer patients?

7. How does the setting of care (e.g. outpatient practice, inpatient, nursing home) and physician reimbursement (salaried, capitation, fee-for-service, concierge) influence communication between physicians and older patients?

Research that encompasses the multiple levels of meaning in cancer care demand qualitative and quantitative approaches to capture the essential communication processes. Ultimately, these research findings must be translated into medical education and training, which will improve care of the older cancer patient.

Communication issues in palliative care

Well-developed communication skills are critical to provide effective palliative care. Duggleby and Raudonis (Duggleby and Raudonis 2006) describe some of the special communication needs in palliative care, including recognition that older and younger patients describe pain differently. Quality of life has a different meaning to older adults and is influenced by their ability to remain in control of their lives and participate in daily activities (Duggleby and Raudonis 2006; Levasseur *et al.* 2009). While these authors acknowledge that communication with older patients in palliative care requires different skills, few studies specifically examine older patient–healthcare professional interactions surrounding palliative care. There is a clear need to develop evidence-based recommendations for older patients (Parker *et al.* 2007).

Communication skills include the ability to direct a patient/family meeting to discuss advance planning and goals of care. About 70% of family physicians who provide palliative care report no training in communication (Alvarez 2006) and doctors in training have been found to be inadequately prepared to deal with end-of-life care decision-making (Gorman *et al.* 2005). Reinke *et al.* (2011) found that clinicians focus on life-preserving treatment for older patients with COPD and avoid discussing end-of-life issues. The authors state that physicians have inadequate training and thus, lack the self-efficacy needed to initiate difficult end-of-life discussions. Caring for older adults with life-threatening illnesses can elicit anxiety about death, feelings of impotence, failure, and guilt in healthcare providers; which, if unrecognized can affect the physician–older adult relationship (Tulsky 2003). Recognizing these feelings as normal and discussing them with colleagues are effective ways of improving communication and care for older adults (Tulsky 2003), as well as providing reassurance to the health professional.

When called to make an inpatient palliative care consultation, the palliative care clinician is often meeting the patient and family for the first time. From the personal experience of two of the authors (RA and MS), one tactic that seems to engage patients is, on the first meeting, to ask open-ended questions that focus on the patient's identity and to listen to the patient's view of his/her current quality of life. This approach often is well-received, allows for exploration of patient goals, and opens up a non-medicalized, 'life-world' perspective that gives the patient permission to present personal values and aspects of his or herself. Understanding patients' motivations can assist clinicians in guiding patients toward choices that are consistent with their values (Pollak *et al.* 2011). Anecdotally, often families, particularly when the older patient is unable to speak for him or herself, have an urgent need to present the elder patient's identity as a way to make certain that their loved one is perceived as an individual who deserves respect and attention.

Summarizing a palliative care encounter for the patients and their families will help them organize their thoughts and should end with questions to check accuracy (Pollak *et al.* 2011). Humour is another strategy, which is unexpected and under-utilized to engage the patient. Humour may play an important role in building therapeutic relationships, relieving tension, and humanizing medical care, including end-of-life care (Dean and Gregory 2004; Dean and Major 2008). A study evaluating the acceptability of humour between palliative care patients and healthcare providers found that the vast majority of participants found humorous interactions with their nurses and doctors acceptable and appropriate regardless of age (Ridley *et al.* 2014).

Even with the increased interest and medical education initiatives that focus on dying and death, discussions about death in the medical encounter are infrequent and uncomfortable for physicians and unsatisfactory for patients. Exploring patient's personal experiences with the end-of-life care of others is important in physician–older adult communication. When older individuals have one or more experiences with the death and dying of loved ones, there is greater readiness to discuss advance care planning (Amjad *et al.* 2014). Older patients need to be reassured by their physicians that they will not be abandoned. Information about the availability and efficacy of current palliative care interventions should be provided. Because death continues to be a taboo subject in medical practice, very few patients are being enrolled in hospice programmes or are being enrolled too late to obtain the full benefit of the programme. In fact, as many older patients are likely to be unaware of programmes such as hospice care, physicians need to inform patients and their families about this service in a timely way.

Common barriers to effective communication with terminally ill patients about dying include a pervasive social and personal denial of death, patients' fears about the dying process and death, and physicians' and other heath professionals' discomfort and anxiety about such discussions. In addition, families may have limited experiences with death and may possess unrealistic expectations about the healthcare system's ability to restore a patient's health, even when the patient has a terminal illness. Overcoming these barriers is very dependent on clinicians' communication skills. Central to this approach is to better understand the meaning of the illness and death for the patient, whatever his or her age might be.

Much of the research has been on communicating about advance directives. Using focus groups of patients with chronic and terminal illness, family members, and health professionals, Wenrich *et al.* (2001) identified other skills for communication with terminal patients, including talking with patients in an honest and straightforward way, being sensitive to when patients are ready to talk about death, picking up non-verbal cues, and creating an appropriate physical environment. In addition, Tulsky (2005) suggests strategies to communicate with hope, including eliciting patients' realistic short-term goals.

When a patient is terminally ill, the team is catapulted into one of the most emotionally significant and inescapable rites of passage in an individual's life. How can the palliative care team access the patient's perspective and that of the family at this crucial time? Attention to the patient's personhood and his/her presentation of self, as described by Greene *et al.* (1994), can enable the patient's identity to emerge. Dy *et al.* (2008) concur that 'personalization' is a key element of patients' satisfaction at the end of life.

It becomes important to reframe the care goals so that patients, families, and healthcare professionals recognize what can be achieved in the patient's remaining days. Care goals at this stage can include pain-management and symptom relief; sharing last words with significant others; giving a loved one permission to die, bringing meaning and closure to one's life; and reassurance that the individuals being left behind will be fine. Understanding the cultural and religious context for care at the end of life is critical for the patient and family comfort, and must be specifically elicited. When older patients do not have family, the significance of the team's involvement is even greater. If an older patient is socially isolated, often recruiting a volunteer to spend time with the patient can be helpful.

Palliative care team communication

When a patient is hospitalized in the depersonalized hospital environment, it can be frightening and lonely. With overburdened physicians, too few nurses, and ever-increasing bureaucratic demands, it is difficult to provide individualized, supportive care. In the contemporary hospital, it is often the palliative care team that enables this level of attentive care to occur.

When a palliative care team has been called in to see a patient, not only must the team communicate well with the older patient and family members, but it must also be skilled in communicating with other members of the patient's care team (e.g. oncologist, primary nurse, social worker, primary care physician, hospitalist, medical resident). Palliative care teams may be formal, as in an academic setting in which often nurses, physicians, and social workers compose the team, or more informal, with appropriate teams forming as needed, for example, consulting with a chaplain, or a psychiatrist. During major family meetings, where goals of care are being discussed, the palliative care team wisely includes the patient's primary care physician whenever possible. After all, part of the purpose of an inpatient palliative care team is to train physicians to better deal with the multiple issues involved in communication, such as discussions about terminal illness, symptom relief, and goals of care. It is ironic, perhaps, but eminently understandable, that 'specialists' (i.e. the palliative care team), sometimes have to be called in to perform duties that all physicians should be aware of and trained in.

Proper preparation for patient/family meetings is an important task of the palliative care team. Preparation requires a comprehensive understanding of the clinical history and the patient's current medical status to have an adept discussion about goals of care with the primary care physician and other appropriate disciplines. The objectives of a family meeting need to be defined in advance (see Chapter 19, 'Communication about coping as a survivor') and the interdisciplinary team members need to be in agreement about the goals. At the start of the conference, a member of the primary care or palliative care team who is working most closely with the patient and family should be present to identify the goals of care meeting and lead the discussion. It is fruitful to ask the patient (if present) and each family member to define his/her understanding of the patient's illness near the start of the meeting. This overall strategy facilitates the patient/family to voice their concerns, thoughts and feelings, and allows staff to gauge the patient/family members' perspectives. Otherwise, the professionals may dominate talk and the critical perceptions of the patient and family remain unspoken (at least until later in the meeting).

Conclusion

Attending to communication issues is critical for effective geriatric medical care in all stages of the continuum through health and disease. Given the often negative perceptions of the elderly and the great heterogeneity of this population, it is imperative that health professionals assess each older patient as an individual. The impact of a cancer diagnosis and treatment, as well as a terminal illness, has a powerful effect on the lives of older people. Health professionals who care for the elderly with sensitivity to their personhood, their medical status, and psychosocial needs will have a profound influence on the quality of older patients' lives.

References

Adelman RD, Greene MG, Charon R (1987). The physician-elderly patient-companion triad in the medical encounter: The development of a conceptual framework and research agenda. *Gerontologist* **27**, 729–34.

Adelman RD, Greene MG, Chacon R (1991). Issues in physician-elderly patient interaction. *Aging and Society* **11**, 127–48.

Adelman RD, Greene MG, Ory MG (2000). Communication between older patients and their physicians. *Clin Geriatr Med* **16**, 1–24.

Alvarez MP (2006). Systematic review of educational interventions in palliative care for primary care physicians. *Palliat Med* **20**, 673–83.

Amjad H, Towle V, Fried T (2014). Association of experience with illness and end of life care with advance care planning in older adults. *J Am Geriatr Soc* **62**, 1304–9.

Bouchardy C, Rapiti E, Fioretta G, et al. (2003). Undertreatment strongly decreases prognosis of breast cancer in elderly women. *J Clin Oncol* **21**, 3580–7.

Cobbs El, Duthie EH, Murphy JB (eds) (1999). *Geriatrics Review Syllabus: A Core Curriculum in Geriatric Medicine*, 4th edition. Kendall/Hunt, Iowa, IA.

Costa Jr PT, Williams TF, Sommerfield M, et al. (1996). *Recognition and Initial assessment of Alzheimer's Disease and Related Dementias*. Clinical Practice Guideline No.19. US Department of Health and Human Services, Public Health Service. Agency for Healthcare Policy and Research, AHCPR Publication No. 97-0702. Rockville, MD.

Dean RA, Gregory DM (2004). Humor and laughter in palliative care: an ethnographic investigation. *Palliat Support Care* **2**, 139–48.

Dean R, Major J (2008). From critical care to comfort care: the sustaining value of humour. *J Clin Nurs* **17**, 1088–95.

Duggleby W, Raudonis B (2006). Dispelling myths about palliative care and older adults. *Semin Oncol Nurs* **22**, 58–64.

Dy S, Shugarman L, Lorenz K, et al. (2008). A systematic review of satisfaction with care at the end of life. *J Am Geriatr Soc* **56**, 124–9.

Elkin E, Lee S, Casper E, et al. (2007). Desire for information and involvement in treatment decisions: Elderly cancer patients' preferences and their physicians' perceptions. *J Clin Oncol* **25**, 5275–80.

Extermann M, Hurria A (2007). Comprehensive geriatric assessment for older patients with cancer. *J Clin Oncol* **25**, 1824–31.

Frankel R (1990). Talking in interviews: a dispreference for patient-initiated questions in physician-patient encounters. In: Psthas G (ed.). *Studies in Ethnomethodology and Conversation Analysis*. The Interactional Institute for Ethnomethodology and Conversation Analysis and University Press of America, Washington DC, WA.

Fuchshuber P (2004). Age and cancer surgery: judicious selection or discrimination? *Ann Surg Oncol* **11**, 951–2.

Gazmararian J, Williams M, Peel J, et al. (2003). Health literacy and knowledge or chronic disease. *Patient Educ Couns* **51**, 267–75.

Gorman TE, Ahem SP, Wiseman J, et al. (2005). Residents' end-of-life decision making with adult hospitalized patients: a review of the literature. *Acad Med* **80**, 622–33.

Greene MG, Adelman RD, Charon R, et al. (1986). Ageism in the medical encounter: An exploratory study of the doctor-elderly patient relationship. *Lang Commun* **6**,113–24.

Greene MG. Hoffman S. Charon R, et al. (1987). Psychosocial concerns in the medical encounter: A comparison of the interactions of doctors with their old and young patients. *Gerontologist* **27**, 164–8.

Greene MG, Adelman RD, Charon R, et al. (1989). Concordance between physicians and their older and younger patients in the primary care medical encounter. *Gerontologist* **29**, 808–13.

Greene MG, Adelman RD, Rizzo C, *et al.* (1994). The patient's presentation of self in an initial medical encounter. In: Hummert M *et al.* (eds). *Interpersonal Communication in Older Adulthood*. Sage Publications, California, CA.

Greene MG, Adelman RD (1996). *Responsiveness of Physicians and Older Patients to Self-Initiated and Other-Initiated Topics in First Medical Visits*. Presented at the 5th Kentucky Conference on Health Communication. Lexington, KY.

Greenfield S, Blanco DM, Elashoff RM, *et al.* (1981). Patterns of care related to age of breast cancer patients. *JAMA* **257**, 2766–70.

Gulden Peter J, III (2007). Battling ageism in cancer negligence cases: many people view the elderly as having little to live for and even less to offer society. Uncovering these assumptions is step one in achieving justice for an older client whose cancer went undiagnosed or undertreated for too long. The Free Library (May 1). Available at: http://www.thefreelibrary.com/Battling ageism in cancer negligence cases: many people view the...-a0164421031 (Last accessed August 8, 2016).

Hagerty R, Butow P, Ellis P, *et al.* (2005). Communicating prognosis in cancer care: a systematic review of the literature. *Ann Oncol* **16**. 1005–53.

Haigh BK, Haight BS (2007). *The Handbook of Structured Life Review*. Health Professions Press, Baltimore, MD.

Haight BK, Webster J (1995). *The Art and Science of Reminiscing: Theory, Research, Methods, and Applications*. Taylor & Francis Group, Washington DC, WA.

Haug M, Ory M (1987). Issues in older patient-provider interactions. *Res Aging* **19**, 3–44.

Hazzard W (1994). Introduction: the practice or geriatric medicine. In: Hazzard WR, Bierman EL, Bass JP, *et al.* (eds). *Principles of Geriatric Medicine and Gerontology*, 3rd edition. McGraw Hill, New York, NY.

Higashi R, Tillack A, Steinman M, Harper M, Johnston B (2012). Elder care as 'frustrating' and 'boring': Understanding the persistence of negative attitudes toward older patients among physicians-in-training. *J Aging Stud* **26**, 476–83.

Hurria A, Cleary TA, Adelman RD (2006). Cancer in the frail elderly. In: Muss HB, Hunter CP, Johnson KA (eds). *Treatment and Management of Cancer in the Elderly*. Informa Healthcare/Taylor& Francis, New York, NY.

Koenig C, Ho E, Yadegar V, Tarn D (2012). Negotiating complementary and alternative medicine use in primary care visits with older patients. *Patient Educ Couns* **89**, 368–73.

Levasseur M, St-Cyr Tribble D, Desrosiers J (2009). Meaning of quality of life for older adults: Importance of human functioning components. *Arch Gerontol Geriatr* **49**, e91–100.

Litvak D, Arora R (2006). Treatment of elderly breast cancer patients in a community hospital setting. *Arch Surg* **141**, 985–90.

Marvel MK, Epstein RM, Rowers K, *et al.* (1999). Soliciting the patient's agenda: have we improved? *JAMA* **281**, 283–7.

Mira J, Orozco-Betran D, Perez-Jover V, *et al.* (2013) Physician patient communication failure facilitates medication errors in older polymedicated patients with multiple comorbidities. *Fam Pract* **30**, 56–63.

Nordin AJ, Chinn DJ, Moloney I, *et al.* (2001). Do elderly cancer patients care about cure? Attitudes to radical gynecologic oncology surgery in the elderly. *Gynecol Oncol* **81**, 447–55.

Orange JB, Ryan EB (2000). Alzheimer's disease and other dementias: implications for physician communication. *Clin Geriatr Med* **16**, 153–73.

Parker S, Clayton J, Hancock K, *et al.* (2007). A systematic review of prognostic/end-of-life communication with adults in the advanced stages of a life- limiting illness: patient/caregiver preferences for the content, *style,* and timing of information. *J Pain Symptom Manage* **34**, 81–93.

Peake M, Thompson S, Lowe D, Pearson M (2003). Ageism in the management of lung cancer. *Age Ageing* **32**, 171–7.

Penson R, Daniels K, Lynch T (2004). Too old to care? *Oncologist* **9**, 343–52.

Pollak KI, Childers JW, Arnold RM (2011). Applying motivational interviewing techniques to palliative care communication. *J Palliat Med* **14**(5), 587–92.

Prohaska TR, Glasser M (1996). Patients' views of family involvement in medical care decisions and encounters. *Research on Aging* **18**, 52–69.

Reinke L, Slatore C, Uman J, *et al.* (2011). Patient–clinician communication about end-of-life care topics: is anyone talking to patients with chronic obstructive pulmonary disease? *J Palliat Med* **14**, 923–8.

Ridley J, Dance D, Pare D (2014). The acceptability of humor between palliative care patients and health care providers. *J Palliat Med* **17**, 472–4.

Stewart MA, Brown JB. Weston WW, *et al.* (1995). *Patient-Centered Medicine: Transforming the Clinical Method*. Sage Publications, California, CA.

Townsley C, Selby R, Siu L (2005). Systematic review of barriers to the recruitment of older patients with cancer onto clinical trials. *Journal of Clinical Oncology* **13**, 3112–24.

Tulsky JA (2003). Doctor-patient communication. In: Morrison RS, Meier DE (eds). *Geriatric Palliative Care*. Oxford University Press, New York, NY.

Tulsky 1 (2005). Beyond advance directives: importance of communication skills at the end of life. *JAMA* **294**, 359–65.

Wenrich MD, Curtis R, Shannon SE, *et al.* (2001). Communicating with dying patients within the spectrum of medical care from terminal diagnosis to death. *Arch Intern Med* **161**, 868–74.

West C (1984). *Routine Complications Troubles Talk Between Doctors and Patients*. Indiana University Press, Bloomington, IN.

Yancik R (1997). Cancer burden in the aged. *Cancer* **80**, 1273–83.

CHAPTER 53

Communicating with children when a parent is dying

Cynthia W. Moore and Paula K. Rauch

Introduction to communicating with children when a parent is dying

Concerns about dependent children are prominent, and distressing, for the many parents diagnosed with a life-threatening illness. Concerns commonly identified include the impact of the parent's own altered physical and emotional functioning on the child's day-to-day routine and emotional well-being, as well as how to simultaneously protect children from distress, and keep them informed about the illness. And, even in the early stages of illness, many parents consider how children would cope in the event of their death and are aware that children worry about that possibility as well (Muriel *et al.* 2012; Asbury *et al.* 2014). Like adults, children experience a range of concerns about the parent's illness. Latency age children worry about the side effects of treatment, the parent's possible death, changes in the parent's appearance, and the potential for separations from the child. Adolescents worry, as well, about making mistakes in the parent's care, the well parent's functioning, their own risk for cancer, and how to make meaning of the illness (Grabiak *et al.* 2007; Thastum *et al.* 2009; Bradbury *et al.* 2012).

Thus, helping parents feel prepared to talk with children about their illness and possible death, at any stage of illness, has the potential to alleviate distress in both parents and children. This chapter provides suggestions about how clinicians can support parents' open communication with their children, drawing on the authors' clinical experience from over a decade of providing parent guidance to patients treated in an academic cancer centre in Boston.

Review of the literature

Patients who are parenting minor children experience some unique challenges, resulting in increased strain for them (Bultmann *et al.* 2014). Compared to survivors without children, young mothers report more fear of cancer recurrence and a sense that the illness intrudes more in their lives (Ares *et al.* 2014). Parents reporting high levels of distress about the impact of the illness on children also have more symptoms of depression and anxiety, and poorer quality of life (Muriel *et al.* 2012).

Children's adjustment is affected by parental cancer. Over a 21-year period, children of cancer patients in Finland used more specialized psychiatric care than peers (Niemela *et al.* 2012). Children with an ill parent are at risk for symptoms of anxiety and depression, irritability, intrusive thoughts, somatic complaints,

difficulty concentrating in school, and poorer school performance (Nelson and While 2002; Visser *et al.* 2005; Watson *et al.* 2006; Rainville *et al.* 2012). While the stage of a parent's illness, type of cancer, and other illness-related variables do not predict children's distress, illness-related disability predicts worse adjustment in children, partly through its impact on role redistribution in the family (Pakenham and Cox 2012; Bultmann *et al.* 2014).

A parent's depression or anxiety heightens a child's risk for adjustment problems; depression combined with poorly defined family roles further heightens risk for internalizing problems (Watson *et al.* 2006; Bultmann *et al.* 2014; Gotze *et al.* 2014). Parental depression seems to impact children's symptoms partially through its negative effect on family cohesion, or sense of 'we-ness' (Watson *et al.* 2006; Lindqvist *et al.* 2007; Pakenham and Cox 2012). A family's ability to solve problems flexibly predicted less adolescent distress, and warm and supportive parenting was associated with fewer internalizing symptoms in 8–16-year-old children in families dealing with parental cancer, but not in families without illness (Lindqvist *et al.* 2007; Vannatta *et al.* 2010).

Communication and children's adjustment

Family communication style relates to children's adjustment to parental cancer. Adolescents who feel there is open communication between family members have less anxiety and fewer externalizing problems (Watson *et al.* 2006; Lindqvist *et al.* 2007). Adolescents with negative feelings about family communication, or who tend not to share feelings with parents, reported more intrusive thoughts about the parent's illness, greater efforts to avoid thinking about it, and more overall distress. Further, communication was poorer when the parent had recurrent disease or was receiving more intensive treatment (Huizinga *et al.* 2005).

Further studies on communication about parental cancer are needed to clarify whether the family's general communication style, which is what is typically assessed, translates consistently to communication about cancer in particular. In addition, too little and too much information about cancer might negatively affect children; if this were so, the linear models commonly used to test the relationship between open communication and child functioning may obscure some important information.

Content of family communication about illness

Interviews with parents further clarify the communication challenges they face. Choosing whether, when, and how to share news of a cancer diagnosis with children is one of a parent's first, and most difficult, decisions. Parents base these decisions on their wish to protect children and maintain a sense of normalcy (Asbury *et al.* 2014), and there is variability in the extent to which children are told about the illness. In a group of children whose mothers had breast cancer, 19% were unaware of the diagnosis even after the mother's surgery or radiation therapy (Barnes *et al.* 2002). Older children received more information sooner. Mothers who talked more openly believed the child had a right to know, wanted to keep the child's trust, and hoped that talking would alleviate the child's anxiety. Those who disclosed less wanted to avoid facing difficult questions, including questions about death, wished to protect the child, to preserve special family occasions, and believed that the child would not understand the illness (Barnes *et al.* 2000).

While parents want very much to protect children from worrisome news, children themselves seem to want information. A qualitative study of 8-15 year olds indicated their desire for a clear understanding of their parent's illness, even though they realized such conversations could be difficult (Thastum *et al.* 2008). Interviews with adolescents with a mother with breast cancer indicated that a major concern was whether she would survive (Kristjanson *et al.* 2004). Bereaved adolescents overwhelmingly believe they should have been told that a parent was going to die imminently, within hours or days. Strikingly, 43% of them had not realized that the death was imminent up to a few hours before the loss (Bylund-Grenklo *et al.* 2014).

These studies emphasize the value that parents and children place on open communication about illness. Yet the fact that individual adolescents' need for information varied, depending on family and personal characteristics, poses a challenge in translating these results to family interventions. It may be that an individualized parent or family guidance approach is better suited to meeting the unique needs of each child in a family, than a group 'one size fits all' model.

A recent review found that helping children to understand the parent's somatic illness and medical treatments was a consistent priority for interventions (Diareme *et al.* 2007). However, this need is not fully yet fully met, as healthy parents who wanted to talk with a health professional about how and when to tell children when their parent would die, were rarely offered such a conversation (Aamotsmo and Bugge 2014). The remainder of this chapter is focused on helping health professionals to feel comfortable providing just that kind of support.

Children's reactions to parental illness and death: A developmental model

Conversations with children about parental illness must be developmentally appropriate, or they risk being confusing or mis-attuned to children's real worries. Highlights of children's understanding of, and reactions to, illness based on stage of development are summarized in Table 53.1.

Across age groups, it is important to maintain regular routines and expectations to promote children's sense of security. Additionally, children will benefit from having family time that feels 'normal' and which is not always focused on the parent's illness. Parents may need help in recognizing the many ways that reminders of illness impinge on their child's life, and in learning how to retain a sense of normality.

Children at any age may have temporary fluctuations in their behaviour or mood following a change in a parent's medical status. However, these are usually not expected to last more than a few weeks or to cause significant ongoing impairment. Should a child exhibit difficulty in more than one setting (home, school/daycare, with peers), or for more than several weeks, a conversation with the paediatrician, and perhaps an evaluation with a mental health professional, would be warranted.

Guidelines for talking about a parent's terminal illness and death

Although the approach to talking to children about illness and death must take into consideration the child's developmental level, certain general goals guide most of these conversations. Conversations should balance warmth and openness, with care not to overwhelm a child with more than s/he needs to know. In timing the conversation, the goal is to prevent the child both from being caught unawares by significant events, and from being made too anxious for too long about events far in the future. Often, a child's questions in response to a 'news bulletin' provide a guide for further discussion.

Family conversations about a parent's chronic illness have different goals at different times, but address a number of common themes. Most families will find they need to share information about the diagnosis, treatment progress, and changes in prognosis; to discuss how treatment will affect a child's day-to-day life; to problem-solve around some area of family life that isn't working well; and simply to provide reassurance and an opportunity for children to express their feelings. Some families will also need to discuss a parent's impending death, or address children's worries about a parent's death, even when the parent is medically stable.

When these conversations are handled sensitively, they teach children a number of important lessons. Open communication signals to children that they are a valued part of the family, worthy of being included in age-appropriate decision-making. This feeling of 'family as team', on which each member has an important role to play, may reduce a child's sense of isolation. Parents are encouraged to have conversations that actively inquire about, and validate, children's feelings and reactions to illness, whether positive or negative. Children need to feel confident that their worries will not be taken lightly, and that adults will do their best to help them manage their worries. Finally, allowing children to hold on to hope, even when a death is imminent, may be more helpful than working too hard to help the child see 'the truth'.

Talking about initial diagnosis

Parents frequently express concern about having the first conversation with children in which they confirm a cancer diagnosis. They worry that their children will feel overwhelmed with fear or sadness, and that they will be unable to cope with their children's feelings. This fear can inhibit communication, so it is important to help parents set the stage for these conversations. Children tend to feel most comfortable hearing distressing news when they are in a comfortable place, usually home, where they can react without fear of embarrassment. There is no single 'just right' time to talk, but parents may plan the conversation for a time when there will be time for talking as a group, as well as individually with each child. Ideally, the child will be free after the conversation to make some

Table 53.1 Children's conceptualization of parental illness and death

Child's understanding and reactions	Guidance for parents
Infants and toddlers (0–2 years)	
◆ Aware of parent's absence, but not the reasons ◆ Sensitive to disruptions in their routine and caregivers' distress	◆ Provide consistent caregivers, routines, and settings
Preschoolers (3–5 years)	
◆ Aware of the absence of a loved person ◆ Explanations for illness and death are often inaccurately self-centred or self-blaming ('I got mad at Daddy, and made Daddy sick') ◆ Egocentric questions are common ('When can you play with me again?') ◆ Limited concept of time creates need to tie events in the future to concrete markers (a birthday, Halloween) ◆ Concrete thinkers, so euphemisms like 'Mummy is in Heaven now', are misunderstood ◆ Death understood as prolonged separation; may believe the deceased is alive elsewhere ◆ Do not appreciate that death is irreversible, and may offer 'solutions' to death, such as trying a new medicine or replacing old batteries	◆ Explore child's understanding of the illness and/or death; dispel guilt by correcting misconceptions and reassuring the child that nothing they did caused the illness or death ◆ If a parent is withdrawn, explain that the parent is sad or worried, and why, and that the child did not cause the adult's distress ◆ Provide concrete descriptions of death (his body does not work anymore: he can't see, hear, or feel anything; his heart stopped pumping and he stopped breathing) ◆ Be patient in repeating that the deceased will not come back ◆ Maintain consistent caregivers, preschool attendance, play dates, meal times, and bedtime rituals during illness and after a death
School-age children (6–12 years)	
◆ Simple cause and effect logic promotes curiosity about causes of illness and death, but may have significant gaps in understanding, e.g. may believe that cancer is contagious, or cancer is always caused by smoking ◆ May believe that stress causes or maintains illness, and be extremely concerned about 'stressing out' the parent with less-than-perfect behaviour, poor school performance, or even talking about worries ◆ Worry about the health of other important adults ◆ Understand that death is final and irreversible, but do not fully appreciate that it is universal ◆ Better understand the physical aspects of death, but may struggle to comprehend the spiritual aspects ◆ May experience guilt about things they did or did not do with or for the deceased	◆ Provide a simple explanation of the diagnosis and treatment of an illness, and clear, accurate information about causes of death ('Mom's cancer had spread to so many places in her body, and there just weren't any medicines that helped anymore') ◆ Dispel misconceptions regarding causes of illness or death, as well as contagion ◆ Maintain predictable routines and expectations ◆ Maintain school as an island of normality ◆ Somatic complaints are common; ask for updates from school about frequency of visits to the nurse ◆ Help put guilt and other concerns in perspective by thinking together about the entire relationship rather than only the recent past
Adolescents (13–18 years)	
◆ New capacity for abstract reasoning promotes adult-like worries (e.g. about family finances, the well-being of siblings) as well as questions about justice, and the meaning of life and suffering ◆ Egocentrism and emotional immaturity may still cause them to focus on the personal effects of illness or loss in ways that can feel selfish to adults ◆ Understand that death is final, irreversible, and universal ◆ May feel anxious about their own mortality, e.g. susceptibility to a heritable illness ◆ Sensitive about how a loss sets them apart from peers ◆ Conflictual relationships with either parent may produce resentment, guilt, or regrets, that complicate adaptation to the illness and grief	◆ Provide information about the illness and treatment, and clear, accurate information about causes of death ◆ Remember that adolescents may seek information from other sources, such as the internet, and encourage them to check the accuracy of this information with parents ◆ Respect adolescent's wish for privacy and control over dissemination of information about an illness or loss, as much as seems reasonable ◆ Encourage conversations and relationships with appropriate non-parental adults ◆ Do not expect adolescents to assume adult responsibilities ◆ Watch for evidence of risk taking behaviour or substance abuse in response to the illness or death

choice about what to do next—whether calling a friend, engaging in a solo activity, or engaging with the parent.

Often parents struggle with whether to simply tell children that they are 'sick' or whether to specify the name of the illness. They fear burdening their children, especially when the child has experienced a cancer-related death. Parents are reassured to learn that, frequently, their own worries are different than their children's. The word 'cancer' may not carry the same frightening connotation for children as for adults.

Children are likely to overhear conversations between parents and doctors, friends, and other family. Without direct communication, it is difficult to know what the child has heard but isn't talking about. An atmosphere of openness allows parents to feel more confident that their children will ask questions, rather than keep concerns private.

Parents may find it easiest to begin by recapping any unusual events from the past weeks, explaining the events, and checking with children about their understanding and reactions:

You might remember that I've had a few doctors' appointments in the past couple of weeks, and that sometimes you've gone to a friend's house after school since I haven't been home. The doctors have been trying to understand why I have [whatever symptom may have initiated the process]. They just told me that I have something called [breast, colon, etc.] cancer. I am feeling sad, and wish I didn't have [—], but there are treatments that my doctors expect will [cure, contain] the cancer. I'm going to do everything I can to get better. You will probably have questions and feelings about this and I want us to talk about them together as they come up.

For a younger child, a parent might simply say:

I am sick with something called cancer. I'm going to be visiting the doctor a lot and taking medicine to get better. Some days, Mrs Smith will bring you to preschool instead of me.

Talking about a change in treatment

To an adolescent or a school age child, the parent can say something such as:

My doctors told me recently that the medicine I've been taking/treatment I've been getting isn't working to shrink the cancer. It turns out the cancer has spread, or metastasized. I'm upset about that because I had hoped this treatment would really help. But, my doctor has suggested a new kind of medicine that I'm hopeful will work better.

Parents can go on to let the child know when and where the new treatments will occur, and how this will affect the child's routine.

Some children will ask, 'But what if this medicine doesn't work, either?' Parents may want to be hopeful, while acknowledging the uncertainty:

Well, that's a possibility, but right now I'm optimistic that this new medicine [or treatment] will help a lot. If it turns out that this doesn't help, I'll work with my doctors to figure out another kind of treatment that might work better. And, I'll let you know how this goes.

They may also want to underscore their confidence in their medical team, so that the child is less likely to feel worried that better care would be found elsewhere.

Talking about the end of active treatment

Learning that active treatment options have been exhausted is extremely painful, and parents may struggle with whether to share this information with their children. With younger or very anxious children, as long as the parent is not facing death within a few months, it may be better to wait. But for adolescents and children who ask many questions, a conversation may be helpful. Parents might say:

You know I have tried quite a few different kinds of treatments for cancer—radiation, several chemotherapy medicines, surgery, more chemotherapy—and none of them worked as well as we hoped. The cancer has continued to spread [or grow]. My doctors just told me that we have run out of treatments that might even slow down the cancer. I will still go see them, but the medicine they will be giving me is just to make sure I am comfortable and not in too much pain.

Or with a younger child:

You probably remember that I have tried several different kinds of medicine to get better from cancer. None of them has been able to keep the cancer from getting worse. I just found out from my doctors that there aren't any more medicines to even try that could make my cancer better. So now the medicine I take will just be to make sure I don't have too many aches and pains.

Soon after this point, adults may also need to discuss the possibility of a referral to a hospice, home care with hospice, or inpatient treatment. It may be helpful to talk with older children about how these different options would look and to elicit their feelings and concerns about the options. For example, some children have great difficulty seeing a parent in a hospital bed at home. A temperamentally inflexible child may be unsettled by the frequent comings and goings of nurses. On the other hand, some anxious children prefer that everyone stay under one roof together and are reassured by frequent check-ins with the ill parent.

Talking about imminent death

Adults often wonder about how to facilitate children's saying goodbye to a dying parent, and at what age such a conversation becomes appropriate. In part, it depends upon what is meant by 'saying goodbye' and the dying parent's ability to be responsive to the child. For a toddler or preschool child, saying goodbye might mean giving the parent a kiss and saying 'night-night' as he has every evening, without awareness that this may be the last time he receives a kiss in return. For a 6–12-year-old child, it might mean telling the parent the best and worst parts of her day, and hearing in return the parent's love and pride in her. For an adolescent, saying goodbye might entail simply saying, 'I love you' to a parent with whom the adolescent had argued frequently.

If children are made aware that a parent is not likely to survive much longer, these kinds of final conversations with the parent become more likely. Parents, in return, can say how much they love the child and also that they forgive the child for any conflict or difficulties in the relationship and recognize that the child loves them in return. Ideally, these conversations will happen gradually, rather than in one afternoon. While there is no definitive time at which to tell a child that a parent will die, parents will want to do so early enough so that talking is not prevented by sudden declines in cognitive function or mental status. However, telling children too far in advance can serve to heighten anxiety, establish an expectation for good behaviour over an impossibly long period of time, and be confusing for a child who sees the parent continuing to function reasonably well. Sharing feelings aloud can be encouraged by simply saying that it is important to do so in case things do not go as everyone hopes. It is often unclear how much longer a parent will have the capacity for these conversations, so adults can suggest to children that time with the ill parent is precious and it is important for them to say what needs to be said soon.

Not all children will want to, or should, see a parent who is close to death. If caring adults take the time to try to understand and alleviate any concerns the child may have, the child may be amenable to visiting, but should never be forced. Children express concerns about being in the hospital and feeling frightened of the strange people and equipment there; fear that they will have trouble remembering a parent as healthy if they see the parent looking extremely ill; and fear that they will be embarrassed if they cry in front of other people outside the immediate family. Often, providing very clear descriptions of what the child may see, hear, and experience, reminding children that they may leave the parent's room at any time with a designated adult, limiting other visitors while children are there, and normalizing a variety of emotional responses, will allow the child to feel well enough prepared.

Talking about death with children

Death is commonly referred to euphemistically. We speak of someone 'passing on' or 'passing away', 'being called to be with God', 'going to Heaven' or 'going to live in the sky', or 'being taken by the angels'. Even when adults disagree about the spiritual meaning of death, we share a common understanding that death is the end of biological life. Children lack this shared understanding and thus rely on clear explanations from adults about what has occurred. Once again, development plays an important role in the child's ability to comprehend and process the news of a parent's death (see Table 53.1). Hearing death described solely in spiritual terms may be confusing for children, as it was for a five-year-old who resolved to become an astronaut so he could visit his father who now 'lives in the sky'.

In addition to a clear description of the death, children may need reassurance that adults are available to care for them and to love them, that much about life will remain constant, and that they will not always feel so sad. Their questions may range from the concrete ('What will happen to Mum's clothes and credit cards?') to the philosophical ('Do you think Dad somehow knew it when I got that goal in hockey?').

Talking about the funeral

Adults can prepare children for a funeral by describing what they are likely to see and hear during the rituals, and the kinds of emotions that may be expressed by mourners. For example, the child may see a large wooden box, called a casket or coffin, in the middle of the church. The casket (coffin) holds the dead body. People may be crying during the service because they are sad and miss the person who died.

Family members may disagree about whether younger children should attend a parent's funeral. It may be helpful to provide them with the option of leaving the service early, by identifying in advance an adult to stay with each child. Families may also wish to take the opportunity presented by having many friends and relatives together to request that stories about the deceased be put in writing. These create a legacy of memories of the parent that children may appreciate even more as they get older.

Challenges to professionals

Talking with patients about their children can be emotionally draining. However, enormous gains in rapport and trust can accrue from asking about, and addressing, parenting concerns, precisely because these are such affect-laden issues. Clinicians can start by making the effort to ask parents about their children, to learn a bit about child development, and to identify or create some resources for these families.

References

Aamotsmo T, Bugge KE (2014). Balance artistry: The healthy parent's role in the family when the other parent is in the palliative phase of cancer- Challenges and coping in parenting young children. *Palliat Support Care* **12**, 317–29.

Ares I, Lebel S, Bielajew C (2014). The impact of motherhood on perceived stress, illness intrusiveness and fear of cancer recurrence in young breast cancer survivors over time. *Psychol Health* **29**, 651–70.

Asbury N, Lalayiannis L, Walshe A (2014). How do I tell the children? Women's experiences of sharing information about breast cancer diagnosis and treatment. *Eur J Oncol Nurs* **18**, 564–70.

Barnes J, Kroll L, Burke O, Lee J, Jones A, Stein A (2000). Qualitative interview study of communication between parents and children about maternal breast cancer. *Br Med J* **321**, 479–82.

Barnes J, Kroll L, Lee J, Burke O, Jones A, Stein A (2002). Factors predicting communication about the diagnosis of maternal breast cancer to children. *J Psychosom Res* **52**, 209–14.

Bradbury AR, Patrick-Miller L, Egleston B, et al. (2012). Perceptions of breast cancer risk, psychological adjustment and behaviors in adolescent girls at high-risk and population-risk for breast cancer. *Cancer Res* **72**, 1931–2.

Bultmann JC, Beierlein V, Romer G, Moller B, Koch U, Bergelt C (2014). Parental cancer: Health-related quality of life and current psychosocial support needs of cancer survivors and their children. *Int J Cancer* **135**, 2668–77.

Bylund-Grenklo T, Kreicbergs U, Uggla C, et al. (2014). Teenagers want to be told when a parent's death is near: A nationwide study of cancer-bereaved youths' opinions and experiences. *Acta Oncol* **54**, 944–50.

Diareme S, Tsiantis J, Romer G, et al. (2007). Mental health support for children of parents with somatic illness: A review of the theory and intervention concepts. *Families, Systems, and Health* **25**, 98–118.

Gotze H, Ernst J, Brahler E, Romer G, von Klitzing K (2014). Predictors of quality of life of cancer patients, their children, and partners. *Psychooncology* **24**, 787–95.

Grabiak BR, Bender CM, Puskar KR (2007). The impact of parental cancer on the adolescent: an analysis of the literature. *Psychooncology* **16**, 127–37.

Huizinga GA, Visser A, van der Graaf WT, Hoekstra HJ, Hoekstra-Weebers JE (2005). The quality of communication between parents and adolescent children in the case of parental cancer. *Ann Oncol* **16**, 1956–61.

Kristjanson LJ, Chalmers KI, Woodgate R (2004). Information and support needs of adolescent children of women with breast cancer. *Oncol Nurs Forum* **31**, 111–19.

Lindqvist B, Schmitt F, Santalahti P, Romer G, Piha J (2007). Factors associated with the mental health of adolescents when a parent has cancer. *Scand J Psychol* **48**, 345–51.

Muriel AC, Moore CW, Baer L, et al. (2012). Measuring psychosocial distress and parenting concerns among adults with cancer: The Parenting Concerns Questionnaire. *Cancer* **118**, 5671–8.

Nelson E, While D (2002). Children's adjustment during the first year of a parent's cancer diagnosis. *J Psychosoc Oncol* **20**, 15–36.

Niemela M, Paananen R, Hakko H, Merikukka M, Gissler M, Rasanen S (2012). The prevalence of children affected by parental cancer and their use of specialized psychiatric services: the 1987 Finnish Birth Cohort study. *Int J Cancer* **131**, 2117–25.

Pakenham KI, Cox S (2012). Test of a model of the effects of parental illness on youth and family functioning. *Health Psychol* **31**, 580–90.

Rainville F, Dumont S, Simard S, Savard MH (2012). Psychological distress among adolescents living with a parent with advanced cancer. *J Psychosoc Oncol* **30**, 519–34.

Thastum M, Johansen MB, Gubba L, Olesen LB, Romer G (2008). Coping, social relations, and communication: a qualitative exploratory study of children of parents with cancer. *Clin Child Psychol Psychiatry* **13**, 123–38.

Thastum M, Watson M, Kienbacher C, et al. (2009). Prevalence and predictors of emotional and behavioural functioning of children where a parent has cancer: a multinational study. *Cancer* **115**, 4030–9.

Vannatta K, Ramsey RR, Noll RB, Gerhardt CA (2010). Associations of child adjustment with parent and family functioning: Comparison of families of women with and without breast cancer. *J Dev Behav Pediatr* **31**, 9–16.

Visser A, Huizinga GA, Hoekstra HJ, Van der Graaf WT, Klip EC, Pras E (2005). Emotional and behavioral functioning of children of a parent diagnosed with cancer. *Psychooncology* **14**, 746–58.

Watson M, St James-Roberts I, Ashley S, et al. (2006). Factors associated with emotional and behavioural problems among school age children of breast cancer patients. *Br J Cancer* **94**, 43–50.

Education and international initiatives in communication training

Section editor: Barry D. Blutz

CHAPTER 54

Facilitating communication role play sessions: Essential elements and training facilitators

Ruth Manna, Carma L. Bylund, Richard F. Brown, Barbara Lubrano di Ciccone, and Lyuba Konopasek

Rationale for role play

Effective communication between a clinician and patient is the essential component of quality medical care. Many effective communication skills training (CST) programmes for healthcare professionals, as described by Kurtz and colleagues, have relied on small group role play sessions as a key part of their training (1998). In facilitator-led role play sessions, learners act out simulations of consultations, frequently using an actor taking the role of the patient. In such sessions, learners are able to exercise the use of new skills within the safe environment of a confidential and constructive practice session. Without such practice and feedback on communication skills, a learner's sustained behaviour change in clinical settings is improbable (Kurtz *et al.* 1998; Lane and Rollnick 2007).

The success of CST programmes is dependent on adept facilitation, wherein skilled facilitators not only engage learners and conduct role play sessions in a learner-centred fashion, but also provide quality feedback when debriefing the role play exercise with each learner. In order to ensure a high standard of instruction, facilitators must be trained to effectively lead these sessions.

In this chapter, we begin by describing common variations on role play sessions, highlighting the important elements. Next, we delineate the essential components of facilitating skills practice in a role play session. Third, we outline processes that are helpful in conducting train-the-trainer programmes and in sustaining a core of competent facilitators. Finally, we end by identifying areas for future research and continued development in facilitation.

Role play variations

Role play sessions provide an ideal and appropriate opportunity for the learner to practice new skills by performing the desired behaviour. There are different variations in how role play sessions are managed. The principles discussed in this chapter are applicable to different types of communication training situations. Two important variations of role play are the size of the group and who plays the role of the patient (learner or actor). Playing and debriefing the role of patient can be valuable in training clinicians in patient-centred communication techniques. Whatever form the role play session takes, the skills practised remain very similar and few changes in teaching strategy are required; these teaching strategies are shared in this chapter

Small group vs. large group role play sessions

We use the term 'small group role play' to describe 2–3 learners working with a facilitator and a simulated patient. The term 'large group role play' or 'fishbowl' describes training with a role play demonstrated in front of an entire training group, often in a larger room. Both styles are examples of experiential learning.

Small group sessions are usually preferable for skills acquisition, as they allow each learner dedicated time in the role of the clinician. It is useful to consider practical considerations, such as resources, the skill level of learners, and the specific learning objectives when designing a CST session and choosing which type of role play session to use. For example, a module on conducting a family meeting as described by Gueguen *et al.* (2009) would involve a group of simulated patients to play a family; it is unlikely most CST programmes have the resources and space to support several small group sessions of this nature, and therefore a large group role play might be more realistic.

Rather than practising skills, fishbowls are particularly useful for demonstrating and analysing skills. The focus on analysis may be preferable for training experienced learners rather than novices, as experienced practitioners bring a wealth of practical knowledge to the group, as they have all previously struggled with these communication issues. Fishbowls give more people the opportunity to observe a specific encounter and participate in the feedback session. This allows the group, rather than just the instructor, to influence the learning and the attitudes of participants.

Actors versus learners as simulated patients

In any role play session, it is necessary to have a 'patient' for the learner to interact within the simulated consultation. In some training sessions, actors are hired to play the patient's role; in others, fellow trainees play that role. For clarity in this chapter, we use the term simulated patient (SP) to denote the person playing the role of the patient, whether that be an actor or another learner. It is critical to the success of any role play session that the scenario and environment are as authentic as possible, so that the learners are able to suspend disbelief and fully engage in the role play. Actors are generally preferable as they can be trained ahead of time to play a role in a particular way, and perhaps more importantly keep the learner engaged by not breaking out of the patient role. Keeping the role play as realistic to a routine clinical interaction will allow the learner freedom to fully explore the use of new skills without distraction. Actors are likely better equipped to accurately portray a patient in distress, or any other emotion. Such skills are imperative for the learner to be confronted with when the communication goal might be responding empathically to patients.

As previously acknowledged, using and training actors involves significant resources (e.g. money and time). However, the importance of this time and effort is equally important to spending similar time in training the facilitators of the CST programme. Not only do actors provide a realistic platform where the learner can engage and exercise new skills, trained actors can also provide an excellent opportunity to give the learner feedback from the patient's perspective at the close of the role play.

Essential elements of facilitating role play sessions

Just as there are different variations the size and shape of a role play sessions, there are also variations in facilitation. Commonly, a single facilitator manages a small group role play session. Other times, a co-facilitation model may be used. Despite the need for extra resources, there are many advantages to co-facilitating small group role play sessions. Facilitators frequently bring different areas of expertise to the group, which can lead to the learners having a better educational experience. Facilitators often complement each other's strengths—whereas one may be good at structuring learning and giving feedback, another may excel at helping learners stretch themselves by trying new things. Finally, facilitators can act as a backup to each other, ensuring that all the important facilitation tasks are completed.

With either variation, a competent facilitator (or facilitator team) provides the foundation for successful communication training. The facilitator's goal is to achieve a consistent and reliable experience for learners across role play groups. The aim is to create a learner-centred experience, and this is achieved by prioritizing the learner's agendas and needs. The processes of CST and the corresponding facilitation skills that we have adopted are based on principles of adult learning theory. Adult learners need to understand the reason why they should learn something even before starting to learn it, and they need to be actively engaged, not only in the theoretical, but in the participatory and practical settings as well. Optimal learning conditions that satisfy many of these principles include: self-initiation; self-direction; realistic learning solutions; internal motivators; problem-centred organization; a variety of resources; and the opportunity to receive and offer feedback (Green and Ellis 1997).

Guidelines and role play rules can be effective in helping to set expectations and standards for the group. Here are some useful training rules (Bylund et al. 2008):

◆ **Confidentiality.** Reinforce the rule that 'what happens in the group stays in the group' and discourage discussions outside the role play. Any role play effort is safe, as it is a laboratory environment and the learner has the freedom to explore the use of new skills without judgement or ridicule (McClelland 1965). Also, any simulated interaction need not be shared with any learner's supervisor in terms of performance issues or progress. This protects the learner from any possible 'failed' role play where the interaction did not go well.

◆ **Stopping.** Only the facilitator or the learner active in the role play can stop the role play at any time. When the facilitator stops the role play, it is not indicative of poor performance, but often will represent a natural break in the conversation or other necessary stop due to time. Letting the learner know this in advance eases anxiety by setting up proper expectations about the role play.

◆ **Feedback.** Starting with the learner, the facilitator solicits positive (reinforcing) feedback first and also manages constructive alternative suggestions.

◆ **Flexibility.** Learners should feel free to make adjustments to written role play scenarios in order to meet their goals.

◆ **The practice principle.** Re-running a particular segment is not remedial or punitive. Instead, role play is an opportunity to try new skills and to compare different methods of communication.

Sequence of strategies for facilitating small group role play

In this section, we outline a series of quality strategies for facilitation of small group role play. These strategies are based on MSK's Comskil facilitation guidelines (Bylund et al. 2008), which were developed based on best practices in literature and other training materials (Kurtz et al. 1998; Baile et al. 1999; Fryer-Edwards et al. 2006). Here, we outline a series of tasks that facilitators in their Comskil programme should demonstrate in group sessions. The basic teaching tasks that facilitators use during group sessions fall into the following categories:

1. start the session;

2. structure the group's learning;

3. run the role play;

4. facilitate the feedback process; and

5. close the session.

Start the session

The facilitator introducing role play and establishing a safe and stimulating learning environment has an important task that contributes to a smooth role play session. Fryer-Edwards et al. (2006) explain this can be done through making introductions, reviewing the rules and processes of role play and giving feedback, normalizing anxiety, and requesting a volunteer to begin the role play.

Structure the group's learning

The facilitator should take several preparatory steps to structure learning. Learners should be given time to read copies of the role play scenario and discuss any questions that they might have. If necessary, adjustments can be made to the role play scenario as written.

Eliciting individual learning goals is a significant part of structuring the group's learning. During the goal-setting, the facilitator will ensure that the learner has reviewed the role play scenario and identified specific skills that s/he would like to practice. Successful goal-setting should not be overwhelming or uncomfortable; instead it should help learners to identify their own 'learning edge', which has been defined by Fryer-Edwards and colleagues as 'the place where the learner can work that will be challenging but not overwhelming' (2006, p. 640).

The facilitator should check in with the SP privately prior to the start of the role play to communicate any changes of scenario or any specific instructions (e.g. the intensity of emotion desired or a particular cue to be given).

Run the role play

After checking that the learner is ready, the facilitator should start the role play. During the role play, the facilitator should carefully observe and take notes. The facilitator should also note the amount of time that has passed and look for the appropriate stopping place. Factors influencing the decision to stop a role play include if the learner's objective has been met and whether enough data has been gathered for meaningful feedback. Generally, this is about three to four minutes. Exceptions to this may include, if the learner's goal has been accomplished early on or, alternatively, if the goal is more complex (i.e. explaining a complicated, randomized clinical trial).

When the role play segment is ended, the facilitator should instruct the SP whether to stay in the room for the feedback discussion (usually only relevant if the SP is an actor). If the learner chooses to replay the segment again and the SP is present for the feedback discussion, it may impact the way the SP plays the character. The SP leaving the room promotes a more standardized approach. However, well-trained SPs can give valuable feedback. It can be helpful to direct the SP to comment from the patient's perspective on specific discussion points brought up by the group, or ask specific questions to how a certain comment or question from the learner during the interaction was received.

Facilitate the feedback process

Facilitating feedback is most critical to learning through role play. The facilitator's task is to create a supportive, stimulating, learner-centred environment, in which all group members' opinions are valued. The facilitator should first ask the learner to give feedback on his or her own performance in order to promote self-assessment. Starting with the positive feedback is recommended (e.g. 'What do you think you did well in that consultation?') (Baile *et al.* 1999). Often learners respond only negatively for their self-assessment, so it may take a second prompt by the facilitator to encourage the learner to list what went well for him/her in the interaction. Also, a good question to ask is whether or not the learner feels his or her learning goal was achieved. The facilitator should ask the learner to identify what problems or challenges he or she faced in the interaction; the facilitator can then elicit the help of the group in coming up with ways to address the problem or challenge. Throughout the feedback process, the facilitator should reinforce the communication skills that were taught in the earlier didactic session through reinforcing and naming what was observed (Baile *et al.* 1999).

Members of the group should generally be invited to give feedback before the facilitator gives feedback. The facilitator should work to maintain a balance of positive and constructive feedback during this time. Focusing on positive behaviours may seem counter-intuitive to group members, but the reinforcement of such behaviours is critical for the learner who is playing the role of

clinician, as well as the observing learners. Of note, the facilitator should be encouraged to ensure the balance of both positive and negative assessment. Hearing constructive criticism can be very productive in changing communication behaviour, while hearing positive appreciation can reinforce continued communication skill use. Levin and colleagues (2010) highlight the importance in the sensitivity of providing feedback in role plays. Less skilled facilitators might deliver feedback too critically or less empathically.

Using the SP as one of the key members of the feedback process can be very successful. However, it is recommended to spend initial time and effort in training the actors in giving quality feedback; this will help focus the comments provided on the learner's specific communication behaviour and uttered skills, rather than more general statements of, 'you were very nice to me'. Now, the learner is able to walk away knowing that something s/he has identifiably done or said has made the patient feel a certain way.

Some CST programmes have the resources to offer video playback as part of the learning process. Video-recording the role plays and reviewing specific sections in the feedback session are valuable in allowing learners to observe and reflect upon their own performance. Suggested strategies include selecting specific portions of the video recording to show examples, pausing the video to ask questions (e.g. 'What did you think when the patient said that?'), and observing non-verbal communication. For programmes without a video-recording resource, this would be an opportunity to ask the SP this specific question and prompt similar discussion.

As facilitators manage the role play session, it is recommended to pay attention to any created awkward moments in the small group. For example, at times during feedback sessions, a learner who was observing may make an inappropriate critical comment or a conflict may arise. This has the potential to become a 'critical incident' and must be responded to quickly (Finlay 2000). An excerpt from the MSK Facilitator Training Booklet states:

> Occasionally, a learner will become acutely distressed as a result of role-play and feedback. We term this a 'Critical Incident' because of its potential to demoralize and impede learning—a harmful outcome. Facilitators carry the key responsibility to both recognize and respond to such an event. The aim is to ameliorate the distress and re-establish a constructive learning environment as quickly as possible.
>
> Empathic support for the learner is the key strategy to be applied by the facilitator should the learner appear distressed. For instance, the facilitator might state, 'I sense you were upset by what occurred. How did you feel?' or 'I sense you are discomforted by those comments—they seemed too critical.' When learners experience the support of a facilitator in this manner, they are likely to rally and work constructively with feedback that was clumsy or insensitive. A skilled facilitator will turn awkward moments prophylactically into creative opportunities, keep the learning environment safe and prevent major critical incidents from occurring.

Text extracts from Finlay I, 'Rules of role play—guidance for tutor', in *Diploma in Palliative Medicine*, Cardiff University, Copyright © 2000, reproduced with permission of the author.

After sufficient feedback has been given through group discussion, the facilitator's task is to provide a segue to the next role play segment in a learner-centred manner. In some cases, the learner may want to replay the segment, trying out some of the suggestions that were given. A facilitator might say, 'You've heard a couple of suggestions for doing that differently. Would you like to try it over using some of these ideas?'. The process of replaying a segment of a consultation more successfully can be a significant learning moment. Alternatively, the learner may choose to move forward with the consultation, picking up where s/he left off. The facilitator should ensure that the SP and learner understand the next role play and then cycle through the tasks of running the role play, and facilitate the feedback process again.

Paying close attention to the amount of time available in the role play session, and ensuring that each learner (in small group sessions) has a chance to take the role of the physician, is a difficult yet important task. When it is time for a new learner to take the role of the doctor, the facilitator should go back to the task of structuring the group's learning and then cycle through the tasks again. Time management of a small group session can be assisted by using a co-facilitation approach, as one facilitator can really focus and structure the session according to equal time spent on each learner in the group.

Facilitators should be flexible and adaptable to the group's needs. Flexibility usually relates to identifying learning goals (and the various forms or styles of learning goals as expressed by the learner) and responding to them. For instance, in one role play session on discussing prognosis in our programme, members of a small group decided that they wanted to see how a patient would respond with varying prognoses. As each learner took a turn as the physician, s/he offered a different prognosis—ranging from a 10% chance of cure to a 90% chance of cure. A few other examples of such flexibility are as follows:

◆ Instead of having a third learner do the same role play scenario that two learners before have done, the group can work together to come up with a way of adjusting the role play.

◆ A learner may be encouraged to offer up a real-life scenario that he or she has found particularly problematic.

◆ The facilitator may have the SP play the emotion differently for each learner (e.g. highly emotional versus muted).

◆ If one learner is struggling with a portion of the consultation and another learner who has been observing has an idea about how to handle it, the facilitator can switch learners for a few moments for the observing learner to demonstrate.

Close the session
The final task is to provide closure to the end of the role play session. The facilitator can do this by summarizing some of the important points in the group's learning, asking group members to state what they found to be the most useful new skill they learned, and taking time to discuss any questions from the group (Fryer-Edwards *et al.* 2006). Additionally, this is a good time to 'de-role' the SP (if a professional actor), by taking them out of role, introducing them, and thanking them for their time. Especially in cases where the SP has been asked to stay in role during feedback, this is an opportunity to normalize relationships, particularly if there has been a tense encounter between the SP and a learner as part of the role play (e.g. anger module). Relating out of the context of the role play is important to avoid persistent negative feelings, as well as remain consistent to representing a safe learning environment in CST.

Training and sustaining competent facilitators

As facilitators play such a key role in the success of CST programmes, we strongly recommend the value in training facilitators

to comfortably manage role play sessions. Not only will the quality of the role play practice benefit from the facilitator's comfort in giving and managing feedback, the teaching experience is also crucial in reinforcing and naming communication skills and behaviour for each learner.

We also propose that more attention be given to continued assessment and development of facilitators.

Training facilitators
A commonly used method of training facilitators for CST programmes is a train-the-trainer model. This model is grounded in the education literature and often referred to as 'the cascade model'. One group trains another group, who then trains another group; thus, the education is 'cascading' downward (Bax 2002).

Effective facilitator training programmes follow a basic principle of first ensuring that the facilitator trainee is trained in the *content* of the workshop that they will be facilitating and then in the *process* of facilitation. Train-the-trainer workshops can range in time intensity, depending on what facilitators are asked to do. For example, the NewYork-Presbyterian Hospital had residency training directors come together for a full day of training to learn how to lead two different one-hour communication seminars with their residents or fellows. Other training programmes, such as the programme at MSK, invites facilitator trainees to first participate in the full training programme (18 hours) as learners, and then to participate in a separate three-hour workshop on training facilitators (Bylund *et al.* 2008). Participating as learners in training also adds to credibility as a facilitator, because they can relate first-hand to the anxiety or apprehension that a learner might feel. Thus, future facilitators have an opportunity to observe how effectively facilitators conduct the small group session, establish learning goals, and manage feedback.

As the content of what a facilitator may teach will vary from programme to programme, the remainder of this section is focused on the facilitator training workshop itself: the process of training facilitators in the essential elements of good facilitation.

We recommend that, where possible, a two to three-hour workshop be set aside to focus solely on the facilitation process. In order to train effective facilitators, sufficient time must be given to explain and demonstrate important facilitation tasks, as well as allowing facilitator trainees some time to practice and give feedback. As such, this final workshop should mimic other communication training workshops—providing a didactic session, as well as small group practice time, including opportunities to observe and analyse video-recorded sessions.

In the MSK programme, the main objectives covered in the facilitator training module are to: understand the basic principles of the adult learning theory; understand the essential components of experiential communication skills training; understand the tasks and skills needed to run an effective CST role play session; and, practise the tasks and skills needed to run an effective CST role play session. The didactic comprises a detailed discussion of the Comskil facilitator tasks. To illustrate each of these tasks, we show videos of a simulated small group role play session. Following the didactic portion of the training, we move into small groups—each group having a facilitator trainer and two to three facilitator trainees. Just as learners in CST programmes have opportunity to role play, each facilitator trainee also gets a chance to practice facilitating a small group, with his or her fellow trainees playing the roles of learners. The facilitator trainer performs a higher-order facilitation process, occasionally stopping the small group session and leading a feedback session on the facilitator trainee's performance as a facilitator. This workshop has improved facilitators' feelings of self-efficacy in their ability to facilitate role play (Bylund *et al.* 2008). With a large group of facilitator trainees, the fishbowl technique may be useful in teaching the skills of observation and giving feedback around communication skills.

In experienced CST programmes, such as the Comskil programme, facilitators have provided feedback on wishing for further support, such as advanced training opportunities. The Comskil programme partnered with colleagues at Hamad Medical Corporation (Qatar) and University of Newcastle (Australia) to survey the emphasized wishes from experienced facilitators for useful areas of advanced training. Topics such as time management, managing feedback, and cultural sensitivity or language barriers within a small group were among the top concerns for experienced facilitators (defined as regularly facilitating more than twice a year). New work is emerging on creating a booster training session for facilitators to focus on these tasks.

Facilitator feedback and assessment

The end of the training module for facilitators should not mark the end of their training. Instead, we view the process of training as lasting through the trainee's first few experiences as a facilitator. Novice facilitators need support and feedback as they work towards achieving competence as facilitators. Several strategies that we have found useful in supporting facilitators include:

- ◆ Pair up novice facilitators with more experienced facilitators in a co-facilitator model. The novice facilitator can then take a turn at facilitating one or two learners, without being responsible for the entire session.

- ◆ Conduct briefing and debriefing sessions with facilitators before and after the workshops. Briefing sessions allow time to review facilitator guidelines and role plays for the current module. Debriefing sessions are a time to discuss any problems that may have been faced by the facilitators and to brainstorm possible solutions.

- ◆ At each session provide copies of facilitator tasks and possible learner question prompts.

- ◆ Provide support with video equipment, if applicable.

Assessing novice facilitators' performance and giving them feedback is also a means of support. For instance, in one MSK programme, we audio-recorded novice facilitators three times during their first nine times facilitating. We coded these audio recordings, using a coding system we developed based upon the tasks described above (Bylund *et al.* 2009). Feedback letters that describe strengths and offer areas of improvement were then provided to the facilitators before their next training session.

Future areas of research and development for facilitation skills

As CST programmes become more integrated into all levels of medical education, there should be ample opportunities for further research and development into facilitating skills practice in role play sessions. Three particular areas we see for growth

include: examining different methods of training and supporting facilitators; identifying the impact of using a co-facilitator model; and establishing measures for treatment fidelity in CST intervention studies.

First, it is unclear if facilitators' improvement over time is due to practice alone, or if periodic feedback can assist in improving facilitation skills. If feedback is helpful, questions about the frequency, method, and content of the feedback should be explored. Second, much of the work written about facilitation assumes a single facilitator model. However, in some programmes, the supply of facilitators is sufficient to use a co-facilitator model. For instance, a programme may choose to use a co-facilitator model that pairs a medical or surgical facilitator with a psychiatrist or psychologist facilitator. Questions regarding the added benefit of using co-facilitators and how to best train facilitators to work in such a model could be explored.

Finally, in terms of researching CST as an intervention, future work should prioritize the issue of treatment fidelity—ensuring that all subjects in an intervention are getting reliable and valid treatments (Borelli *et al.* 2005). Since multiple facilitators are often involved in a training programme, systems for ensuring competence and adherence to the facilitation model are key.

Conclusion

Effective communication skills training relies on quality role play work. Facilitators for such role play work need to be trained in providing a learner-centred approach to this activity. Effective facilitation includes beginning and structuring the session, running role play, managing balanced feedback, and closing the session. In providing valuable CST, the focus on facilitators should not be overlooked. Through continued support, feedback, and assessment, facilitators can hone their skills and provide standardized, competent training.

References

Baile WF, Kudelka AP, Beale EA, *et al.* (1999) Communication skills training in oncology. Description and preliminary outcomes of workshops in breaking bad news and managing patient reactions to illness. *Cancer* **86**, 887–97.

Bax S (2002). The social and cultural dimensions of trainer training. *J Educ Teach* **28**, 165–78.

Borelli B, Sepinwall D, Ernst D, *et al.* (2005). A new tool to assess treatment fidelity and evaluation for treatment fidelity across 10 years of health behaviour research. *J Consult Clin Psychol* **73**, 852–60.

Bylund CL, Brown RF, di Ciccone BL, *et al.* (2008). Training faculty to facilitate communication skills training: Development and evaluation of a workshop. *Patient Educ Couns* **70**, 430–6.

Bylund CL, Brown RF, Lubrano di Ciccone B, *et al.* (2009) Assessing facilitator competence in a comprehensive communication skills training programme. *Med Educ* **43**, 342–9.

Finlay I (2000). Rules of role-play—guidance for tutors. In: *Diploma in Palliative Medicine*. Cardiff University, Cardiff, UK.

Fryer-Edwards KA, Arnold RM, Baile W, Tulsky JA, Petracca F, Back A (2006). Reflective teaching practices: an approach to teaching communication skills in a small-group setting. *Acad Med* **81**, 638–44.

Green M, Ellis P (1997). Impact of an evidence-based medicine curriculum based on adult learning theory. *J Gen Int Med* **12**, 742–50.

Gueguen JA, Bylund CL, Brown RF, Levin TT, Kissane DW (2009). Conducting family meetings in palliative care: Themes, techniques and preliminary evaluation of a communication skills module. *Palliat Support Care* **7**, 171–9.

Kurtz S, Silverman J, Draper J (1998). *Teaching and Learning Communication Skills in Medicine*. Radcliffe Medical Press Ltd, Abingdon, UK.

Lane C, Rollnick S (2007). The use of simulated patients and role-play in communication skills training: A review of the literature to August 2005. *Patient Educ Counsel* **67**, 13–20.

Levin T, Horner J, Bylund C, Kissane D (2010). Averting adverse events in communication skills training: A case series. *Patient Educ Counsel* **81**, 126–30.

McClelland DC (1965). Towards a theory of motivation acquisition. *Am Psychol* **20**, 321–33.

CHAPTER 55

The role of the actor in medical education

Paul Heinrich

Introduction to the role of the actor in medical education

The world of medical education has been transformed over the past 40 years through the introduction of role play simulation to teach and assess clinical and communication skills. From the beginning, members of the public have been brought in to play the roles of patients. Howard S. Barrows began to use 'programmed patients' in the early 1960s and, in a sustained creative burst, pioneered most of the subsequent applications of the method (Wallace 1997). Programmed patients were employed to teach, demonstrate, assess in laboratory and clinical practice settings, and to provide constructive feedback to medical students. The technique was extended by a number of research clinicians, such as Paula Stillman (Stillman *et al.* 1976) and Robert Kretzschmar (1978), who involved members of the public as patient instructors of basic clinical skills and as gynaecological teaching associates (GTAs) in pelvic examinations. The technique spread extensively through the United States and into a number of other countries including Canada, the United Kingdom, Australia, the Netherlands, Switzerland, Israel, the Ukraine, Russia, Spain, Brazil, and China (Wallace 1997).

These surrogate patients have undergone a number of name changes that reflect the variety of functions that they fulfil, including programmed patients, professional patients, simulated patients, pseudo patients, standardized patients, patient partners, and patient instructors. They are most commonly referred to as SPs, an abbreviation that covers the more general term of simulated patient and the standardized patient for examination purposes.

A large number of papers have documented communication training programmes utilizing SPs and have reported on student satisfaction with the method (McManus *et al.* 1993; Baerheim and Malterud 1995; Greenberg *et al.* 1999; Razavi *et al.* 2000; Smith *et al.* 2002; Rosenbaum and Ferguson 2006; Bosek *et al.* 2007). Others have described the approaches taken to recruitment, training, and the effect on the SPs of repeat performance, especially when undertaken over a prolonged period and in simulation of intense scenarios (Naftulin and Andrew 1975; Meier *et al.* 1982; Davies 1989; Woodward and Gliva-McConvey 1995; Woodward 1998; McNaughton *et al.* 1999; Bokken *et al.* 2004).

Numerous researchers have questioned the need to restrict the role of the SP to professional actors and SPs are now routinely recruited from a wide pool, which includes retirees, past patients, nurses, and drama students (Barrows 1987). Variety in the recruitment pool has been shown to be justified beyond financial considerations, as the performance demands are not always advanced and many of the simulation tasks are well within the grasp of many people.

The role of SP as patient is by definition an acting role, requiring at least a basic level of acting—the ability to enter into a hypothetical reality for a period of time, the ability to reproduce appropriate behaviour according to a predetermined script, and the readiness to access one's personal repertoire of behaviour to act as you would were you to find yourself in that particular situation. More demanding roles require higher levels of acting usually associated with professional actors, such as moving into situations beyond personal experience and empathically recreating experiences as someone other than oneself. Many of the discussions over whether SP performance is actually acting or not (Davies 1989; Barrows 1993; Woodward and Gliva-McConvey 1995; Woodward 1998; McNaughton *et al.* 1999) consider acting only as that of the higher levels.

The universal designation of SP implies a uniform style of performance and obscures the fact that an actor working within an assessment context performs quite differently than someone who is called upon to demonstrate a skill or to respond in an emotionally authentic manner.

This chapter proposes a taxonomy of five different modes of performance that have developed in medical education, namely: assessment, audit, experiential learning, demonstration, and instruction. These distinctions are significant in that each task leads to a distinctive mode of performance, which then determines the nature of the subsequent decisions that need to be made in relation to recruitment, training, performance, and feedback.

Each role play mode comprises three players who work together in what we might call a simulation triad.

Simulation triad

All five modes of performance comprise three distinct roles.

1. Actor. The role of a patient, performed by an SP, is an acting role. Based on a recognizable clinical reality either actual (Barrows 1987) or classic, the performer possesses the discipline and understanding to control and direct their actions in line with predetermined guidelines and the ability to reproduce

this behaviour over successive occasions. Many members of the public are comfortable and capable of carrying out simpler repertoires, such as memorizing a short list of symptoms and providing questions and answers for clinical examinations. Those who can perform these tasks have at least moderate levels of acting ability, and simply act as they themselves would if they found themselves in the situation. Professional actors are usually employed for longer and more demanding roles.

2. A role player, usually a learner or examinee, who acts as they would in their professional life. The role player is almost always aware that the patient is an actor and that they are performing within a hypothetical situation. Clinical training, knowledge acquisition, and past experience are sufficient to enable the role player to carry out the designated task. This role, which requires the imagination to act as one does in real life, only becomes acting proper if students are asked to make an imaginative leap and pretend to be clinicians with experience and knowledge beyond their present capacities.

3. A watching educator or group of educators who design the simulation, set the rules and criteria of behaviour, observe the actions of the actor and role player, and provide feedback of one kind or another. This feedback may be in the form of a formative or summative assessment at the conclusion of the performance; facilitation of the learning process; or post-performance guidance in video review of the consultation.

The mode of performance determines the nature of each of these three roles and the interaction among them. The selected mode also sets in motion a series of decisions that affect, among other things, the design of the scenario; the choice of casting of the actor; the training of the actor; the role and preparation of the role player; the role and preparation of the educator; the nature of feedback and debriefing subsequent to performance; and the sustainability of performance over time. As these factors are largely determined by the mode and its underlying purpose, it is important first to clarify the nature of each mode of performance before discussing some of the implications for design and training.

Assessment

Since their inception, SPs have been used in medical education to assess clinical and communication skills, either as separate activities or in tandem. The practice has become widespread in North America through the impetus of Barrows, Stillman, and others (Stillman *et al.* 1976; Wallace 1997), and the inspiration of early education centres such as the Morchand Center at Mt Sinai. The Association of American Medical Colleges (AAMC) and the American Medical Association (AMA) have recommended the use of SPs, and national examinations of clinical competency have been established by the Medical Council of Canada (MCC) and the National Board of Medical Examiners (NBME) in the United States. The Macy Foundation provided financial support in setting up eight consortia for propagation of the technique and for mutual support (Rethans *et al.* 1991; Morrison and Barrows 1994), and the Association of Standardized Patient Educators (ASPE), internet networking, and annual SP trainer conferences have fostered strong ties among medical schools with SP programmes.

Actors performing as SPs in an assessment capacity work within frameworks requiring standardization of roles and reliable reproducibility, so that all students are given the same communication challenge. The actors must be able to:

1. work within scenarios that significantly prescribe their behaviour;

2. repeatedly reproduce the same role;

3. recover quickly with minimal rest periods between encounters;

4. maintain focus; and

5. rate students according to predetermined criteria on some form of checklist or rating scale.

The interaction may be brief and focused on the performance of a clinical skill, or it may extend up to an hour as a simulation of a full consultation with a patient. Extended simulation demands of the actor a conscious grasp of the many performance factors at play in reproducing a realistic recreation of real life, which is the study domain of the professional actor.

The educator takes the role of objective assessor and views the encounter either in real time as a passive observer in the room, through a viewing mirror from another room, or on videotape at a later time. The students attempt to match their behaviour to skill sets that are taught as appropriate responses to the encounter.

Audit

Audit is a special case of assessment. Instead of bringing a doctor in to an educational centre to assess clinical or communication skills, educators send the actors into the doctor's own clinical practice in the guise of an actual patient (Burri *et al.* 1976; Rethans *et al.* 1991; Baerheim and Malterud 1995; Beullens *et al.* 1997; Glassman *et al.* 2000). Doctors usually volunteer for a future visit by an SP as a follow-up to communication skills training workshops. Barrows tested this practice of actor as undercover agent and found it to be effective (1987).

Ideally, in an audit situation, the medical professional has given consent for the exercise well beforehand so that the visit takes place within a low index of suspicion. Audit mode is a form of 'invisible theatre' (Boal 1985) in which the doctor is unaware of the artifice, and depends for its success on careful planning and thorough preparation. The device requires that the clinician be unable to differentiate between the actor and other patients in the practice. Actors need to be well-cast to match closely the social types and stereotypical behaviour of the patient population in question, and they need to appear with realistic props, which include perfectly realized documentation.

Professional actors are ideal for this kind of performance, as they are already trained to be aware of the large number of performance factors at play in recreating realistic performance and to be able to manipulate their behaviour to match the expectations of the clinician. However, with longer training and good casting, non-professionals are able to manage the illusion as standard interactions between doctors and patients fall within fairly prescribed boundaries. The actors do not need to enter into the persona of someone other than themselves. They simply need to act as they would were they in that situation with that medical history.

The educator's main focus is that of auditor or inspector. Unlike other modes, the educator cannot be present at the interaction or view it at a later period, but is represented in the encounter by the actor as undercover agent. Feedback is based on carefully prescribed criteria that determine the actor's script for action and the nature of the items in the actor's report on the interaction.

Experiential learning

Whereas assessments measure skills already acquired, experiential learning creates an environment in which students extend their expertise. The learning event may take the form of an encounter with an individual student, a small group, or a 'fishbowl' interaction with 20 or more participants. The performance takes place within a contained environment designed for safety of exploration; the opportunity for learning from one's own interaction with the actor and the observation of one's peers; time to temporarily step out from the interaction to receive feedback; and the opportunity to test out heretofore untried decisions and actions. Experiential learning facilitates gaining confidence and skill to expand one's personal repertoire, or to personalize a line of action sanctioned as professional best practice.

The educator's role is that of facilitator of the students' learning. The scope of the workshop depends largely upon the facilitator's own understanding of the learning process, experience in the role of a facilitator, and comfort with ambiguity and uncertain outcome, in that no two learners will come up with exactly the same solution to a situation. Maximizing the experience for the learners is the key focus for the facilitator and the choices made by the role player are the cues for educational intervention.

The emphasis of performance is marked less by standardization and reproducibility as by the ability to improvise within clearly defined boundaries, with a major focus on authentic personal response to the students' words and actions.

Demonstration

SPs often perform within demonstration mode, either live and in real time before an audience of medical students or professionals, or in a video-recorded interaction as part of a training module as a trigger for discussion. Demonstration usually takes one of four forms:

1. The clinician produces exemplary behaviour as a model for imitation and study.

2. The performance is cautionary, portraying behaviour that produces disastrous consequences.

3. The simulated consultation can be a finely nuanced 'slice of life'. The actors' performance shows something of the complexity of clinical practice with scope for possible improvements in various places. These dramatizations provide rich interactions that reward close observation and reflection.

4. The performance could be in any one of a number of comic modes that laughably render inappropriate behaviour which is self-evidently inadequate and unsupportable.

Professional actors and traditional approaches to scripting and rehearsal are most appropriate for this kind of performance. The scriptwriter may be a clinician with a dramatic sensibility or a non-medical scriptwriter with close access to a clinician experienced in the particular interaction. The script can also be workshopped with the actors from a rough scenario outline. Experience at the Pam McLean Centre of the University of Sydney has demonstrated that medical professionals are able to play the role of the doctor on camera if well-cast and if workshopped into the role. Workshopping reduces the tendency to the wooden or stereotypical behaviour often displayed by doctors thrust with a script before lights and cameras.

Instruction

As early as the 1970s, Stillman recruited members of the public as subjects upon whom students could practise routine, specific, physical examination skills (1976). Around this time, Kretzschmar also introduced the use of GTAs for pelvic examinations (1978). These patients were trained to identify clinical best practice, as exemplified by experienced physicians, and used those criteria to assess student practice. Both Stillman and Kretzschmar quickly expanded the role to include the communication skills used in conjunction with the examinations. Patients playing this role of student instructor are trained in specific clinical examination and communication skills.

Within a short period of time, researchers established three main streams of patient instructors:

1. Healthy members of the public who were able to act as subjects for routine examination skills, where physical findings were not necessary;

2. Patients with stable chronic findings, such as aortic stenosis, asthma, or arthritis (Wallace 1997);

3. SPs who are able to simulate physical findings. Barrows reported that SPs could realistically simulate such findings as lid lag, lid ptosis, wheezing, shortness of breath, carotid bruit, loss of hearing and vision, Babinski sign, and asymmetrical deep tendon reflexes (1987).

Professional actors have traditionally not been necessary for this mode of performance, even when simulation of symptoms is required. The motivation to be involved in the teaching of young doctors is a strong prerequisite for this kind of SP. The roles of actor and educator fuse in this mode, with the educator imparting some of their knowledge to the actor who is able to stand in as proxy. The educator functions as recruiter, trainer, and supervisor.

The rest of the chapter examines the implications of the mode of performance for recruitment, preparation and training, performance, feedback and debriefing, and the effects on the actors.

Recruitment

Barrows identifies only two essential requirements for an SP—intelligence and motivation (1987). Intelligent and motivated applicants most likely possess a third necessary factor: a basic level of comfort with performance.

Professional actors are valuable recruits in several capacities. They are trained to identify the many dynamics of performance at play in common human interactions. In assessment situations that are complex, multifaceted, and of lengthy duration, they can apply these insights to the medical consultation and reproduce an interaction with a high degree of similarity over many performances. In audit situations, they do not need to be schooled in the basics of performance and can quickly learn the nature of the interaction and the criteria by which they are to assess the behaviour of the clinician. The major drawback of the use of actors in audit is financial. In experiential learning workshops they are skilled in authentic interaction with a partner; in accessing and reproducing true emotional states at will; in recognizing and describing the impact of their partner's behaviour; and in producing convincing recreations of a range of patient types and responses. In demonstrations, they can play both patient and clinician roles.

Recruits from the world of medicine and nursing present a mixed bag. In general, clinicians and educators are not a first choice as SP for most modes. In assessment or learning, the educator or clinician may be known to the student and may hinder the student's ability to accept the simulated reality. Even where the educator is unknown, medical knowledge will often affect their ability to empathize and respond as a patient would. Most medical students already have acquired the same problem of medicalization. In the case of demonstrations of communication skills, many doctors and nurses can be rehearsed into playing the clinical role. The role is already known to them through extended practice in real life, and the rehearsal task involves making their usual behaviour known to them so that they can reproduce it comfortably. Our experience shows that many clinicians can reproduce an appropriate version of exemplary behaviour, and the more skilled can manage slice of life. Clinicians tend to drop into comic mode if they portray cautionary behaviour, perhaps as a form of self-protection from the criticism of peers. A small percentage of clinicians with natural abilities as performers are able to play across the spectrum.

Simpler assessment situations can be more than adequately performed by acting students, amateur actors, or members of the public who are comfortable with public interaction. Such scenarios require little more than comfort with performance, alert minds, the ability to learn a simple script of words and actions and to repeat them accurately over many encounters, and a lack of personal agenda from past negative experiences with the medical world. As instructors, the possible need for physical findings or the readiness to expose oneself for pelvic or genital examination limits the pool. Actors or artist models are a potential source for the latter. Non-professionals can perform as auditors, provided that they are chosen for their fit to the population profile of the relevant clinicians' practice, are naturally comfortable with performance, and are given more extensive training than would be required by professional actors.

Typecasting is a safe and wise option in most cases, given that interactions are brief and initial impressions are powerful. Gender, age, ethnic background, physique, or personality type may be an essential requirement to produce the illusion of clinical reality. Clinically inessential elements of the patient's personal and social history can be left to the actor, as long as the actor's choices do not lead the interaction in a direction counter to the purpose of the exercise.

Training for performance

Rehearsals can mostly be relatively short, as the actor, whether lay person or professional actor, does not rehearse to become a character in any rounded sense but as themselves-as-patient in a brief and focused encounter. Inexperienced SPs require longer rehearsal because of the need to be orientated to the mode of performance and to learn their role.

In all cases, the nature of the performance and the desired outcomes determine the training of the actor. Instruction focuses on the specific elements of the examination or history, assessment criteria, and learning how to give an experiential tutorial. Audit requires extensive preparation, especially where non-professionals are recruited as SPs, because invisible theatre demands a cool head acquired through command of the many variables of performance. Experiential learning explores the range of options possible in an open interaction where the actor follows the lead of the student. In experiential learning, there is greater latitude in training as facilitators vary greatly in their approach and objectives, and standardization is relinquished in favour of student-centred learning. Training for assessment differs from that for experiential learning in that the actor's behaviour needs to be far more prescribed, with specific actions and words being rehearsed. The interaction is more formal and less reactive to the individual style of the student. These prescriptions are particularly at play in the clinical examination setting and put performance within reach of a large pool of potential SPs. In assessment of a full consultation, the frame can loosen but still not reach the flexibility of performance of most experiential learning workshops, due to the demand for standardized responses.

In most cases, SPs follow scripts that are produced from the point of view of the patient and written in plain language. Scripting requires conscious effort by educators to abandon their own medical view of the events. In the case of demonstration, the script is either provided as a written text or workshopped by the director and actors into final form. All other modes are improvisational, scenario-based performance, the fixed elements of which are determined by the purpose of the exercise. Scenario-based scripts take the form of units of action to be played more or less in a prescribed sequence, with a small number of verbatim elements. In most modes, the script is built on an illness narrative that proceeds from presenting symptoms through significant events up to the role play consultation, including any prior interactions with other clinicians. The actor rehearses the overall shape and direction of the interaction, essential sequences of history-giving and questioning, and specific questions, or verbatim wording where required.

In instruction, the scripting depends upon the degree to which the SP teaches the skill or responds to the students' actions. The script for the former lays down a series of actions, and for the latter provides responses to a menu of possible stimuli from the student.

Training needs to incorporate some level of medicalization of the actor for two reasons. Patients gradually become medicalized through experience with the medical system. A patient may have personal knowledge of medications, tests, scans, operations, and may have read booklets, or researched on the internet. The actor needs this information in order to play the part with any conviction and credence. However, even where a patient is informationally naïve, it is important for the actor not to be so, especially in experiential learning settings. Many scenarios require the actor to recognize what kind of difficulties students are likely to experience, how well students are performing in relation to approved standards, and information that they, the patient, are not being given. The more professional the actors, the more likely they can internalize this knowledge and direct their performance while their characters respond in ignorance of these facts.

Feedback

Training also needs to include rehearsal of feedback, which provides another source of complexity and adds further levels of concentration to the performance. In most modes, the actors must split their focus to carry out three simultaneous tasks: remain spontaneously open to the interaction with their partner; direct their performance in accordance with the overall script; and remain alert to the specific behaviours to be reported in feedback. This third task alters according to the mode of performance. For example, in assessment and audit, the feedback required will include a checklist, rating scale, or report in which the clinician's behaviour is judged according to objective, predetermined criteria. These criteria need to be communicated clearly to the actors and practised in rehearsal. Checklists require of the actor a sudden and major shift in focus from subjective performance to detached critique; clarity and practice are required.

In instruction, feedback is of two kinds—objective matching of the student's actions to a model of clinical best practice, and subjective response to how the student handles, relates to, and communicates with the SP.

In experiential learning, feedback takes place in three ways:

1. The actor's responses within the interaction through words and body language provide immediate feedback to the role player and observers of the impact of the role player's actions. This form of feedback is the most direct, yet is most often left out of discussions on feedback.

2. The actor is able to give feedback in character during timeout breaks to guide the student in assessing their performance and directing it forward.

3. After the interaction, the SP can give general feedback according to broad guidelines set out by the facilitator.

In this setting, feedback takes the form of considered and constructive response to the choices of the role player, rather than the objective assessment of successful performance of external criteria of the examination setting. Feedback can include any number of factors, such as the impact of a role player's manner and language, whether they block or facilitate communication, their ability to elicit personal concerns, or the extent to which they share ownership of the consultation.

On method acting

The debate over the relative merits and safety of method acting versus technique approaches to SP performance (Naftulin and Andrew 1975; Davies 1989; Woodward and Gliva-McConvey 1995; Woodward 1998; McNaughton *et al.* 1999) is a little overstated as most modern actors borrow skills from a wide range of sources. Method is mostly an internal approach to performance, while technique refers to working from outside behaviour to inner motivation. For instance, an actor wishes to pick up and drink a glass of water. Using method, the actor reminds himself that he is thirsty, remembers how dry his mouth is when thirsty, and recreates that sense of dryness as he reaches over to pick up the glass to quench his thirst. Using technique, the actor allows his gaze to pass over the glass while he talks with the doctor. When, a moment later, he reaches out for the water and drinks it, his noticing of the glass provides sufficient motivation for his action and the doctor accepts that he is thirsty. Method has real value as a rehearsal technique; however, it is not always intended for use in performance itself. For instance, an exercise such as emotional memory (Stanislavski 1984) is a valuable rehearsal technique by which the actor goes back to personal trauma to obtain empathic access to emotions experienced by patients on receiving bad news. Once the actor has accessed the emotion in rehearsal, technique is often sufficient to trigger the emotional reality in performance. Constant return to one's own library of distress can become very emotionally draining. Lack of experience or training in acting may be responsible for reports

of distress after intense or emotional performances (Naftulin and Andrew 1975; Woodward and Gliva-McConvey 1995; Woodward 1998; McNaughton *et al.* 1999; Bokken *et al.* 2004, 2006).

However, the fact remains that the more intense and demanding roles as an SP can take their toll. In general, professional actors tend to possess the techniques and resources to safely enter and debrief from their roles. Cool down after acting is an intrinsic part of the performance process. Less experienced performers would benefit from opportunities offered by educators for times of debriefing afterwards. The repeated impact of emotionally intense roles or of scenarios that demand that the actor vicariously experience emotional pain or existential turmoil over their own mortality is still unknown, and the capacity of actors to manage these roles over an extended period of time varies. Capacity over the long term is probably a function of a number of variables and not just acting style alone. A wise course is to provide the actor as wide a range of roles as possible.

Conclusion

Various studies have exhibited confusion as to whether medical simulation should even be considered acting. Acting is often erroneously interpreted purely as the aesthetic drama of the stage. In fact, drama constitutes a continuum from games and simple role play to professional acting, and medical simulation falls within the scale of this continuum. The patient role is always an acting role, which is one-third of the simulation triad of actor, role player, and educator. The tasks of each of these three players, and the relationships among them, change according to the demands of the specific performance. Some of the patient roles are playable by untrained members of the public, while other, more demanding roles require actors who are trained to recreate complex behaviour.

This chapter distinguishes among five different modes of performance that have developed in medical education. Actors perform in:

1. assessment;

2. audit;

3. experiential learning;

4. demonstration;

5. instruction mode.

Recognition of these distinctions clarifies the nature of the decisions that need to be made in relation to recruitment, training, performance, and the specific kind of feedback required within each mode. It is hoped that this proposed taxonomy of performance may contribute clarification for future uses of medical simulation.

References

Baerheim A, Malterud K (1995). Simulated patients for the practical examination of medical students: intentions, procedures and experiences. *Med Educ* **29**, 410–13.

Barrows H (1987). *Simulated (Standardized) Patients and Other Human Simulations.* Health Sciences Consortium, Chapel Hill, NC.

Barrows H (1993). An overview of the uses of standardized patients for teaching and evaluating clinical skills. *Acad Med* **68**, 446–51.

Beullens J, Rethans J, Goedhuys J, Buntinx F (1997). The use of standardized patients in research in general practice. *Fam Pract* **14**, 58–62.

Boal A (1985). *Theatre of the Oppressed.* pp. 126–47. Theatre Communications Group, New York, NY.

Bokken L, van Dalen J, Rethans J (2004). Performance-related stress symptoms in simulated patients. *Med Educ* **38**, 1089–94.

Bokken L, van Dalen J, Rethans J (2006). The impact of simulation on people who act as simulated patients: a focus group study. *Med Educ* **40**, 781–6.

Bosek M, Li S, Hicks F (2007). Working with standardized patients: a primer. *Int J Nurs Educ Scholarsh* **4**, 1–12.

Burri A, McCaughan K, Barrows H (1976). The feasibility of using the simulated patient as a means to evaluate clinical competence of practicing physicians in a community. In: the proceedings of the Fifteenth Annual Conference on Research in Medical Education: pp. 295–9. Association of American Medical Colleges, Washington DC, WA.

Davies M (1989). The way ahead: teaching with simulated patients. *Med Teach* **11**, 315–20.

Glassman P, Luck J, O'Gara E, Peabody J (2000). Using standardized patients to measure quality: evidence from the literature and a prospective study. *Jt Comm J Qual Improv* **26**, 644–53.

Greenberg L, Ochsenschlager D, O'Donnell R, Mastruserio J, Cohen G (1999). Communicating bad news: a pediatric department's evaluation of a simulated intervention. *Pediatrics* **103**, 1210–17.

Kretzschmar R (1978). Evolution of the gynecology teaching associate: an educational specialist. *Am J Obstet Gynecol* **131**, 367–73.

McManus I, Vincent C, Thom S, Kidd J (1993). Teaching communication skills to clinical students. *BMJ* **306**, 1322–7.

McNaughton N, Tiberius R, Hodges B (1999). Effects of portraying psychologically and emotionally complex standardized patient roles. *Teach Learn Med* **11**, 135–41.

Meier R, Perkowski L, Wynne C (1982). A method for training simulated patients. *J Med Educ* **57**, 535–40.

Morrison L, Barrows H (1994). Developing consortia for clinical practice examinations: the Macy Project. *Teach Learn Med* **6**, 23–7.

Naftulin D, Andrew D (1975). The effects of patient simulations on actors. *J Med Educ* **50**, 87–9.

Razavi D, Delvaux N, Marchal S, De Cock M, Farvacques C, Slachmuylder J (2000). Testing health care professionals' communication skills: the usefulness of highly emotional standardized role-playing sessions with simulators. *Psychooncology* **9**, 293–302.

Rethans J, Drop R, Sturmans F, van der Vleuten C (1991). A method for introducing standardized (simulated) patients into general practice consultations. *Br J Gen Pract* **41**, 94–6.

Rosenbaum M, Ferguson K (2006). Using patient-generated cases to teach students skills in responding to patients' emotions. *Med Teach* **28**, 180–2.

Smith P, Fuller G, Kinnersley P, Brigley S, Elwyn G (2002). Using simulated consultations to develop communication skills for neurological trainees. *Eur J Neurol* **9**, 83–7.

Stanislavski C (1984). *An Actor Prepares*, pp. 155–81. Theatre Arts Books, New York, NY.

Stillman P, Sabers D, Redfield D (1976). The use of paraprofessionals to teach interviewing skills. *Pediatrics* **57**, 769–74.

Wallace P (1997). Following the threads of an innovation: the history of standardized patients in medical education. *Caduceus* **13**, 5–28.

Woodward C, Gliva-McConvey G (1995). The effect of simulating on standardized patients. *Acad Med* **70**, 418–20.

Woodward C (1998). Standardized patients: a fixed-role therapy experience in normal individuals. *J Construct Psych* **11**, 133–48.

CHAPTER 56

The Oncotalk/Vitaltalk model

Robert M. Arnold, Anthony L. Back, Walter F. Baile, Kelly A. Edwards, and James A. Tulsky

Introduction to the Oncotalk/Vitaltalk model

In 2002, we received funding from the National Cancer Institute to develop a new teaching model for communication skills at the end of life, aimed at medical oncology fellows. Using this model, originally named Oncotalk, and now called Vitaltalk, we taught more than 200 oncology fellows trained in the United States over a five-year period. Subsequently, we have developed similar programmes to train faculty in critical care, nephrology, cardiology, and neonatology. In developing the programme, we utilized key educational principles, some of which had been used in other communication skills training, others of which evolved as a result of the unique demands of the teaching context. Given our primary audience of oncology fellows, we paid particular attention to how we structured the programme to ground the learning in practical, patient-care challenges that reflected the fellows' clinical experiences. Throughout the course of development, implementation, and evaluation, we learned important lessons that can be taken up and tested further by other communication skills educators (Edwards-Fryer et al. 2006). This chapter describes common evidence-based principles used in developing an advanced communication skills programme based on our Oncotalk experiences, identifies unique aspects of the learning context within an intensive retreat structure, and illustrates the lessons learned that can be tested in other settings. The aim is to provide tools and frameworks to facilitate teaching communication skills within oncology and other training programmes that prepare clinicians to work with seriously ill patients.

Why Oncotalk?

A variety of studies document shortcomings in communication between physicians and patients with advanced cancer (Barclay et al. 2007). First, the literature suggests that oncologists do not often talk to patients with advanced cancer about palliative care (Gattellari et al. 2002). Even when discussions occur, poor quality frequently undermines their usefulness. Tulsky et al. found that physicians who do talk about advanced care planning focus largely on treatments, rarely give patients enough information to make informed decisions, and neglect more general values and goals (Tulsky et al. 1998; Roter et al. 2000).

Deficiencies in communication are common. For example, a variety of studies show that oncologists rarely discuss issues surrounding quality of life with patients who have advanced cancer (Detmar et al. 2001). It is, therefore, no surprise that most oncologists inaccurately assess patients' emotional distress (Ford et al. 1994). When patients express negative emotions, their doctors typically respond by changing the subject, by providing reassurance, or by providing cognitive information (Pollak et al. 2007).

Oncologists' communication skills are suboptimal, at least in part, because they receive little training in this area. A survey of more than 3,200 American Society of Clinical Oncology members found that few had formal training in end-of-life care or communication skills (Baile et al. 2000). More recently, fellows revealed that only 15% had any exposure to communication skills training (Hoffman et al. 2004). While the American Council of Graduate Medical Education includes communication skills as a core competency for all oncology fellows, little of this education relates to communication with patients having advanced cancer (Weissman and Block 2002). Oncology fellows reported, in one study, that they felt more capable talking about chemotherapy side effects than discussing ending chemotherapy and focusing on quality of life (Buss et al. 2007). While fellows routinely have difficult conversations with seriously ill patients, only 56% of them report being observed and given feedback on these conversations by their attending physicians (Buss et al. 2007).

A number of important organizations recommend improved communication skills at the end of life. The National Cancer Institute designated cancer communication as an 'extraordinary scientific priority' in 2002 and developed a Health Communication and Informatics Research Branch. Two Institute of Medicine reports—one focusing on cancer care and one on palliative care—emphasize the importance of communication skills in shared decision-making (Hewih and Simme 1999). Finally, the National Institute of Health State of the Science in End-of-Life Care summary statement concluded that 'effective communication is critical' to improving outcomes in end-of-life care (State of the Science Conference Statement 2004). This combination of empirical data and institutional reports reinforces broad support for training programmes like Oncotalk.

Evidence-based principles for teaching communication skills

A Cochrane systematic review of communication skills training for healthcare providers working with cancer patients and their families concluded that: communication skills do not reliably improve with experience alone; and training programmes using appropriate educational techniques are effective in improving skills (Fellowes *et al.* 2004). Studies of oncologists, internists, and family medicine physicians demonstrate that after communication skills training, doctors discuss more psychosocial issues, use more open-ended questions, are better able to elicit patients' values and feelings, and attend to distress (Roter *et al.* 1995; Fallowfield *et al.* 2002; Delvaux *et al.* 2005).

A theory of teaching communication skills

At the centre of the Oncotalk design, for both intervention and evaluation, is self-efficacy theory (Bandura 1982). In self-efficacy theory, the impetus for change resides in the individual's efficacy expectations. These expectations reflect the learner's beliefs about his/her ability to perform the task. Efficacy expectations are acquired from four sources: performance accomplishments; vicarious experience; verbal persuasion; and emotional state (Maguire and Faulkner 1988; Carroll *et al.* 1995; Fellowes *et al.* 2004; Kurtz *et al.* 2005).

Based on this theoretic model and the Cochrane review, we chose the following design features for the Oncotalk intervention:

1. Brief didactic sessions to provide specific communication models.

   A systematic review of continuing medical education indicates that traditional lecture-based conferences have little direct effect on changing physician performance. That being said, it is still necessary to provide a cognitive map for the upcoming skill practice. Didactics are minimized and focus on both the rationale for, and demonstration of, specific skills. Thus, Oncotalk limits didactics to 30-minute blocks, in which specific skills are identified and illustrated.

   After talking about skills, faculty must demonstrate them. First, given that we are asking the participants to practice in front of their colleagues, we believed that it was important that we also demonstrate our willingness to practice in front of others. Second, hearing about the skills in a didactic lecture is very different from watching them being operationalized. Third, this demonstration allows us to emphasize the importance of close observation when giving feedback.

2. Skill practice with group feedback.

   Previous studies indicate that demonstration of new skills is not sufficient. Successful programmes have the participant try new behaviours and receive immediate feedback on their performance. Oncotalk focuses more than 75% of its time on skill practice within a small group of fellows, allowing them to receive immediate feedback from their peers, and see how other fellows interact with patients.

   The skills practice takes two forms. The majority of time is spent with the learner seeing the patient as if it were an actual encounter ('a scrimmage'). The goal is to make the situation realistic so that the learner experiences the emotionality of the encounter. Recently, we have begun to have learners practice specific skills in drills. In these short encounters, we ask the learner to practice a specific skill such as an empathic response to a question. The faculty moves around the room asking each learner a question ('Does this mean there is nothing more to do?'), and the learner is expected to respond empathically. The focus is less on realism and more on practice.

3. Use of simulated patients.

   The use of simulated patients allows the participant to learn, in an environment approximating clinical practice, the exact skills that they will use in clinical practice. In addition, using simulated patients allows the participant to rewind and try the same scenario in different ways. Finally, simulated patients can be trained to provide immediate feedback on his or her experience of the clinician's behaviour. Oncotalk uses five simulated patient cases, in which the patient story unfolds over four visits, allowing the learners to give bad news, negotiate treatment goals, and talk about end-of-life issues.

4. Focusing on the trainees' needs.

   Allowing the participants open time to focus on self-identified skills and challenges is key. Research in adult learning indicates that learning must be relevant to a valued task, immediately transferable, and participant-centred. Didactics and structured skill practice target participant goals, but some open space is used to address unique participant challenges. Oncotalk does this in two ways. First, trainees are asked to identify their learning goals before every practice session. Second, open sessions, in which fellows role play their most difficult patients, are scheduled to allow fellows to name and work on encounters that are particularly important and challenging to them.

5. Attend to trainees' attitudes and emotions.

   Successful courses address physician attitudes and emotions, as well as knowledge and skill deficits. Caring for oncology patients, particularly dying patients, can elicit strong feelings in the physician. Most courses spend some time focusing on emotional issues, either by integrated discussion within the skill practice sessions, or as a separate reflective session on specific emotional issues. In addition to talking about fellows' emotions during practice sessions, Oncotalk includes specific reflective exercises to help fellows think about the type of doctor they want to become and how communication skills practice fits into their professional identity.

6. Because of the complexity of the teaching and the challenging nature of the learning, we chose an intensive retreat as the primary educational intervention for teaching communication skills. While possible to do in shorter sessions over a longer time period within the healthcare setting, removing fellows from their daily work routine allows them to leave their pagers behind and encourages them to focus on learning. Oncotalk is scheduled in an intensive two-to-three-day block of time.

The Oncotalk/Vitaltalk programme populates these principles with specific core content (Back *et al.* 2003).

Core cognitive maps in end-of-life communication

While details in the literature on communication skills in end-of-life care vary, we can identify a core set of common communication skills. Our objective in the didactic sessions is to provide the fellows with a cognitive overview of these core skills. Then in the skills practice session, they can practise the skills, including for when predictable and unpredictable challenges arise.

We emphasize a foundation with three basic skills in our first session. 'Ask tell ask' requires that participants assess the patient's experience prior to giving information and then, after the information is provided, inquire about what the patient heard. Second, encouraging the patient to tell the story is taught using open-ended questions and phrases such as, 'Tell me more'. Finally, we provide several tools for responding with empathy using the acronym NURSE: **N**ame the emotion, show that you **U**nderstand the emotion, **R**espect the patient's experience, use **S**upportive statements, and **E**xplore the patient's experience (Smith and Hoppe 1991).

The foundational skills are repeated throughout the task-specific communication skills training. Following a trajectory of illness, we begin with the task-specific skill of giving bad news. We teach this skill using both the SPIKES (**S**etting, **P**reparation, **I**nformation, **K**nowledge, **E**mpathy, **S**trategy) and GUIDE (**G**et ready, **U**nderstand, **I**nform, **D**eepen, and **E**quip) acronyms (Baile *et al.* 2000; Vitaltalk app, iTunes). Trainees find these acronyms helpful as it gives them a structured way to think about an emotionally difficult task. These acronyms rely heavily on the core skills taught in the first session:

1. Assessing the patient's perception before giving the bad news.

2. Empathizing with the patient's emotional reaction before going on to make a plan.

Giving bad news is central to talking about transitioning from curative to palliative goals of care. Talking about transitions requires that an oncologist be able to give bad news and then help the patients come up with other goals in the time that they have remaining. This requires skills, such as first recognizing the transitions discussion as a bad news discussion and then employing specific communication strategies, such as hoping for the best, preparing for the worst (Evans *et al.* 2006), and attending to loss and the shift in expectations using wish statements (Back *et al.* 2003).

Finally, like most clinicians who work with seriously ill patients, oncologists must learn to talk about dying in an explicit fashion. Talking about dying requires the learners to integrate the skills outlined above, including the ability to integrate giving bad news while attending to strong emotions and the ability to assess the patient's fears, concerns, and hopes. We explicitly speak about how these skills integrate to achieve two new communication challenges: talking about goals of care and making a treatment recommendation that matches those goals; and saying goodbye to a patient (Back *et al.* 2004).

Teaching using simulated patients

One of the ways we emphasize the developmental aspects of skills is to use a simulated patient case study. Each patient's story unfolds over four sessions, and the participant is given a specific task at each (see Table 56.1). Using the time-series case studies has many advantages. First, by working with the same patient over an illness trajectory, it allows the participants to develop a relationship with the patient making the emotional work more realistic. Second, because each day focuses on a specific skill in a specific order, participants learn basic skills before moving on to complex ones. Finally, by having five distinct patients, we can ensure that the participants experience (either directly or vicariously) a diverse set of patients. For example, the patients respond to bad news with different emotional responses—anger, sadness, disbelief, frustration, and being overwhelmed—each of which require a different response from the participant.

The Oncotalk experience

Between April 2002 and June 2007, 180 medical oncology fellows, mostly in the second and third years of their fellowship, were asked to participate in three-and-a-half-day intensive communication

Table 56.1 Communication skills curriculum based on illness trajectory

Session	Content focus	Skills practice with simulated patient
1	Developing a relationship / Dealing with uncertainty	A 47-year-old female with breast cancer after lumpectomy, chemotherapy, radiation one year ago, seen for routine surveillance, notes some back pain
2	Giving bad news	One week later: bone scan ordered last visit shows multiple metastases; CT shows liver metastases
3	Discussing goals of care	Three years later: now having received multiple chemotherapy regimens, with disease progression on therapy
4	Discussing do-not-resuscitate orders	Two months later: at home with hospice, told nurse she 'wants everything'

Reproduced with permission from Back AL *et al.*, 'Efficacy of communication skills training for Giving Bad News and Discussing Transitions to Palliative Care', *Archives of Internal Medicine*, Volume 167, Number 5, pp. 453–50, Copyright © 2007 American Medical Association. All rights reserved.

skills retreats. We ran two courses a year and included 20 participants per retreat, allowing us to run small groups with a 1:5 faculty to participant ratio. Based on our sample size calculations, evaluative data were collected on 120 participants, distributed in training programmes across the United States (Back *et al.* 2007).

The evaluation includes both self-evaluation measures of competence and satisfaction, as well as a comparison of pre-retreat and post-retreat encounters with standardized patients (see Back *et al.* 2003 for a complete description of the methods). Each participant completes two pre-retreat and two post-retreat simulations—one focusing on giving bad news, and the other on goals of care when things are not going well. The evaluative standardized patient encounters are audiotaped and analysed for behaviour change by independent and blinded coders. The investigators developed a coding instrument consisting of a set of observable behaviours for each communication task. The codes are intended to represent best practice communication behaviours that could be recognized by coders with adequate inter-rater reliability. The task-specific codes for bad news, for example, are based on the literature and the SPIKES acronym. Finally, as part of the audio tape evaluation, we ask the coders to guess whether the tape they are listening to is pre- or post-intervention (Back *et al.* 2007).

The participants' evaluations of Oncotalk have been overwhelmingly enthusiastic. For example, they rated the statement, 'I would recommend this training to other fellows' a mean of 4.95 on a 5-point Likert scale. All components of the retreat were highly rated.

Respondents clearly learned skills that they did not know prior to the retreat. For example, of the participants who, prior to the retreat, did not respond empathically after giving bad news, 73% did so after the retreat. In response to the required standardized patient statement, 'I'm really scared', 100% of the participants who had not responded empathically to this cue in the pre-test were able to do so post-retreat. We also measured whether participants were able to use empathic statements. Post-retreat, both the number and the types of empathic responses markedly increased. Participants acquired a median of six new communication skills related to giving bad news (Back *et al.* 2007).

Similar improvements were found in participants' skills in discussing goals of care when the patient is not doing well. In post-retreat encounters, participants demonstrated statistically significant skill acquisition in the following areas: assessing and understanding; discussing the overall clinical picture; responding to emotion; and asking about worries, fears, and concerns. Again, a large number of participants improved their skills. For example, when the standardized patient hears that palliative chemotherapy is no longer working and asks 'Isn't there anything more you can do?', 92% of the participants pre-retreat did not include an empathic or an 'I wish' statement in their response. Post-retreat, approximately a third used one of these responses (Back *et al.* 2007).

Finally, blinded coders were able to correctly identify pre- or post-retreat participants in 91% of the bad news and 70% of the transition audio recordings (Back *et al.* 2007).

Subsequently, many individual oncology fellowships have begun teaching Oncotalk (University of Indiana, University of Pittsburgh, Beth Israel Deaconess, Mt. Sinai School of Medicine, and Duke University). The feedback from these programmes has been very positive (Back *et al.* 2007).

What we learned from Oncotalk

In developing and implementing Oncotalk, we learned a number of important and somewhat unexpected lessons about how to teach communication skills. First, we learned about the importance of trust in the small group. In early renditions of Oncotalk, we had participants spend time in both small groups of five, where they practised skills, and larger groups of ten, where they did their reflective exercises. Participants felt more comfortable talking about their emotions and worries in the small groups because they had spent time as a cohort and had taken risks together. In our follow-up teaching sessions, we paid more attention to the importance of trust within the group. Now, all teaching, reflective exercises, and follow-ups take place in the same five-person small groups.

Second, in teaching these sessions, we began to see a common developmental learning process. Participants have to first recognize an emotion in the encounter (the patient seems emotional), then name this emotion (the patient's emotion is sadness), and finally they need to be able to respond empathically to the patient's emotion ('You seem really sad'). While many communication skills programmes emphasize the words to say to patients, developing a sense of the learning trajectory helped us target our feedback and learning experiences to move a participant towards responding genuinely to a patient's needs. Different insights will move participants along the trajectory at a different pace. Some insights are instrumental, meaning that the conversation can move forward after trainees respond to a patient's emotion in a genuine way; others involve a shift in how the participants come to see their responsibility to develop a therapeutic alliance with the patient. Either insight helps move them forward towards recognizing and responding to emotions.

Third, we noticed that as learners focused on one skill, other skills may be ignored. Thus, for example, we noticed that as fellows focused on attending to emotions, their ability to process patients' cognitive information may decrease. This seemed to be a developmental learning process as with increased empathic ability, their ability to pay more attention to the other things that are happening in the interview increased. Focusing on one skill at a time and only

then focusing on skill integration helped the learner from being overwhelmed.

Fourth, we were impressed by the importance of participants' own emotions in learning communication skills. Most of the participants knew how to give bad news, and they could quickly tell you the cognitive steps involved in SPIKES. However, in the process of having to give the news, even to standardized patients, they got tripped up by their own emotions. Sadness led them to hedge or to provide false reassurance, or their anxiety led them to move quickly into a treatment plan before the patient was ready to hear it. It was critical for us to acknowledge the trainee's sadness and the powerlessness in preventing the progression of cancer. Once the faculty attended to his or her own sadness, they were better able to cope with the patient's sadness. To a certain degree, we were role modelling how to be empathetic regarding emotion. Moreover, by normalizing their emotions, we allowed them to be more comfortable in feeling emotions when talking about death and dying. Finally, some trainees worried about being overwhelmed by the patient's emotions and, as a result, blocked discussion of difficult topics. The use of simulated patients allowed us to take a time-out for discussion if the participant seemed overwhelmed.

Fifth, our Oncotalk experience helped teach us the importance of positive feedback and reflection. For decades, sociologists have commented on the punitive and negative teaching methods used in medical education. To a certain degree, the participants came to Oncotalk wanting to learn what 'they did wrong'. This meant that they did not appreciate their strengths in communicating with patients and, therefore, could not make a conscious effort to use them when stuck. Once a participant saw that they were viewed by others as calm and empathic, they could be more intentional in using these skills when a patient got upset. In addition, once the participants recognized their strengths, they were more willing to identify their own weaknesses.

This lesson of emphasizing the positive occurred in the other sessions as well as within the skill practice sessions. For example, initially in the didactics, we role played bad encounters and asked the participants to comment on what could have been done differently. Based on the feedback, we realized that many of the participants had never had the skills of a good communication encounter described. They needed a positive role model to demonstrate and name each of the skills that one uses in a difficult discussion. We, therefore, modified the curriculum and focused on role plays that illustrated how the encounters should go.

The reflective sessions also changed over time to emphasize positive experiences. In the initial Oncotalk retreats, our reflective sessions dealt with loss or participants' most difficult encounters. These sessions elicited little discussion and received the most negative feedback of the entire retreat. Therefore, about half-way through the sessions, we changed the exercises to focus on the positive aspects of healing. For example, rather than have them talk about the most difficult death, we asked them to talk about the last time they felt like a healer. By focusing on the positive aspects of communication, the participants got in touch with why they went into oncology in the first place and how they could utilize their clinical skills to promote more healing. Following this change, the sessions received better participant evaluations.

Finally, Oncotalk helped us see the importance of skills practice that enables participants to experience success. Participants often want to practice the hardest situation possible, what we called 'cases from hell'. The problem is that it is very hard to experience success in these situations. Regardless of what the participant does, the case goes badly, decreasing self-efficacy and confidence. We, therefore, focused on helping the participant identify their 'learning edge' (i.e. work that would be challenging for the participant, but not overwhelming). The goal was to encourage the participant to choose to work on a skill in which they have yet to achieve competency, but not one where they are unlikely to succeed. By succeeding, they learned how the new skills positively impacted the simulated patient, which in turn encouraged them to try the skills again.

These teaching skills helped us envision the process of oncology communication skills learning as a series of steps resulting in a positive feedback loop:

◆ The participant hears feedback about strengths from the group.

◆ The participant identifies a salient skill that requires work.

◆ The participant practises these skills in a small group with trusted colleagues.

◆ The participant achieves some success in learning the new skill.

◆ The participant reflects on his/her progress and revises the learning goal based on the session (Edwards-Fryer et al. 2006).

Conclusion

Over a five-year period, we trained 10% of America's oncology fellows in an elective course held in Aspen. Oncotalk represents a successful model of a residential communication skills course, and given the behaviour change outcomes, represents a benchmark for this kind of teaching model.

Oncotalk, however, is only the first step. Subsequently, we started a non-profit organization, Vitaltalk (vitaltalk.org), to nurture healthier connections between patients and clinicians. Using the Oncotalk methods, we are developing courses for other specialties involved in caring for seriously ill patients (neonatology, paediatric, and adult intensive care, cardiology, and nephrology). These courses are designed to be integrated into fellows' training.

A number of factors need to be addressed before oncological communication training can be scaled to serve more healthcare professionals. The first factor is the most difficult: faculty teaching capacity. There are few oncology faculties with training in the communication skills required to conduct this teaching. To meet this need, we conducted a follow-up project entitled Oncotalk Teach, designed to begin training a cohort of oncology faculty who would use Oncotalk principles in communication teaching at their home institutions, using real time clinical encounters. We also held two train-the-trainer retreats for faculty interested in teaching Oncotalk at their institutions. The advantage of training a cadre of local communication experts is that communication can be required during fellows' clinical training, much like other important educational objectives.

Other barriers may impede teaching oncologists communication skills: the course is relatively expensive; requires time off from clinical responsibilities; and requires the commitment from training programmes to prioritize this aspect of education for oncologists in training. We are building mobile applications and courses to bring communication skills to more learners. The challenge is to determine what can only be taught face-to-face and what can be taught at a distance.

Oncotalk has shown that we can improve fellows' communication skills. The next generation of courses needs to build on this success to ensure that all oncologists are skilled in communicating with their cancer patients.

References

Back, A, Arnold RM, Quill T (2003). Hoping for the best, preparing for the worst. Ann Int Med 138, 439–44.

Back A, Arnold RM, Tulsky J, et al. (2003). Teaching communication skills to medical oncology fellows. J Clin Onc 21, 2433–6.

Back AL, Arnold RM, Tulsky JA, et al. (2004). On saying goodbye: acknowledging the end of the patient-physician relationship with patients who are near death. Ann Intern Med 142, 682–5.

Back AL, Arnold RM, Baile WF, et al. (2007). Efficacy of communication skills training for giving bad news and discussing transitions to palliative care. Arch Int Med 167, 453–60.

Baile WF, Buckman R, Lenzi R, et al. (2000). SPIKES-A six-step protocol for delivering bad news: application to the patient with cancer. Oncologist 5, 302–11.

Bandura A (1982). Self-efficacy mechanism in human agency. Am Psychol 37, 122–47.

Barclay JS, Blackhall LJ, Tulsky JA (2007). Communication strategies and cultural issues in the delivery of bad news. J Palliat Med 10, 958–77.

Buss M, Lessen DS, Sullivan AM, et al. (2007). A study of oncology fellows' training in end-of-life care. J Supp Onc 5, 237–45.

Carroll JG, Lipkin M, Nachtigall L, et al. (eds) (1995). A Developmental Awareness for Teaching Doctor–Patient Communication Skills. The Medical Interview, pp. 388–96. Springer, New York, NY.

Delvaux N, Merckaert I, Marchal S, et al. (2005). Physician communication with a cancer patient and a relative: a randomized study assessing the effects of consolidation workshops. Cancer 103, 2397–411.

Detmar SB, Muller MJ, Wever LD (2001). The patient–physician relationship; patient–physician communication during outpatient palliative treatment visits: an observational study. JAMA 285, 1351–7.

Edwards-Fryer K, Arnold RM, Baile W, et al. (2006). Teaching communication skills: a qualitative study of reflective teaching practices. Acad Med 81, 638–44.

Evans W, Tulsky J, Back A, et al. (2006). Communication at times of transitions: how to help patients cope with loss and re-define hope. Cancer J 12, 417–24.

Fallowfield L, Jenkins V, Farewell V, Saul J, Duffy A, Eves R (2002). Efficacy of a Cancer Research UK communication skills training model for oncologists: a randomized controlled trial. Lancet 359, 650–6.

Fellowes D, Wilkinson S, Moore P (2004). Communication skills training for health care professionals working with cancer patients, their families and/or careers. Cochrane Database Syst Rev (2): CD003751.

Ford S, Fallowfield L, Lewis S (1994). Can oncologists detect distress in their out-patients and how satisfied are they with their performance during bad news consultations? Br J Cancer 70, 767–70.

Gattellari M, Voigt KJ, Butow PN, et al. (2002). When the treatment goal is not cure: are cancer patients equipped to make informed decisions? J Clin Oncol 20, 503–13.

Hewih M, Simme JV (eds) (1999). Ensuring Quality Cancer Care. National Academy Press, Washington DC, WA.

Hoffman M, Ferri J, Sison C, et al. (2004). Teaching communication skills: an AACE survey of oncology training programs. J Cancer Educ 19, 220–4.

Kurtz S, Silverman J, Draper J (2005). Teaching and Learning Communication Skills in Medicine, 2nd edition. Radcliffe Medical Press, Oxford, UK.

Maguire P, Faulkner A (1988). Improve the counseling skills of doctors and nurses in cancer care. Br Med J 297, 847–9.

Pollak KI, Arnold RM, Jeffreys A, et al. (2007). Oncologist communication about emotion during visits with advanced cancer patients. J Clin Oncol 25, 5748–52.

Roter DL, Hall JA, Kern DE, *et al.* (1995). Improving physicians' interviewing skills and reducing patients' emotional distress. A randomized clinical trial. *Arch Intern Med* **155**, 1877–84.

Roter DL, Larson S, Fischer GS, *et al.* (2000). Experts practice what they preach: a descriptive study of best and normative practices in end-of-life discussion. *Arch Int Med* **160,** 13477–85.

Smith RC, Hoppe RB (1991). The patient's story: integrating the patient- and physician-centered approaches to interviewing. *Ann Intern Med* **115**, 470–7.

State of the Science Conference Statement (2004). *Improving End-of-Life Care*, National Institutes of Health. Available at: http://consensus.nih.gov/2004/2004EndOfLifeCareSOS024html.htm [Online].

Tulsky JA, Fischer GS, Rose MR, et al. (1998). Opening the black box: How do physicians communicate about advance directives? *Ann Int Med* **129**, 441–9.

Weissman DE, Block SD (2002). ACGME requirements for end-of-life training in selected residency and fellowship programs: a status report. *Acad Med* **77**, 299–304.

CHAPTER 57

The Swiss model

Friedrich Stiefel, Jürg Bernhard, Gabriella Bianchi,
Lilo Dietrich, Christoph Hürny, Alexander Kiss,
Brigitta Wössmer, and Céline Bourquin

Introduction to the Swiss model

The Swiss communication skills training (CST) for oncology clinicians was initiated in 1998 by the Swiss Cancer League (SCL), which mandated a national task force[1] to elaborate a concept for a CST for oncology physicians and nurses (Kiss 1999). In order to learn about key elements of existing CST, the task force, together with the SCL, organized a meeting with three invited experts—Leslie Fallowfield and Peter Maguire from the United Kingdom, and Darius Razavi from Belgium—who presented their models by means of interactive workshops; chiefs of service and head nurses from different oncology centres participated in this meeting. Based on these experiences, the task force developed a concept for a national CST for oncology clinicians.

Initially, a 'train-the-trainers' course was organized for the members of the task force, allowing them to experience the CST as participants and to gain insight into its dynamics. Following a pilot CST, organized in the German, French, and Italian parts of Switzerland for local chiefs of oncology services and head nurses, the Swiss CST was implemented; it was officially endorsed by the Swiss Society of Medical Oncology (SSMO), and sponsored by two pharmaceutical companies that were willing to financially support this training during the first years.

In 2005, the SSMO declared this CST to be mandatory for physicians specializing in oncology. Meanwhile, 687 physicians and nurses working with cancer patients received training.

Setting of the Swiss communication skills training

Several times a year, a CST for up to ten participants is organized by two of the trainers. The trainers have extensive experience in psychooncology; their professional background is psychiatry, psychology, internal medicine, and nursing, and all of them have been trained in psychoanalytic, systemic or cognitive-behavioural psychotherapy, or in psychosomatic medicine and supervision. The CST starts with a two-day course, followed by four to six individual supervisions, and ends with a full day course, focusing on depression in cancer care, six months later. The training is based on case discussions, role plays, and video-analyses of participants' interviews with a patient simulated by an actor (for reasons of research, each participant was filmed at the beginning and the end of the training; meanwhile, participants are only filmed prior to training). The Swiss CST provides only a very limited amount of theory; it is mainly based on interactivity and practical exercises by means of the abovementioned case presentations, role plays, analyses of video sequences, and guided imagery.

Objectives of the Swiss communication skills training

The training focuses on four elements of communication: (i) structure, (ii) exchange of information, (iii) emotions, and (iv) relational aspects. While these elements are interdependent and occur simultaneously, for didactic reasons they will be discussed separately and illustrated by examples (Stiefel 2006).

Structure

The training aims to raise participants' awareness of structural elements of the consultation, such as the setting (time, space, participants, and so on), negotiation of the patient's and clinician's agenda, announcement of transitions to new topics during the interview, and regular intermediate syntheses of what has been discussed. The example in Box 57.1, taken from a CST, illustrates the difficulty of a nurse to follow a coherent structure, changing topics rapidly, and without announcing the transitions.

Box 57.1 Structure—chaotic and transitions not announced

Nurse: Before you receive chemotherapy, we will give you a medication to help with the nausea.

Patient: ... good.

Nurse: Chemotherapy is not always associated with nausea, but we would like to prevent it, that's why we prescribe you this medication ... Where do you work?

Patient: I own a small factory ...

Nurse: The chemotherapy should be well-tolerated; we only give you this medication as a precaution.

Patient: OK.

Box 57.2 Exchange of information—jargon, lack of checking

Physician: You describe what sounds like a paraneoplastic phenomenon.

Patient: Can't we do something, where does it come from?

Physician: Paraneoplastic syndromes have different origins. It is difficult to treat.

Patient: But I thought that I have only cancer …

Physician: Paraneoplastic symptoms may be related to immunological responses induced by your cancer.

Patient: Immunological responses?

Physician: Yes, immunological responses, leading to paraneoplastic syndromes induced by cancer, very rare …

Exchange of information

Participants of the training learn that different types of questions (closed, open and leading questions) have different functions within a consultation. They are brought to understand that non-verbal expression of time pressure can hamper exchange of information, while a concentrated interest in the patient can facilitate the exchange of information. Training also focuses on using language that can be understood by the patient; limiting the amount of information provided; checking patient comprehension; and identifying anxiety or other sources of a diminished capacity of the patient to retain information. Box 57.2 illustrates an exchange of information characterized by medical jargon, which may not be understood by the patient.

Emotions

The CST teaches how emotions of the patient can be perceived (verbal and non-verbal expression) and how they can be contained in an empathic manner. Participants learn to distinguish between a cognitive expression (communicating information) and an emotional expression (communicating a feeling), and learn how to respond accordingly. Box 57.3 illustrates how a clinician fails to recognize this distinction and then responds with a cognitive, medical answer, instead of providing empathic support.

Box 57.3 Emotions (deception)—failure to let the patient develop his perspective and failure to provide empathic support

Physician: To summarize, the results show that the cancer has come back.

Patient: But I thought that I was cured!

Physician: I told you two years ago …

Patient: That doesn't make sense, I don't want any further treatment.

Physician: I would suggest a new chemotherapy …

Patient: With the same results?

Physician: Chemotherapy may reduce the tumour mass and prolong your life.

Patient: I don't know; this is so unexpected.

Physician: Palliative chemotherapy could have a positive impact.

Box 57.4 Relational aspects—projection of anxiety and introduction of a consultant without clarifying concerns

Patient: I do understand. The operation was only partly successful and now chemotherapy seems necessary?

Physician: That's correct.

Patient: (sighs) My kids are still small and …

Physician: We do have psychooncologists, they could be of help.

Patient: I would like first to think about everything.

Physician: I just thought that maybe you feel lonely and the kids …

Patient: No, my husband is very supportive.

Relational aspects

Relational aspects of the interview are important, but difficult for participants to perceive. Relational aspects are discussed by viewing and analysing selected video sequences and role plays. Sequences characterized by abrupt transitions from one topic to another; an escalation of an underlying relational dynamic; inadequate non-verbal expressions or stagnation in a topic are used to illustrate relational aspects of communication. Participants recognize that effective communication is not concerned with the question 'who is right?' and are trained to let the patients express their views and to accept that different views can co-exist. Box 57.4 illustrates how the anxiety of a clinician, projected on to the patient, leads to the proposition of a consultant instead of first clarifying the patient's needs.

While improvements with the first three elements (structure, exchange of information, and containing emotions) can be obtained within the first two days of the training, relational aspects are more easily discussed in individual supervision.

Observations from the Swiss communication skills training

Communication difficulties in the videotaped interviews are identified by an unbalanced focus on medical issues, a predominance of closed questions, abrupt transitions from one topic to another, interruptions of the patient, premature or inadequate comforting, or avoidance of patients' concerns. For each participant, different sequences of their filmed interviews are selected and discussed.

With regard to the different elements of the interview, we observe the following difficulties during the training. Interviews are 'understructured' (e.g. when talking to anxious patients) or 'overstructured', with the consequence that the patient is deprived of the possibility to exist as an individual. Information is not adapted to the patient's needs: clinicians show difficulties distinguishing between cognitive and emotional expressions of the patient; questions are answered without clarifying underlying concerns; and the comprehension of the provided information is not checked. Emotions of the patient are not identified or are avoided, and helplessness exists as to how to respond to an irritated, anxious, or sad patient. Inadequate relational reactions from clinicians are linked to specific situations, such as the limits of medical treatment, transition between curative and palliative treatment or the patient's refusal to comply with prescriptions; in such moments, clinicians are subjected to pressure and may lose the capacity to continue to support the patient and respond with empathy.

Specific features of the Swiss model: Interdisciplinary training, individual insight-oriented supervision, and mandatory training

Interdisciplinary training is a key element of the Swiss CST. Working with both nurses and physicians allows the opportunity not only to practise interdisciplinary communication, which is often a major problem in daily clinical care, but also to recognize the specific challenges and responsibilities of each profession through the case discussions and video-recorded interviews, thus often raising a respectful attitude towards each other.

We have observed differences between professions with regard to communication skills. In general, physicians have a good capacity to structure the interview, to adequately provide medical information, and to assume leadership during the consultation. On the other hand, physicians sometimes structure the interview in a way that hinders the discussion of certain topics, such as prognosis of the disease; they forget to check if the information has been understood by the patient; and have difficulties perceiving the emotional climate, and may react with irritation when confronted with 'difficult' patients. Nurses usually show a good capacity to obtain sensitive information, to facilitate emotional expression and to contain patients who are angry, anxious, or depressed. On the other hand, they are sometimes troubled by emotional contagion, have a hard time to refocus on medical matters or to end the consultation, while taking the blame when a patient is irritated by the disease, its treatments, or the physicians.

However, working with participants of different professional backgrounds also has disadvantages. If, for example, a professional group is overrepresented, specific topics of the minority may be neglected and some participants may feel inhibited to discuss sensitive issues in front of the other profession.

After the initial two-day training, participants attended four to six individual supervisions over the next six months. In the French and Italian parts of Switzerland, supervision is provided either in the trainer's office or, more rarely, in the oncologist's office. In the German part of Switzerland, most supervision is conducted over the phone due to geographical distances. Participants wish to discuss very different issues in the supervision; some like to work on audio or video-recorded consultations, while others demand to reflect on difficult cases or ask for 'live supervision', with the supervisor being present in the medical consultation.

Often participants present a 'difficult patient' and then, through supervision, recognize that the problem they encounter is related to their own communicational difficulties. For example, a young oncologist who worked in a palliative care unit presented the case of a 55-year-old man with brain metastases who asked for another MRI. After the oncologist replied that 'this was not necessary any more', the patient refused to speak to him for three days. During supervision, the oncologist recognized that instead of clarifying the underlying concerns of the patient's question, he had responded with a 'medically correct', but empathically inadequate, answer.

Sometimes supervision may also lead to a reflection on a participant's personal issues that are affecting communication. For example, an oncologist presented the case of an elderly patient suffering from advanced breast cancer, who complained about pain, but at the same time refused analgesic treatment; the oncologist became so angry that he started shouting at her, feeling very guilty afterwards. During supervision, the clinician first realized that this 'unreasonable behaviour' of the patient may have had a hidden meaning (preservation of autonomy, fears associated with pain medication, and so on). Once the clinician realized these possible sources of the patient's behaviour, he was able to reflect on his own strong emotional reaction. He reported that he not only felt angry, but also very anxious when he shouted at the patient, and linked his reaction to his own medical history of melanoma three years ago: 'I would certainly not be alive any more if I had not followed the doctor's advice and facing a patient not following medical advice had certainly provoked a great deal of anxiety in me'. During follow-up supervisions, he became more and more aware of how his own medical history affected his psychological state and interfered, as in the case he presented, with his clinical work. The case was finally understood as a collusion (a reaction of the clinician, which is shaped by an unconscious and unresolved problem he shares with the patient): both were struggling with dependency/independency issues, manifested in the patient by the refusal to accept pain medication, and in the physician by the refusal to integrate that he himself had recently been a patient. These insights and the experience of the supervision with a mental health professional motivated this oncologist to enter psychotherapy.

The 'narcissistic deconstruction' that participants experience when confronted with their filmed interview in CST sometimes leads to a crisis situation, which stimulates a reflection on (professional) identity. In individual supervision, participants start to discuss sensitive issues and some of them link their own (biographical) elements with difficulties in daily clinical work. Individual supervision is, therefore, a cornerstone for the identification and analysis of relational aspects of communication and allows participants to recognize that communication is a co-construction, which demands not only technical skills, but also the willingness to reflect on oneself and one's own relational patterns. The confronting experience in CST is certainly a key element for change and improvement of skills; for some participants, however, it represents too much of a challenge to face. We have observed on rare occasions that participants experienced great difficulties in the training and were left quite distressed. While most of the vulnerable participants seem to benefit from training, for a minority, the experience can be counterproductive. However, we still lack a procedure to exclude these clinicians from CST and to offer them a more adequate alternative.

Until the decision of the SSMO to declare CST as mandatory for specialization in oncology, participation was voluntary. Since then, some of the clinicians enter the training with ambivalent feelings and sometimes explicitly declare that they are only participating because CST has become mandatory. However, even these ambivalent participants generally engage actively in the CST and we observe that defensive oncologists quite often turn from passive resistance to motivated participation, and then benefit a great deal from training. The fact that the CST is mandatory, therefore, allows otherwise refractory physicians to gain a more constructive perspective with regards to communication in cancer care. It also provides a powerful signal of the SSMO to the medical community, to the patients and to society as the whole, indicating that communication matters for oncology clinicians. We are, therefore, very grateful to the SSMO for their support and the trust by declaring this CST as mandatory for oncology physicians.

A systematic evaluation of the level of satisfaction of oncologists with the Swiss CST before (2000–2005) and after (2006–2012) it became mandatory shows that levels of satisfaction with the CST were high, and satisfaction of physicians participating on a voluntary or mandatory basis did not significantly differ for the majority of the 18 examined items (e.g. conceptualization of the content, level of information, practical relevance, or usefulness for own individual professional activity) (Bourquin et al. 2014).

Research

The Swiss CST in oncology has been investigated by means of different scientific projects, all financially supported by the Swiss Cancer Research foundation and/or Swiss Cancer League. One project (Langewitz et al. 2010) evaluated the videos before and after CST, and focused on clinician–patient interactions. The videos of the 258 nurses and physicians who participated in the Swiss CST were analysed with the Roter Interaction Analysis System (RIAS), which yields categories under which patient and professional utterances can be summarized. Furthermore, it reports on the emotional climate of the interview, using global ratings. Interviews were also analysed with the Observing Patient Involvement Scale (OPTION), which assesses to what extent professionals involve patients in decision-making. A total of 54,692 utterances were analysed; the largest part of the interviews consisted of the exchange of information (36,677 utterances). The following results were observed: nurses showed a significant increase in the proportion of empathic statements (1.6% vs. 3.2%) and of reassuring statements (2.3% vs. 3.4%), a decrease in medical information provided (17.8% to 13.3%), and an increase in closed and open questions concerning psychosocial information (2.8% to 4.0%); (simulated) patients speaking with the nurses showed a decrease of medical information provided and an increase of reported lifestyle information (8.1% vs. 6.7%; 3.3% vs. 5.7%). In physicians, an increase in checking/summarizing utterances (1.8% vs. 2.3%) and an increase in patients' explicit agreement statements (3.6% vs. 4.7%) were observed. In addition, after training, the length of patients' speech without being interrupted by the nurses increased (3.7 to 4.3 utterances), but not when speaking with physicians (2.8 vs. 2.9 utterances). The authors concluded that there were many significant improvements in nurses on various dependent variables, but for the physicians, the outcome was more limited.

Another project focused on psychodynamic aspects of CST (Favre et al. 2007; Bernard et al. 2010). The aim was to investigate if clinicians' defence mechanisms are modified by CST, based on the hypothesis that this is the underlying process of skills improvement. Operating without conscious effort and triggered by anxiety-provoking situations, defences contribute to the individual's adaptation to, and protection from, stress (Perry 2001). Usually described in patients (for example, as denial when facing threatening news), defences operate in any individual and thus also in clinicians under distress. In patients, different types of defence mechanisms have been described (Vaillant 1992) and classified depending on their degree of adaptation to, or distorting of, reality, ranging from 'immature defences', such as projection or denial, to 'mature defences', such as displacement or intellectualization (Vaillant 1992; Perry and Cooper 1989). While patient's defence mechanisms have been studied extensively in psychotherapy research (Despland et al. 2009a), they have never been investigated in clinicians, not even in psychiatrists or psychotherapists (Favre et al. 2007; Bernard et al. 2010). As in patients, clinicians' defences diminish their ability to integrate all aspects of a given situation, and thus may hamper the working alliance with the patient and the recognition of patient's needs—especially when immature defences are triggered. A clinician might then be perceived by the patient as detached and less empathic. Based on our impression, after CST most clinicians feel more secure (or less anxious) when facing patients in interviews and, therefore, less defensive, they seem better prepared to encounter the patient, to perceive his emotions, and to respond empathically. In a first step of this project, a sample of 114 videos (57 videos pre- and 57 videos post-CST) were compared to 112 videos of a control group (56 videos using the same actors and the same scenarios as in the CST group, 56 videos 6 months later, no training). The videos were evaluated with the Clinician Defence Mechanism Rating Scale (DMRS-C) (10), which identifies a total of 30 defence mechanisms assigned to seven hierarchical levels: mature, obsessional, other neurotic, narcissistic, disavowal, borderline, and action defences. Each level includes three to eight individual defences, which can be weighted according to the level of maturity and summed up to an overall defensive functioning score (ODF). Results showed: a high number (mean = 16, SD = 6) and a high variety (all hierarchical levels were observed) of defences triggered by the 15-minute interviews; no evolution difference (ODF) with regard to defences between groups; but an increase of mature defences after CST for clinicians with an initial higher level of defensive functioning.

A follow-up project (Stiefel et al. 2009; Meystre et al. 2013), based on the same pre-post controlled trial, aimed to evaluate the impact of CST on working alliance and to identify specific communication elements related to working alliance. Alliance was evaluated with the widely use Working Alliance Inventory-Short Revised Form (WAI-SR) (Hatcher and Gillaspy 2006), observer version, which consists of 12 items rated on a five-point Likert scale assessing three aspects of collaborative features: (i) patient's agreement on the tasks of the treatment; (ii) patient's agreement on the goals of the treatment; and (iii) quality of interpersonal bond between patient and clinician. Verbal communication was analysed with the RIAS. The following results were obtained: working alliance did not improve with CST, but relevant links between alliance and some interaction process categories of the RIAS were observed; for example, the more positive talk and psychosocial counselling in the interview, the higher the alliance was rated; the more biomedical information the clinicians provided, the lower the alliance was rated; and negative talk and patients' questions were negatively correlated with alliance.

Finally, a project (Stiefel and Singy 2007; Singy et al. 2012) investigated the impact of CST on clinicians' linguistic strategies. Utterances produced by clinicians, as well as words used by simulated patients and clinicians of the aforementioned sample (CST group and control group) were analysed using the content analysis software LaComm, developed by Razavi and colleagues (Liénard et al. 2010). The software performs, in a single-stage process, a twofold analysis of clinician and patient discourse. Discourse of clinicians is analysed by (i) identifying utterances reflecting different communication strategies, which are regarded as sets of statements produced to achieve a communication goal, and (ii) classifying the words of these utterances, depending on their meaning, into categories of distinct topics. Given that no specific strategies are expected from the patients, their discourse is only classified into topic categories. The results showed that changes after CST were observed only on the level of words and topics investigated. Words in relation to certain topics significantly increased with CST; trained clinicians more often used precise diagnostic terms, such as *carcinoma* or *malignant*, and relatively fewer terms which are vague, like *nodules* or *cells*; they also used more frequently words related to secondary processes and self-motivation, which reflect the patient's experience of illness, and work and leisure-related words, thus giving room to the patient's subjectivity and fostering the therapeutic alliance.

These projects have led to further related studies, supported by the Swiss Cancer Research foundation and/or Swiss Cancer League and by the Swiss National Science Foundation (SNF). These studies have various objectives; for example, to assess if results of the project on defence mechanisms, mentioned above, can be replicated with real patients and to define the relationship between clinicians' defence mechanisms and patients' satisfaction and information recall (Despland *et al.* 2009b, 2011), to better understand how oncologists and advanced cancer patients communicate in a real-world setting, what aspects of communication advanced cancer patients value, and what factors determine the quality of communication from their perspective (Stiefel and Bourquin 2014), to evaluate whether an undergraduate CST with individual supervision (one-to-one teaching) improves medical students' skills in breaking bad news in oncology, and enhances skills in breaking bad news compared to standard small group teaching (Berney *et al.* 2011), and to develop a specific end-of-life(EOL)-CST for clinicians caring for dying patients, based on clinicians' self-perceived training needs (Stiefel and Singy 2012). The findings of these studies contribute to continuous improvement of the Swiss CST.

Recommendations for communication skills training

Based on the Swiss experience, in 2009 the Swiss Cancer League organized a European consensus meeting on CST. Recommendations taking into consideration a systematic review and a meta-analysis (Moore *et al.* 2001; Barth and Lannen 2011) were developed, agreed upon, and outlined in a position paper (Stiefel *et al.* 2010). This position paper states (i) that CST is required at under- and postgraduate levels of education, and (ii) should be based on learner-centred courses, role plays with structured and constructive feedback, and (iii) that implementation of such training should be evaluated with validated assessment instruments or measures.

Acknowledgement

We would like to express our gratitude to Maya Andrey, former head of the Division of Psycho-Social Issues of the Swiss Cancer League, for her initiative and support in the development and organization of this Swiss CST.

Note

1 The initial task force consisted of: M. Andrey, J. Bernhard, A. Bischoff, L. Dietrich, Ch. Hürny, A. Kesselring, A. Kiss, F. Stiefel, M. Tomamichel, and B. Wössmer.

References

Barth J, Lannen P (2011). Efficacy of communication skills training courses in oncology: a systematic review and meta-analysis. *Ann Oncol* **22**, 1030–40.

Bernard M, de Roten Y, Despland JN, *et al.* (2010). Communication skills training and clinicians' defences in oncology: An exploratory, controlled study. *Psychooncology* **19**, 209–15.

Berney A, Stiefel F, Schmid Mast M, *et al.* (2011). Pregraduate training for medical students on breaking bad news in oncology. *Swiss Cancer Research foundation/Swiss Cancer League*; Grant 02776-02-2011.

Bourquin C, Stiefel F, Bernhard J, *et al.* (2014). Mandatory communication skills training for oncologists: enforcement does not substantially impact satisfaction. *Support Care Cancer* **22**, 2611–14.

Despland JN, Bernard M, Favre N, *et al.* (2009a). Clinicians' defences: an empirical study. *Psycho Psychother-T* **82**, 73–81.

Despland JN, Stiefel F, de Vries M, *et al.* (2009b). Communication in cancer care: the relationship between clinician's defense mechanisms, patient satisfaction and information recall. *Oncosuisse*; Grant 02338-02-2009.

Despland JN, Stiefel F, de Vries M, *et al.* (2011). Communication in cancer care: the relationship between clinician's defense mechanisms, patient satisfaction and information recall. *Swiss Cancer Research Foundation/Swiss Cancer League*; Grant (continuation) 02828-08-2011.

Favre N, Despland JN, De Roten Y, *et al.* (2007). Psychodynamic aspects of communication skills training: a pilot study. *Support Care Cancer* **15**, 333–7.

Hatcher RL, Gillaspy JA (2006). Development and validation of a revised short version of the Working Alliance Inventory. *Psychother Res* **16**, 12–25.

Kiss A (1999). Communication skills training in oncology: a position paper. *Ann Oncol* **10**, 899–901.

Langewitz W, Heydrich L, Nübling M, *et al.* (2010). Swiss Cancer League communication skills training programme for oncology nurses: an evaluation. *J Adv Nurs* **66**, 2266–77.

Liénard A, Merckaert K, Libert Y, *et al.* (2010). Is it possible to improve residents breaking bad news skills? A randomized study assessing the efficacy of a communication skills training program. *Br J Cancer* **103**, 1717.

Meystre C, Bourquin C, Despland JN, *et al.* (2013). Working alliance in communication skills training for oncology clinicians: a controlled trial. *Patient Educ Couns* **90**, 233–8.

Moore PM, Wilkinson SSM, Rivera Mercado S (2001). Communication skills training for health care professionals working with cancer patients, their families and/or carers. *Cochrane Database Syst Rev* **2**, CD003751. *See also:* Moore PM, Rivera Mercado S, Grez Artigues M, Lawrie TA (2013) . Communication skills training for healthcare professionals working with people who have cancer (Review). *Cochrane Database Syst Rev* **3**, CD003751.

Perry JC, Cooper S (1989). An empirical study of defence mechanisms: I clinical interview and life vignette ratings. *Arch Gen Psychiat* **46**, 444–52.

Perry JC (2001). A pilot study of defences in psychotherapy of personality disorders entering psychotherapy. *J Nerv Ment Dis* **189**, 651–60.

Singy P, Bourquin C, Sulstarova B, Stiefel F (2012). The impact of communication skills training in oncology: a linguistic analysis. *J Canc Educ* **27**, 404–8.

Stiefel F (ed.) (2006). *Communication in Cancer Care: Recent Results in Cancer Research*. Springer Verlag, Berlin, Heidelberg, Germany.

Stiefel F, Singy P (2007). Effects of communication skills training on oncology clinicians' communication styles and defence mechanisms.

Swiss Cancer Research Foundation/Swiss Cancer League; Grant 02035-02-2007.

Stiefel F, de Roten Y, Despland JN, *et al.* (2009). Effects of communication skills training on oncology clinicians' defence mechanisms, communication outcomes and working alliance. *Swiss Cancer Research Foundation/Swiss Cancer League*; Grant 02353-02-2009.

Stiefel F, Barth J, Bensing J, *et al.* (2010). Communication skills training in oncology: a position paper based on a consensus meeting among European experts in 2009. *Ann Oncol* **21**, 204–7.

Stiefel F, Bourquin C (2014). Communication in cancer care: what is good for the patient?—the cancer patient perspective. *Swiss Cancer Research Foundation/Swiss Cancer League*; Grant 3459-08-2014.

Stiefel F, Singy P (2012). Communication skills in end-of-life care. *Swiss National Science Foundation*; Grant 406740-139248.

Vaillant GE (1992). *Ego Mechanisms of Defence*. American Psychiatric Press, Washington, WA.

CHAPTER 58

The United Kingdom general practitioner and palliative care model

Simon Noble and Nicola Pease

Introduction to the United Kingdom general practitioner and palliative care model

Within the United Kingdom, the general practitioner (GP) will manage the care of the majority of patients with life-limiting and terminal disease. Even those patients with complex problems requiring specialist palliative care involvement are likely to receive the majority of their care at home or within the community healthcare system, with their GP as key healthcare worker. The consultation is at the heart of general practice and communication skills, underpinning the UK General Practitioner Vocational Training Scheme (GPVTS). To attain membership of the Royal College of General Practitioners (RCGP), trainees are required to undertake learning methods during their training programme as outlined in the RCGP Curriculum (RCGP 2010), which include:

- video analysis of consultations;
- random case analysis of a selection of consultations;
- sitting in with GPs and other healthcare professionals in practice to observe different consulting styles;
- GP trainer to sit in with specialty registrar to give formative feedback;
- patients' feedback on consultations, using satisfaction questionnaires or tools.

While the GPVTS offers exposure opportunities to develop generic communication skills within the primary care setting, the breadth of possible consultations and clinical scenarios will only offer limited depth of experience with respect to specific specialties. Furthermore, the time restraints in the primary care consultation encourage brevity, and such skills developed for GP settings may not be transferable to specialist palliative care.

The Cardiff University model

Since its development in 1987, the Cardiff University postgraduate course has offered specialist palliative care education to meet the needs of specialists and of GPs with a developing specialist interest.

It has evolved to become an internationally recognized and quotable qualification, with alumni in over 30 countries. In recognition of the needs of children with life-limiting illness, a paediatric option has also been developed. The course utilizes a web-based portfolio e-learning system and is available to physicians, nurses, pharmacists, social workers, physiotherapists, occupational therapists, pastoral workers, dieticians, and other allied healthcare professionals, reflecting the multiprofessional approach to learning and patient care.

Communication skills training makes up an integral part of the course that initially requires close supervision and support. For this reason, the course includes two 'face-to-face' residential modules to address the fundamentals of communication skills before empowering the adult learner to further progress their skills through self-directed learning. Combinations of interactive teaching experiences are used in communication skills training, where the evidence, rationale, and 'toolkit' for good communication can be explained. This is followed by an opportunity to explore and practise such tools in a safe, learning environment using role play. The outline for the teaching programme is discussed below and consists of five core sections:

- Introduction to the process of communication.
- Analysis of the consultation.
- The Cardiff six-point toolkit.
- Role play.
- Reflection on real world experience/portfolio learning.

Introduction to the process

The introduction occurs early within the course as part of the first residential module and is given as an interactive lecture. Participants will need sufficient time prior to the course to reflect on relevant pre-course material and as an opportunity for facilitators to address any concerns that are raised. For many participants, the communication skills component of the course is the one that gives them most cause for concern; an interactive lecture engaging the whole class can be reassuring for candidates to see that their concerns are shared by others.

The importance of good communication should be discussed and participants may wish to explore the consequences of a bad consultation. Various aspects of healthcare-related communication can, and should, be discussed including: the consent process; the role of communication in advance care planning (for adults and children); the identification and exploration of psychosocial issues; written communication, either to the patient, other healthcare professionals, or carers; and information leaflets including a discussion on their limitations.

The Cardiff six-point toolkit

The Cardiff six-point toolkit developed in recognition of the fact that many participants have limited experience with role play and find the experience quite stressful. The toolkit attempts to break down the bare essentials of the palliative consultation. It offers six key techniques or tools that should be applied to any consultation and developed as individual skills to improve the role play and real world consultation. These are listed below and discussed in further detail after:

+ listening;

+ reflection;

+ summarizing;

+ question style;

+ comfort;

+ language.

Depending upon the experience and confidence of the individual, and at the discretion of facilitator, participants may focus on several tools in one role play scenario. For the less confident individual, a role play that has the objective of focusing on only one of the tools can still produce significant developments. This is most marked when focusing on tools 1, 2, and 3. For example, a participant who does not know what next to say in a consultation for whatever reason, be it nervousness or unsure of what question to ask next, may be encouraged to summarize the consultation thus far, thereby demonstrating to the patient that they have been listened to and allowing clarification of key points.

Tool 1: Listening/use of silence

One of the key tools that can be used in teaching communication skills is the appropriate use of silence, which will facilitate active listening. Silence is a valuable tool in communicating. It helps by:

+ allowing the patient time to assimilate news;

+ demonstrating that the patient is being listened to;

+ giving the patient time to react;

+ giving the patient time to ask questions.

Communication studies suggest that doctors do not listen to their patients enough and interrupt patients' dialogue early, thus creating a barrier to communication. In addition, early interruption may result in relevant facts being missed from the patient's history (Fletcher 1980; Beckman and Frankel 1984). Furthermore, the use of silence is essential for consultations where bad news has just been broken. A useful illustrator exercise in the group setting is to have all participants raise their hands. The facilitator then keeps

talking, during which they inform the group that at some point s/he is going to suddenly stop talking. Participants are then asked to lower their hand when they begin to feel uncomfortable. In practice, 50% of the group usually drop their hand within 15 seconds, with the remainder following over the next 20 seconds. When the facilitator then asks participants whether they feel that 15 seconds is enough time for a patient to take on board bad news, they realize that when they are uncomfortable with the silence, this will impact on the time patients have to assimilate bad news.

In the initial stages of the consultation participants should be encouraged to:

+ Allow the patient to talk. This is best achieved by the role play facilitator, instructing the participant to avoid interrupting the patient and allowing them to tell the whole story.

+ Engage in active listening. This involves the avoidance of interrupting and the continuation of dialogue with short words of encouragement such as 'I see', 'Yes', 'Go on', or merely by maintaining eye contact and using appropriate body language such as nodding. Scenarios that can be used to explore the use of listening skills may include breaking bad news, dealing with anger, or managing the distressed patient.

If you give a patient bad news or a lot of difficult information, it is inevitable that there will be silence. You will hear silence, but for the patient opposite you there is nothing but noise. It's just all internal. They need a bit of time to sort it out in their head and if you talk too soon during the silence, it will interrupt them (Dalton and Noble 2005).

The judicious use of silence can allow the patient to feel more in control of the consultation, and to set the pace and direction of the topics to be covered. As a general rule, the patient should have about 80% of the consultation time to talk with the doctor or nurse speaking for about 20% of the time. Unfortunately, the reverse is often seen in practice, with the healthcare professional dominating the conversation and not allowing the patient time to say whatever is uppermost on their mind.

Tool 2: Reflection

Good use of reflection is important. It really makes the patient feel you are listening to them (Dalton and Noble 2005).

This technique is particularly useful for participants new to communication skills training, who get stuck and do not know what to say next. Reflecting back what a patient has just said may help and will encourage the patient to proceed with their story. It also demonstrates that they are being listened to and helps to develop rapport. In addition, it is a technique that can be used to encourage dialogue at times when the patient may be finding it difficult to go on because of their feelings. Reflection can also be used to pick up on key words said by a patient and signal that they are being followed up on.

Tool 3: Summarizing/recapping

Another technique that can be practised is summarizing. It is useful to encourage candidates to do this, especially when they are unsure where to go with the consultation or if their mind goes blank.

Just by recapping with: 'So what you're saying is …' makes you feel that you are being taken seriously (Dalton and Noble 2005).

Going back over the patient's story with them demonstrates to the patient that they have been listened to. It also offers them a chance to clarify anything that may have been missed. Often, they will then pick up on something and direct the consultation towards their agenda.

Tool 4: Question style

The question style is crucially important. As a general rule, the more open the question the greater the amount of information obtained. So the open questions, such as 'How have things been?', allows the patient to tell the doctor anything at all about what has been happening—ranging from medical details of the condition to social catastrophes, other family illness, and so on. Focused questions do just as the name describes, they focus down onto a particular area and then explore it further: 'Can you tell me more about your pain?'; then further direct questions may have a place such as: 'Does the skin over the area feel very sensitive?'. Of course, the style of question must fit the occasion—using focused or direct questions too early leaves the patient feeling interrogated, but unable to express the real issues that are troublesome.

Multiple questions (double-barrelled questions) and leading question styles are best avoided in all consultation settings. Multiple questions, as their name suggests, are a series of questions asked in one statement; they are often confusing for the patient, as they are not sure which part to answer first. For example: 'The pain that you mentioned, is that a new pain or has it been there for some time? Do the painkillers make it any better?'. Leading questions often direct the consultation to the wrong answer, thereby providing misinformation to the healthcare professional. For example: 'On the new pain killers, how much better is your pain?'.

Tool 5: Comfort

The concept of comfort encompasses many facets to the effective consultation. First and foremost, it reminds participants of the importance of preparation for the consultation. The more they develop their communication skills, the more comfortable they will be in communicating.

It also highlights the importance of the setting in which communication occurs. Experienced communicators will recognize that a sensitive consultation needs to take place in a quiet place, free from interruptions and disturbances. The physical environment of the consultation should avoid barriers, such as a desk or computer, between the doctor and patient; should avoid sitting the patient in the glare of bright light from a window or lamp; and should ensure that the patient has as comfortable a chair as the healthcare professional.

Participants must also be encouraged to understand that discussing upsetting or bad news is likely to evoke strong emotions. Bad news, by definition, is going to upset the receiver. Participants may feel guilty that they have made the patient cry and may feel compelled to say something to 'make it better'. However, such remarks often come across as banal and patronizing, just as a mother says 'There there, don't cry' to a child.

Such words provide false reassurance; they may stem the flow of tears and distress in the immediate term, but will lead to further problems later, such as mistrust or lack of confidence in physicians. In general, 'jollying along' makes the professional feel better, but blocks the patient's ability to communicate.

Tool 6: Language

When discussing language, it is often considered under the broad categories of verbal and non-verbal language. Every person communicates a great deal by the way they look, their expression, their body posture, and their overall demeanour—indeed it is said that about 80% of communication is non-verbal (Finlay and Sarangi 2005). The remainder is made up of the language used to speak, whether that language is spoken, written, or in another form. In the context of a consultation it is verbal communication that often receives most attention, with relatively little attention being paid to the non-verbal.

All healthcare professionals must guard against using jargon and remain aware of the settings in which they are most likely to use it:

- tacit vocabulary;
- fear of causing distress;
- as a barrier.

Tacit vocabulary

The majority of medical education is conducted solely among clinical peers, and complex medical words or abbreviations become commonplace in their vocabulary. Sometimes when professionals relax in a consultation, they find themselves using jargon, which they no longer consider abnormal or specialist. Exercises that encourage candidates to focus on using vocabulary raised by the patient can help to develop insight into the way that everyday speech of a professional can be quite incomprehensible to a patient.

Fear of causing distress

People are sometimes worried about using words such as 'cancer' and may be tempted to use euphemisms to avoid causing distress. Once again, this may avoid immediate distress but leads to problems later on.

Patients require uncomplicated words brought sympathetically, which is something that participants can explore within the context of role play and reflection.

As a barrier

Jargon and complex words are frequently used as a barrier to further communication between doctor and patient. By using medical words, doctors establish that they have a greater knowledge and expertise, thereby exerting their position of superiority over the patient. When professionals become nervous or unsure, they often resort to the communication style in which they feel most comfortable.

Role play

Role play using either actors or colleagues as patients, has long been a useful tool for developing communication skills (Mansfield 1991). Within the Cardiff model, it is done as a small group of learners with one trained facilitator and the participants playing the role of patients. Small numbers of participants promote a cohesive group, help students feel safe, and ensure that everyone has the opportunity to role play. Students generally become supportive and constructive and view their 'turns' at role play as an opportunity to develop further. Discussions of difficult issues/encounters lead to personal growth and adjustment. The learning and teaching becomes increasingly learner-centred and increasingly complex communication situations can be introduced without the risk of the student feeling overwhelmed or inadequate (Lipkin and Williamson 1995).

Role play allows people to be prepared for situations that they rarely encounter; the skills for breaking bad news or dealing with anger are best learned prior to such an encounter in practice. Role play affords the learner the luxury of a second try at a difficult encounter and the group process often enhances learning.

There are several basic principles that should underpin any such learning session:

◆ clearly established rules of role play;

◆ strict adherence to confidentiality;

◆ safe environment;

◆ avoidance of role playing situations that are potentially distressing for learners in the initial learning sessions;

◆ option to call 'time-out' at any point;

◆ opportunity for all learners to participate;

◆ non-confrontational feedback;

◆ time for those involved to 'come out of role' after a session;

◆ review of learning points and de-brief at end of each session.

A formative learning approach is useful during the role play sessions as it helps focus both participants and observers on the principles and techniques of communication. Establishing learning needs and outcomes with the group is a useful way of planning the session. When learning needs are being defined, it is helpful for the student to think about the activities and skills that need to be improved and then to write the learning outcomes in these terms. This will help the learner to be able to demonstrate that learning has occurred—a process that is becoming increasingly important in the current climate of revalidation of professional groups in some countries, such as the United States and the United Kingdom. An example of some learning outcomes for communication skills teaching are given in Box 58.1.

It should be noted that the assessment schedule for a simulated consultation covers many of these areas, so the assessment is explicitly matched to the learning outcomes.

Within the role play setting, facilitators must be prepared to give feedback and, where appropriate, feedback can also be given by other observers. Pendleton's method is one of the safest ways to give feedback singly or involving other participants. It involves the application of four enquiries (Pendleton et al. 1984):

◆ Asking the learner what went they felt they did well or were particularly happy with.

◆ Asking other learners what they observed to be done well.

◆ Asking the learner what they felt could be improved.

◆ Asking the other learners what they felt could be improved.

This approach to feedback has the merit of first highlighting what was done well, thereby reinforcing good practice and offering positive suggestions for improvement. Those members of the group

---

Box 58.1 Cardiff course communication learning outcomes

At the end of the module the students will be able to:

◆ demonstrate non-verbal ways of:
  • facilitating a patient feeling comfortable and safe
  • opening up a communication
  • helping a patient to disclose their problems
◆ demonstrate the use of open questions;
◆ demonstrate the use of focused questions;
◆ demonstrate the process of checking that a patient has understood information;
◆ apply the process of closure of a consultation;
◆ demonstrate a stepwise approach to breaking bad news;
◆ demonstrate respect of the patient and the patient's concerns;
◆ list potential barriers to communication with patients, with patients' families and with colleagues;
◆ suggest ways to overcome barriers to communication;
◆ reflect on their own communication style;
◆ analyse the processes they use in a consultation.

---

who are not role playing should take an active part in the appraisal system to observe and learn from peers. More recently the Calgary–Cambridge approach to communication skills teaching has been developed as a facilitation tool. It encourages a far more agenda-led approach to communication skills, encouraging learners to focus on those specific areas of the consultation that they otherwise avoid through lack of confidence.

The skills to facilitate such sessions are very sophisticated, so training the trainers is strongly recommended before embarking on this teaching style. Most learning of value will occur from the role play itself and the feedback session, but summative assessment can highlight particular areas of weakness. Selected videotaped consultations can complement role play. Box 58.2 illustrates a suggested marking scheme for the palliative care consultation—it is used in the Cardiff Diploma/Master's course in palliative medicine.

Reflective practice/portfolio learning

An opportunity to explore and practice such tools within the safe confines of a learning environment is invaluable prior to bringing these skills to the real world. Within the Cardiff model, participants are required to submit two video recordings of consultations from their own practice. The first, submitted in the year one of study, should feature a real patient from their day-to-day practice. The following year requires a more complex consultation reflecting the progress made over the year. The consultation should cover one of the following scenarios: collusion, denial, handling uncertainty, or interprofessional relations. In view of the complexities of such scenarios and the logistics of recoding such an encounter, candidates are allowed to use an actor patient for this consultation.

Box 58.2 Summative marking schedule for palliative care consultation*

1. Puts patient at ease.
2. Establishes problems sufficiently to erect hypothesis.
3. Prioritizes problems/hypothesis.
4. Checks back on problem list agreement.
5. Elicits fears/concerns.
6. Elicits beliefs/concepts/attitudes.
7. Establishes physical/psychosocial relationship of complaints.
8. Explores physical issues appropriately.
9. Evolves plan acceptable to patient.
10. Checks back that plan is understood/agreed.
11. Overall non-verbals facilitate.
12. Overall verbals appropriate.
13. Overall patient appears comfortable/safe.
14. Overall respects patient's pace.
15. Overall closes interview well.

*Marks are given in each section out of ten, five being a pass mark.

Reproduced courtesy of Dr Nikki Pease and Professor Ilora Finlay.

Candidates are required to provide a critique of their own consultation using the form shown in Table 58.1. Examiner's marks take into account the views of the participants in identifying whether they have identified their own learning needs and have been able to achieve them through the self-critique of the video recording. This process is essential if the training given on the course is to successfully promote lifelong learning. It is not enough to train people in communication skills; they must be trained to continue to further develop and hone how they talk with patients and their families throughout their career. The self-critique has developed from the self-directed portfolio learning model, which relies heavily on reflective practice.

Table 58.1 Reflective critique form

Part	Content
1	Your previous knowledge, reflections, and experience in consultations of this type (10 marks)
2	Key learning areas identified from the critique of this consultation (10 marks)
3	How will your clinical practice change as a result of this learning? (10 marks)
4	The resources used to reflect on the communication style within this consultation and explain of how they have influenced practice (10 marks)

Reproduced courtesy of Dr Nikki Pease and Professor Ilora Finlay.

Portfolio learning is now widely recognized as a valuable learning tool, as it provides a record of learning and also acts as a stimulus to reflection. Portfolio learning is designed to provide a chronological record of the learning process of the student. The learning process is self-directed; the learner chooses the areas within a subject of particular interest. In the context of adult learners, this enables each participant to meet their own individual learning objectives. Those unaccustomed to this learning style often require gentle support and supervision, as it differs greatly from their previous technical-rational learning experiences. The beauty and simplicity of a reflective portfolio, which allows the learner to determine format, learning objectives, and emphasis to the learner, may be seen by some as too unstructured and challenging. Most physicians are new to the relative lack of prescribed formal structure in the portfolio. Depending upon the experience of the educational supervisor, even the method of presenting the portfolio can be relaxed if the reasons are clear. The learner should be encouraged to develop the portfolio in a similar way to an artist's portfolio, reflecting their freedom of creativity in presentation. Most successful portfolios consist of the elements described in Box 58.3.

Within the realms of self-directed learning, the portfolio will act both as a tool for learning and as evidence to the supervisor that learning has taken place. It is important that adult learners have feedback on their progress. This can sometimes be difficult with portfolio marking, since the scope and form of portfolios may differ greatly. Formative assessment between the supervisor and student, in an informal setting, is essential; it enables the supervisor to give constructive feedback to the student and provide support, especially to those new to the concept of portfolio learning. The supervisor will need to identify those students who require more frequent feedback sessions and extra support. Summative assessment can help the student identify areas of learning that they

---

Box 58.3 Elements for a successful portfolio

- Factual case histories around which the learning usually occurs.
- References to items that have influenced the clinical decision-making process and have been foci of learning.
- References to diverse sources (e.g. text-book reading, literature search, lay press, conversations with colleagues).
- A record of the clinician's own decision-making processes, including details of decisions made and how the student came to them.
- Documentation of how the student felt at the time: sources of stress or doubts are as useful as the outcome, since the personal feelings of the learner will influence how they were able to approach a problem.
- Ethical considerations.
- Illustrative items such as photographs, drawings, quotations, poetry, etc., may clarify points being made.
- Some form of indexing is important, so the learner and supervisor can follow the learning process and refer to specific items at a later date.

Table 58.2 Summative portfolio mark schedule

	Score
Contextual description of case	5%
Biological issues of the case	5%
Individual issues of the case	5%
Team-working	10%
Clarity of presentation	10%
Decision-making logic	20%
Attribution of evidence	20%
Critical analysis	15%
Index and discretionary marks	10%
Total	**100%**

Reproduced courtesy of Dr Nikki Pease and Professor Ilora Finlay.

may wish to consider in the future. Examples of a mark schedule, as used at Cardiff University for a general portfolio, are given in Table 58.2.

A suggested framework for participants to formulate a critique around their video-consultation is outlined in Table 58.1. In addition, Box 58.4 contextualizes the consultation for the course examiner to better enable them to understand the background to the video recording.

Conclusions

Over the coming years, GPs in the United Kingdom will be responsible for more patients with advanced cancer and terminal disease. In addition to medical developments and advances in healthcare, GPs will need to engage in an ongoing development of their communication skills, in particular with respect to difficult scenarios around end-of-life care. The models described above deliver an evidence-based template of training, supported by a simple toolkit with which to empower GPs to enhance their communication skills throughout their professional careers.

Box 58.4 Background to consultation

Reason for consultation

Relevant background information (e.g. previous consultations with this patient or information from a referral letter).

Explain the presence of anyone else present (if not stated on the video).

Physical findings relevant to profession, if any.

Working diagnosis (if relevant to profession).

Management plan (provide information regarding any prescription given, test ordered, or other action taken that is not made completely clear from the tape).

Overview (in approximately 50 words outline the setting of the consultation, what was achieved, and what issues may arise later).

References

Beckman HB, Frankel RM (1984). The effect of physician behaviour on the collection of data. *Ann Intern Med* **101**, 692–6.

Dalton HR, Noble SIR (2005). *Communication Skills for Final MB: A Guide to Success in the OSCE*. Churchill Livingstone, London, UK.

Finlay IG, Stott NCH, Marsh HM (1993). Portfolio learning in palliative medicine. *Eur J Cancer Care* **2**, 41–3.

Finlay IG, Sarangi S (2005). *Oral Medical Discourse, Communication Skills and Terminally Ill Patients*. Encyclopaedia of Language and Linguistics, 2nd edition. Elsevier, Oxford, UK.

Fletcher C (1980). Listening and talking to patients. I: The problem. *Br Med J* **27**, 845–7.

Kurtz S, Silverman J, Draper J (1998). *Teaching and Learning Communication Skills in Medicine*. Radcliffe Medical Press, Oxford, UK.

Lipkin M Jr, Williamson P (1995). Teaching interviewing using direct observation and discussion of actual interviews (Ch. 35). In: Lipkin M Jr, Putnam SM, Lazare A (eds). *The Medical Interview. Clinical Care, Education and Research*. Springer-Verlag, New York, NY.

Mansfield F (1991). Supervised role-play in the teaching of the process of consultation. *Med Educ* **25**, 485–90.

Pendleton D, Schofield T Tate P, Havelock P (1984). *The Consultation: An Approach to Learning and Teaching*. Oxford University Press, Oxford, UK.

Royal College of General Practitioners (2010). Statement 2.01 The GP Consultation in Practice (Revised May 2014). RCGP London, UK.

CHAPTER 59

The Belgian experience in communication skills training

Isabelle Merckaert, Yves Libert, and Darius Razavi

Introduction to the Belgian experience in communication skills training

In the last two decades, communication skills training programmes, designed for healthcare professionals working in cancer care, have been the focus of several research endeavours of our research group based in Belgium. The efficacy of designed programmes has been tested in studies using a controlled design. Studies varied in the type of teaching method, the length of training, and the outcome measures considered. Four programmes will be detailed in this chapter in terms of rationale and results. The conclusion will build upon these experiences to develop recommendations and discuss where we may go from there.

Training programmes

Four training programmes have been tested for their efficacy. The aim of the first randomized, controlled trial was to determine the optimal duration of a training programme in order to ensure long-term training effects and transfer in the clinical practice. The duration of the training programme was chosen according to recommendations made at the time of the development of the programme and according to results of programmes developed previously. A 105-hour communication skills training programme for nurses was, therefore, designed. This amount of time allowed each nurse enough time to test the proposed communication strategies in role plays (Razavi et al. 2002; Delvaux et al. 2004; Canivet et al. 2014).

The second study involved physicians working in cancer care. The aim of this study was to assess the impact on physicians' communication skills of a 40-hour communication skills training programme, utilizing a two-day basic training programme followed by six three-hour consolidation workshops (Razavi et al. 2003; Delvaux et al. 2005). The duration of the basic training programme was chosen according to results of previous studies that had showed the usefulness of short training programmes designed for physicians. Consolidation workshops were considered in order to further improve the communication skills learned during the basic training programme. It had been suggested that consolidation follow-up sessions may be required to facilitate maintenance of newly acquired skills and transfer into the clinical practice.

The aim of the resident study was to assess the efficacy of the Belgian Interuniversity Curriculum—Communication Skills Training (BIC-CST) (Bragard et al. 2006; Liénard et al. 2010a; Merckaert et al. 2013). The BIC-CST programme included 30 hours of communication skills training and 10 hours of stress management training (Bragard et al. 2006). Residents were chosen because optimal communication skills should be acquired as early as possible during physicians' curriculum before they become rooted in habits. The main topic addressed in the training was breaking bad news (BBN) in two- and three-person interviews. Physiological arousal was assessed to study residents' engagement to use newly acquired skills, despite the stressfulness of a BBN task. At that time available studies on BBN emphasized the stressfulness of the BBN task (Hulsman et al. 2010). To our knowledge, no study had investigated physicians' physiological and psychological arousal responses during BBN and none had investigated the impact of training in this regard.

Finally, the latest study assessed the efficacy of a 38-hour communication skills training programme designed to train an entire multidisciplinary radiotherapy team (Gibon et al. 2013; Merckaert et al. 2015). Training an entire team was chosen in order to promote transfer in the clinical practice. Team members targetted by the training programme were secretaries, nurses, physicians, and physicists. Training was divided in two modules: a 16-hour patient-oriented training was carried out among members of the same discipline—for example, nurses came together to carry out role playing and to practice communication skills that might be called upon in their specific discipline. The training also consisted of 22 hours of interdisciplinary, team-oriented communication skills modules, in which at least one member of each discipline was present. These modules included role playing exercises, designed to improve members' ability to address situations that may arise during radiotherapy sessions and to improve communication with both colleagues and patients.

Study designs and training techniques

All of the studies used a randomized, pre-post design. The rationale behind the samples included in the successive randomized studies was based on the investigators' wish to determine the threshold of training programme efficacy, not only as regards improvements in communication skills but also as regards improvements in participants' attitudes and stress levels, and in patients' satisfaction. The aim of the different studies was also to assess transfer of learned skills to the clinical practice.

The training programmes developed by our group were based on adult theory for complex learning. They were learner-centred, skills-focused, practice-oriented, and tailored to participants' needs. Training was organized in small groups of up to 12 participants in the nurse study and was reduced to six participants in the subsequent studies. Organizing training in smaller groups allowed participants to more intensively practice the learned skills in the role plays. Training included a cognitive, a behavioural, and a modelling component.

The cognitive component of learning focused on lectures and hand-outs providing evidence of current needs in healthcare professional communication skills and reasons for these. For example, the 105-hour nurse training programme included 30 hours of theoretical information about basic communication components, psychosocial dimensions associated with cancer diagnosis and treatments, coping with patients' and their relatives' uncertainties and distress, detecting psychopathologic reactions, and discussing death and euthanasia. The subsequent studies drastically reduced the amount of theoretical information (max 2 hours) given in order to focus on the behavioural component of learning.

The behavioural component was based on role plays. Role plays allow participants to practice the suggested skills in a protected environment, where trials are encouraged and errors are experienced. In the 105-hour training programme for nurses, every participant had the opportunity to participate in four role plays. These role plays were videotaped and feedback was delivered from the video recordings (Delvaux et al. 2004). While this type of role-play allows viewing and reviewing the sequence of interactions, it does not allow the participant the opportunity to try the suggested skill(s). Skill trial had to be planned for one of the next role play sessions. In the subsequent studies, role plays with immediate feedback were used. Such role plays allowed participants to immediately test the suggested skills in the 'protected' environment of the role-play. Pre-defined role plays were planned in the first sessions in the two physicians' studies. The next sessions focused on role plays based on clinical problems brought up by the participants. In the team study, all role plays were based on clinical problems brought up by the participants, in order to facilitate transfer of learned skills to participants' everyday practice. In all studies, participants were asked to play the role of the patient in at least one session. This was done in order to allow them the opportunity to experience the impact of communication skills used by colleagues.

Modelling was achieved through health professionals' observation of the skills used by their colleagues in the role plays. This allowed them to observe the positive and negative consequences of using specific communication skills for patients and professionals.

Taught skills

The choice of the skills taught was based on results of studies indicating the positive impact of using specific communication skills on patients' disclosure of concerns. Communication skills promoting patients' disclosure of concerns are important because they allow healthcare professionals to respond to patients concerns and needs in terms of information and support that can be provided. They are also the basis of a patient-centred communication. Though there are many different definitions, patient-centredness can be defined as healthcare professionals' behaviours that enable the patient to express his/her perspective on illness, treatment, and health-related behaviour, his/her symptoms, concerns, ideas, and expectations (Levenstein et al. 1986; Smith and Hoppe 1991). Healthcare professionals should use facilitating behaviours—behaviours that aim to elicit the patient's perspective on illness and treatment, such as assessment skills (open and open-directive questions, assessing, checking, summarizing), information skills (appropriate information), and supportive skills (acknowledging, appropriate reassurance giving, empathy, or educated guesses). They should also avoid inhibiting or blocking behaviours—behaviours that restrain the patient from expressing his or her view, such as leading or multiple questions, premature information, or reassurance (Zandbelt et al. 2007).

Outcome measures

Three different approaches have been used for measuring changes in participant communication behaviours: measuring participant-based outcomes, assessing behavioural changes in the use of communication skills both in simulated interviews and in actual patient interviews, and measuring patient-based outcomes.

Participant-based outcomes can be proximal measures directly related to healthcare professionals' behaviour in the observed consultation (i.e. increased confidence, comfort in interaction, reported use of specific skills) or distal measures concerning the more general functioning of healthcare professionals (e.g. attitudes, burnout, stress, physiological arousal). In terms of participant-based outcomes, we decided in our studies to focus on changes in distal measures. This allowed us to observe the impact of the training programmes on the general functioning of healthcare professionals. In the physician study, we assessed physicians' ability to detect patients' distress (Merckaert et al. 2005; Merckaert et al. 2008). Indeed, research suggests that physicians have a limited ability to detect patient distress and often tend to underestimate the level of distress that they experience (Sollner et al. 2001; Cepoiu et al. 2008; Mitchell et al. 2011). In the residents' study, we investigated the impact of the communication skills training programme on residents' physiological arousal (measured through changes in heart rate and salivary cortisol levels) in a breaking bad news task (Meunier et al. 2013). Given the complexity and duration of the breaking bad news task, it was considered that heart rate and salivary cortisol changes reflect resident physiological arousal in the context of emotional and cognitive demands of a task and their task engagement. Trained subjects were expected to show an elevated physiological arousal, which is an indicator of their engagement to respond adequately to the task using newly learned communication skills while maintaining step-by-step attention to the task challenges.

The *behavioural assessments* of communication skills rely on audio or video recordings of medical interviews (whether simulated or actual patient interviews) before and after training, and on the objective coding of behaviours using an interaction analysis system. Our first studies used the Cancer Research Campaign Workshop Evaluation Manual (CRCWEM) (Booth and Maguire 1991), which is an utterance-by-utterance analysis assessment tool. The CRCWEM rates the form, function, content, and emotional level of each utterance from transcripts of audio- or video-recorded consultations. In the physician study, a new coding (coders identified whether the utterance was addressed to the patient, the relative, or to both) was added in order to analyse three-person interviews

(Delvaux *et al.* 2005). Raters were specifically trained to ensure concordance of ratings. Moreover, to ensure a quality control and to avoid rating conflicts, raters were systematically supervised by a rater coordinator. This was done through regular sessions where rating problems were discussed. For the nurses' study, a new coding system was also used to analyse the simulated interview transcripts in terms of pain management (Canivet *et al.* 2014). PainComCode (Pain management Communication Coding system), which was specifically developed for this study, includes a total of 12 communication strategies derived from recommendations found in the literature about (i) basic communication skills in oncology, (ii) pain assessment for nursing practice and evidence-based analgesia, and (iii) patient-centred communication. The coding system does not involve coding all the utterances in the interview but focuses on identifying and categorizing utterances dealing with pain management. Behavioural analysis is a time-consuming and cost-intensive process, however, it is required in order to ascertain training effects in an objective, non-self-report fashion.

In order to diminish the costs of behavioural analysis and to avoid interrater reliability issues, our different studies also used different computer content analysis techniques. The nurse study used a computer-assisted content analysis programme called PROTocol ANalyser (PROTAN) (Hogenraad *et al.* 1995), which allows to count the number of words corresponding to word categories defined by dictionaries. PROTAN was used to tag both patients and nurses emotional words found in the transcripts of audio-recorded simulated and actual patient interviews (Razavi *et al.* 2002). Moreover, a communication content analysis software, LaComm (Centre de Psycho-Oncologie, Brussels, Belgium; http://www.lacomm.be/) was developed and used in the residents' and the radiotherapy teams' study. This software analyses verbal communication (in medicine in general and in oncology/radiotherapy in particular) utterance-by-utterance and identifies turns of speech and the type and content of utterances. LaComm provides counts of turns of speech, utterance types, and content. LaComm was used because it is sensitive to change (Gibon *et al.* 2016) and avoids interrater reliability problems. A validation study has shown that the sensitivity to change of the LaComm is similar to the sensitivity to change of the Cancer Research Campaign Workshop Evaluation Manual (Booth and Maguire 1991). Finally, as the residents' study focused on breaking bad news, the three phases of bad news delivery (pre-delivery, delivery, and post-delivery) were tagged and their length was measured (Liénard *et al.* 2010a; Merckaert *et al.* 2013).

The third approach involves measuring *patient-based outcomes*, which can be proximal measures (such as patient perception of physician behaviour or patient satisfaction with the interview) or distal measures (such as compliance with treatment, anxiety, or quality of life). As far as we know, studies have mainly focused on proximal measures and few programmes to date have included patient-based distal measures. In terms of patient-based outcomes, several of our studies focused on proximal measures: patient perception of nurses' and physicians' behaviour, and satisfaction with nurses' and physicians' behaviour (Razavi *et al.* 2003; Delvaux *et al.* 2004; Delvaux *et al.* 2005; Liénard *et al.* 2010b; Merckaert *et al.* 2015). Changes in patients' anxiety pre-post interview are another proximal measure that has been considered in the physician study (Liénard *et al.* 2006; Liénard *et al.* 2008). It should be recalled at this level that interaction analyses are objective observational measures of nurse or physician behaviours, while patient perception of nurse or physician behaviours reflects the effects of those communication skills on patients. The two types of measures are thus complementary, as they allow evaluating the effect of communication skills training programmes at different levels.

Factors associated with learning

Another important issue to be reported here is the identification in one of our studies of a factor that could mitigate the impact of learning. In our physician study, we assessed the predictive value of a participant characteristic on their ability to learn new communication skills. It is widely recognized that educational interventions may be more effective for people with an 'internal' locus of control (LOC) (who believe that life outcomes are controlled by their own characteristics or actions) compared to people with an 'external' locus of control (who believe that life outcomes are controlled by external forces such as luck, fate, or others). Therefore, we tested the hypothesis that physicians with an 'internal' LOC would demonstrate communication skills acquisition to a greater degree than those with an 'external' LOC (Libert *et al.* 2007). As it was expected, learned communication skills are more frequent among physicians with an 'internal' LOC compared to the frequency of learned skills among physicians with an 'external' LOC, either in two-person or three-person simulated interviews.

Conclusion

In the last two decades, several communication skills training programmes, designed for healthcare professionals working in oncology, have been tested by our research group in Belgium. The main aim of the training programmes described here was to promote the knowledge and use of communication skills to improve patient care. Results of these studies have allowed us to draw some conclusions with regards to training effects and intervention techniques.

First of all, it should be underlined that all our programmes were learner-centred, skills-focused, practice-oriented, and tailored to the participants' needs. In particular, the use of role plays based on clinical cases brought up by the participants, and the use of immediate feedback appears to be acceptable for trainees and effective. These techniques allowed healthcare professionals to receive feedback about their specific communication difficulties and have promoted transfer to the clinical practice. Trainers should choose the more difficult clinical cases brought up by participants and start from there. Trainers should, also, be able to provide rapid and immediate feedback to each participant. Communicating is a behaviour highly rooted in habits and therefore needs a lot of practice in order to really modulate these habits. Providing room for physician to engage in the learning process by limiting the number of participants in a training group is the key. Finally, trainers should be careful to promote role playing. Case discussions are useful but they may often be a way for participants of avoiding to engage in role playing exercises.

Second, it should be noted that all of the programmes led, as expected, to changes in the way participants communicated with patients both in simulated and in actual patient interviews. Changes observed in simulated interviews were in general more numerous than changes in participants' everyday clinical practice. This difference in terms of changes observed highlights the usefulness of simulated interviews, where a high emotional level may be induced and maintained. The complexity of such simulated tasks allow us to observe a wide range of learned skills. It is not surprising that a training duration effect was found. Our different studies showed, however, that the transfer of some skills—for example, skills addressing relatives' concerns and needs—remain limited, even after a training programme. Training programmes focusing on patient-centred communication skills acquisition seem to produce little change in more distal participant-based outcomes, such as detection of distress or burnout, or on patient-based outcomes, such as patients' or their relatives' anxiety.

Third, one of our training programmes allowed us to study the physiological correlates of residents' communication skills' acquisition in the context of a simulated breaking bad news task. After training, the physiological arousal levels of trained residents are high compared to the levels recorded in untrained residents. This higher residents' physiological arousal—which is associated with higher self-efficacy and satisfaction about their performance in the task, with less stress to communicate and with an improvement in their communication skills—may be an indicator of their engagement in performing the communication task. Centring one's communication on patients' concerns and needs certainly implies that healthcare professionals make a conscious choice towards exposing themselves to potential sources of distress (patients' fears, anxiety, uncertainty, suffering, loss of hope …). Communication disengagement may certainly be an automatic protective psychological reaction of professionals in this context. This reaction may however also be a source of suffering for professionals, as it may result in less professional satisfaction. Our training programmes focused on helping professionals to learn the skills needed to be able to engage in highly emotional communication tasks. Focusing role plays on problems brought up by the participants allows them to develop self-efficacy and promotes transfer of learned skills to the clinical practice. Facilitators should certainly be aware of the numerous contexts where professionals tend to disengage in order to help them cognitively engage themselves in the communication, while maintaining an appropriate emotional distance in order to avoid being overwhelmed by their patients' suffering. It should be underlined that the type of engagement in clinical practice may be quite different at the start and at the end of the training. The type of engagement associated with pleasure to communicate and skills mastery later in some clinician career is certainly quite different also. The process underlying learning and transfer to clinical practice includes at least three phases: a knowledge-building phase, where professionals learn to cognitively analyse the phases inherent to highly complex communication tasks such as breaking bad news and develop the skills needed to tackle the different phases; a trial and error phase, where they can practice the skills in the secure context of the role plays; and a continuous self-assessment phase, where they learn to optimally adjust their communication to patient needs and concerns in the context of an interview's specific agenda. Research is needed to better study the impact of different levels of communication skills acquisition on outcomes such as patient information, satisfaction, relation building, and so on.

Fourth, some results of our communication skills training programmes on patients should be stressed. In all of the studies described in this chapter, changes in trainees' communication skills were observed and patients interacting with trained professionals reported changes in their perception of these professionals' communication, or in their satisfaction with their communication skills. These impacts highlight that cancer patients may be able to perceive and appreciate their healthcare professionals' communication skills. This type of results validates the usefulness of communication skills training programmes for healthcare professionals.

Finally, assessment tools used in our first studies led to solid conclusions about behavioural changes. It should be underlined that the use of interaction-process analyses was cost-intensive. A first way to reduce this cost has been to develop a computer-assisted systems of interaction analyses. Such a system has been developed for French transcripts (Gibon *et al.* 2016). Another positive impact of such systems could be to provide healthcare professionals with an annotated feedback of their consultation, which may further facilitate their communication skills learning.

The results of our studies confirm the usefulness of communication skills training programmes for healthcare professionals working in cancer care. To be effective, training should include learner-centred, skills-focused, and practice-oriented techniques; be organized in small groups; and be at least 20 hours long. The development of communication skills training programmes designed for nurses and physicians can thus be recommended to all healthcare professionals dealing with cancer patients and their families.

References

Booth C, Maguire P (1991). *Development of A Rating System to Assess Interaction Between Cancer Patients and Health Professionals*, Report to Cancer Research Campaign, London, UK.

Bragard I, Razavi D, Marchal S, et al. (2006). Teaching communication and stress management skills to junior physicians dealing with cancer patients: a Belgian Interuniversity Curriculum. *Support Care Cancer* **14**, 454–61.

Canivet D, Delvaux N, Gibon AS, Brancart C, Slachmuylder JL, Razavi D (2014). Improving communication in cancer pain management nursing: A randomized controlled study assessing the efficacy of a communication skills training program. *Support Care Cancer* **22**, 3311–20.

Cepoiu M, Mccusker J, Cole MG, Sewitch M, Belzile E, Ciampi A (2008). Recognition of depression by non-psychiatric physicians—a systematic literature review and meta-analysis. *J Gen Int Med* **23**, 25–36.

Delvaux N, Merckaert I, Marchal S, et al. (2005). Physicians' communication with a cancer patient and a relative: a randomized study assessing the efficacy of consolidation workshops. *Cancer* **103**, 2397–411.

Delvaux N, Razavi D, Marchal S, Bredart A, Farvacques C, Slachmuylder JL (2004). Effects of a 105 hours psychological training program on attitudes, communication skills and occupational stress in oncology: a randomised study. *Br J Cancer* **90**, 106–14.

Gibon AS, Durieux JF, Merckaert I, et al. (2016). Development of the Lacomm, a French Medical Communication Analysis Software: A study assessing its sensitivity to change. *Patient Educ Couns*, doi:10.1016/j.pec.2016.08.005.

Gibon AS, Merckaert I, Liénard A, et al. (2013). Is it possible to improve radiotherapy team members' communication skills? A randomized study assessing the efficacy of a 38-h communication skills training program. *Radiother Oncol* **109**, 170–7.

Hogenraad R, Daubies C, Bestgen Y (1995). Une théorie et une méthode générale d'analyse textuelle assistée par ordinateur: le Système PROTAN (PROTocol ANalyser). [Unpublished document]. Psychology Department, Université Catholique de Louvain, Louvain-la-Neuve, Belgium.

Hulsman RL, Pranger S, Koot S, Fabriek M, Karemaker JM, Smets EM (2010). How stressful is doctor-patient communication? Physiological and psychological stress of medical students in simulated history taking and bad-news consultations. *Int J Psychophysiol* **77**, 26–34.

Levenstein JH, Mccracken EC, Mcwhinney IR, Stewart MA, Brown JB (1986). The patient-centred clinical method. 1. A model for the doctor-patient interaction in family medicine. *Fam Pract* **3**, 24–30.

Libert Y, Merckaert I, Reynaert C, *et al.* (2007). Physicians are different when they learn communication skills: influence of the locus of control. *Psychooncology* **16**, 553–62.

Liénard A, Merckaert I, Libert Y, *et al.* (2010*a*). Is it possible to improve residents breaking bad news skills? A randomised study assessing the efficacy of a communication skills training program. *Br J Cancer* **103**, 171–7.

Liénard A, Merckaert I, Libert Y, *et al.* (2010*b*). Transfer of communication skills to the workplace during clinical rounds: impact of a program for residents. *PLoS One* **5**, e12426.

Liénard A, Merckaert I, Libert Y, *et al.* (2006). Factors that influence cancer patients' anxiety following a medical consultation: impact of a communication skills training programme for physicians. *Ann Oncol* **17**, 1450–8.

Liénard A, Merckaert I, Libert Y, *et al.* (2008). Factors that influence cancer patients' and relatives' anxiety following a three-person medical consultation: impact of a communication skills training program for physicians. *Psychooncology* **17**, 488–96.

Merckaert I, Delevallez F, Gibon AS, *et al.* (2015). Transfer of communication skills to the workplace: impact of a 38-hour communication skills training program designed for radiotherapy teams. *J Clin Oncol* **10**, 901–9.

Merckaert I, Libert Y, Delvaux N, *et al.* (2005). Factors that influence physicians' detection of distress in patients with cancer: can a communication skills training program improve physicians' detection? *Cancer* **104**, 411–21.

Merckaert I, Libert Y, Delvaux N, *et al.* (2008). Factors influencing physicians' detection of cancer patients' and relatives' distress: can a communication skills training program improve physicians' detection? *Psychooncology* **17**, 260–9.

Merckaert I, Liénard A, Libert Y, *et al.* (2013). Is it possible to improve the breaking bad news skills of residents when a relative is present? A randomised study. *Br J Cancer* **109**, 2507–14.

Meunier J, Merckaert I, Libert Y, *et al.* (2013). The effect of communication skills training on residents' physiological arousal in a breaking bad news simulated task. *Patient Educ Couns* **93**, 40–7.

Mitchell AJ, Hussain N, Grainger L, Symonds P (2011). Identification of patient-reported distress by clinical nurse specialists in routine oncology practice: a multicentre UK study. *Psychooncology* **20**, 1076–83.

Razavi D, Delvaux N, Marchal S, *et al.* (2002). Does training increase the use of more emotionally laden words by nurses when talking with cancer patients? A randomised study. *Br J Cancer* **87**, 1–7.

Razavi D, Merckaert I, Marchal S, *et al.* (2003). How to optimize physicians' communication skills in cancer care: results of a randomized study assessing the usefulness of posttraining consolidation workshops. *J Clin Oncol* **21**, 3141–9.

Smith RC, Hoppe RB (1991). The patient's story: integrating the patient- and physician-centered approaches to interviewing. *Ann Int Med* **115**, 470–7.

Sollner W, Devries A, Steixner E, *et al.* (2001). How successful are oncologists in identifying patient distress, perceived social support, and need for psychosocial counselling? *Br J Cancer* **84**, 179–85.

Zandbelt LC, Smets EM, Oort FJ, Godfried MH, De Haes HC (2007). Patient participation in the medical specialist encounter: does physicians' patient-centred communication matter? *Patient Educ Couns* **65**, 396–406.

CHAPTER 60

Communication in cancer care in Europe and EU policy initiatives

Luigi Grassi and Luzia Travado

Introduction to communication in cancer care in Europe and EU policy initiatives

Communication in cancer settings is an extremely significant component of person-centred care. This is particularly so for the doctor–patient relationship when exchanging information about diagnosis, prognosis, and treatment-related decisions across the trajectory of the disease. With respect to this, it is clearly demonstrated that cultural and social factors have a specific role in influencing communication in oncology (Butow and Baile 2012). It is a fact that culture moulds both the patients' and communities' attitudes towards cancer care health professionals, institutions, cognitive, emotional, and behavioural responses to cancer and cancer treatment, as well as the patient's attitudes towards illness and suffering, decisions about treatment, and the whole organization of care (Surbone 2012). For these reasons, identification and negotiation of different styles of communication, decision-making preferences, roles of family, gender issues, and issues of mistrust, prejudice, and racism, becomes a significant component of clinical activity and a major challenge for oncologists practicing in Europe where significant cultural differences exist.

In this chapter we will present some of the main aspects of communication, taking into account the cultural differences between northern and southern European countries and the multiculturalism determined by the recent immigration phenomena in Europe. Also this chapter will discuss the main initiatives promoted over the last 10 years by European institutions regarding communication skills training in cancer care.

Communication issues and cultural aspects in European countries

Differences between northern and southern European countries

Several studies have shown significant differences in communication styles between healthcare professionals and cancer patients, according to geographical parts of Europe. The main finding suggests northern European countries (e.g. Scandinavian countries, United Kingdom, Germany) traditionally follow the tendency to openly communicate with cancer patients and their families with an attempt to create a shared decision-making process with regard to treatment. In contrast, Southern Europe communication styles around a cancer diagnosis, treatment, and prognosis has been more problematic. For example, paternalistic attitudes by physicians is common and is seen as an attempt to minimize the amount of medical information given to their patients so as to protect them ('the less you know, the less you worry'). A second reason is related to the different characteristics of the family. For example, southern European countries have been characterized as being more family-centred (extended families) than northern European countries. The repercussion of this in cancer settings is reflected in a marked tendency of southern European families to need to protect their relatives and to play a role in decision-making when dealing with medical illnesses. In Italy, for example, it was common in the 1980–1990s, to not tell cancer patients all of the facts about their clinical situation. More recently, because of the research, a shift has taken place indicating that the percentage of cancer patients who are informed and aware of their diagnosis has increased, with the majority of cancer patients correctly being informed of their diagnosis. However, even today about half of cancer patients are still not aware of their prognosis, with challenges existing in how to balance the exchange of information between patients and the families. This is even more apparent in situations where patients have been diagnosed and are being treated in advanced phases of their cancer. In a recent multicentre study, 87% of the patients were aware of their diagnosis, while 49% of those with metastatic cancer thought they were curable (Costantini et al. 2015). Similar findings have been shown in Portugal, where about 70% of cancer patients know the extent of their diagnosis, but in palliative care settings, only one-third of doctors tend to disclose the extent of the cancer diagnosis out of a concern that too much information might 'damage the patients psychologically' (Travado 2013).

Multiculturalism in Europe

Because of the large-scale immigration, a new challenge is developing in Europe. The incidence of cancer in this immigrant population and the consequent treatment needs will likely present new communication challenges. In the last 30 years, communication training and research has focused attention on the impact of cultural diversity and multiculturalism in clinical settings. In particular, research has addressed the impact of racial and ethnic minorities where health disparities are related to socioeconomic disadvantage and the difficulty of integrating their cultural model into the dominant model (Kagawa-Singer *et al.* 2010). The different cultural representations of illness and suffering (including language, thoughts, communications, actions, customs, beliefs, values, race, ethnicity, and religion) influence the whole of oncology care, from communication of diagnosis to decisions about treatment, from physical and psychological assessment to end-of-life care.

Several studies in recent years have been carried out by examining the differences related to the interpretation of cancer and cancer treatment according to culture. Research about the need to consider cultural backgrounds of different populations (e.g. African, Asian) in communication and psychosocial assessment is increasingly being presented. We are beginning to see the way cultural norms are influencing the way patients express their needs physically and emotionally to physicians, or to challenge physicians when their needs are not met (Grassi *et al.* 2015a). Therefore, psychological concerns related to worry about children and burdening the family, body image and sexual health concerns, beliefs about illness, gender roles, family obligations (e.g. self-sacrifice), as well as language barriers should be monitored when assessing patients from different cultural groups.

Physicians' issues

Several variables related to physicians' personalities and individual characteristics are also important in communication in cancer settings. In a southern European study, low psychosocial orientation and burnout symptoms (i.e. emotional exhaustion, depersonalization, and poor personal accomplishment in their job) were found to be associated with lower confidence in communication skills and higher expectations of a negative outcomes (Travado *et al.* 2005). As a consequence, physicians' burnout and stress negatively influences empathy and the capacity to give reassurance. Thus communication performance in the patient consultation is negatively affected. In fact, not only is the amount of information, but how communication occurs is extremely important in oncology. Having an 'empathic professional' is preferred by cancer patients than having a 'distanced expert'. Thus, 'affective' communication, in addition to 'effective' communication, should be the standard in cancer settings. In line with this, a European study showed that perceiving a physician as supportive, and interested in all aspects of the person, including emotional issues, has been associated with cancer patients' lower level of distress and better adjustment. In contrast, physician disengagement is associated with hopelessness and higher distress (Meggiolaro *et al.* 2015). Specific attitudes, behaviours and skills (e.g. capacity to impart confidence, being empathic, providing a 'human touch', relating on a personal level, being forthright, being respectful, and being thorough) are necessary components for effective/affective communication in cancer care, and in severe medical conditions (Grassi *et al.* 2015b).

Communication skills training experiences in Europe

Given these differences between northern and southern European countries, training in communication has become a priority in

Europe, with cancer care health professionals asking for help in improving their communication and relational skills with their patients and families.

Several training models on communication skills (CSTs) have been developed for European countries, with the objective to develop better strategies in communicating with seriously ill patients and their families. The seminal work of Peter Maguire and colleagues has had a profound impact in CST literature in oncology. Their model is based on the role that knowledge and skill deficits, self-efficacy, outcome expectancy beliefs, and perceived support plays in the ability and willingness of health professionals to assess their patients' concerns. The model has been applied to guide the development of a revised approach to brief and problem-focused workshops (Maguire and Faulkner 1994). Leslie Fallowfield and her team (Fallowfield and Jenkins 2006) also carried out a series of significant investigations, pointing out the impact of CST in improving the relationship between oncologists and cancer patients. As a result, several studies showed significant changes in oncologists' communication skills training programmes. This led to positive shifts in attitude towards patients' psychosocial needs and a more patient-centred care. CSTs using behavioural, cognitive, and affective strategies not only make the interviewing style more effective, but also have been observed to alter attitudes and beliefs of healthcare providers. This increases the likelihood that such skills can be transferred to the clinical setting. The use of focused and open questions, expressions of empathy, and appropriate responses to patients' cues are significantly increased after CSTs, with enduring effect and high likelihood of integration of key communication skills into clinical practice. Also CSTs significantly improve team awareness, knowledge of teams' clinical trials portfolios and clarity about clinical trial(s) to be conducted in oncology settings (Jenkins *et al.* 2010).

Interesting and clinically significant changes and adaptations have also been made according to the country and the relative cultural derived factors. In Francophone speaking countries, such as Belgium, significant results were obtained by Darius Razavi and his team (Merckaert *et al.* 2005) in the last 20 years. Razavi's CST model involves cognitive (e.g. theoretical information), experiential (e.g. case-history discussions), behavioural (e.g. role playing exercise), and supportive (e.g. stressor identification) techniques as key components for good communication skills. Several studies have shown that CST has had significant effects on attitudes including self-concept and the level of occupational stress of healthcare providers. In more recent studies, CST has been shown to facilitate transfer of team-member learned communication skills to clinical practice and improved patients' satisfaction with care (see Chapter 59 'The Belgian experience in communication skills training' and Chapter 17 'Communicating with relatives in cancer care' for more details). Therefore, in the experience of the authors, a core curriculum on CST is mandatory in cancer settings and junior and senior oncologists, as well as other healthcare professionals (e.g. nurses should participate in CST).

In southern European countries, some CST models such as SPIKES have been adapted and modified to fit with the Mediterranean cultural context. In this regard, a specific educational and experiential model (12 hours divided into two modules) involving formal teaching (e.g. journal articles, large group presentations), practice in small groups (e.g. small group exercises and role playing), and discussion in large groups was developed in southern European countries, namely Italy, Portugal, and Spain (Southern European

Box 60.1 Key elements of European CST consensus meeting

Setting, objectives, and participants

- CST is required at all the levels of professional education and in the post-graduate setting should consist of a mandatory basic course and advanced courses on specific objectives (e.g. discussing treatment options, end-of-life issues, identifying and treating emotional distress).

- A course of at least three days appears necessary to ensure transfer of skills into clinical practice' (although no evidence for the optimal length of CST in oncology with regard to effectiveness, some evidence for a dose–response relationship is available).

- Supervision and periodic booster sessions are a promising add-on.

- Courses may be mono-disciplinary or multidisciplinary according to the goal to be achieved.

- Courses should be given in small groups (4–6 persons per facilitator), which allows active participation and promotes interactivity.

- Content and pedagogic tools.

- Learner-centred courses meeting individual and group needs must be run by trained and competent facilitators.

- Role play with structured/constructive feedback on communication skills is essential.

- Specific goals—relationship building, emotion handling, discussing complex information—may be achieved via group discussion, role play and/or didactic material including prepared videos with patients or actors (Stiefel *et al.* 2010).

Organization

- Trainers should be healthcare professionals with credibility and experience in an oncology setting.

- Trainers must have passed an accredited train-the-trainer course with assessment of key competencies, such as knowledge in establishing confidentiality rules and group safety, utilization of a learner-centred approach, provision of opportunities for group to resolve problems, handling of conflicts and criticism, responding appropriately to comments made and individual reactions, meeting individual and group objectives, time keeping, self-awareness, and experience in handling group dynamics.

- Participation in accredited CST programmes should be supported by professional societies and place of work and awarded credits for medical education.

- Patient organizations should be encouraged to support the recommendations of the consensus meeting.

- CST must have financial support (unrestricted grants) from a variety of funding sources to ensure sustainability (Stiefel *et al.* 2010).

Outcome

- Validated assessment measures should be used to permit consistency and comparability across studies.

- All outcomes, whether objective or subjective, must be tightly linked to course aims and content.

- Assessment of long-term impact is needed to evaluate maintenance of skills (Stiefel *et al.* 2010).

Future directions and research

- Establishment of a European Institute for fostering CST and quality assurance of programmes and faculty.

- Future research.

- Use existing databases to further develop standardized, validated, reliable, and responsive outcome measures.

- Investigate head-to-head comparison of existing interventions.

- Involve cancer patients in the definition of outcome measures.

- Evaluate different delivery methods of CST (e.g. e-learning).

Text extracts reproduced from Stiefel F *et al.*, 'Communication skills training in oncology: a position paper based on a consensus meeting among European experts in 2009,' *Annals of Oncology*, Volume 21, Issue 2, pp. 204–7, Copyright © 2010, by permission of Oxford University Press.

Psycho-Oncology Study—SEPOS). The objective in this case was to improve the ability of oncologists to detect emotional disturbances in cancer patients (e.g. depression, anxiety, and adjustment disorders) (Grassi *et al.* 2005). Data have shown that the training course was well-accepted by most participants, who expressed general satisfaction and a positive subjective perception of the utility of the course for clinical practice. Other specific experiences have been developed in Italy by Costantini, Grassi, and Baile, who adapted the SPIKES-Oncotalk model and set up a CST which included formal lectures, small group work, role play, and interviews with simulated patients. Preliminary studies showed that these CSTs were effective in improving self-efficacy, knowledge of communication skills, favourable changes in attitudes towards disclosure of medical information, and assessing patients' concerns and fears (Costantini *et al.* 2009; Lenzi *et al.* 2011). Other initiatives were also developed in Portugal, namely a pilot training programme at National level conducted under the Portuguese National Cancer Control Programme for cancer physicians (Travado 2013). This programme adapted the SEPOS model tested in Portugal and introduced a new module on 'communicating bad news'. A two-DVD set on 'Communication and Relationship Skills for Health Professionals' (Reis and Travado 2006), providing illustrative teaching material on basic and advanced communication techniques and how to break bad news to patients using SPIKES protocol, was used both as a workshop supportive tool and for self-learning. The results of this programme showed significant improvements (p <0.001) in communication skills after the workshop; the participants rated it as very useful for their clinical practice, confirming its relevance for physicians' training (Travado 2013).

In a consensus meeting, based on European experts' opinions, a series of key components necessary for CST communication training programmes in European countries have been proposed (Stiefel *et al.* 2010) (Box 60.1). The improvement of cultural competence for multicultural settings in cancer settings has also become a necessity in Europe. Cultural (and linguistic) competence implies having the capacity to function effectively within the context of the cultural beliefs, behaviours, and needs presented by patients from different countries. As well, the flexibility of being able to make a major shift in communication framework is seen as essential (Surbone 2013). With respect to this, it has been indicated that healthcare professionals should be trained in developing programmes that include a cultural and diversity sensitivity for staff, reflecting the communities being served (Box 60.2) (Teal and Street 2009).

European Union policy initiatives in communication in oncology

Communication skills training in oncology is seen as a fundamental aspect of comprehensive and high-quality cancer care. The endorsement by cancer patients' organizations, and political institutions, is a definite sign that communication skills training is being embraced. The European Cancer Patient Coalition (http://www.ecpc.org) is in fact an example of an organization that has been very active in lobbying within the European Parliament to focus attention to cancer patients' needs and policies in Europe. The importance of a multidisciplinary and integrated approach in cancer care has also embraced the inclusion of psychological variables and related-communication issues. As a result, a number of initiatives have taken place under the umbrella of the Portuguese and Slovenian EU Presidencies (Gouveia *et al.* 2008; Coleman *et al.* 2008). The important role of psychosocial oncology in cancer care and communication skills training (Grassi and Travado 2008), were recognized. A Resolution document on reducing the burden of cancer in Europe was signed by all the European Member States (EPSCO Council 2008), which has resulted in the development of a cancer control and care action plan by the European Partnership for Action Against Cancer (EPAAC: www.epaac.eu). The main aim of the partnership is for all European Member States to have integrated cancer plans to reduce cancer by 15% in 2020. Within this framework, two important deliverables gave special visibility to

---

Box 60.2 Culturally competent communication skills that can be useful in multicultural settings in oncology (Teal and Street 2009)

◆ **Non-verbal behaviours**: reflect the physician's respect, concern and interest in the patient's well-being (active listening, focusing on the patient, and moderating culturally variable aspects of the interaction such as eye contact, touch, physical space, facial expressiveness, and the use of gestures).

◆ **Verbal behaviour skills**: asking about and assessing the patient's problems, showing understanding, acknowledging, reflecting, and calibrating emotions to help form a connection.

◆ **Recognition and exploration of potential cultural differences**: evaluation of the patient's community and family; skills and abilities that aid the patient and his/her family in dealing with the illness; factors that contribute to understanding health issues (e.g. education, mental acuity, familiarity with disease); aspects of the patient's environment that influence his/her ability to care for him/herself (e.g. socioeconomic factors, structural environment, stressors); and emotional implications of illness).

◆ **Incorporation of and adaptation to cultural knowledge**: integrating a patient's cultural values or beliefs into the encounter; awareness and ability to adapt communication behaviours to maximize the patient's comfort; reconcile misunderstandings; be responsive to the patient's values.

◆ **Negotiation and collaboration**: operating with awareness and adaptability to negotiate a shared understanding with the patient; reaching agreement on how the patient's symptoms will be prioritized, diagnosed, and treated; discussing the meaning of screening and assessment and the risks and benefits of different treatment options in ways that are individualized to the patient's socio-cultural and biomedical context.

Adapted from *Social Science and Medicine*, Volume 68, Issue 3, 'Critical elements of culturally competent communication in the medical encounter: a review and model,' pp. 533–543, Copyright © 2008 Elsevier Ltd, with permission from Elsevier, http://www.sciencedirect.com/science/journal/02779536

---

psychosocial oncology and CST: (i) the publication of the European Guide for Quality National Cancer Control Programmes, included Psychosocial Oncology Care as an important area for cancer care and service planning in integrated cancer care, highlighting the need for healthcare professionals to undergo CST (Travado and Dalmas 2015); and (ii) the Psychosocial Oncology Action Plan (http://www.epaac.eu/healthcare) with the main aim to implement a training strategy to improve psychosocial care and communication skills among healthcare providers in Europe (Travado and Borras 2013), as a way to foster and improve psychosocial cancer care.

More specifically the Psychosocial Oncology Action Plan conducted a mapping of needs and resources in communication skills and psychosocial oncology care (PSOC) in European countries (Travado and Borras 2013), and developed an educational training tool in these areas including CST. This was successfully piloted in Romania. This action was a breakthrough in European mainstream cancer care and it was carried out with the support of the

International Psycho-Oncology Society (IPOS), among other European partners (http://www.epaac.eu/healthcare).

Preliminary data from the mapping of needs and resources in communication skills and psychosocial care in Europe from the Psychosocial Oncology Action Plan under the healthcare work-package (WP7) of the *European Partnership on Action Against Cancer* is available elsewhere (Travado and Borras 2013; Travado *et al.* 2015). In summary, of the 27 European countries in the study, nine (33%) referred to having CST for healthcare professionals, and 17 countries (63%) reported providing CST during medical education. In terms of training priorities, CST for doctors and nurses was referred to as important by 18 countries (67%).

All these initiatives are extremely significant, but more resources and energy should be dedicated to improving the effectiveness in communication in healthcare providers.

Conclusions

The differences in cultural backgrounds among European countries and the more recent changes due to immigration phenomena in Europe strongly indicate that cultural issues should be taken into account regarding communication skills training in the cancer settings.

A patient and family-centred approach becomes essential so that cultural values and beliefs of the patient and the family are incorporated in the therapeutic relationship with healthcare providers.

Thus, as a practical consequence, it is mandatory in Europe to develop specific CSTs for oncology healthcare professionals, by considering both the 'traditional culturalism' between European countries (the historically and culturally-based difference between Latin and Anglo-Saxon cultures) and multiculturalism (the existence, acceptance, or promotion of multiple cultural traditions in European countries due to immigration from non-European countries). However, although we have witnessed progress in Europe in the last decade concerning CST inclusion in formal and continuing medical education, communication skills training is not yet a part of the core curriculum, nor is this training mandatory. Continuous efforts are still needed at academic and policy levels to make CST mandatory as a recognized core-competence for clinical practice in the healthcare professions. In a rapidly changing globalized and post-modern Europe, it will be important to monitor how language and cultural sensitivity imbedded in communication skills training will impact cancer care.

References

Butow P, Baile W (2012). Communication in cancer care: a cultural perspective. pp. 11–20. In: Grassi L, Riba M (eds). *Clinical Psycho-Oncology: An International Perspective*. Wiley, Chichester, UK.

Coleman MP, Alexe DM, Albreht T, McKee M (2008). *Responding to the Challenge of Cancer in Europe*. Slovenian Institute of Public Health, Ljubljana, Slovenia.

Costantini A, Baile WF, Lenzi R, *et al.* (2009). Overcoming cultural barriers to giving bad news: feasibility of training to promote truth-telling to cancer patients. *J Cancer Educ* 24, 180–5.

Costantini A, Grassi L, Picardi A, *et al.* (2015). Awareness of cancer, satisfaction with care, emotional distress, and adjustment to illness: an Italian multicenter study. *Psychooncology* 24, 1088–96.

EPSCO Council (2008). Council Conclusions on Reducing the Burden of Cancer, 2876th Employment, Social Policy, Health And Consumer Affairs Council meeting, Luxembourg, June 10, 2008. Available

at: http://www.eu2008.si/en/News_and_Documents/Council_Conclusions/June/0609_EPSCO-cancer.pdf [Online].

Fallowfield LJ, Jenkins V (2006). Current concepts of communication skills training in oncology. pp. 105–12. In: Stiefel F (ed.). *Communication in Cancer Care*. Springer-Verlag, Berlin Heidelberg, Germany.

Jenkins VA, Anderson JL, Fallowfield LJ (2010). Communication and informed consent in phase 1 trials: a review of the literature from January 2005 to July 2009. *Support Care Cancer* 18, 1115–21.

Gouveia J, Coleman MP, Haward R, *et al.* (2008). Improving cancer control in the European Union: conclusions of the Lisbon round-table under the Portuguese EU Presidency, 2007. *Eur J Cancer* 44, 1457–62.

Grassi L, Donovan KA, Nanni MG, Jacobsen PB (2015*a*). Cross-cultural Considerations in Screening and Assessment. pp. 411–18. In: Holland JC (ed.). *Handbook of Psycho-Oncology*, 3rd edition. Oxford University Press, New York, NY.

Grassi L, Caruso R, Costantini A (2015*b*). Communication with patients suffering from serious physical illness. pp. 10–12. In: Balon R, Wise TN (eds). *Clinical Challenges in the Biopsychosocial Interface: Update on Psychosomatics for the 21st Century*. Advances in Psychosomatic Medicine Series, Basel, Karger, Switzerland.

Grassi L, Travado L, Gil F, Campos R, Lluch P, Baile W (2005). A communication intervention for training southern European oncologists to recognize psychosocial morbidity in cancer. *J Cancer Educ* 20, 79–84.

Grassi L, Travado L (2008). The role of psychosocial oncology in cancer care. pp. 209–29. In: Coleman MP, Alexe DM, Albreht T, McKee M (eds). *Responding to the Challenge of Cancer in Europe*. Slovenian Institute of Public Health, Ljubljana, Slovenia.

Kagawa-Singer M, Valdez A, Yu MC, Surbone A (2010). Cancer, culture and health disparities: time to chart a new course? *CA Cancer J Clin* 60, 12–39.

Lenzi R, Baile WF, Costantini A, Grassi L, Parker PA (2011) Communication training in oncology: results of intensive communication workshops for Italian oncologists. *Eur J Cancer Care (Engl)* 20, 196–203.

Maguire P, Faulkner A (1994). *Talking to Cancer Patients and Their Relatives*. Oxford University Press, Oxford, UK.

Meggiolaro E, Berardi MA, Andritsch E, *et al.* (2015). Cancer patients' emotional distress, coping styles and perception of doctor-patient interaction in European cancer settings. *Palliat Support Care* 9, 1–8.

Merckaert I, Libert Y, Razavi D (2005). Communication skills training in cancer care: where are we and where are we going? *Curr Opin Oncol* 17, 319–30.

Reis JC, Travado L (2006). Communication and Relationship Skills for Health Professionals and Introduction to the Breaking Bad News Protocol [two-set DVD]. Psicolis, Lisbon, Portugal. Available at: http://www.psicolis.com [Online].

Stiefel F, Barth J, Bensing J, *et al.* (2010). Communication skills training in oncology: a position paper based on a consensus meeting among European experts in 2009. *Ann Oncol* 21, 204–7.

Surbone A (2010). Cultural competence in oncology: where do we stand? *Ann Oncol* 21, 3–5.

Surbone A (2012). Bioethical challenges: understanding cultural differences and reducing health disparities. pp. 199–210. In: Grassi L, Riba M (eds). *Clinical Psycho-Oncology: An International Perspective*. Wiley, Chichester, UK.

Surbone A (2013). From truth-telling to truth in the making: a paradigm shift in communication with cancer patients. pp. 3–13. In: Surbone A, Zwitter M, Rajer M, Stiefel R (eds). *New Challenges in Communication with Cancer Patients*. Springer-Verlag, Berlin, Germany.

Teal CR, Street RL (2009). Critical elements of culturally competent communication in the medical encounter: a review and model. *Soc Sci Med* 68, 533–43.

Travado L, Grassi L, Gil F, *et al.* (2005). Physician-patient communication among Southern European cancer physicians: the influence of psychosocial orientation and burnout. *Psychooncology* 14, 661–70.

Travado L (2013). Communication skills training of physicians in Portugal. In: Surbone A, Zwitter M, Rajer M, Stiefel R (eds). *New Challenges in Communication with Cancer Patients*. Springer-Verlag, Berlin, Germany.

Travado L, Borras J (2013). Psychosocial care in Europe: Preliminary results from a survey conducted under the psychosocial oncology action of the European Partnership for Action Against Cancer. *Psychooncology* **22** (Suppl. 3), K-5, 36.

Travado L, Dalmas M (2015). Psychosocial oncology care. pp. 35–9. In: Albreht T, Jose M, Moreno M, Jelenc M, Gorgojo L, Harris M (eds). *European Guide for Quality National Cancer Control Programmes*. National Institute of Public Health, Ljubljana, Slovenia.

Travado L, Reis JC, Watson M, Borras J (2015). Psychosocial oncology care resources in Europe: a study under the European Partnership on Action Against Cancer [EPAAC]. *Psychooncology*: doi: 10.1002/pon.4044. [Epub ahead of print]

CHAPTER 61

Communication skills training in Arab countries: Opportunities and challenges in the Qatar experience

Carma L. Bylund, Stephen Scott, and Khalid Alyafei

Healthcare communication in Arab countries

Although the literature and scholarly work in the Western world has long recognized the importance of good healthcare communication in improving patient outcomes, less attention has been paid to this issue in Arab countries. In the past few years, however, there has been a growing interest in provider–patient communication, particularly around the topic of breaking bad news to a patient and family (Al-Abdi et al. 2011).

Key differences between the West and Eastern/Arabic cultures impact healthcare communication, particularly around giving bad news. Salem and Salem focus specifically on Muslim cultures, and describe these differences as falling under three categories: healthcare decisions; patient's perspective of bad news; and patient's illness (Salem and Salem 2013). These authors explain that in Muslim cultures, healthcare decisions are often seen as being led by the family rather than the individual, as in the West. In the West, patients are seen to have the right to be given bad news with the belief that this will help them to better make decisions about their care. In Middle Eastern cultures, there is more of a concern that a patient's knowledge of his illness will lead to psychological disruption and low self-esteem; however, some patients may accept illness because of their faith. Finally, the experience of illness is considered to be more of an individual event in the West, whereas it is seen as a family event in Muslim cultures. Of course, we must keep in mind that these are cultural generalizations and real life is not so black-and-white. A more nuanced approach would allow for individual and family differences within these cultures.

Due to some of the cultural differences and the growing recognition of the importance of good communication, there have been many calls for improved communication skills training in the Arab world, with at least two published examples of training programmes. In Saudi Arabia, 168 physicians, interns, and medical students participated in a day-long workshop on communication. Using lecture, video, and role play, topics such as breaking bad news and conflict management were discussed (Al-Umran and Adkoli 2009). As another example, a randomized control trial of communication skills training with residents in Syria found no effect on the satisfaction with the physician–patient relationship of middle and lower-class mothers giving birth in a highly crowded hospital (Bashour et al. 2013). The authors concluded that without structural changes in the delivery of care, training individuals in communication skills may not have an impact on improving communication quality.

Although there has been no systematic report of which we are aware, it seems that communication skills training is lacking in many medical schools in the Arabian Gulf region. In our survey of 164 medical residents in Qatar from 2013 to 2015, 62% reported not having received any communication training during medical school.

From our review of the literature and our experience teaching communication skills across the continuum of medical education, we have identified several challenges in communication that may present in Arab countries.

Disclosure of diagnosis

In the West a patient's right to know is considered paramount to good healthcare. Although many physicians practising in Arab cultures also believe in patient autonomy as an ethical principle, and hospitals have patient rights' policies, this principle may come into conflict with local and family cultures. Cancer is likely the most relevant example for this type of family non-disclosure. Several recent studies in the Arab world have shown that patients with cancer are unlikely to have been told of their disease. The majority of cancer patients in Pakistan and Saudi Arabia are not informed of their diagnoses (Aljubran 2010; Jawaid et al. 2010). Many cancer patients report wanting information about their disease (Al-Amri 2009; Jawaid et al. 2010). Not surprisingly, research shows that family members may be a significant barrier to disclosure (Oksuzoglu et al. 2006). Although not informed by their doctors, most come to know they have cancer while receiving cancer treatments or experiencing adverse side effects (Atesci et al. 2004; Jawaid et al. 2010). Even though they may come to know or suspect their diagnosis, the patient often does not disclose this knowledge to the family.

Collusion often occurs with best intentions. Family members are worried that the reaction of the news of cancer by the patient will be so severe that he or she will become depressed and give up on trying to live. Patients may also be trying to protect their family members from having to have difficult conversations about the end of life.

Non-disclosure can also occur in other types of medical situations. For example, a father may ask the doctor not to tell the mother about an unborn or newborn child's condition, stating that he is worried about how the mother will react to the news. Or an individual may hide a diagnosis of HIV/AIDS where there is concern about the family's reaction.

Working with families

As described earlier, Western models of health view illness as an individual experience, while Arab or Eastern cultures view illness as a family experience. Challenges in working with families include family non-disclosure as discussed above, but can also extend to other times in the disease trajectory.

Physicians in our communication courses often express frustration at the logistical difficulties of managing large number of family members at a doctor's visit, inpatient room, or surgery recovery room. The complexity of communicating information or having a discussion about treatment options is multiplied when many well-meaning family members are there, with their own questions and concerns. Family members who are not at a visit may call a doctor later, asking for an update, for more information, or clarification. Although such challenges are also present in the West, they seem to be more pronounced in Arab countries where family size is large and family often has precedence over the individual.

When family members have conflict over treatment options, the clinician may be put in the middle of the opposing views. These conflicts over health decisions may just be one manifestation of deep, long-rooted patterns of conflict in a family. For instance, a brother and sister who have not spoken to each other in years due to an estrangement may be reluctant to meet together with the doctor to discuss treatment options for their elderly mother who has had a stroke.

One solution to some of these difficulties is for one family member to be named as the spokesperson and decision-maker, if the patient is incapacitated. For most Arabic communities living in Qatar, the most senior male family member is traditionally the one to take this role. For expatriate patients with no family in country, the patient's home country's embassy may help with decision-making and contacting family abroad.

Language

Qatar, Saudi Arabia, and other Arabian Gulf countries have multinational populations, which can produce a complicated setting for healthcare communication (Elzubier 2002). With a myriad of languages being spoken by both physicians and patients, for each to communicate in their native tongue is often a challenge. In addition, culturally-held health beliefs may impact both the communication and adherence to care (Elnashar et al. 2012). Having trained interpreters to help patients receive culturally competent healthcare in their own language is important (see Chapter 41). This ideal is more difficult to achieve in multinational developing countries where a significant proportion of the population is made up of immigrant workers from a variety of countries, especially when the countries have multiple languages.

At least three specific challenges are present in terms of the language of the learner in many of the communication skills training interventions in Qatar and other Arabian Gulf countries. We have a poor understanding of the transfer of communication skills from the classroom to working with patients when communication skills trainings are most frequently conducted in English. Medical students for whom English is a second language may have more trouble acquiring these skills in English (Hashim et al. 2013). In the teaching of communication skills, complex language and idioms can be confusing. In our own work, we have had to change some of our teaching vocabulary to be more simple and clear. For instance, terms like: 'modular blueprint', and 'take stock', have been replaced with 'module summary' and 'shift agenda'. Furthermore, when many physician–patient encounters are conducted in Arabic due to the local population, whether the skills taught in English translate easily into Arabic is unknown. One study has shown that Arabic speaking medical students taught communication skills in English report less confidence in taking a patient history in Arabic than English (Mirza and Hashim 2010). Finally, the meanings of certain words may translate or be understood differently based on language or culture. For example, whereas in English the phrase, 'I'm sorry' is often interpreted as an expression of sympathy, the Arabic equivalent of 'Ana asif' may bring with it a connotation of culpability and blame.

In the case study below, we highlight how some of the issue of language and understanding may present challenges.

Dr Amira, a medical oncology fellow, is the daughter of a Saudi father and British mother. Amira lived in Saudi Arabia as a young girl, but completed her secondary and medical schooling in England. She subsequently completed a residency training programme in Ireland. For her fellowship training programme, Amira decided to return to her Arabian roots and accepted a position in an Arabian Gulf Country.

In her first year of fellowship training, Amira cared for a local woman, Noor, who was suffering from metastatic breast cancer. Over the course of several months, the two women developed a friendship. One evening, after finishing her outpatient clinic, Dr Amira went in to see Noor, who had been hospitalized due to some side effects from palliative chemotherapy treatment.

Dr Amira was surprised to find Noor alone, and in tears, when she arrived. Remembering everything she had learned in her communication training courses in medical school and residency, she pulled up a chair next to Noor's bed and asked her why she was crying. Noor begin to talk about how she knew she was going to die, even though no one in her family, including her husband Omar, would talk with her about it. She said she felt very sad that she was leaving behind a young son who would not remember much about his mother. She knew extended family members had already been discussing a suitable new wife for Omar.

Amira felt so much emotion as she listened to Noor. Tears came to her own eyes as she thought about what Noor was going through. After Noor had disclosed these feelings, Amira took a deep breath and tried to communicate her empathic feelings: 'Oh, Noor, this must seem so unfair for you to be suffering like this.' Noor immediately turned her head away, and told Amira she wanted her to leave. Confused, Amira left Noor, but didn't understand what went wrong.

The next day, Amira was informed by her attending physician that Noor's family had filed a complaint with the Hospital Management about Amira. The complaint stated that Amira was trying to get Noor to question her religious beliefs and God's will for her.

Amira was really upset by this and spent many days thinking about what had gone wrong.

Qatar

Qatar is a small country in the Middle East with a land size of 11,437 sq km. Approximately a half million population lived in Qatar a decade ago. Since that time, the country has made huge investments in many projects to develop and improve services in all aspects, especially in industrial, health, and education. To do so has required opening many job opportunities for people to come and work in Qatar. Now there are more than two million people from different countries living in Qatar, and more than 65 different nationalities. The population with the majority are Indians (24%) and Nepalese (17%), and Qataris themselves representing only (12%). The largest proportion of the population is men (75%). This extreme demographic shift has been taking place over the past 10 years and has led to Qatari geographical changes.

The population today consists of people from all over the world with more than 60 different languages and different cultures and backgrounds, which form quite a challenge in communication, especially when patients are seeking medical advice in a busy healthcare centre without the interpreter or relatives who speak the other languages.

The main language in Qatar is Arabic, though in the public hospital the language of communication is English. There are approximately 3,000 doctors from different countries, backgrounds, and training are working today in Hamad Medical Corporation, the public healthcare system. Often the staff members working in a particular area will need to translate. Some staff members speak more than one language, which can help in communication with non-Arabic/non-English speakers. However, a large number of the expatriate population speak only their mother tongue, and some speak non-fluent Arabic or English; this can lead to miscommunication and poor health compliance.

One author on this chapter (KA) is a Qatari physician who has practised in Qatar for many years, and has led educational programmes for his colleagues. From his experience, understanding patients' cultures, beliefs, and background is challenging for the healthcare providers. In some cultures, a patient may suffer from serious illness but will remain quiet and may not go to hospital until the illness has progressed. In other cases, the patient may not give all information, especially about symptoms that are related to psychiatry or sexual illness. Some patients may not say anything because they don't want to upset their family. Some families will not allow a male physician to speak or examine a female patient. Other families interfere in a patient's care and refuse to tell a patient of his diagnosis in order to not upset him or her. There may be a patient who comes to clinic and get treatment, not knowing about the diagnosis or treatment because of family request, especially in case of malignancy. All these are considered challenges for conducting successful communication with patients and form a barrier related to mistrust, expectations of care, including preferences for or against treatment plans, diagnostic testing, and procedures. The patient's ability to comprehend what is prescribed may influence the healthcare providers' decisions.

Communication skills training in medical school

Weill Cornell Medicine in Qatar (WCM-Q) was established as the first medical school in Qatar in 2001. It is a branch of Weill Cornell Medicine in New York (WCM-NY), and it offers an integrated programme of pre-medical (two years) and medical studies (four years) leading to the Weill Cornell MD. All instruction is in English. It admits students in accordance with the admissions standards of WCM-NY, delivers the same curriculum, and uses the same student assessment methods. An essential component of this curriculum is communication skills training, which formally begins in the first year of the four-year medical school programme as part of a longitudinal doctoring course that embeds clinical skills training, small group skills practice, clinical experiences, and formal evaluation both in clinical settings and through observed encounters with standardized patients. Training continues through the second year, reinforcing communication skills training while adding components of the physical exam and clinical reasoning. In the third and fourth year, additional communication skills training is provided through clerkship-based seminars and objective structured clinical examinations (OSCEs) in more advanced or context specific communication skills; for example, communicating in emergencies, breaking bad news, anticipatory guidance in pregnancy, smoking cessation and behaviour change, cultural competency, and interprofessional communication.

Since 2005, WCM-Q has had an active clinical skills centre to enhance clinical skills training and simulated encounters for medical students. Since 2010, the centre has also provided communication skills training and simulated patient encounters for residents and trainees from local affiliate institutions, including the Hamad Medical Corporation. It has also conducted interprofessional education (IPE) sessions in partnership with local allied health programmes in nursing, pharmacy, and other fields since 2012.

As may be anticipated, the medical school communication skills curriculum is aligned with models developed outside the Middle East and North Africa (MENA) region, including Kalamazoo (Brunett et al. 2001) and the Accreditation Council for Graduate Medical Education (ACGME) interpersonal and communication skills competencies (Rider and Keefer 2006). In part due to the desire by the sponsoring institutions to ensure quality and rapid development of the medical school, the initial curriculum was largely imported while acknowledging that important aspects, such as particular physician–patient communication, would require ongoing development and adaptation. Several challenges and areas for further study may be highlighted.

With Qatar's highly diverse patient population (as outlined here), students must learn to interact with patients whose primary language is different from theirs from their earliest clinical experiences. Through cultural competency training, students learn to consider and explore the unique dimensions of each patient, receive instruction in the use of interpreters, and consider resources for addressing individual patient needs. Students themselves usually speak at least one other language besides English (and often two or three besides English); however, it may not include Arabic or the language of the patient they encounter. Professional interpreter services are sometimes available, but often a proxy (i.e. peer, nurse) is used, or simply not available. Student experience confirms that while concepts in effective communication are clear to them as taught in the classroom and during simulated encounters, and also generally perform well in these settings (i.e. scores on OSCE encounters are comparable to their US counterparts, and most students sit and pass the United States Medical Licensing Examination (USMLE) Step 2 Clinical Skills Exam), they experience difficulty and struggle at times to find the right words or strategies to be able to effectively employ these concepts in clinical encounters.

Students often encounter challenges in observing and practising skills in the clinical setting. In most settings in Qatar and other MENA countries, a clinician resides and sees patients in a single office room, without other office space or exam rooms. Schedules are often packed, and clinicians may see more patients per session (i.e. 20 or 30 patients in a half-day session for an adult internal medicine clinic, compared to 12–16) than might be anticipated in a Western context. When a learner and other professionals are present, there may be reduced privacy and confidentiality for the patient. With the challenges of space, time, and other professionals who are completing their duties, the learner may have fewer opportunities to move beyond the observer role, unless the clinician intentionally permits the learner to conduct portions of the encounter while being observed. These challenges appear to be reduced in the inpatient settings, where learners can see the patient at the bedside apart from the team or attending.

Impacts of gender and culture on patient–physician communication are encountered early, as the first-year communication skills curriculum includes training on eliciting a sexual history. These are sensitive topics in the Middle East and in Qatar, and appropriate training of medical students in this region to address these important topics has not been well studied. In an exploratory qualitative review of perceptions of sexual history-taking among first-year medical students in Qatar and New York through written reflective essays completed as a course assignment (unpublished), we found that students in Qatar more often commented on sexual history-taking as being taboo. For example, one student wrote:

> I wasn't looking forward to taking a sexual history, since there is so much taboo associated with the act … this highlights the detrimental effect that the taboo around sex in the region has in providing good medical care to the local patients. Instead of asking how many sexual partners they have had, [my preceptor] would ask if they were married to more than one wife. He would not ask about sex outside of wedlock, as that may be taken as an insult by the patient … He explained that doctors are willing to ask more direct questions [about] sex, but that the society's perceptions of sex prevents them from doing so.

Qatar students also were more likely to highlight or recommend strategies that use vague language or hints, or attempt to soften the impact of potentially sensitive or embarrassing questions, such as framing or providing additional background to the patient about the nature and reason for questions about sexual history. For example, another student wrote:

> He usually just asks, 'How are things with your family?' and that would imply sexual function … He usually refers to these topics indirectly so that, unless the patient was facing the problem, [s/he] would say, 'All is well, Alhamdulillah'.

Qatar students were also more likely to highlight the importance of patient autonomy and confidentiality, and might defer or avoid asking about questions about potentially important elements of the sexual history; for example, if a male family member were present and did not agree to be excused, or avoiding any question that might imply an unmarried woman could be pregnant. Further important contextual elements that inform these approaches include that polygamy is legal and commonly practised, and homosexual acts and heterosexual acts outside of marriage are punishable by law. It is our observation that though sexual health is an important component of overall health, it is often not elicited, a finding that has been documented and is not unique to the Middle East (Wimberly et al. 2006; Loeb et al. 2011; Auwad and Hagi 2012). Students who have learned about and can demonstrate the ability to elicit a sexual history in a controlled setting may not see effective models in a clinical setting and consequently encounter challenges in developing their own approaches.

Communication skills training for residents and physicians

Hamad Medical Corporation (HMC) is the primary public healthcare provider in Qatar and consists of nine hospitals. In 2008, leaders at HMC recognized that there was a need to improve communication among healthcare providers and patients both to improve the quality of care, as well as to contribute to the ACGME competency-based medical education programmes for residents and fellows.

The Department of Medical Education partnered with the Comskil training programme at Memorial Sloan Kettering Cancer Center to provide train-the-trainer courses and curriculum through the initial stages of the programme implementation. (See Chapter 3 for a description of the Comskil training model.) The Comskil training modules were originally designed for cancer clinicians, and oncologists were the first priority at HMC. This focus came as a result of Qatar's National Cancer Strategy, which was developed to guide the improvement of cancer care in Qatar. One of the recommendations in this strategy was that cancer physicians and nurses participate in communication skills training to improve communication with patients. In addition, many of the challenging communication situations faced by cancer clinicians are also present in medicine, paediatrics, emergency, surgery, and other specialties. The course was modified to meet the needs of multidisciplinary physicians at HMC.

Currently the course is a two-day course, covering seven modules, and falls under the Department of Medical Education's Center for Professionalism and Communication in Healthcare. The course follows best practices of regular engagement in facilitator-guided small group role play work with simulated patients. We regularly offer communication skills workshops and have trained more than 850 doctors. It is a required course for residents and fellows, as well as for physicians who are being promoted to consultant.

Although the core skills and methodology for teaching remain the same as in the Memorial Sloan Kettering Cancer Center Comskil training programme (Bylund et al. 2011), we have made modifications to the curriculum to make it more culturally sensitive. Didactic sessions use literature from the Middle East and the Arab World, while role play scenarios use a mix of nationalities and names to represent the multinational population. We are in the process of replacing demonstration videos with locally made videos with HMC doctors. The course includes the following topics: Breaking Bad News; Shared Decision-Making; Responding to Patient Anger; Discussing Prognosis; Discussing End-of-Life and DNR. In addition, to help physicians better work with their fellow employees or family or community members who often act as interpreters, we teach a module called Working with Untrained Interpreters. Finally, we address issues of family non-disclosure and working with families as raised in the beginning of the chapter in this final module on Conducting a Family Meeting.

Also guided by the Qatar National Cancer Strategy, we have worked closely with the Department of Nursing Education and Research to implement a communication skills training programme for oncology nurses. To be consistent with the curriculum and methodology of the training of physicians, we again partnered with the Memorial Sloan Kettering Cancer Center to train the facilitators and implement the curriculum, using the Comskil training programme for nurses. The programme is currently being implemented with oncology nurses, but will later be disseminated to nurses in other disciplines. This curriculum consists of three modules: Responding Empathically to Patients; Discussing Death and Dying; and End-of-Life Goals of Care.

Important to the success of any institutionally-based communication skills training programme are the core resources of standardized patients and small group facilitators. Due to the large volume of participants in the course, we have more than 60 physicians and nurse educators who help with the training through teaching didactics and running small groups. We regularly conduct facilitator training courses for new facilitators and advanced facilitator training courses for current facilitators. We also have developed a strong programme of standardized patients, mostly staff nurses at HMC with interest and talent in acting. They have undergone training about our curriculum, playing the patient role, and giving feedback.

Conclusion

Challenges in Arab countries for healthcare communication result predominantly from multicultural populations and from cultural differences with the West. We believe that through education and communication training interventions, a culture of patient-centred communication can be further developed and quality healthcare can be improved. Our experience has been that the vast majority of physicians, residents, and medical students are quite open to the principles and practices of communication skills training. Indeed, the large number of former participants who have joined the group of instructors in the HMC programme speaks to the enthusiasm for improvement in quality healthcare communication.

References

Al-Abdi SY, Al-Ali EA, Daheer MH, Al-Saleh YM, Al-Qurashi KH, Al-Aamri MA (2011). Saudi mothers' preferences about breaking bad news concerning newborns: a structured verbal questionnaire. *BMC Med Ethics* **12**, 15.

Al-Amri AM (2009). Cancer patients' desire for information: a study in a teaching hospital in Saudi Arabia. *East Mediterr Health J* **15**, 19–24.

Al-Umran KU, Adkoli BV (2009). Experience of a workshop on communication skills in health professional education. *J Family Community Med* **16**, 115–18.

Aljubran AH (2010). The attitude towards disclosure of bad news to cancer patients in Saudi Arabia. *Ann Saudi Med* **30**, 141–4.

Atesci FC, Baltalarli B, Oguzhanoglu NK, Karadag F, Ozdel O, Karagoz N (2004). Psychiatric morbidity among cancer patients and awareness of illness. *Support Care Cancer* **12**, 161–7.

Auwad WA, Hagi SK (2012). Female sexual dysfunction: what Arab gynecologists think and know. *Int Urogynecol J* **23**, 919–27.

Bashour HN, Kanaan M, Kharouf MH, Abdulsalam AA, Tabbaa MA, Cheikha SA (2013). The effect of training doctors in communication skills on women's satisfaction with doctor-woman relationship during labour and delivery: a stepped wedge cluster randomised trial in Damascus. *BMJ Open* **14**, 3.

Brunett PH, Campbell TL, Cole-Kelly K, *et al.* (2001). Essential elements of communication in medical encounters: The Kalamazoo Consensus Statement. *Acad Med* **76**, 390–3.

Bylund CL, Brown RF, Bialer PA, Levin TT, Lubrano Di Ciccone B, Kissane DW (2011). Developing and implementing an advanced communication training program in oncology at a comprehensive cancer center. *J Cancer Educ* **26**, 604–11.

Elnashar M, Abdelrahim H, Fetters MD (2012). Cultural competence springs up in the desert: the story of the center for cultural competence in health care at Weill Cornell Medical College in Qatar. *Acad Med* **87**, 759–66.

Elzubier AG (2002). Doctor-patient communication: a skill needed in Saudi Arabia. *J Family Community Med* **9**, 51–6.

Hashim MJ, Major S, Mirza DM, *et al.* (2013). Medical students learning communication skills in a second language: Empathy and expectations. *Sultan Qaboos Univ Med J* **13**, 100–6.

Jawaid M, Qamar B, Masood Z, Jawaid SA (2010). Disclosure of cancer diagnosis: Pakistani patients' perspective. *Middle East J Cancer* **1**, 89–94.

Loeb DF, Lee RS, Binswanger IA, Ellison MC, Aagaard EM (2011). Patient, resident physician, and visit factors associated with documentation of sexual history in the outpatient setting. *J Gen Intern Med* **26**, 887–93.

Mirza DM, Hashim MJ (2010). Communication skills training in English alone can leave Arab medical students unconfident with patient communication in their native language. *Educ Health (Abingdon)* **23**, 450.

Oksuzoglu B, Abali H, Bakar M, Yildirim N, Zengin N (2006). Disclosure of cancer diagnosis to patients and their relatives in Turkey: views of accompanying persons and influential factors in reaching those views. *Tumori* **92**, 62–6.

Rider EA, Keefer CH (2006). Communication skills competencies: definitions and a teaching toolbox. *Med Educ* **40**, 624–9.

Salem A, Salem AF (2013). Breaking bad news: current prospective and practical guideline for Muslim countries. *J Cancer Educ* **28**, 790–4.

Wimberly YH, Hogben M, Moore-Ruffin J, Moore SE, Fry-Johnson Y (2006). Sexual history-taking among primary care physicians. *J Natl Med Assoc* **98**, 1924–9.

Research in cancer communication

Section editor: Barry D. Blutz

CHAPTER 62

Evaluating communication skills training courses

Lyuba Konopasek, Marcy Rosenbaum, John Encandela, and Kathy Cole-Kelly

Introduction to evaluating communication skills training courses

Across the continuum of medical education, the focus is shifting from the teacher and the curriculum to the learner and the evaluation of educational outcomes. In the field of communication skills training, educators are now carefully examining the outcomes of their programmes. While the effect of many communication skills training programmes have been measured exclusively with questionnaire surveys of learner satisfaction, a number of other outcome measures are essential to consider in planning effective evaluation strategies. These include surveys of self-efficacy, demonstration of skills, patient satisfaction surveys, and health outcomes. In this chapter, we will identify assessment strategies used for communication skills training, describe how to design an effective evaluation methodology, and consider how outcomes have been measured in the oncology communication skills training literature.

Evaluation is broadly defined as the use of social research methods to systematically investigate the quality and effects of an intervention, activity, or programme (Rossi *et al.* 2004). In education, the object of evaluation may be individual learners, educational interventions, or educational policy, and other social structures affecting education. For the sake of this chapter, we will concentrate on evaluation of learners and interventions.

Educational interventions to be evaluated can be a single instructional or training activity (e.g. a lecture or training demonstration to teach a clinical skill), a set of such activities (e.g. all educational endeavours that occur within a clinical rotation), or an entire curriculum or training programme (e.g. the medical education curriculum or residency programme). Each of these levels of activity depends on the same set of social research methods that help determine how and how well the intervention has been implemented (a focus on process); and how and how well it has achieved its intended results (a focus on outcomes). The most effective approach to determine how well an educational intervention has attained its desired outcomes is to consider the aggregate results of individual learner evaluations.

Evaluation of communications training programmes should produce data that are valid and reliable. The validity of a measure or assessment is the extent to which it measures what is intended to be measured. For example, faculty ratings of learners' skills to communicate with patients provide a valid measure to the extent that these ratings actually reflect how well learners communicate with patients. Similarly, evaluation of training should meet standards of reliability with consistent results no matter who uses the assessment approach and when it is used. Though new measures or instruments may be available, it is typically recommended that educators locate reliable measures already existing for assessing communication skills. As a precaution, the assessment tool should be implemented under conditions that are similar to the conditions in which the tool was initially tested.

It is also important that assessment approaches be feasible, especially given the resource and time constraints that confront medical educational programmes. To be feasible, an assessment approach should require a reasonable amount of time, training, materials or technology, and financial cost.

Perhaps most important, assessments should yield information that will be useful to the trainees and to programmes as a whole. A good test of usefulness is asking these questions of any evaluation:

1. Will learners know how well they perform and what they need to do to improve as a result of assessment findings?

2. Will trainers know how to improve training and curriculum as a result of the findings?

Assessment methods and evaluation system design

The design of a programme evaluation system should be considered at the beginning of planning for a curriculum or teaching module. Rather than being an afterthought, the development of the evaluation system should proceed in parallel with curricular planning and design. Evaluation should also be closely linked to the content, the learning objectives, the process, and the instructional methodology.

Other issues to consider when developing a programme assessment plan include use of control groups, recruitment, and randomization of participants, method of observation, blinding of subjects and raters, use of validated instruments, and timing of assessment. A 2004 Cochrane review of communication skills training for healthcare professionals working with people who have cancer found that most studies measured changes in physician attitudes and/or knowledge rather than actual behaviour (Fellowes *et al.* 2004). While increasing number of RCTs have been done in the past decade (Moore *et al.* 2013), most reports do not use control groups. Also, in the majority of studies, subjects have self-selected to attend the training; thus, personal motivation may be a confounding factor. It is difficult to double-blind the study subjects to allocation in behavioural interventions such as communication skills training (Smith *et al.* 2007). The blinding of raters is possible, although not always done. Finally, the sustainability of training effect needs to be considered. In most studies, the impact of the intervention is generally measured immediately after training. Some authors have also measured effects from one to six months, and up to twelve months later (Gulbrandsen *et al.* 2013).

One way of assuring that many of the above evaluation standards are met is to closely align evaluation plans with corresponding curriculum and programme plans. A useful tool in helping to build such congruence is the logic model, which is a graphic depiction of the basic programme or curriculum organization (WK Kellog Foundation 2004). A logic model consists of related components:

◆ *Inputs* or resources that are needed in order to implement a programme or curriculum. Inputs commonly consist of funding, materials, equipment, and programme or instructional staffing.

◆ *Activities* are the actual instructional and programme processes that are implemented. These can be workshops, classes, computer-based training programmes, and so on.

◆ *Outputs* are the immediate results or products of activities as experienced by participants of these activities, such as the trainees of a communications training programme.

◆ *Outcomes* are the desired results or changes in knowledge, attitudes, behaviours, or skills among participants or trainees that should come about as a result of taking part in the programme or curriculum.

Sketching out exactly how a programme or curriculum will operate by using a set of inputs to deliver activities and outputs, and how these will influence desired outcomes among trainees, provides a framework for evaluating the total curriculum/programme and its results. An example of a communications training logic model and its corresponding evaluation plan is shown in Figure 62.1.

Desired outcome measurements need to be considered explicitly in developing an evaluation system. Kirkpatrick has defined four levels of evaluation related to educational interventions and ways to assess their impact (Hutchinson 1999) (see Fig. 62.2). These levels progress from Level 1, measuring learner reactions; to Level 2,

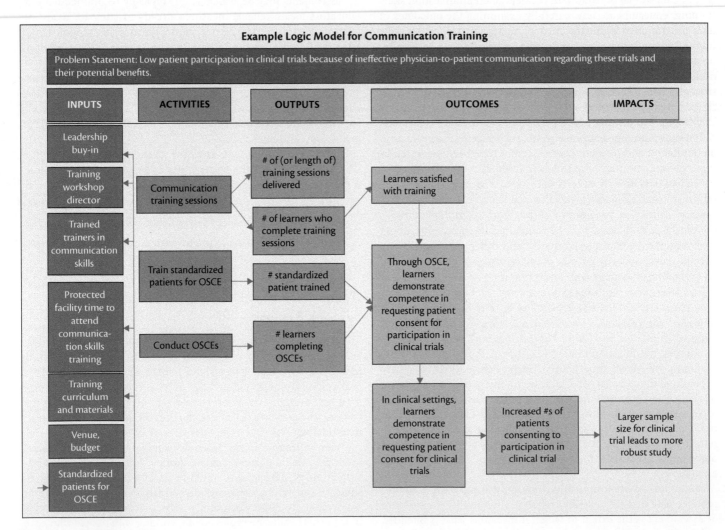

Fig. 62.1 A sample logic model.

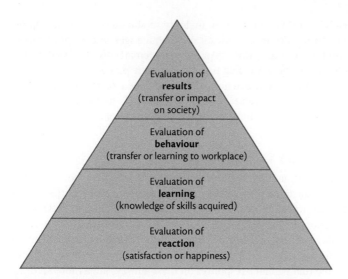

Fig. 62.2 Kirkpatrick's hierarchy of levels of evaluation (Hutchinson 1999). Reproduced from *The British Medical Journal*, Hutchinson, L., 'Evaluating and researching the effectiveness of educational interventions,' Volume 318, pp. 1267–1269, Copyright © 1999 British Medical Journal Publishing Group with permission from BMJ Publishing Group Ltd. Source: data from Kirkpatrick DI, 'Evaluation of training' pp. 87–112, in Craig R and Bittel I (Eds.), *Training and development handbook*, McGraw-Hill, New York, USA, Copyright © 1967.

measuring learning as indicated by change in attitudes, knowledge, and/or skills; to Level 3, measuring changes in learner behaviours; and finally to Level 4, measuring the intervention's impact on society (e.g. the effect on healthcare outcomes, such as adherence and patient satisfaction). For purposes of this chapter, we will examine each of these evaluation levels, examples of types of measures used for each level in specific relation to communication skills training, advantages and disadvantages of types of measures for each level, and will present some examples of evaluation studies using multiple levels.

Kirkpatrick's Level 1

In Level 1, the learner's reaction to the training is evaluated. These types of measures examine participants' views on the learning experience, its organization, presentation, content, teaching methods, and quality of instruction. In other words, did the participants like the training? Instruments that measure at this level have often been called 'smile sheets' and are the focus of many communication skills programme evaluations. They often take the form of Likert scales focused on different aspects of training programme content and organization, supplemented with opportunities for open-ended comments.

Advantages of using this type of assessment method include identification of learners' reaction to training method and content with minimal effort in developing and implementing evaluation instruments. Assessment of trainee reactions can be easily conducted using paper-based surveys at the end of a training programme or paper and/or web-based surveys administered at some point after training has been completed. Delayed administration of this type of programme evaluation allows for an assessment of trainees longer-term satisfaction with programme content and structure. The disadvantages of relying solely on trainee reactions for evaluation include that a positive result of learners liking an educational intervention does not ensure learning, satisfaction ratings can be influenced by the selection criteria for participants, and measures of satisfaction

by participants who want to learn a particular subject may not be generalizable. A final limitation is that smile sheets focus attention on evaluation of the teacher and instructional methods, rather than on the learner, and impact on learning. Thus, while they are easy to administer, give the instructor immediate feedback, and look valid because quantifiable data is generated, Level 1 evaluations should not be the only measure of a module's impact.

Kirkpatrick's Level 2

Level 2 addresses changes in learner's attitudes, knowledge, and/or skills, as measured both through self-assessment and assessment of knowledge and skills by others. Steinert and others have adapted Kirkpatrick's model to distinguish between changes in attitudes (Level 2A) and changes in knowledge and/or skills (Level 2B) (Steinert *et al.* 2006).

Level 2A

Level 2A evaluations focus on learners' self-efficacy and changes in attitudes towards learning or using a specific skill. Self-efficacy is assessed by asking learners if they perceive a change in specific knowledge or skill domains following training. For example, Baile evaluated two half-day communication skills workshops with satisfaction questionnaires (Level 1), as well as Level 2A self-efficacy measures (Baile *et al.* 1999). In addition to finding that participants were satisfied with the workshops, Baile found that participants felt that learning objectives were met, and that they had greater confidence in communicating bad news. Fujimora used Baile's 21-item scale before and after training to demonstrate Japanese oncologists' increased confidence in communicating with patients (Fujimori *et al.* 2014). Self-efficacy can also be measured using a retrospective pre-test and post-test survey, where participants are asked to compare their skills prior to the training with skills after the training. Level 2A evaluations can also measure attitudes towards communication skills; for example, learners' perceptions of the importance of a particular communication skill, as well as plans to use this skill (Jenkins and Fallowfield 2002). Parle asserted that attitudes, such as self-efficacy and outcome expectancy towards skills, are essential to the maintenance and development of communication skills (Parle *et al.* 1997). Thus, advantages of this type of evaluation include understanding the learner's attitude towards a new skill, which is an important pre-requisite to applying it in clinical practice. The limitation is that this level of evaluation does not assess actual knowledge, skills, or behaviours. In fact, physicians have been found to be imprecise assessors of their own clinical competence particularly if they have deficits. Type 2A outcomes might be most useful when linked with higher Kirkpatrick outcomes. In a randomized controlled trial (RCT), Gulbrandsen demonstrated that a 20-hour training could promote improvement in self-efficacy correlated with improvement in performance as measured by analysis of videotaped encounters (Gulbrandsen *et al.* 2013).

Level 2B

Level 2B evaluations include measurement of knowledge and skill level by others through written exams and/or observed simulated patient encounters with standardized checklists, for example, objective structured clinical exams (OSCEs). When viewed in aggregate, data on individual learner performance can yield valuable information for programme evaluation. As with all Level 2B evaluations, this is only a measure of the impact of an educational intervention if pre- and post-intervention measurements of knowledge or skills are compared. While written exams can provide information on achievement of certain stated learning objectives related to knowledge, such as learning a new conceptual framework for a communication skill, observed encounters with simulated patients are considered a high-fidelity method for measuring the skills related to communication (Duffy *et al.* 2004), identifying learners' ability to put content into practice in a simulated situation. OSCEs also allow for control of variables that cannot be controlled in actual clinical encounters. This is especially important in programme evaluation in which OSCEs are used to measure specific tasks that have been taught. While many OSCE stations are designed to focus primarily on the process of communication and interpersonal skills, it is possible to challenge learners with increasingly complex content. Hodges demonstrated that OSCE stations with more challenging content, such as difficult emotional situations, can be created with acceptable reliability (Hodges *et al.* 1996). Most programmes have used single, focused, simulated patient (SP) encounters to test specific skills before and after the training (Maguire *et al.* 1996). Multiple station OSCEs control better for case specificity. In an RCT of the effect of communication skills training on improving oncologists' palliative care transition skills, Goelz developed three scenarios for each of two SP stations to be used pre- and post-intervention to avoid sequence effect (Goelz *et al.* 2011). In this study, positive effects in skills in transitioning to palliative care, basic communication skills, and communicating with family members were demonstrated in the intervention group. Disadvantages of using SPs include labour and cost intensity, the challenge of rater reliability, and the potential for trainees' perception that they are less realistic than actual encounters. Also, while this level of evaluation may measure what a learner is capable of achieving, either in a written exam or a simulated patient exam, it does not measure actual behaviour change in clinical practice (Maguire 1999).

Back's evaluation of Oncotalk, a communication skills retreat workshop for oncology fellows, is an excellent example of the use of SPs for measuring the efficacy of training (Back *et al.* 2007). Participant communication skills were measured before and after a training intervention by analysing audio-recorded, standardized, patient encounters. The audiotapes were assessed by blinded coders using a validated coding system. Back's decision to not use a separate cohort of individuals as a control was informed by a number of studies, which demonstrated that communication skills do not improve in control arms (Fellowes *et al.* 2004). Back's study clearly demonstrated an increase in the use of taught skills with SPs, but stopped short of evaluating the impact of the workshops on physician behaviour in the live clinical encounter.

Kirkpatrick's Level 3

Level 3 evaluation assesses the actual change in communication behaviours in the context of patient care. As communication is a behavioural skill, assessment of actual communication behaviour is considered one of the most accurate measures of the impact of training programmes. A variety of approaches have been used to assess changes in communication behaviours related to cancer care: observation of encounters with patients by others (live, audio-recorded, or videotaped); use of unannounced patients to assess behaviours; and use of real patients to assess behaviours. Disadvantages of assessing communication skills in patient encounters include costs and logistical challenges associated with gathering this type of data, inability to standardize the encounter to assure certain communication challenges and opportunities, and the additional time required to systematically analyse the data. Observing between five to nine different patient encounters per measurement time can help solve the problem of variability in these interviews (Hulsman *et al.* 1999). Tested tools are available to assess changes in communication behaviours in cancer care (Stubenrauch *et al.* 2012).

Kirkpatrick's Level 4

Level 4 evaluations measure change in patient care outcomes related to the education intervention. Approaches to measuring the impact of training on healthcare outcomes include changes in patient satisfaction and changes in healthcare outcomes measured by chart review. Patient surveys of physician and nursing communication skills are now increasingly being used. Many authors have suggested that patients' responses on these surveys are a more accurate reflection of the physicians' skills than observed encounters with skills checklists. Others have pointed out that patient satisfaction scores may be positively skewed (Parle *et al.* 1997; Gulbrandsen *et al.* 2013). The importance of looking beyond changes in behaviour to patient outcomes is illustrated by Brown's study in which a one-day experiential workshop on seeking informed consent for cancer clinical trials led to some changes in physician behaviour, as measured by audio-recorded patient interviews (Brown *et al.* 2007). These changes, while statistically significant, did not lead to any significant patient outcomes. Fujimora designed an RCT studying both Level 2 physician outcomes of self-efficacy and assessment of skills in an SP encounter and Level 4 patient satisfaction outcomes (Fujimori *et al.* 2014). Of note, although the intervention group demonstrated uniformly positive effects on physician confidence and performance, the patient outcomes were more mixed: patients in the intervention group reported less psychological distress and more trust, but no difference in perception of communication skills. The author reports that this may be due to a ceiling effect with patients reporting a high level of satisfaction at baseline (Fujimori *et al.* 2014).

Planning for assessment

In planning for assessment, it is also critical to select appropriate instruments for measuring programme effect. Skills checklists of observed behaviours in interactions with peers, SPs, or real patients are essential for assessing communication and interpersonal skills explicitly in Level 2B, Level 3, and even some Level 4 evaluations. Checklists can be standard observation instruments, examining general communication skills, or study-specific instruments, which focus on the behaviours taught in the training programme (Hulsman *et al.* 1999). Examples of standard communication skill observation instruments include the Calgary–Cambridge Observation Guide (Kurtz *et al.* 2003) and the Four Habits Model (Krupat *et al.* 2006). Communication skills evaluation instruments vary considerably in content, psychometric properties, and usability (Schirmer *et al.* 2005), and need to be selected carefully. In programme evaluation, skills checklists should link closely with learning objectives and the conceptual communication skills framework that is being taught. In a review of the communication objectives and behaviours addressed in the communication skills literature, Cegala found that many studies did not specify behaviours taught, and in several studies there was a mismatch between objectives and instruments used (Cegala and Lenzmeier Broz 2002). Checklists generally describe a skill and are linked to an evaluation component that is either a numeric (Likert) scale of ratings for low to high ratings or merely headings (e.g. done, not done, or does not apply). Some checklists include anchoring statements to help the observer best define the numeric rating. Many checklists provide space for a brief narrative or general comments. Some checklist forms request respondents to record the time the skill was done or could have been done (e.g. an empathic opportunity), so that when the learner observes his/her interview, the specific time when that skill was done or could have been done is apparent. The rater of the checklist may be a peer, a senior learner, a faculty member, a trained simulated patient, or a real patient. Makoul's communication assessment tool is an example of a checklist that has been validated as an instrument for patients' assessment of physicians in live encounters (Makoul *et al.* 2007). Observations used for coding may be live, video-recorded, or audio-recorded. Analysing audio-recorded encounters is limited by the inability to assess non-verbal cues. Ensuring familiarity and comfort in using the scale, and inter-rater reliability are critically important if it is to serve as the basis for programme evaluation. Of note, in a review of 14 evaluation studies of communication skills training programmes for clinically experienced physicians, Hulsman found positive training effects in only half or less of observed behaviours (Hulsman *et al.* 1999). Positive training effects may also be obscured by high performance levels prior to the training, another potential bias for self-selected participants (Hulsman *et al.* 1999). An additional potential limitation is that many checklists emphasize thoroughness and, therefore, present long lists of questions or items; thus, experienced clinicians whose approach is more focused may actually receive a lower score because they have not asked all of the questions on the list, even if they have communicated effectively.

As we have described, Kirkpatrick's model can be useful for guiding evaluation of training programmes (Bylund *et al.* 2011). While the model is not meant to be hierarchical, the rigour of the information gleaned in general increases as we move up the levels. In addition, the labour and cost intensity of different levels appears to increase as we move up the levels, with smile sheets being easiest to implement, while measurement of actual behaviour and patient outcomes is more intense. Many programme evaluations report using a combination of assessments at different levels to develop an overall picture of the reactions to training, plus impact of training on knowledge, attitudes, behaviour, and outcome. Several studies described below illustrate assessment strategies that employ multiple Kirkpatrick levels and thus yield different kinds of information to inform programme efficacy and development.

Fujimori's RCT which studied changes in physician confidence (Kirkpatrick Level 2A), performance with SPs with a validated checklist (Kirkpatrick Level 2B) and patient satisfaction and levels of psychological distress (Kirkpatrick Level 4) before and after communication skills training demonstrates the advantage of this type of approach. Fallowfield's study of the effect of a three-day course and written feedback on communication skills included ratings made by researchers, doctors, and patients, as well as evaluations on multiple Kirkpatrick levels (Fallowfield *et al.* 2003). Measured outcomes addressed several of Kirkpatrick's levels: physician satisfaction (enjoyment, relevance to practice) and confidence (Level 1); ratings of observed behaviours in practice (Level 3); and patient satisfaction (Level 4). One limitation of her study was that in using live

unscripted patients, not all behaviours taught could be observed or evaluated, especially if the circumstances for using them are rare and not likely to occur over just 6–10 encounters. Furthermore, if the behaviours are not observed both before and after the intervention, it is difficult to assess if there has been a change as a result of the programme.

Butow's 2008 study of the effect of a communication skills programme to increase oncologists' skills in eliciting and responding to emotional cues assessed doctor behaviour through videotaped SP encounters (Kirkpatrick Level 2) and evaluated physician burnout and satisfaction through questionnaires as secondary outcome measures. An acceptability survey was completed six months after the intervention and was very positive, with all doctors utilizing the patient information, believing that the training provided them with useful information, and finding that practising skills was useful. However, the SP data revealed no significant change in the number of behaviours demonstrated. Thus, while the physicians' high level of acceptability is certainly important for intended behaviour change, it does not guarantee it. This study illustrates the need to evaluate at multiple levels.

Summary and implications

This chapter has provided an overview of approaches to evaluating communication skills training programmes. This review has several important implications for future design of communication skills training evaluation. First, the majority of training evaluations reported in the literature have tended to limit measures to Kirkpatrick's Levels 1 and 2, likely reflecting the relatively lower cost required in these types of evaluations. Evaluators should be encouraged to consider how to better measure the impact of training programmes on actual behaviour and/or healthcare outcomes for a more rigorous understanding of both the shorter and longer term impacts of the educational programme. Second, choice of evaluation methods should be based on overall curriculum design and objectives. For example, if the objective of the training is to change attitudes, a pencil and paper measure of attitudes may suffice; however, if the objective is to change learner behaviour, the impact of training is best measured using SP or actual patient encounter observations. Third, use of methods that measure impact of training on more than one level can provide a more in-depth picture of the effects of training on attitudes, knowledge, behaviour, and skill. Fourth, while we have emphasized the importance of learner and programme evaluation for assessing the impact of training, evaluation also serves the purpose of increasing learners' and practitioners' perceptions of the value and importance of the skills being assessed. As an example, the incorporation of explicit assessment of learner communication skills through OSCEs as part of high stakes national licensing exams in Canada, the United Kingdom, the United States, and other countries, has stimulated an increased emphasis on the importance of these skills among learners, educators, and practitioners. Evaluation measures can also provide essential feedback for individual learners on how they can improve their communication skills and can provide feedback to help guide curriculum development and revision. Finally, evaluation of communication training interventions can provide the basis for scholarship that can be disseminated to academic colleagues interested in designing, assessing, and improving their own communication skills training programmes. Designers and implementers of communication skills training programmes should be encouraged to use rigorous programme evaluations and to disseminate their results in the literature.

References

Back AL, Arnold RM, Baile WF, et al. (2007). Efficacy of communication skills training for giving bad news and discussing transitions to palliative care. *Arch Intern Med* **167**, 453–60.

Baile WF, Kudelka AP, Beale EA, et al. (1999). Communication skills training in oncology. Description and preliminary outcomes of workshops on breaking bad news and managing patient reactions to illness. *Cancer* **86**, 887–97.

Brown RF, Butow PN, Boyle F, Tattersall MHN (2007). Seeking informed consent to cancer clinical trials; evaluating the efficacy of doctor communication skills training. *Psychooncology* **16**, 507–16.

Bylund CL, Brown RF, Bialer PA, et al. (2011). Developing and implementing an advanced communication training program in oncology at a comprehensive cancer center. *J Cancer Educ* **26**, 604–11.

Cegala DJ, Lenzmeier Broz S (2002). Physician communication skills training: a review of theoretical backgrounds, objectives and skills. *Med Educ* **36**, 1004–16.

Duffy FD, Gordon GH, Whelan G, et al. (2004). Assessing competence in communication and interpersonal skills: the Kalamazoo II report. *Acad Med* **79**, 495–507.

Fallowfield L, Jenkins V, Farewell V, Solis-Trapala I (2003). Enduring impact of communication skills training: results of a 12-month follow-up. *Br J Cancer* **89**, 1445–9.

Fellowes D, Wilkinson S, Moore P (2004). Communication skills training for health care professionals working with cancer patients, their families and/or carers. *Cochrane Database Syst Rev* **2**, CD003751.

Fujimori M, Shirai Y, Asai M, Kubota K, Katsumata N, Uchitomi Y (2014). Effect of communication skills training program for oncologists based on patient preferences for communication when receiving bad news: a randomized controlled trial. *J Clin Oncol* **32**, 2166–72.

Goelz T, Wuensch A, Stubenrauch S, et al. (2011). Specific training program improves oncologists' palliative care communication skills in a randomized controlled trial. *J Clin Oncol* **29**, 3402–7.

Gulbrandsen P, Jensen BF, Finset A, Blanch-Hartigan D (2013). Long-term effect of communication training on the relationship between physicians' self-efficacy and performance. *Patient Educ Couns* **91**, 180–5.

Hodges B, Turnbull J, Cohen R, Bienenstock A, Norman G (1996). Evaluating communication skills in the OSCE format: reliability and generalizability. *Med Educ* **30**, 38–43.

Hulsman RL, Ros WJ, Winnubst JA, Bensing JM (1999). Teaching clinically experienced physicians communication skills. A review of evaluation studies. *Med Educ* **33**, 655–68.

Hutchinson L (1999). Evaluating and researching the effectiveness of educational interventions. *BMJ* **318**, 1267–9.

Jenkins V, Fallowfield L (2002). Can communication skills training alter physicians' beliefs and behavior in clinics? *J Clin Oncol* **20**, 765–9.

Krupat E, Frankel R, Stein T, Irish J (2006). The Four Habits Coding Scheme: validation of an instrument to assess clinicians' communication behavior. *Patient Educ Couns* **62**, 38–45.

Kurtz S, Silverman J, Benson J, Draper J (2003). Marrying content and process in clinical method teaching: enhancing the Calgary-Cambridge guides. *Acad Med* **78**, 802–9.

Maguire P, Booth K, Elliott C, Jones B (1996). Helping health professionals involved in cancer care acquire key interviewing skills—the impact of workshops. *Eur J Cancer* **32A**, 1486–9.

Maguire P (1999). Improving communication with cancer patients. *Eur J Cancer* **35**, 2058–65.

Makoul G, Krupat E, Chang CH (2007). Measuring patient views of physician communication skills: development and testing of the Communication Assessment Tool. *Patient Educ Couns* **67**, 333–42.

Moore PM, Rivera Mercado S, Grez Artigues M, Lawrie TA (2013). Communication skills training for healthcare professionals working with people who have cancer. *Cochrane Database Syst Rev* **3**, CD003751.

Parle M, Maguire P, Heaven C (1997). The development of a training model to improve health professionals' skills, self-efficacy and outcome expectancies when communicating with cancer patients. *Soc Sci Med* **44**, 231–40.

Rossi PH, Lipsey MW, Freeman HE (2004). *Evaluation. A Systematic Approach*, 7th edition. Thousand Oaks, California, CA.

Schirmer JM, Mauksch L, Lang F, et al. (2005). Assessing communication competence: a review of current tools. *Fam Med* **37**, 184–92.

Smith S, Hanson JL, Tewksbury LR, et al. (2007). Teaching patient communication skills to medical students: a review of randomized controlled trials. *Eval Health Prof* **30**, 3–21.

Steinert Y, Mann K, Centeno A, et al. (2006). A systematic review of faculty development initiatives designed to improve teaching effectiveness in medical education: *Med Teach* **28**, 497–526.

Stubenrauch S, Schneid EM, Wunsch A, et al. (2012). Development and evaluation of a checklist assessing communication skills of oncologists: the COM-ON-Checklist. *J Eval Clin Pract* **18**, 225–30.

WK Kellog Foundation (2004). *Using Logic Models to Bring Together Planning, Evaluation, and Action: Logic Model Development Guide*. WK Kellog Foundation, Battle Creek, MI.

CHAPTER 63

Qualitative approaches to clinician–patient communication

Felicia Roberts

Introduction to qualitative approaches to clinician–patient communication

In *The Country Doctor*, Kafka's central character laments that writing a prescription is easy, but coming to an understanding with people is hard (Muir and Muir 1952). If the practice of medicine were as simple as sending a clear message, then the practitioner's job would be reduced to correctly formulating the right words. The reality, however, is that patient care is not simply about message transmission; it is about a dynamic interplay of information, emotions, expertise, goals, beliefs, and so on. To study the artful management of the complexities of healthcare communication, qualitative approaches are highly productive and can stimulate new insight because 'how' may be a more relevant question to begin with, than 'how much'.

In oncology and palliative care, as in any medical domain, both physicians and patients have concerns, regarding preferred treatments trajectories, and outcomes of the medical visit. Whether or not these preferences are realized during a consultation, patients come away with information about the nature and course of their illness, as well as with recommendations on how, or whether, to proceed with treatment. Physicians, from their side, face the tension of maintaining the delicate balance between informative yet hopeful communication (Helft 2006), deftly navigating the line between recommending yet avoiding guarantees (Roberts 1999). For those concerned with understanding these kinds of communication tensions in the practice of oncology and palliative medicine, the inductive and interpretive approaches presented in this chapter, along with several illustrative research examples, will prove useful. Necessarily, reference will be made to a wider scope of research than just those studies that focus on face-to-face communication because empirical work based on actual clinical interactions is still relatively scarce in the oncology setting (Beach and Anderson 2003). The final sections of the chapter reflect on the special ethical challenges facing researchers engaged in field-based studies, and a brief discussion is offered concerning the trade-offs between reliability and validity in qualitative research.

Unique contribution of qualitative methods for studying clinician–patient communication

Engaging in health communication research presumes a wide range of goals: to discover something new or to understand a phenomenon more fully; to make the world better in some way; or to advocate for a position in a manner that is acceptable to a community of practitioners, scholars, or policy makers. Regardless of the research goal, each person engaged in the process brings preconceptions of how the world works, what constitutes knowledge, and what is the most appropriate way to find answers to his or her individual questions.

What distinguishes the qualitative study is its commitment to understanding lived experience by privileging the dialogic nature of human life. From this vantage point, understanding is created in concert with others; it is not the result of a correct message being sent down a correct channel. Hence the lament of Kafka's country doctor who recognizes that it is our discursive involvement with others that produces the challenges of everyday life. For doctors, as for all of us, meaning is created socially; we cannot produce understanding in isolation. Ironically, it is that very essence of creating meaning through talk that can also lead to misunderstanding or missed opportunities for connection. If it were as simple as writing prescriptions, medical visits would be much shorter.

Taking a qualitative approach, the researcher is committed to being reflexively aware of his or her own meanings as an analysis emerges of the participants' orientations. The aim is to reconstruct participant sense-making practices, not to confirm a theoretical concern of the researcher. In addition to providing rich interactional detail, qualitative approaches can also serve as groundwork for further exploration and informed development of testable hypotheses.

Representative approaches and relevant empirical studies

In this section, data collection techniques and interpretive approaches are discussed with examples from relevant empirical healthcare research. The goal is to present a variety of frameworks that share grounding in terms of basic field techniques for data collection (observation, interviews, recordings) but which differ in scope, focus, or fundamental philosophy. First, field-based frameworks are presented that draw on an approach of observing and describing real entities. Gubrium and Holstein (1997) have termed this the 'naturalist idiom' in qualitative research, because it adheres to a belief in a discoverable truth, one which will 'truly' represent participant lives. Included here are ethnography, grounded theory, and conversation analysis.

In contrast to these naturalistic approaches, postmodernism is also briefly presented because it offers a different philosophical basis, one which highlights paradoxes, disrupting the traditional sense of a shared or monolithic truth that can be captured and represented. The value of this form of scholarship is that it can provide openings for new insight, offering a way into understanding the healthcare setting that would be inconceivable from more traditional vantage points.

Whatever the philosophical grounding (e.g. naturalist vs. postmodern) researchers using these approaches are generally interested in patients' and practitioners' beliefs, practices, and understandings of health and illness. They are attempting to derive participants' understandings from the researcher's detailed observation, description, and analysis of behaviour and artefacts.

Ethnography

'Ethnographic methods' has become an umbrella term for a wide array of procedures for data collection, analysis, and description of findings. Under this heading, interviewing and focus groups will be discussed, though these techniques are not unique to ethnographic studies.

For studies of medical interaction, an ethnographic approach can provide a wide scope, taking in a setting as large as an oncology unit as a unique culture, or studies can be more focused on particular segments of that culture. There is a long tradition of ethnographic work in medical settings, beginning with a description of medical student life (Becker et al. 1961) and the groundbreaking work that enabled an understanding of hospitalized dying as an orchestrated process (Glaser and Strauss 1965).

In this descriptive tradition, Linnard-Palmer and Kools (2005) examined nurses' attitudes and interactions in the context of paediatric oncology. Using field interviews and observations, the researchers addressed the ethical complexities embedded in nurses' interactions with parents who refuse treatment for their children. Inman (1991) likewise uses multiple field methods (observations, interviews, gaze interaction charting, and analysis of childrens' drawings) to examine the child's view of their cancer experience. Using a more traditional ethnographic approach, observing patients and families over several years from the clinic to their homes and even to some funerals, The et al. (2000) excavated underlying patterns of communication that result in cancer patients' false optimism about recovery. While these field studies used recording technologies, the effort was primarily to record interviews with participants, not necessarily the medical visit itself.

Interviewing

In many field-based approaches, interviewing is a core technique; it is a conversation with a purpose that primarily benefits the researcher, not the participant. Interview studies are common in patient–provider research and are valuable for exploring perceptions, attitudes, and beliefs.

Types of interviews can be delineated based on the depth and range of the conversation and the type of relationship one has with the participant (Guest et al. 2013). 'Ethnographic interviews' are those conversations that can just happen when the researcher is in the study setting and something serendipitously prompts a question related to the research project. In contrast, 'informant interviews' are designed with a purpose and participants comment on their experiences, possibly several times to discuss various topics of interest to the researcher. These can be open-ended conversations, but they are entered into with a general purpose in mind. Further along the continuum, 'respondent interviews' are brief, stand-alone interactions that generally have pre-set questions in a particular order. These are the least naturalistic and may provide only superficial, even socially desirable responses; nonetheless, the approach can be quite valuable for exploratory work. Because of the relative ease and confidentiality afforded by individual interview protocols, this type of study tends to predominate in healthcare research. For example, Kelly et al. (2003) interviewed 24 doctors on the topic of cancer patients' wish to hasten death (WTHD). Because the researchers had access to measures of patients' wishes, it was possible to associate the physician's responses with levels of WTHD in their patients. The authors clearly point to the need for more research on actual interactions where these issues are discussed.

Focus groups

Focus groups provide a format for understanding the world of the patient or the practitioner through their own stories, accounts, and experiences. Zimmerman and Applegate (1992) use this technique to examine the ways in which hospice teams communicate, providing insight into coordination and challenges for these healthcare providers. On the patient side, Davey et al. (2010) use focus groups to explore the experience of African American breast cancer patients in terms of their accounts of navigating the healthcare system. What these exemplars indicate is that, in contrast to individual interviews, and contrary to conventional assumptions, focus groups provide a setting in which people are more likely to disclose their health or professional concerns (see Wilkinson 1998 for a review). Whereas an individual may be reluctant to disclose deeper feelings to a researcher who does not share their experience, the focus group encourages people to share in a supportive atmosphere, potentially stimulating deeper thinking, and a broader spectrum of response.

Focus groups have been used in a wide variety of health research and allow researchers to observe, if not wholly natural and spontaneous discussions, then at least the process of how beliefs are expressed in concert with others. In addition to possibly promoting disclosure, the focus group format provides a more natural setting for group discussion. Since the participants often share some health or professional concern, this approach can help researchers get deeper and more detailed insight into issues, concerns, and understandings that might otherwise be missed in individual interviews.

Grounded theory

Grounded theory is a research strategy for inductively developing concepts and theories, primarily on the basis of in-depth interviews and field observations (Birks and Mills 2013). The approach, instantiated first by Glaser and Strauss (1965) was motivated from an interest by medical sociologists to grasp the actor's viewpoint. In this particular case, as the researchers attempted to describe and understand the process of dying in a hospital setting.

In grounded theory, analysis proceeds as a coding process that is intended to open up an initial understanding and allow core categories to emerge. The purpose is not to deconstruct an interaction into countable units, but to understand and integrate what is available from interviews and observations. As analysis proceeds, there is a movement away from literal meanings and towards the relationships among concepts. Over time, grounded theory has evolved in two directions: one characterized by a more agnostic stance towards data, and the other by a more question or theory-driven approach. Regardless of the strand that one follows in a grounded theory approach, the focus is always on discovery as opposed to hypothesis testing. While the notion of 'hypothesis' is used in an informal way in grounded theory, it develops in terms of plausibility, not testability.

Clair (1990) used this approach to study the end of life among oncology patients in a hospital setting. From data collected in the oncology unit, the researcher inductively generated the concept of 'regressive intervention', demonstrating how physicians withdraw, whether abruptly or gradually, once the patient has been re-cast, by the physician's diagnosis, from the sick role to the dying role. While medical staff are still expected to maintain humane, palliative treatment, the patient relies less and less on medical staff, and families become more accountable for the patient's activities. Likewise, using a grounded theory and thematic coding approach to the study of recorded clinic interactions (Audrey et al. 2008) and family conferences (Curtis et al. 2005), studies of palliative and end-of-life care have begun to examine decision-making and 'missed opportunities' for support and provision of information.

Sandgren (2012) used a grounded theory approach to examine how patients, their relatives, and nurses manage uncertainty in both hospital and home palliative care contexts. Using a novel secondary data approach (re-coding interviews and observations from prior field studies) Sandgren addresses the question of what participants' main concern is at this transitional stage, where new roles, values, and attitudes may be hovering under the surface of normalized behaviour. Knowing how to act and behave in this novel, unresolvable end-of-life stage was a core problem for patients and families. The process of deciphering unwritten rules, or figuring out what the unspoken expectations and values were in this new phase, emerged as a key for understanding patterns of behaviour that affect quality of care and quality of life

Conversation analysis

Conversation analysis (CA) has been highly productive for bringing to light the endogenous order and interactional dilemmas in oncology visits. Unlike ethnographic and grounded theory approaches, which can be based on field observations and interviews, CA is predicated on capturing naturally occurring interactions in real time. Researchers using a CA approach are not engaged in describing contexts or in deriving concepts and theories through inductive coding; they are working to discern patient and clinician perspectives and practices as evidenced through embodied action and interaction. Using close transcription of audio and video-recorded materials, the conversation analyst attends to the details of verbal and non-verbal behaviour to see how the participants pursue and co-create an understanding of the situation, including what information, concerns, or behaviours are treated as relevant (or not) within the interaction. Because recordings of actual interactions (as opposed to reported, scripted, or observed/described) are replete with the details of an encounter, researchers have greater access to the momentary contingencies that participants orient to in their activities together. It is thus possible to discern how they accomplish many facets of the work of the clinic through face-to-face interaction, allowing researchers to closely view and describe the visible processes of 'coming to an understanding' (in Kafka's terms).

Several lines of research in the oncology setting have provided insight into clinical tasks, recommendations, and presentation of clinical trials, as well as issues of psychosocial importance. Early research made it clear that health practitioners risk meeting with resistance from their clients when there is a failure to properly justify the advice or recommendation (Costello and Roberts 2001). Indeed, the final formulation of a treatment recommendation can be accounted for by the conversational actions of both participants, including the shaping that occurs when patients subtly resist an initial formulation. Additionally, patients' poor understanding of the risks and benefits of cancer treatment has been partly explained by an examination of the inherently equivocal nature of those recommendations (Roberts 1999), because an unavoidable tension persists between oncologists' presentation of recommendations and their avoidance of guarantees. Moreover, it has been suggested that oncologists' talk about clinical trials is shaped in such a way that it may contribute to differing rates of enrolment (Roberts 2002).

Moving beyond the study of clinical tasks, Beach et al. (2005) and Maynard et al. (2016) analyse sequences of talk that could be overlooked as oblique to the main agenda of the oncology visit: patients' embedded disclosure of fears during history-taking, and oncologists' orientation to 'appreciation sequences', which occur after reports of test results or recommendations. Both of these interactional phenomena, seemingly ancillary moments relative to other goals of the clinical visit, are actually moments of great potential in terms of providing an 'in' to discuss matters of end of life or other matters of emotional consequence. Without close and repeated examination of actual physician–patient interaction, using techniques from CA, these small, but rich moments of potential connection with psychosocial issues would be lost.

Postmodernism

Postmodernist and critical modernist scholarship, like other interpretive approaches, emphasizes the discursive or social construction of reality. Data collection techniques, such as examination of texts, participant observation, and interviews, are shared with other qualitative approaches. However, in postmodern scholarship, the underlying assumption is that there is no single, observable truth, and a patient's experience of disease is shaped by belief systems and cultural norms along with the physical reality. As Lupton (2003) argues, the value of postmodern and critical modernist approaches for understanding healthcare is their insistence on examining paradoxes. For example, the military and sports metaphors that predominate in Western medicine (Erwin 1987; Seale 2001), along with a belief in the individual will for overcoming adversity, clearly shapes the practice of informing patients. The dominant ideology is for patients to 'fight' their disease; however, the dark side of this metaphor is that cancer patients may experience being at war with themselves, which has implications for the patient's sense of rationality (Pinell 1987).

As spotlighted in postmodern and critical research, explorations of metaphor and ideology provide points of departure for thinking about the ways in which attitudes and behaviours are shaped, and how patients and clinicians strive to make sense of health and illness within paradoxical webs of meaning.

Ethical issues in field-based qualitative research

In qualitative field studies, there is usually an ongoing and interactive relationship between the researcher and the setting's participants. Thus, issues of rapport, confidentiality, and consent can be particularly delicate matters where the biomedical and social overlap seamlessly. And the ethical challenges can be emergent and unpredictable. Seeing documents or overhearing conversations that might otherwise have been guarded by participants is bound to occur in busy, public domains. This can be particularly sensitive in medical settings where, perhaps naïvely, staff believe they are doing a good job of protecting patient confidentiality.

The sensitive nature of medical settings also raises the critical question of the incorporation of follow-up with participants who may have been observed or interviewed at vulnerable moments. Polit and Hungler (1995) address this dilemma in the context of how parents cope with a child's terminal illness. Since such a study would require a potentially painful probing of parents' emotional states, the researcher must consider not only whether the benefit of such knowledge would assist in the design of effective strategies for helping parents, but also what the long-term result of making such demands on parents would be. Once the child has died, what is the researcher's responsibility to the parents? Protection of subjects must, therefore, be broadly construed and considered integral to follow-up, as well as to implementation.

An additional complexity of field research in medical settings is that social and medical settings are permeable; people who were not expected, and, therefore, were not part of a consent process, can enter a scene. Thus, the ability to easily obtain informed consent is undermined. In envisioning projects, researchers should consider the possibility of such contingencies and plan accordingly. Post hoc consent may be possible, but is often untenable. Furthermore, some locations are considered public (e.g. corridors) and would be exempt from consent procedures, while others (e.g. patient rooms) may be considered private. For those collecting audio or video-recorded data, an additional consent form is warranted that outlines possible uses of the recorded data beyond research team meetings (e.g. for use in classrooms, at conferences, in electronic journals). Participants should initial those uses to which they consent; this would constitute full and open disclosure concerning the use of recordings. Clearly, the complexities of attaining informed consent are many, and must be balanced against the potential social and scientific benefits to be gained.

Finally, though not an ethical issue at first glance, researchers must 'consider the possible consequences of their culturally ascribed identities for the ethics and politics of conducting research' (Lindloff and Taylor 2002, pp. 141–2). The physical characteristics, social attributes, and degree of insider knowledge are among the 'ambiguous gifts' that fieldworkers can carry unwittingly into a scene, establishing 'axes of difference and similarity' with other participants (Lindloff and Taylor 2002, pp. 141–2). Again, the researcher's reflection and monitoring of these dimensions both in planning and implementation are necessary for considering the ethical challenges of field-based studies.

For those interested in healthcare communication research in cyberspace, Jones (1994) lays out ethical issues that are relevant for that medium where what is considered public, private, and deceptive becomes even more challenging.

Validity and reliability

Scholars differ in their opinions of whether or not reliability and validity are relevant concepts for qualitative research. From a social constructionist perspective, the argument is that the transient and contingent nature of human interaction renders any concern for reliability irrelevant. Validity is probably more relevant, since a particular interaction or event may be accurately analysed, but rare enough that it would be hard to find another just like it for comparison. Although the process of collecting instances and comparing them provides for a grounded claim about a particular action or behaviour, it is also the case that 'one' is a number and that analysis of a particular case holds value (Schegloff 1993) and can be built upon for developing further insights.

However, Silverman (1993) warns that if qualitative researchers are not mindful of issues of reliability and validity then they are at risk of engaging in the romanticism of nineteenth-century thinkers and chroniclers. In that tradition, observers may have selected data for its dramatic or exotic qualities, or because it fit an idealized pre-conception of the culture being studied. Therefore, Silverman suggests formulating hypotheses and testing assumptions through triangulation, and checking for participant validation.

Conclusion

Misunderstandings or missed opportunities for connection, whatever their root cause, can haunt patients and practitioners as they strive to make sense of a complicated interpersonal world within the medical organization. The value of qualitative and interpretive methods for studying medical communication resides precisely in the ability of the researcher to discern practices and beliefs that may give rise to misunderstandings. These participant orientations and behaviours are not necessarily available at a conscious level, and may only be available through systematic observation and interpretive analysis. In addition to gathering patient and clinician narratives about their experiences and beliefs (through interviews and focus groups), a great deal can be learned from systematic observation and recording of actual interactions (ethnographic and conversation analytic approaches), which can capture details of the dynamic, transactional nature of communication. Greater attention to theory development that is grounded in inductive analysis and interpretive procedures (such as grounded theory) can bring to light the interdependent relationship of practitioner and patient, in terms of the larger social context. Critical and postmodernist approaches help to uncover paradoxes and power dynamics that can bring to the surface the webs of social and cultural meaning in which we manoeuver with little awareness.

To better understand patient–clinician communication is to better understand the ongoing, situated processes that constitute communication. How are recommendations made and justified, how is advice given and received, and therefore what opportunities are naturally open within the interaction for exploration of psychosocial issues or end-of-life discussions? These kinds of questions imply understanding of the communication process, not just its outcomes. By definition a process is a series of activities, but in human terms, these activities rarely have discreet, discernible boundaries. Qualitative methods lend themselves especially well to understanding this fluid, socially constructed process of communication.

References

Audrey S, Abel J, Blazeby JM, *et al.* (2008). What oncologists tell patients about survival benefits of palliative chemotherapy and implications for informed consent: qualitative. *BMJ* **337**, a752.

Becker H, Geer B, Hughes E, Strauss A (1961). *Boys in White: Student Culture in Medical School.* Chicago University Press, Chicago, IL.

Beach WA, Andersen J (2003). Communication and cancer? Part I: The noticeable absence of interactional research. *J Psychosoc Oncol* **21**, 1–23.

Beach WA, Easter DE, Good JS, Pigeron E (2005). Disclosing and responding to cancer 'fears' during oncology interviews. *Soc Sci Med* **60**, 893–910.

Birks M, Mills J (2013). *Grounded Theory: A Practical Guide.* Sage Publications, Thousand Oaks, CA.

Clair JM (1990). Regressive intervention: the discourse of medicine during terminal encounters. *Adv Med Sociol* **1**, 57–97.

Costello BA, Roberts F (2001). Medical recommendations as joint social practice. *Health Commun* **13**, 241–60.

Curtis JR, Engelberg RA, Wenrich MD *et al.* (2005). Missed opportunities during family conferences about end-of-life care in the intensive care unit. *Am. J Respir Crit Care Med* **171**, 844–9.

Davey MP, Kissil K, Nino A, Tubbs C (2010). "They paid no mind to my state of mind": African American breast cancer patients' experiences of cancer care delivery. *J Psychosoc Onc* **28**, 683–98.

Erwin D (1987). The militarization of cancer treatment in American society. pp. 201–27. In: Baer H (ed.). *Encounters with Biomedicine: Case Studies in Medical Anthropology.* Gordon and Breach, New York, NY.

Glaser WA, Strauss MR (1965). *Awareness of Dying.* Aldine Publishing, Chicago, IL.

Gubrium JF, Holstein JA (1997). *The New Language of Qualitative Method.* Oxford University Press, New York, NY.

Guest G, Namey EE, Mitchell ML (2013). *Collecting Qualitative Data: A Field Manual for Applied Research.* Sage Publications, California, CA.

Helft PR (2006). An intimate collaboration: prognostic communication with advanced cancer patients. *J Clin Ethics* **17**, 110–21.

Inman CE (1991). Analyzed interaction in a children's oncology clinic: the child's view and parent's opinion of the effect of medical encounters. *J Adv Nurs* **16**, 782.

Jones RA (1994). The ethics of research in cyberspace. *Internet Res* **4**, 30–5.

Kelly B, Burnett P, Badger S, Pelusi D, Varghese FT, Robertson M (2003) Doctors and their patients: a context for understanding the wish to hasten death. *Psychooncology* **12**, 375–84.

Lindlof TR, Taylor BC (2002). *Qualitative Communication Research*, 2nd edition. Sage Publications, Thousand Oaks, CA.

Linnard-Palmer L, Kools S (2005). Parents' refusal of medical treatment for cultural or religious beliefs: an ethnographic study of health care professionals' experiences. *J Pediatr Oncol Nurs* **22**, 48–57.

Lupton D (2003). *Medicine as Culture*, 2nd edition. Sage Publications, London, UK.

Maynard DW, Cortez D, Campbell TC (2016). 'End of life' conversations, appreciation sequences, and the interaction order in cancer clinics. *Patient Educ Couns* **99**, 92–100.

Muir W, Muir E (1952). *Selected Short Stories of Franz Kafka.* p. 152. Random House, New York, NY.

Pinell P (1987). How do cancer patients express their points of view? *Sociol Health Illn* **9**, 25–44.

Polit DF, Hungler B (1995). *Nursing Research: Principles and Methods.* Lippincott, Philadelphia, PA.

Roberts F (1999). *Talking About Treatment: Recommendations for Breast Cancer Adjuvant Therapy.* Oxford University Press, New York, NY.

Roberts F (2002). Qualitative differences among cancer clinical trial explanations. *Soc Sci Med* **55**, 1947–55.

Sandgren A (2012). Deciphering unwritten rules. Grounded Theory Review, 11/2: Posted on Nov 28, 2012. (online, open-access journal). Available at: http://groundedtheoryreview.com/2012/11/28/deciphering-unwritten-rules/ [Onlnc].

Schegloff EA (1993). Reflections on quantification in the study of conversation. *Res Lang Soc Interact* **26**, 99–128.

Seale C (2001). Sporting cancer: struggle language in news reports of people with cancer. *Sociol Health Illn* **23**, 308–29.

Silverman D (1993). *Interpreting Qualitative Data: Methods For Analysing Talk, Text and Interaction.* Sage Publications, Thousand Oaks, CA.

Taylor K (1988). Physicians and the disclosure of undesirable information. pp. 441–63. In: Lock M, Gordon D (eds). *Biomedicine Examined.* Kluewer, Dordrecht, the Netherlands.

The AM, Hak T, Koeter G, *et al.* (2000). Collusion in doctor-patient communication about imminent death: An ethnographic study. *BMJ* **321**, 1376–81.

Wilkinson S (1998). Focus groups in health research: exploring the meanings of health and illness. *J Health Psychol* **3**, 329–48.

Zimmerman S, Applegate JL (1992). Person centered comforting in the hospice interdisciplinary team. *Commun Res* **19**, 240–63.

CHAPTER 64

Issues in coding cancer consultations: Interaction analysis systems

Phyllis N. Butow

Introduction to issues in coding cancer consultations

It is now well-accepted that effective communication is critical at all phases of cancer care. Therefore, a range of communication guidelines have been developed, and communication skills training is widely endorsed at both the undergraduate and postgraduate levels. Such guidelines and training should be evidence-based, promoting communication that is proven to produce improved patient and doctor outcomes. Furthermore, the efficacy of such training, and the extent to which guidelines are implemented in routine clinical practice, should be demonstrated. These goals require valid and reliable methods for documenting how patients and health professionals communicate with each other.

Coding health-professional-patient encounters

Systems analysis deconstructs a system into its component pieces for the purpose of studying how well those component parts work and interact to accomplish their purpose (Bentley and Whitten 2007). Interaction analysis systems (IAS) analyse communication between the doctor, patient, family, and other health professionals in a qualitative and/or quantitative fashion. IAS typically describe task-oriented and/or socioemotional behaviours. IAS differ in their clinical focus (e.g. general practice or specialty), extent of coverage (whole consultation or specific behaviours only), and communication modes encoded (verbal, non-verbal, or both) (Ong *et al.* 1995). Which IAS is best for a particular situation depends on the research or clinical question being explored, the communication model or theory utilized and the resources available for analysis. In this chapter, we will explore some of the advantages and disadvantages of different IAS systems in different settings.

Interaction analysis systems—whole consultation

Ong *et al.* (1995) conducted a systematic review of the literature in this area in 1995 and identified 12 whole consultation IAS systems.

Since 1995 three new systems have emerged: CN-LOGIT (later renamed CANCODE) (Butow *et al.* 1995), The Medical Interaction Process System (MIPS) (Ford *et al.* 2000) and the Siminoff Communication Content and Affect Program (SCCAP) (Siininoff 2011). The most commonly applied IAS is the Roter Interaction Analysis System (RIAS), including in oncology (Ong *et al.* 1998). Only the RIAS, MIPS, CANCODE, and SCCAP have been assessed for both reliability and validity. These systems are described in some detail, below.

The Roter Interaction Analysis System

The RIAS is derived loosely from social exchange theories related to interpersonal influence, problem solving, and reciprocity, and was originally developed for the family medicine context. The RIAS codes every doctor and patient utterance into one of 37 mutually-exclusive and exhaustive categories. In the RIAS, *utterances* are defined as the smallest distinguishable speech segment to which a classification may be assigned. Utterances may vary in length from a single word to a lengthy sentence. The RIAS captures *socioemotional behaviours* (e.g. agreement, showing concern, reassurance); and *task-oriented behaviours* (e.g. giving directions, asking medical/therapeutic questions, giving lifestyle/feelings-related information). These categories can be combined to reflect the total amount of talk in broader categories. Additionally, global ratings of anger, anxiety, dominance, interest, responsiveness, and warmth are allocated. More detail about the RIAS is provided in the next chapter.

The RIAS is widely used and therefore there is a plethora of comparative data available. It has been shown to be reliable and valid, with training, in a variety of medical settings (Ong *et al.* 1998). It records number of events, not time spent and therefore may not fully reflect the balance between different components in the consultation (although it is perfectly possible to time speech units and this was demonstrated recently in a study which used the computer software The Observer Base Package and Observer Video Analysis to both time and apply sequence analysis to RIAS data (Eide *et al.* 2004). Because the RIAS allows only one code per unit of speech, multidimensional aspects of communication behaviours may be lost, and it does not code non-verbal behaviour. Furthermore, by necessity, the RIAS picks up very general aspects of the consultation.

Codes are limited, and focus on general communication skills. If the researcher, educator, or clinician is seeking to capture or provide feedback about specific communication behaviours (such as the provision of particular information items, or responses to individual emotional cues) the RIAS will not be helpful. Finally, coding the whole consultation using the RIAS is a lengthy process, and this is true of all of the whole consultation systems described below.

The Medical Interaction Process System

The Medical Interaction Process System (MIPS) is a coding system adapted from the RIAS, designed specifically for the cancer setting. The system captures not just the linguistic (syntax) level, but also the paralinguistic (e.g. tone of voice) and kinesic (e.g. body language) levels of behaviour. Videotape data is the ideal basis for coding using the MIPS, however the system can be used on audiotaped interviews. Each utterance is assigned one content code and one mode of exchange, and may either be doctor or patient initiated. Paralinguistic elements are encompassed by 12 affective categories. Kinesic behaviour can be captured by 11 global body language ratings such as shoulder position (twisted versus square) and posture (closed versus open) alongside the main coding system. The coding format allows consultations to be coded in sequence for detailed analysis and individual feedback. The MIPS allows for parallel coding, thus avoiding major coding conflicts and providing a multidimensional view of the consultation. The MIPS has convergent validity, intercoder reliability (Butow et al. 1995), and criterion validity (Ford and Hall 2004), and has been used to evaluate communication skills training (Fallowfield et al. 2003). However, the global affective and non-verbal ratings are less reliable than the verbal frequency categories (Ford and Hall 2004).

Cancode

CANCODE is a computer-based method composed of: (i) microlevel analysis in real time, retaining the sequence of events; (ii) event counts; and (iii) macrolevel analysis of consultation style and affect. Each utterance is coded for: (i) *source* (doctor, patient, or third party); (ii) *process* (e.g. open and closed questions, initiated statements); (iii) *content* (e.g. diagnosis, prognosis, social matters); and (iv) *emotional tone* (e.g. friendly/warm, tense/anxious). Codes are entered into a software package while listening to the audiotape in real time. The computer calculates the time spent for each individual code, combination of codes, and the total consultation, as well as the number of times each code or combination of codes appears. This interaction analysis system has good validity and inter- and intrarater reliability (Ong et al. 1995; Brown et al. 2001; Dent et al. 2005). CANCODE (like the MIPS) has greater specificity and sensitivity than the RIAS for coding cancer consultations because it was developed specifically for this setting. It is multidimensional and allows time to be captured as well as the number of exchanges.

Siminoff communication content and affect programme

The SCCAP (Siminoff and Step 2011) was designed to capture relational as well as instrumental communication, as well as important contextual features. Relational communication enables people to make interpersonal connections. In the SCCAP, this is captured by measuring instances of confirmation and disconfirmation, immediacy or personal closeness, affiliation (friendliness and support),

and social influence that contributes to decision-making. Content and communication type can be coded for every utterance, supplemented by coding of questions and overall ratings of affect. SCCAP is designed to be used with audiotape data. The reliability and validity of the SCCAP has been demonstrated in large samples of coded data from oncology consultations with women diagnosed with breast cancer, and conversations about tissue donation with the families of deceased patients (Siminoff and Step 2011).

The characteristics and utility of the four whole consultation interaction analysis systems (RIAS, MIPS, CANCODE, and SCCAP) are summarized in Table 64.1.

Specific behavioural coding systems

Some coding systems look for specific behaviours within a consultation, rating them as present or absent. Sometimes an overall qualitative rating is also applied (such as basic/extended, or poor/good). Such coding systems record aspects such as: response to emotion (Del Piccolo et al. 2011), information giving (Koedoot et al. 2004), shared decision-making (Elwyn et al. 2005), and patient-centred care (Brown et al. 2001; Street et al. 2005). Some of these are described below.

The Verona Coding Scheme for Emotional Sequences (VR-CoDES) was developed to allow precise and detailed coding of patient emotional cues, and the physician behaviours preceding and following them (Del Piccolo et al. 2011). The VR-CoDES have been shown to correlate highly with patient identification of emotional cues after watching a video of their own consultation (Eide et al. 2011), suggesting that meaningful emotion is captured. The VR-CoDES-P (coding specifically physician responses) codes the degree of explicitness (yes/no) and space (yes/no) that is given by the health provider to each cue/concern expressed by the patient. The system can be further subdivided into 17 individual categories, and is being increasingly used to code oncology consultations.

Koedoot and colleagues (2004) developed a coding system to capture the adequacy of information given by oncologists to cancer patients when proposing palliative chemotherapy. Twenty-six items of information within six categories were coded as *issue not mentioned, issue just mentioned once*, or *issue explained more extensively*. Applying this system, they found that medical oncologists mentioned or explained the disease course (53%), symptoms (35%), and prognosis (39%) to some patients. Most patients were told about the absence of cure (84%). Watchful-waiting was mentioned to only half of the patients, either in one sentence (23%) or explained more extensively (27%). The authors concluded that patients were currently inadequately informed of their treatment options.

Elwyn and colleagues (2005) developed OPTION, a coding system designed to measure the extent to which health professionals involve patients in treatment decisions. It was created for the GP setting, but is applicable to the oncology setting. Twelve items are rated on a five-point scale, (0 = the item is not observed; 1 = a minimal attempt is made to exhibit the behaviour; 2 = the behaviour is observed and a minimal skill level achieved; 3 = the behaviour is exhibited to a good standard; 4 = the behaviour is exhibited to a very high standard). OPTION has been shown to have good inter- and intrarater reliability and to be sensitive and specific (Elwyn et al. 2004, 2005). It has been used to demonstrate the impact of communication skills training in involving patients in decision-making (Elwyn 2004).

Table 64.1 Comparison of RIAS, MIPS, CANCODE, and SCCAP

Interaction analysis system	Interaction type/ Interview situation	Observational medium	Coding flexibility	Communication levels	Usefulness as a teaching tool	Usefulness as a research tool
Roter Interaction Analysis System (RIAS) (Fallowfield et al. 2003)	Originally developed for doctor–patient interaction in general practice, but applicable to the cancer consultation	Traditionally direct coding of audiotapes, but sequential coding of videotape possible using The Observer Base Package (Elwyn et al. 2009)	One code per utterance. Records number of events, but not necessarily in sequence unless computer package used. Coding conflicts more likely	Socioemotional and task focused categories at the linguistic and, paralinguistic levels with global affective ratings. No non-verbal	Content items are very broad with only general communication categories and in this respect the system is less useful as a teaching tool	Proven reliability and validity. Widely used in process outcome research in a range of settings with a resulting large volume of comparable research data
Medical Interaction Process System (MIPS) (Butow et al. 1995)	Specifically developed for the analysis of doctor–patient interactions in the oncology consultation	Sequentially coded from videotapes and/ or audiotapes using specially designed coding sheet	System allows for parallel coding of utterances and incorporates the content and process of an interaction. Each unit assigned at least one content code and one mode	Linguistic, paralinguistic, affective, and limited global non-verbal. Specific interviewing behaviour items	Items relate to specific interviewing skills including responses to patients' cues thus providing useful information for teaching purposes and individual feedback	Good reliability and validity. Useful tool for evaluating the impact of UK communication skills workshops. Increasingly being used for cancer specific communication research in Canada
CANCODE (formerly CN-LOGIT) (Ong LML et al. 1995)	Computer-based interaction analysis system developed for the analysis of doctor–patient interactions in the oncology consultation	Sequentially coded in real time from audio or videotape directly into a computer software programme	Each unit of speech has four codes: source, process, content, and emotional tone. Can record frequency as well as time length for particular codes	Microlevel analysis, event counts, and macrolevel analysis of the consultation. Linguistic, affective, and paralinguistic. No non-verbal	In general, a good evaluation tool, but more specific communication skills and narrower content categories would be useful	Reliability and validity good in the cancer setting. Used successfully in studies to describe and characterize the Australian cancer consultation and promote patient participation
Siminoff Communication Content and Affect Program (SCCAP) (Ford et al. 2000)	Computer-based interaction analysis system developed for coding instrumental and relational communication in generic health care contexts	Sequentially coded in real time from audio directly into a computer software programme	Each unit of speech is coded for content and communication type. Questions are coded when they occur. Subjective coding of emotions	Linguistic, paralinguistic, affective No non-verbal	In general a good evaluation tool with a focus on relational communication	Reliability and validity good in the cancer setting. Used successfully in studies of breast cancer patients and organ donation discussions

Street *et al.* (2005) have developed a coding system to capture patient-centred care. Patient participation is coded (asking questions, assertive responses and expressions of concern or other negative emotions) as well as physician partnership building (encouraging patient involvement affirmations or accommodating active participation) and supportive talk (verbal behaviours that validate or support the patient's emotional or motivational state). First an instance of one of these behaviours is identified and coded, then the coder transcribes that portion of the dialogue along with three speaking turns before and after the speaking turn that produced the targeted behaviour. Counts of each behaviour are analysed.

A similar measure was developed by Brown and colleagues (Brown *et al.* 2001). The Measure of Patient-Centred Communication (MPCC) measures three aspects of PCC. Component 1 ('exploring both the disease and the illness experience') measures the degree to which the physician explores the patient's symptoms, ideas, expectations, feelings, and the effect of the symptoms on functioning. Component 2 ('understanding the whole person') measures the degree to which the physician explores the patient's family, social network, job, and interests as they relate to the presenting medical concerns. Component 3 ('finding common ground') measures the degree to which the physician explains the findings and involves the patient in generating a diagnosis and treatment plan. Instances of defined behaviours within each component are counted. This has been applied in a number of cancer settings, including radiotherapy.

Discourse analysis

A final approach to interaction analysis is provided by the proponents of discourse analysis. Discourse analysis aims to contribute to the understanding and evaluation of the text of interest, by revealing the meanings behind what is said and not said in the text. At the more sophisticated level of evaluation, linguistic discourse analysis reveals why the text is or is not effective for its own purposes. Analysis at the evaluative levels requires *interpretation* not only of the text itself but also of the context from which the text is drawn and of the systematic relationship between context and text (Eggins 1994). A number of different approaches to discourse analysis exist, but all attempt to move beyond counting behaviours to understanding language as a whole, including what is not said.

The advantages of discourse analysis are that it captures much more subtle aspects of communication, such as power plays, systematic avoidance of certain topics, or discussion of issues, such as prognosis only for certain purposes (such as to assist a treatment decision) and not others (such as to assist with existential crises). However, it is even more time-consuming than other approaches and can generally be applied only to a small number of texts, which limits generalisability.

The impact of visual input on communication coding

Most IAS code verbal behaviours only. However only 7% of emotional communication (how the person is feeling) is thought to be conveyed verbally; 22% is thought to be provided by voice tone, and 55% by visual cues like eye contact and body positioning (Bensing 1991). The cancer consultation is particularly emotionally laden and anxiety provoking for many patients. As a consequence, patients may be very attuned to non-verbal cues. Non-verbal communication leaks (kinesic leakages) can unintentionally convey ambiguous information that causes them further anxiety (DiMatteo *et al.* 1980). Patients are very sensitive to inconsistencies between physician's verbal and non-verbal communication (Friedman 1979).

Two studies have shown that little accuracy is lost in coding consultation content and process by using audiotape only (Weingarten *et al.* 2001; Elwyn *et al.* 2004). However, Dent and colleagues (2005) found that purely non-verbal codes, using Mehrabian's classification (1972) were as sensitive, if not more sensitive, than verbal measures to doctor response to different patient types. Thus, it is probably worthwhile to use both verbal and non-verbal coding if possible.

Automated interaction analysis systems

An increasing trend in the recent literature is to utilize automated coding systems. These employ computers to search for pre-defined word-stems, words or phrases of interest, defined for each research purpose. For example, Razavi and colleagues, have assessed information, support and assessment behaviours in cancer consultations using LaComm, French communication content analysis software, and used the data to assess the efficacy of communication skills training (Gibon *et al.* 2013). These methods have been shown to correlate well with manualized coding (Wallace *et al.* 2014) and to predict patient ratings of doctor–patient communication (Mayfield *et al.* 2014). While still being refined and developed, these systems provide an exciting direction for the future that may offer very cost-effective interaction analysis.

Conclusion

Each IAS system has merits and deficits. For all systems the coding of non-verbal (kinesic) behaviour has yet to be perfected. Automated systems offer promise for the future. In sum, no single system of interaction process analysis can hope to capture every behavioural aspect of an encounter, but some may be more useful than others depending on the task at hand.

References

Bentley LD, Whitten JL (2007). *Systems Analysis and Design for the Global Enterprise*, 7th edition, p. 160. McGraw-Hill Education , Boston, MA

Bensing J (1991). Doctor–patient communication and the quality of care. *Social Science & Medicine* **32,** 1301–10.

Brown JB, Stewart M, Ryan B (2001). Assessing communication between patients and physicians: The measure of patient-centred communication (MPCC). Working Paper Series, Paper #95-2. 2nd Edition. Thames Valley Family Practice Research Unit and Centre for Studies in Family Medicine, Longon Ontario, Canada.

Brown RF, Butow PN, Dunn SM, Tattersall MHN (2001). Promoting patient participation and shortening cancer consultations: a randomised trial. *Br J Cancer* **85,** 1273–9.

Butow PN, Dunn SM, Tattersall MHN, Jones QJ (1995). Computer-based interaction analysis of the cancer consultation. *Br J Cancer* **71,** 1115–21.

Del Piccolo L, de Haas H, Heaven C, Zimmerman C, Finset A (2011). Development of the Verona coding definitions of emotional sequences to code health providers' responses (VR-CoDES-P) to patient cues and concerns. *Patient Educ Couns* **82,** 149–55.

Dent E, Butow P, Brown R, *et al.* (2005). The Cancode interaction analysis system in the oncological setting: Reliability and validity of video and audio tape coding. *Patient Educ Couns* **56,** 35–44.

DiMatteo MR, Taranta A, Friedman HS, Prince LM (1980). Predicting patient satisfaction from physicians' nonverbal communication skills. *Med Care* **18**, 376–88.

Eggins S (1994). *An Introduction to Systemic Functional Linguistics*. Printer Publishers, London, UK.

Eide H, Quera V, Graugaard P, Finset A (2004). Physician-patient dialogue surrounding patients' expression of concern: applying sequence analysis to RIAS. *Soc Sci Med* **59**, 145–55.

Eide H, Eide T, Rustoen T, Finset A (2011). Patient validation of cues and concerns identified according to Verona coding definitions of emotional sequences (VR-CoDES): a video and interview-based approach. *Patient Educ Counsel* **82**, 156–62.

Elwyn G, Edwards A, Hood K, *et al.* (2004). Study Steering Group. Achieving involvement: process outcomes from a cluster randomized trial of shared decision making skill development and use of risk communication aids in general practice. *Fam Pract* **21**, 337–46.

Elwyn G, Hutchings H, Edwards A, *et al.* (2005). The OPTION scale: measuring the extent that clinicians involve patients in decision-making tasks. *Health Expect* **8**, 34–42.

Fallowfield L, Jenkins V, Farewell V, Solis-Trapala I (2003). Enduring impact of communication skills training: results of a 12-month follow-up. *Br J Cancer* **89**, 1445–9.

Ford S, Hall A, Ratcliffe D, Fallowfield L (2000). The medical interaction process system (MIPS): an instrument for analysing interviews of oncologists and patients with cancer. *Soc Sci Med* **50**, 553–66.

Ford S, Hall A (2004). Communication behaviours of skilled and less skilled oncologists: a validation study of the Medical Interaction Process System (MIPS). *Patient Educ Couns* **54**, 275–82.

Friedman HS (1979). Nonverbal communication between patients and medical practitioners. *J Social Issues* **35**, 82.

Gibon A-S, Merckaert I, Liénard A, *et al.* (2013). Is it possible to improve radiotherapy team members' communication skills? A randomized study assessing the efficacy of a 38-h communication skills training program. *Radiother Oncol* **109**, 170–7.

Koedoot CG, Oort FJ, de Haan RJ, Bakker PJ, de Graeff A, de Haes JC (2004). The content and amount of information given by medical oncologists when telling patients with advanced cancer what their treatment options are. palliative chemotherapy and watchful-waiting. *Eur J Cancer* **40**, 225–35.

Mayfield E, Laws MB, Wilson IB, Penstein RC (2014). Automating annotation of information-giving for analysis of clinical conversation. *J Am Med Inform Assoc* **21**, e122–8.

Mehrabian A (1972). Scoring criteria for some categories of nonverbal and implicit verbal behaviour. In: *Nonverbal Behavior*. Aldine & Atherton, Inc., Chicago, IL.

Ong LML, De Haes JCJM, Hoos AM, Lammes FB (1995). Doctor-patient communication: A review of the literature. *Soc Sci Med* **40**, 903–18.

Ong LML, Visser MRM, Kruyver IPM, *et al.* (1998). The Roter interaction analysis system (RIAS) in oncological consultations: psychometric properties. *Psychooncology* **7**, 387–401.

Siminoff LA, Step MM (2011). A comprehensive observational coding scheme for analysing instrumental, affective, and relational communication in health care contexts. *J Health Commun* **16**, 178–97.

Street RL, Gordon HS, Ward MM, Krupat E, Kravitz RL (2005). Patient participation in medical consultations; Why some patients are more involved than others. *Med Care* **43**, 960–9.

Wallace BC, Laws MB, Small K, Wilson IB, Trikalinos TA (2014). Automatically annotating topics in transcripts of patient-provider interactions via machine learning. *Med Decis Making* **34**, 503–12.

Weingarten MA, Yaphe J, Blumenthal D, Menahem O, Margalit A (2001). A comparison of videotape and audiotape assessment of patient-centredness in family physician's consultations. *Patient Educ Couns* **45**, 107–10.

CHAPTER 65

The Roter Interaction Analysis System: Applicability within the context of cancer and palliative care

Debra L. Roter, Sarina R. Isenberg, and Lauren M. Czaplicki

Introduction to the Roter Interaction Analysis System

While references to the patient–physician relationship are found in such early Greek writings as the dialogues of Plato, systematic study of the medical dialogue is a modern phenomenon. Technological advances have made the observation and analysis of large numbers of medical visits feasible, and indeed, the number of empirical studies of medical communication has grown exponentially over the last 30 years. The Roter Interaction Analysis System (RIAS) has emerged over this period as the single most widely used system of medical interaction assessment worldwide. It has been used in over 250 communication studies worldwide and has described communication across a spectrum of medical and healthcare settings, including cancer and palliative care (see https://www.riasworks. com/resources for a full annotated bibliography of RIAS studies).

The purpose of this chapter is to provide a broad overview of the characteristics of the RIAS and to illustrate its contribution to the field of cancer communication by reviewing a selected body of cancer and palliative care studies that have used the RIAS as their primary communication assessment tool.

Conceptual foundations of the RIAS

The RIAS is derived loosely from social exchange theories related to interpersonal influence, problem solving, and empowerment. The social exchange orientation is consistent with health education and empowerment perspectives that recognize the power of the medical dialogue to shape therapeutic relationships and reflect patient and provider roles and obligations.

Conceptually, the communication categories can be broadly viewed as reflecting task-focused and socioemotional elements of medical exchange. Clinicians' task-focused behaviours are defined as technically based skills that comprise 'expertness' acquired through medical education and professional training and for which

a physician is consulted, including history-taking, the conduct of tests and procedures, including the physical exam; and the provision of patient education and counselling across the care spectrum, from diagnosis and treatment, to self-care and prevention. The socioemotional dimension of physician behaviour includes communication with explicit affective content that builds emotional and therapeutic rapport, including social talk, laughter, joking, the expression of empathy, concern, or reassurance, and the exchange of approvals and agreements, as well as criticisms and disagreements. These communication behaviours are not generally regarded as a reflection of 'expertness' acquired in medical school, but are part of the human experience shared by professional and lay people alike (Roter and Hall, 2006).

In many ways, patient and clinician communication may be viewed in a parallel fashion. In this regard, George Engel's insight into the dual nature of patient motivation for seeking a doctor's care is illuminating; '… interpersonal engagement required in the clinical realm rests on complementary and basic human needs, especially the need to know and understand and the need to feel known and understood' (Engel 1988, p. 124). The former can be viewed in task-focused terms, while the 'later may be better understood in socio-emotional terms'. For patients, the need to know may necessitate initiating new and challenging behaviours, such as agenda setting, question asking, and making sense of complex information communicated under time pressure and in unfamiliar terms. And, sometimes the need to be known and understood may require the disclosure of stigmatizing and embarrassing information, along with concerns and fears, laughter and joking, as well as criticisms, and disagreements.

Within this theoretical grounding, the RIAS provides a methodological framework of mutually exclusive and exhaustive coding categories, whereby the contributions to the medical dialogue of both patients and providers may be richly elaborated and finely detailed (Roter and Larson 2002). The source material used for RIAS coding is most often audio or video recordings of the medical encounter; the system does not require or rely upon transcripts for coding. The unit of analysis for code classification is the smallest expression to which a meaningful code can be assigned—generally a complete thought. Every thought expressed by each speaker in the medical dialogue is captured and each is assigned to one of 37 parallel patient and clinician categories. In addition, there are a handful of codes that are clinician specific (i.e. asking for patient opinion, medical, or lifestyle counselling, partnership statements or self-disclosure) or patient-specific (i.e. requesting service).

The codes reflect the content and form of the medical dialogue; form distinguishes statements that are primarily informative (information giving), persuasive (counselling), interrogative (closed and open-ended questions), affective (social, positive, negative, and emotional), and process-oriented (facilitation, orientations, and transitions). In addition to form, content areas are specified for exchanges about medical condition and history, therapeutic recommendations, life-style behaviours, and psychosocial topics relating to social relations, feelings, and emotions. While coding rules and operational definitions of codes are provided in a manual, an interpretive function must also be considered for proper coding. Because coding is done from the spoken record, it is possible to incorporate consideration of the voice and intonation that are used in the delivery of a statement. This is especially important in situations of uncertainty and the coder must decide between categorizing a statement in a task or affect category. For example, the statement 'I hope this is all we'll have to do' may be coded as a statement of concern if the word hope was emphasized and the tone serious. In contrast, the same statement with all words equally stressed and a lighter delivery would likely be coded as reassurance.

In addition to the explicit categories of exchange, coders rate each speaker separately on a six-point scale reflecting the overall affective tone of the visit. The affective dimensions rated include: irritation, anxiety, dominance, interest, friendliness, and engagement. Sadness and emotional distress are rated only for patients, and sympathetic and hurried are rated only for clinicians. The global ratings are made independent of the literal (verbal) content and can be considered a non-verbal marker of emotion conveyed through voice tone.

Since codes are mutually exclusive and exhaustive, they can be used individually or combined to summarize the dialogue in a variety of ways without fear of redundancy. For instance, open or closed questions pertaining to medical history/symptoms, therapeutic regime, psychosocial and lifestyle factors can be tallied separately or combined in various ways to form superordinate categories of open and closed questions within a single topic or across topics (e.g. combining all open and closed questions in the psychosocial and lifestyle domain) or made into ratios (e.g. open to closed questions, biomedical to psychosocial questions, and so on). Similar groupings can be derived from information giving and counselling categories. Other variable combinations represent composites of facilitation, positive and negative talk, emotional expression, orientations, and instructions.

A patient-centredness score can be computed from RIAS codes by combining codes considered to reflect the expression of patients' lived illness experience, characterized by psychosocial and emotional categories of exchange, relative to the language of medicine's disease paradigm dominated by medically-focused categories of exchange. The system also marks five visit phases: opening, history, physical exam, education, and counselling, and closing with specific communication objectives falling within each of these segments of the visit. While the phases of the visit are not directly parallel to the functions of the visit, they capture a functional dynamic that cues both patients and providers to normative expectations for particular communication behaviours. For instance, the opening is useful in attending to social amenities and greetings, as well as establishing the visit agenda and probing the full spectrum of patient concerns. The history segment presents the primary opportunity for patients to tell their story and present details regarding concerns and expectations, while physicians probe symptoms and medical history. The exam segment is dedicated to technical procedures, and perhaps the opportunity for 'laying-on of hands' while the segment of the visit dedicated to patient education and counselling not only allows for clinician education and counselling of the patient about their diagnosis and treatment, but also provides the opportunity for patients to educate providers on their values, preferences, and expectations during the process of treatment decision-making. The closing is the time for summary and planning for follow-up, and sometimes the last opportunity for a patient to convey a problem that had not been addressed earlier in the visit, perhaps out of fear or embarrassment.

A useful framework for organizing the many individual coding categories considers the communication functions of the medical interview to include facilitation and patient activation as a core element, along with more traditionally defined visit functions of data gathering, patient education and counselling, and emotional responsiveness (Roter 2000). Facilitation behaviours include verbal strategies that help patients more fully engage in the medical dialogue and better appreciate the significance and implications of the medical information they receive about their condition and its treatment. These verbal strategies include encouraging patients to speak through verbal and non-verbal cues of interest and attentiveness, checking patient understanding, use of paraphrase and interpretation, and asking the patient directly for their opinion, preferences, and expectations. Table 65.1 displays the four-function framework with physician and patient dialogue examples for each RIAS code.

Cross-cultural and linguistic adaptation

RIAS studies have been conducted in 26 countries and the manual has been translated into more than 15 languages, as well as a number of African languages and dialects. The process of non-English coding has varied somewhat between countries, but routinely begins with RIAS training on the English manual before a translation of it is undertaken. During training, the meaning and nuance of the code categories are discussed to assure that they are considered in light of semantic, cultural, and emotive language characteristics relevant to verbal and non-verbal (voice tone) communication distinct to the second language. The success of language adaptation of the system is in no small part due to the use of local language examples for all code categories taken from recordings of in-country medical visits. An important part of this translation process includes going beyond coding the explicit content of statements to a consideration of vocal qualities that convey affective cues, since these are pertinent to the assigning of codes.

The nature of communication in the variety of cancer contexts

There is a rapidly growing body of studies in which the RIAS has been used to illuminate the communication processes in the

Table 65.1 Functions, code definitions, and dialogue examples of RIAS codes

Medical interview functions	Specific RIAS codes (patient and physician)	Physician dialogue examples	Patient dialogue examples
Data gathering	Open-ended questions re: medical condition/symptoms therapeutic regimen lifestyle and self-care psychosocial topics	What can you tell me about pain? How are the meds working? What are you doing to keep yourself healthy? What's happening with his father?	What can I expect in terms of pain? How would I know if the treatment is working? What else will I be able to do to keep healthy? How do kids handle this kind of thing?
	Closed-ended question re: medical condition/symptoms therapeutic regimen lifestyle and self-care psychosocial topics	Does it hurt now? Do you take your meds? Are you still smoking? Is your wife back?	Will the rash get worse? Will this med make me sleepy? Is there a walking group? Is it ok if my wife calls you?
Information exchange	Biomedical information re: medical condition and symptoms therapeutic regimen	The medication may make you drowsy. You need to take it for 10 days.	I think the medication is making me feel drowsy. I took it for three days and stopped.
	Lifestyle and self-care information	Getting plenty of exercise is always a good idea. I can give you some tips on quitting.	I try to get out to walk every day.
	Psychosocial exchange (including problems of daily living, issues about social relations, feelings, emotions)	It's important to get out and do something daily. The community centre is good for company.	I spend more time alone than I would like.
Emotional expression and responsiveness	Positive talk (specific categories) agreements Jokes/laughter Compliments/approvals	Yes, that's right. You will think I'm a vampire—I need blood again. You look fantastic, you are doing great.	Ok, I'll do that. I don't think I have any more blood Thank you for being such a great doctor.
	Negative talk (specific categories) Disapproval (direct) Criticisms (of others not involved in the visit)	No, stop that it won't help at all. They never have enough openings in that centre.	That med was a waste of money. The receptionist at that centre was so rude.
	Social talk (non-medical, chit-chat)	How about them O's last night?	I'm more of a Colts fan.
	Emotional talk (specific categories) concerns reassurance/optimism empathy partnership legitimation	I'm worried about that. I'm sure it will get better. You seem very angry. We'll get through this together. Anyone would feel that way in your situation.	I'm worried about that. I'm sure it will get better. I can see how harried you are. I know we'll get through this together. I bet everyone reacts this way.
Partnership building and activation	Facilitation (specific categories) asking for patient opinion asking for understanding, checking for understanding back-channels, and cues of interest	What do you think is going on? Do you follow me? Let me make sure I've got it right. Uh-huh, right, go on, hmm.	Do you follow me? Let me make sure I've got it right. Uh-huh, right, go on, hmm.

Source: data from *RIASWorks*, Copyright © 2014 RIASWorks, https://www.riasworks.com/

cancer context and their consequences for patient care and well-being. A review of this literature has identified over 45 papers in which the system has been applied in cancer-related medical care contexts.

A detailed analysis of this literature is beyond the scope of this chapter; however, we will present a selected review of studies to illustrate the varied contribution RIAS has made to this diverse body of work.

Utility in addressing patient outcomes and study objectives

The RIAS has been used in oncology-related contexts to address descriptive, predictive, evaluative, and novel study objectives. Many of these studies were designed to provide a broad quantitative description of the communication experience of cancer patients in ways not previously investigated.

Studies reporting associations between RIAS-based communication codes and patient outcomes can be viewed as indicators of the system's predictive validity, and a variety of outcomes including patient satisfaction, comprehension or understanding, anxiety, and ratings of the decision-making process have all been related to these codes (Dijkstra *et al.* 2013; Roter and Hall 2006; Albada *et al.* 2014). Studies have also used RIAS analysis of cancer communication to explore its effect on physiological indicators of a stress response, such as heart rate and skin conductance level in patients and clinicians. An especially interesting study in this area was conducted by van Dulmen (van Dulmen *et al.* 2007), who examined heart rate changes in medical students after delivery of bad news to a simulated patient. Post-consultation heart rate was higher the more medical information the students had provided and the intensity of eye contact during the simulation; heart rate was lower post-simulation the more often the students had reassured the patient. Another study by Reblin (Reblin *et al.* 2012) explored the physiological responses of study participants with a family history of cancer when receiving educational counselling about their cancer risk and dietary behaviour change recommendations associated with cancer prevention. Heart rate, galvanic skin response (GSR), communication, and participant self-report measures were analysed. Study participants randomized to receive facilitative counselling were more satisfied and had lower heart rate and GSR levels indicative of a lowered stress response than those randomized to receive more directive counselling.

Coding multiple speakers

The system has the ability to distinguish the contribution of multiple speakers, including family members accompanying the patient and medical team members consulting with the treating physician. Most of the descriptive literature reflecting medical exchange is dyadic (patient and clinician); however, it is common for additional participants to be present and to contribute to the conversation in the visit.

Family members are often included in genetic counselling sessions, not only because family members provide social support, but because they may share familial risk for hereditary conditions and much of the prevention counselling directed toward the patient is relevant to them as well. In other instances, family members may accompany patients when news about prognosis, transitions in care, or treatment decisions are contemplated, when medical procedures are to be performed, or when the patient's cognitive abilities are compromised.

An example of coding family member contribution to cancer dialogue is provided by Verhaak *et al.* (2000) in characterizing informed consent exchanges in radiotherapy consultations that included patients and an accompanying family member who may act as a patient proxy. Another, quite different example of multiple speaker coding to capture communication behaviours of hospice nurses, patients, and family caregivers during home visits is demonstrated by Ellington *et al.* (2012), as described more fully below.

Use of visit segments

Few studies have taken advantage of the ability of the RIAS coding software to specify five phases of the visit—the opening, medical history, exam, counselling, and closing. One that did explore the differential impact of communication across visit phases on patient outcome by Eide and colleagues (2003) found that social talk was a positive correlate of patient satisfaction when expressed during the history segment of the visit while psychosocial discussion was a negative correlate of satisfaction, but only when present during the physical exam.

Adaptation of the RIAS to genetic counselling

An emerging area of cancer-related communication is the field of cancer genetics and genetic counselling. In several of these studies, the RIAS category of medical information was split to distinguish between information given in general or population terms (e.g. 'overall one in nine women develop breast cancer') or as personalized estimates (e.g. 'based on your family history, your risk of having the genetic mutation is about 20%') (Roter *et al.* 2006).

Many genetic counselling clients are counselled both before and after genetic testing. Prior to testing personal and family history and other indications for testing are discussed; during post-test counselling test results are delivered and interpreted, risk estimates are given, and personal and family surveillance and treatment recommendations are made. The sequential nature of these visits present an opportunity to assess session communication in relation to outcomes over time, including common indicators of genetic counselling impact like client satisfaction, need fulfilment, anxiety, perceived control of one's condition, information recall, and the assumption of a preferred role in decision-making. These types of studies have the potential to identify areas in which both counsellor training and patient activation and education interventions are warranted.

A rare example of a sequential study was conducted by Albada (2014) to explore changes in client communication between pre-test and post-test counselling for breast cancer associated genetic mutations. The investigators reported that clients were more verbally engaged in follow-up visits compared to first visits and that a positive relationship emerged between client engagement at follow-up and assumption of their preferred role in decision-making, and perceived cognitive, behavioural, and decisional control related to their carrier status and risk of developing breast cancer. A negative relationship was found between session interactivity (operationalized as the number of speaking exchanges per minute) at the post-testing visit, and the assumption of a preferred role in decision-making and information recall; the more conversational exchange, the less likely the patient was able to assume their preferred role and the less information they recalled.

The investigators noted that the clients in their study were well educated and drew a parallel to a similar findings reported in a US study (Roter *et al.* 2007). In that study, genetic counselling sessions that were highly informative were found to use more technical terms, greater general language complexity, fewer and more dense speaking turns, and low dialogue interactivity than less informative sessions. While subjects with adequate literacy tended to learn more in these sessions, subjects with restricted literacy (below 8th grade level) learned less (Roter *et al.* 2009).

Finally, several genetic counselling studies add some form of clinical proficiency assessment to RIAS coding, usually through the use of gold-standard criteria set by experts in the field or a review of the literature. For example, Pieterse *et al.* (2005) developed an 11-topic checklist to assess the comprehensiveness of genetic counselling along with the counsellor's overall communication style. Other studies mark non-verbal behaviours like smiling, nodding, head shaking and eye gaze to better contextualize the association between RIAS codes and client outcomes (Dijkstra *et al.* 2013).

Use of RIAS in palliative care settings

Most RIAS studies have been conducted in the ambulatory care or hospital context but some research has explored its applicability to home settings. One such study, conducted by Ellington (2012) used the RIAS to describe communication behaviours of hospice nurses, patients, and caregivers during in-home visits. The study audio recorded home hospice visits and were able to demonstrate that RIAS is suited to capture the content and process of hospice encounters. The investigators found that patient and family caregiver communication with the hospice nurses varied in focus; caregivers were more active in asking questions and providing information than patients, with the largest portion of their talk devoted to discussion of lifestyle issues. In contrast, patients most frequently talked to the hospice nurse about their physical condition.

Further analysis of this study data by Clayton *et al.* (2014) used the RIAS codes to identify communication antecedents and responses to patient and caregivers' expressions of concern. Antecedent to the articulation of concerns, the nurses used positive emotional statements like reassurance, empathy, compliments, or laughter and joking. The nurses responded to concerns by asking questions, mostly about the patient's physical condition and by expressing concern, empathy, legitimation, and reassurance.

RIAS has also been used to explore differences in patient provider communication when discussing curative treatment versus palliative treatment in the radiotherapy setting. Taking this approach, Timmermans (2006) found that radiation oncologists provided less biomedical information, asked more psychosocial questions, and expressed more concern in palliative consultations relative to curative consultations. Patients in the palliative care visits, however, asked more medically-focused questions about their prognosis and did not express any more concerns compared to patients in the curative consultations. The findings were contrary to the investigators' hypotheses and suggest that patients may be reluctant to express emotional concerns even when their oncologists probed psychosocial and emotional issues in the palliative care context. These type results illustrate how RIAS can be effectively used to differentiate patterns of communication between oncology and palliative care in a very detailed way, with implications for communication intervention directed at both patients and clinicians.

Implications for future research, training, and clinical practice

In 2009, the Swiss Cancer League organized a consensus meeting with communications experts, oncology clinicians, representatives of oncology societies, and patient organizations to consider recommendations regarding the current state of the art and future development and evaluation of communication skills training in oncology (Stiefel *et al.* 2009). Consensus recommendations included making communication skills training required at all levels of professional education and urging the use of common, validated assessment measures to facilitate programme evaluation consistency and comparability across studies.

While the number of palliative care physicians are growing, there are not enough trained clinicians in the field to meet current demand; this gap is likely to widen, especially if the recommendations of the American Society of Clinical Oncology (ASCO) are followed to integrate palliative care services into standard oncology practice for all patients diagnosed with metastatic or advanced cancer (Smith *et al.* 2012).

Address of the primary challenges voiced by both the Swiss Cancer League and ASCO, to expand the oncology and palliative care workforce and establish an evidence base regarding effective clinician training programmes, is necessary to move the care of patients forward, but it is also daunting. RIAS can play a useful role in meeting this challenge by addressing programme effectiveness, generalizability, and comparability of programmes through the use of a common global metric.

Summary and conclusions

As is evident from the studies described in this chapter, the RIAS is sufficiently flexible to capture unique contextual dimensions associated with the variety of medical contexts and circumstance studied. The resource-conservative nature of RIAS makes it logistically possible to analyse relatively large numbers of encounters providing the statistical power necessary to evaluate training and educational programmes. Since RIAS coders work directly from the spoken record, an audio or video recording, it eliminates the very resource-intensive effort necessary for transcription. Not only does RIAS avoid the burden of transcript preparation, but it is also enriched by incorporating voice tone and phrasing cues into coding decisions. High levels of reliability and reasonable coding speed is usually achieved by coders with two to three months of practice. A well-trained RIAS coder can complete basic coding of a medical encounter in approximately four to five times the duration of the session.

Considering the differences in national health systems, the linguistic demands of translation and adaptation, and the cultural diversity represented in so many different national settings, the advantages of a common language-based measurement tool are considerable. RIAS categories are broad enough to capture core communications elements common to a variety of oncology and palliative care contexts, regardless of the national or linguistic nature of the settings, and sensitive enough to provide a detailed and rich descriptive profile of these varied therapeutic encounters.

Note

The website RIASworks.com welcomes visitors interested in posting RIAS-related studies and abstracts and sharing experience in using and adapting the RIAS. Also available on the website is an annotated bibliography of RIAS-based studies organized by clinical setting and country. Information regarding upcoming training sessions is also available on the site.

References

Albada A, Ausems MG, van Dulmen S (2014). Counselee participation in follow-up breast cancer genetic counselling visits and associations with achievement of the preferred role, cognitive outcomes, risk perception alignment and perceived personal control. *Soc Sci Med* **116**, 178–86.

Clayton MF, Reblin M, Carlisle M, Ellington L (2014). Communication behaviors and patient and caregiver emotional concerns: a description of home hospice communication. *Oncol Nurs Forum* **41**, 311–21.

Dijkstra H, Albada A, Klockner Cronauer C, Ausems MG, van Dulmen S (2013). Nonverbal communication and conversational contribution in breast cancer genetic counseling: are counselors' nonverbal communication and conversational contribution associated with counselees' satisfaction, needs fulfillment and state anxiety in breast cancer genetic counseling? *Patient Educ Couns* **93**, 216–23.

Eide H, Graugaard P, Holgersen K, *et al.* (2003). Physician communication in different phases of a consultation at an oncology outpatient clinic related to patient satisfaction. *Patient Educ Couns* **51**, 259–66.

Ellington L, Reblin M, Clayton MF, Berry P, Mooney K (2012). Hospice nurse communication with patients with cancer and their family caregivers. *J Palliat Med* **15**, 262–8.

Engel GL (1988). How much longer must medicine's science be bound by a seventeenth century world view? pp. 113–36. In: White K (ed.) *The Task of Medicine*. The Henri J. Kaiser Family Foundation, Menlo Park, CA.

Pieterse AH, van Dulmen AM, Ausems MG, *et al.* (2005). Communication in cancer genetic counselling: does it reflect counselees' previsit needs and preferences? *Br J Cancer* **92**, 1671–8.

Reblin M, Ellington L, Uchino BN, Roter D, Maxwell A (2012). Communication style affects physiological response in simulated cancer risk reduction interactions. *J App Biobehavioral Res* **17**, 129–56.

Roter D, Ellington L, Hamby Erby L, Larson S, Dudley W (2006). Genetic counseling video project (GCVP): Models of practice. *Am J Med Genet Part C Semin Med Genet* **142C**, 209–20.

Roter DL, Hall JA (2006). *Doctors Talking Patients/Patients Talking With Doctors: Improving Communication in Medical Visits*, 2nd edition. Praeger Publishing, Westport CT.

Roter DL, Larson SM (2002). The Roter interaction analysis system (RIAS): utility and flexibility for analysis of medical interactions. *Patient Educ Couns* **46**, 243–51.

Roter DL (2000). The enduring and evolving nature of the patient-physician relationship. *Patient Educ Couns* **39**, 5–15.

Roter DL, Erby LH, Larson S, Ellington L (2009). Oral literacy demand of prenatal genetic counseling dialogue: Predictors of learning. *Patient Educ Couns* **75**, 392–7.

Smith TJ, Temin S, Alesi ER, *et al.* (2012). American Society of Clinical Oncology provisional clinical opinion: The integration of palliative care into standard oncology care. *J Clin Oncol* **30**, 880–7.

Stiefel F, Barth J, Bensing J, *et al.* (2009). Communication skills training in oncology: A position paper based on a consensus meeting among European experts in 2009. *Ann Oncol* **21**, 204–7.

Timmermans LM, van der Maazen RW, Leer JW, *et al.* (2006). Palliative or curative treatment intent affects communication in radiation therapy consultations. *Psychooncology* **15**, 713–25.

van Dulmen S, Tromp F, Grosfeld F, *et al.* (2007). The impact of assessing simulated bad news consultations on medical students' stress response and communication performance. *Psychoneuroendocrinology* **32**, 943–50.

Verhaak CM, Kraaimaat FW, Staps AC, *et al.* (2000). Informed consent in palliative radiotherapy: participation of patients and proxies in treatment decisions. *Patient Educ Couns* **41**, 63–71.

Index